Overuse Injuries of the Musculoskeletal System

Second Edition

Overuse Injuries of the Musculoskeletal System

Second Edition

Marko M. Pećina
Ivan Bojanić

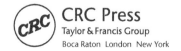

CRC Press
Taylor & Francis Group
Boca Raton London New York

CRC Press is an imprint of the
Taylor & Francis Group, an **informa** business

First published 2004 by CRC Press
This edition published in 2010 by Informa Healthcare

Published 2019 by CRC Press
Taylor & Francis Group
6000 Broken Sound Parkway NW, Suite 300
Boca Raton, FL 33487-2742

First issued in paperback 2019

No claim to original U.S. Government works

ISBN 13: 978-0-367-44668-0 (pbk)
ISBN 13: 978-0-8493-1428-5 (hbk)

Visit the Taylor & Francis Web site at
http://www.taylorandfrancis.com

and the CRC Press Web site at
http://www.crcpress.com

A CIP record for this book is available from the British Library.

Library of Congress Cataloging-in-Publication Data available on application

Preface

It is with pleasure, but also a sense of responsibility, that we present, after an interval of 10 years, the second edition of our book. The implied question is, are the changes in the field that this book covers so important and frequent that a new edition is necessary? The answer is yes.

Overuse injuries of the musculoskeletal system related to athletic activities and recreation or to various professional activities are common occurrences in modern life. Therefore, it is not surprising that overuse injuries are frequently discussed. In recent years, overuse injuries or microtraumatic illnesses have become increasingly recognized as a cause of pain and dysfunction in various parts of the human body. This recognition has been accompanied with a rapidly enlarging body of literature on the subject.

What is the same and what has changed in the second edition of our book? The authors are the same, as is the concept of the book. The second edition continues to probe the origins of these painful syndromes and to propose the possible causes that lead to them. This edition, similar to the preceding one, is intended to provide a quick overview of the definition, etiopathogenesis, clinical picture, diagnostics, non-operative and operative treatment, and the possibility of prevention of the various syndromes.

In addition to presenting the newest discoveries reported in the world medical literature, this book also reveals a wealth of individual cases and experience encompassing pathohistological examinations, imaging modalities, intraoperative photographs, and the results of both conservative treatment and operative procedures.

The second edition of the book has three new chapters. The credit for these new chapters belongs to Alan Ivković, M.D., a resident in our department, and Igor Borić, M.D., M.Sc., a specialist in radiology. Apart from the experience of the senior authors, the enthusiasm of our younger colleague, Alan Ivković, was particularly important in the course of the writing of this book. All chapters from the first edition feature new references and new illustrations, as well as new insights acquired in the intervening 10 years. Because of the continued support and understanding of our publisher, this edition also surpasses the preceding one in graphic design and presentation, for which we are truly grateful, not only for ourselves, but also for the readers of this book.

Marko M. Pećina
Zagreb

The Authors

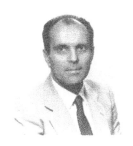

Marko M. Pećina, M.D., Ph.D., is Chairman and Professor of Orthopaedic Surgery and Vice-Dean for Medical Research at the School of Medicine, University of Zagreb, Croatia. He is also Chief of the Department at Zagreb Teaching Hospital Orthopaedic Clinic.

Dr. Pećina is a 1964 graduate of Zagreb University Medical School. He was an assistant lecturer at the "Drago Perovic" Anatomic Institute of Zagreb Medical School from 1966 to 1970. He obtained his M.Sc. degree in experimental biology at Zagreb University Faculty of Natural Sciences in 1969 and defended his Ph.D. in medical science at Zagreb University Medical School in 1970. Dr. Pećina became an assistant lecturer at Zagreb Medical School Orthopaedic Clinic in 1970. He was named senior lecturer in 1978, assistant professor in 1979, associate professor in 1980, and professor of orthopedics in 1984.

Dr. Pećina has visited and worked in many orthopedic institutions around the world for further professional training (Lyon, Bologna, Basel, London, Milwaukee, New York, Baltimore, Los Angeles, Columbus, and others). He has also participated in numerous symposia and conferences in his country and abroad. He is actively involved in professional associations, in particular the Croatian Medical Association and Croatian Orthopaedic Society, where he serves as president. He is also president of the *Croatian Medical Bulletin* council and editor-in-chief of the *Croatian Sports Medicine Journal.* Dr. Pećina is a member of the following international societies: International Knee Society, European Spinal Deformities Society, French Society for Orthopaedic Surgery and Traumatology (Société Francaise de Chirurgie Orthopédique et Traumatologique), European Society of Knee Surgery, Sports Traumatology and Arthroscopy (ESSKA), American Academy of Orthopaedic Surgeons (International Affiliate Member), New York Academy of Sciences, Italian Club of Knee Surgery (Club Italiano di Chirurgia del Ginocchio), Balkan Medical Union (Union Medicale Balkanique), Collège Européen de Traumatologie du Sport, and the International Association of Olympic Medical Officers. He is founder and member of the Croatian Olympic Committee and Chairman of the Medical Commission, and he was chief physician of the Croatian National Team during the Olympic Games in Barcelona in 1992. He is also a member of Société Internationale de Chirurgie Orthopédique et de Traumatologie (SICOT) and is a SICOT national delegate for Croatia and a member of the International Council. Dr. Pećina is an honorary member of the Hellenic Orthopaedic and Traumatologic Society. He is one of the founders of the European Spinal Deformities Society and was vice-president from 1989 to 1992. Since 1993, he has been Assistant Editor of *International Orthopaedics* and a corresponding member of the Editorial Board of *Hip International,* and a member of the Editorial Board of *Acta Chirurgiae Orthopaedicae et Traumatologiae Česhoslovaca.*

For his professional achievements, Dr. Pećina has been awarded numerous tokens of appreciation, including the Balkan Medical Union Award for Scientific Achievement, the Croatian Award of Sports Medicine, and the Croatian Award for Scientific Achievement. He has also received many other diplomas of foreign and domestic associations (International Olympic Committee diploma "H.E. Mr. Juan Antonio Samaranch," SICOT diploma for achievement in orthopedic surgery, ESSKA scientific award for poster presentation, Croatian Medical Academy diploma for the best scientific paper published in 2001, to name a few). He is a regular member of the Croatian Medical Academy and an associate member of the Croatian Academy of Arts and Sciences.

Dr. Pećina is interested in clinical anatomy and applied biomechanics of the locomotor system, knee problems, and sports medicine. He has written more than 400 expert and scientific papers and more than 20 books, including *Tunnel Syndromes. Peripheral Nerve Compression Syndromes,* 3rd ed., published by CRC Press in 2001.

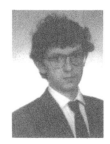

Ivan Bojanić, M.D., M.Sc., is an orthopedic surgeon interested in sports medicine. He is also an assistant lecturer at the Department of Orthopaedic Surgery at the School of Medicine, University of Zagreb, Croatia. Dr. Bojanić obtained his M.D. degree in 1988 from Zagreb University, School of Medicine. He obtained his M.Sc. degree (in biomedicine) in 1991 from Zagreb University, Faculty of Natural Sciences.

Dr. Bojanić is a member of the Croatian Medical Association, the Croatian Orthopaedic and Traumatology Society, and the European Society for Sports Traumatology, Knee Surgery and Arthroscopy (ESSKA). He is editor of the *Croatian Sports Medicine Journal,* chief physician of the Croatian Track-and-Field National Team, and a member of the Medical Commission of the Croatian Olympic Committee. Dr. Bojanić has visited and worked in several orthopedic and sports medicine institutions in Europe for additional professional training. He has participated in international congresses and meetings and has published more than 100 articles. Dr. Bojanić's current major research interests are in sports traumatology, arthroscopy, and knee surgery.

Contents

PART III   Spine

PART V Other Overuse Injuries

Part I

Overview

1 Introduction

I. SIGNIFICANCE OF OVERUSE INJURIES

Athletic activities and recreational exercises are the phenomena of modern civilized societies. The Olympic logo *Citius, altius, fortius* may translate better today as "even faster, even higher, even stronger." If we consider that many sport participants are professionally involved and that sport has become big business and top entertainment in our society, we can understand how sport can place demands on an athlete. At the same time, during the last few decades, recreational exercise has become most people's daily lifestyle. However, as participation in exercise continues to proliferate, so do the concomitant injuries. Injuries to the musculoskeletal system that would not normally happen have become very frequent due to athletic activities.

Acute mechanical injuries are not diagnostic and therapeutic problems as they do not differ from injuries occurring in the average population. Indeed, various studies indicate that approximately 30 to 50% of all sports injuries are caused by overuse. Many physicians do not differentiate between damage and injury and classify all symptoms under injuries. *Injury* may be defined as any damage of the tissue that occurred in a well-defined and limited time span. *Damage* is considered a pathological anatomic entity that cannot be proved (evidenced); in most cases, the patient did not feel and does not even remember when the damage happened. In summary, the main characteristic of an injury is acuteness, whereas damage has a chronic character. Damage of the locomotor system is the result of a series of repetitive microtraumas that overwhelm the tissue's ability to repair itself.[75] Therefore, many authors view it as one of the microtraumatic illnesses, but etiologically and pathologenetically, it would be better to term it an overuse injury.[66]

Whereas overuse of the other major body systems (cardiac, respiratory, renal, nervous, etc.) is relatively easy to test, overuse of the musculoskeletal system is very difficult to prove because there are no morphological and physiological standards with which to compare. The prepathological condition of other major body systems may be objectivized, e.g., electrocardiogram (EKG), electromyoneurography (EMNG), electroencephalogram (EEG), etc., but it is very difficult to establish objective standards for overuse injuries of the musculoskeletal system. The common etiology of all musculoskeletal overuse injuries is repetitive trauma that overwhelms the ability of tissue, including tendons, bursae, cartilage, bone, and especially the musculotendinous unit, to repair itself.

The cause of overuse injuries is much clearer when the biomechanical factors of different sports are analyzed.[16,82] The foot touches the ground soil between 800 and 2000 times on a 1-mile run. The ground-reactive force at midstance in running is 250 to 300% of body weight. A 70-kg runner at 1175 steps per mile absorbs at least 220 tons of force per mile. Therefore, it is not surprising that even the smallest anatomical or biomechanical abnormality of the lower extremities, especially if they are subjected to training errors or some other external factors, may lead to overuse injuries of the lower extremities or the spine.

To understand the genesis of overuse injuries in the upper extremities, one need ponder only briefly the number of times javelin throwers throw their spear, weight lifters lift their weights, or handball or water polo players take a shot at the goal. To cite an example, a swimmer will typically make somewhere in the neighborhood of 4000 overhead strokes during one training session. This adds up to more than 800,000 overhead strokes in just one season and illustrates why approximately 60% of top-class swimmers suffer from overuse injury in the shoulder area.[82] An epidemiological investigation[42] of training and injury patterns in 155 British triathletes showed that the average injury

3

rate was 5.4 injuries per 1000 h of training and 17.4 injuries per 1000 h of competition. Overuse was the reported cause in 41% of the injuries, two thirds of which occurred during running.[42]

One generally tends to equate overuse injuries with professional or recreational athletes (sports-induced overuse injuries). However, physicians should be aware that overuse injuries can also develop in nonathletes and can develop as a result of other human activities,[17,20,28,64] primarily work habits (work-induced overuse injuries). The link between occupation and musculoskeletal disorders has been the focus of numerous research projects, ranging from those simply observing the different pathological findings reported among workers performing particular tasks to the latest studies actually quantifying the "exposure" of workers to physical and psychosocial stimuli.[23,62] An example is the case of an auto mechanic, who typically works for hours, on a daily basis, with a screwdriver and, as a consequence, is at risk for developing lateral (radial) epicondylitis or "tennis elbow." The enormous cost to industry and society is driving many investigators to study the causes and pathologic manifestations of "cumulative trauma disorders," and this research should lead to improved strategies for treating and preventing work-related injuries.[26]

According to Keller et al.[38] computer users experience high rates of injury and disability, broadly termed repetitive strain injury (RSI). With more than 60 million Americans using computers in offices and homes, the potential magnitude of the RSI problem indicates a need for increased attention to prevention and treatment. Pascarelli and Hsu[65] present results of clinical findings in 485 computer users, musicians, and others whose chief complaints were work-related pain and other symptoms. Hyperlaxity of fingers and elbows was found in more than 50%, carpal tunnel syndrome in 8%, radial tunnel syndrome in 7%, cubital tunnel in 64%, shoulder impingement in 13%, medial epicondylitis in 60%, lateral epicondylitis in 33%, and peripheral muscle weakness in 70%. The influence of keyboard design on hand position, typing productivity, and keyboard preference was evaluated by Zecevic et al.[83] comparing two segmented, alternative designs for the linear keyboard. The fixed design incorporated moderate changes in the standard keyboard, changes that promoted a more natural hand position while typing, thereby reducing the potential for cumulative trauma disorders. According to an EMG study of Laursen et al.[48] mental demands during computer work increased muscular activity in the forearm, shoulder, and neck muscles. Increased muscular activity was found in the neck during the use of a mouse vs. the keyboard; this phenomenon may be related to higher visual demands during the use of a mouse than with a keyboard. If we take into account other similarly risk-prone professions such as professional musicians and dancers, computer users, cooks, surgeons, workers on an assembly line, and others, it becomes quite clear that the overuse injury is not just a sports medicine problem but, indeed, a general medical problem.

Lower limb overuse injuries present the greatest source of medical problems during basic military training. The main overuse lower limb injuries are anterior compartment syndrome, stress fractures, Achilles tendinitis, plantar fasciitis, shin splints, and chondromalacia patella.[76] The purpose of the study of Almeida et al.[2] was to identify rates of diagnosis-specific musculoskeletal injuries in 1296 randomly selected male U.S. Marine Corps recruits and to examine the association between patterns of physical training and these injuries. Overuse injuries accounted for 78% of the diagnoses. The results of this controlled epidemiological investigation indicate that the volume of vigorous physical training may be an etiological factor for exercise-related injuries. The findings also suggest that type of training, particularly running, and abrupt increases in training volume may further contribute to injury risk. In addition, numerous studies have indicated that the incidence of repetitive motion disorders in females exceeds that in males.[24]

The most important — and at the same time both diagnostically and therapeutically not completely understood — questions are those dealing with overuse in the musculotendinous functional unit, the area where the muscle inserts into the tendon and the tendon inserts into the bone. La Cava[47] refers to this area as the "mioenthesic apparatus." Other authors use the term *enthesis*, which refers to the area of insertion of the tendon into the bone. The tendon can be inserted either directly or through cartilage, ligament, or membrane (aponeurose). The insertion of the muscle into the tendon forms a more or less sharp angle, which ensures that the direction of the muscle remains relatively constant, despite the fact that the breadth of the muscle is greater than the breadth of the tendon. It is generally believed that, at the area of insertion of the muscle fibers into the tendon, there exists an intermediary zone of adhesive tissue of 10 to 100 mm thickness. Without question the musculotendinous unit has some specific characteristics that differentiate it from the muscle, and it is equally beyond doubt that the musculotendinous unit represents a complete and unique functional unit.

The musculotendinous functional unit suffers the greatest strain during muscle contraction. The force of the muscle is relayed to the ends of the musculotendinous unit where the cross-sectional area is considerably smaller than the cross-sectional area of the muscle. In all cases of longitudinal extension, the maximal forces appear at the ends — in this case, at the musculotendinous unit. The elasticity of the musculotendinous unit is less than the elasticity of the muscle while its fragility is considerably greater, increasing the risk of its injury. Special proprioceptive bodies are located in the musculotendinous unit that enable it to react in accordance with the state of contraction of the muscle fibers or, in other words, in accord with the degree of the mechanical deformation of the muscle.

Because the musculotendinous functional unit has a polymorphic structure, it can be adapted to the multifunctional demands of the musculoskeletal system. The musculotendinous unit is also characterized by its susceptibility to injury, which leads to tissue metaplasia (e.g., calcification) in the tendon. Further, the tendon tissue is bradytrophic, which explains why it is more often affected by pathological changes due to overuse than are other tissues. The changes may affect the musculotendinous area, the tendon itself, its sheath, or the insertion for the bone.[30] The resulting condition is referred to as miotendinitis, tendinitis, paratenonitis, or simply enthesitis, although some authors generally use the term *enthesitis* (and many other names; see Section IV) for changes on the musculotendinous unit (Figure 1.1). Enthesitis is one form of tendon overuse injury that is characterized by pain and discomfort in the area of the tendon–bone junction or osteotendinous junction. According to Jozsa and Kannus[32] none of the names given for this condition fully defines it. Acute forms may display the classic clinical and histological signs of inflammation but no tissue degeneration, whereas in the chronic forms tissue degeneration may be clear but there is no histologically demonstrable inflammation. Mixed lesions can also be found, and the site of the lesion and irritation may sometimes involve the insertion as well as the more proximal area of the tendon belly and tendon bursa. In the chronic forms the histopathologic findings vary considerably with regard to the anatomic site in question.[70]

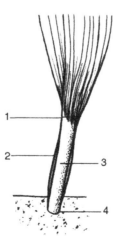

FIGURE 1.1 Possible localizations of pathological changes in the muscle–tendon union. (1) Myotendinitis; (2) paratendinitis or peritendinitis or paratenonitis; (3) tendinitis/tendinosis; (4) enthesitis or insertional tendinopathy.

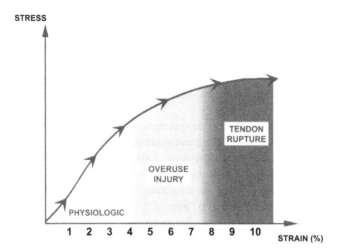

SCHEME 1.1 Development of overuse tendon injuries.

According to current knowledge, "overuse" in tendon injuries implies that the tendon has been strained repeatedly to 4 to 8% of the original length until it is unable to endure further tension, whereupon injury occurs (Scheme 1.1).[19,25,32] The structure of the tendon is disrupted microscopically, macroscopically, or both by this repetitive strain, and inflammation, edema, and pain result.[25] If the damage progresses, tendinosis (i.e., focal area of intratendinous degeneration that is initially asymptomatic), partial tears, and complete ruptures may ensue. In the pathogenesis of overuse injuries, the tendinous tissue becomes fatigued as its basal reparative ability is overwhelmed by repetitive dysfunctional and microtraumatic processes. In other words, when a destructive process of applied stress exceeds the reparative process, overuse injuries result.[7]

When the tendon is overused, the reduction in vascular supply and excessive irritation of nerve ends lead to an aseptic inflammatory reaction, which leads to tissue metaplasia, including cartilage, osteoid, and bone metaplasia. The process is chronic and may last for months with frequent reinflammations, causing a condition with constant complaints. To better understand the etiology of the overuse injuries of the musculoskeletal system, it is essential to understand the pathology of the inflammatory process. Regardless of the injury type, the tissue always undergoes an inflammatory response that encompasses a number of changes of the vascular net, blood, and connective tissue. The inflammatory response is a very complex response, which includes different cell types, numerous enzymes, and many physiologically active substances. Unfortunately, this response has yet to be completely elucidated. The cause of the initiation of the inflammatory response is unknown in many cases. One such example is rheumatoid arthritis. In contrast, the cause may be well known, for example, microorganisms, immunocomplexes, or the by-products of the necrotic tissue. This last cause can be directly and causally correlated to the genesis of the overuse injury and the accompanying tissue damage.

Before we elaborate on the etiology and development of the inflammatory response in overuse injury, it is necessary to elucidate some basic factors concerning this response: vasoactive substances, chemotactic factors, and tissue-damaging agents. Vasoactive substances include prostaglandins, vasoactive amines (histamine, serotonin), anaphylatoxins, and kinins (bradykinin, lysilbradykinin), and it is believed that they cause vasodilation and increased permeability of the blood vessels. The rupture of damaged cells of the tendon releases chemicals that signal other cells to come to the area to help clean up the damaged tissue. Several different molecules that have chemotactic effect have been isolated. Some of them are of bacterial origin, but others originate from the complement system–activated by-products. It has been discovered that leukotriens and kallikreins also have chemotactic effect. Agents that cause tissue rupture are enzymes hydrolases located within the lysosomes of the inflamed cells and enzymes located in the extracellular area (e.g., collagenases, elastases, and cathepsin G).

In overuse injuries, the tendon has been loaded repeatedly and the sum of repetitive force leads to microtraumas that initiate the inflammatory response.[19] The initial vasoconstriction is followed by vasodilation. As a consequence, increase of the intracapillary pressure, increased permeability of the fine vascular net, and release of a fair amount of transudate in the perivascular area occur. Further permeability increase of the blood vessels causes the accumulation of the fluid containing different cell types and many cell compounds (proteins, white blood cells, thrombocytes). The fluid itself is called *exudate*. Chemotactic chemicals act as signals to draw cells involved with the healing process. Polymorphonuclear leukocytes start degradation of the surrounding tissue by activated hydrolases released from their lysosomes. After a few days, they are replaced by monocytes that soon become macrophages. Other cell types, such as lymphocytes, plasma cells, fibroblasts, and mast cells, are also present in the damaged tissue area. Macrophages play the most important role in the inflammatory response by digesting all the by-products of inflammation by the process of phagocytosis or endocytosis and thus help clean up the damaged tissue. This event enables the last phase of the response, the healing phase, to take place.

Although the inflammatory response is necessary to initiate healing, it should last only a short time. If the inflammation is prolonged, we must prevent it from becoming chronic. Only under such circumstances should nonsteroidal anti-inflammatory drugs (NSAIDs) and steroidal anti-inflammatory drugs be used. To clarify the drug effect, we describe the role of prostaglandins in the inflammatory response. Prostaglandins are local hormones derived from arachidonic acid. They are metabolized very quickly, but, other than that, their biological effects have not yet been thoroughly investigated. In the inflammatory response, they cause local vasodilatation and increased vessel permeability resulting in edema of the inflamed tissue. Together with other mediators of inflammation, they stimulate pain receptors and are responsible for pain, the first clinical sign of tendinitis. They stimulate osteoclasts and macrophages and, therefore, cause bone resorption as well. NSAIDs deactivate the enzyme cyclo-oxygenase responsible for the conversion of the arachidonic acid to prostaglandin. Glucocorticoids can also inhibit the biosynthesis of prostaglandins by locking the enzyme phospholipase.

Generally speaking, healing is the body's response to injury. The process may be divided in phases depending on time needed to activate particular healing mechanisms. Connective tissue healing is divided into two broad stages: proliferative and formative. During the former, which lasts approximately 14 days, cells migrate to the area of the tissue damage and new connective tissue is laid down. This new tissue is remodeled during the next formative stage. The formative stage extends from the end of the proliferative stage until the tissue is as near normal as possible. Chvapil[19] further subdivides connective tissue healing into four stages: (1) cell mobilization (inflammatory response), (2) ground substance proliferation, (3) collagen protein formation, and (4) final organization. Stages 1 to 3 are the proliferative stages of healing, and Stage 4 is formative.

During the stage of cell mobilization, the rupture of damaged cells releases chemotactic substances that initiate an increase in vessel permeability and act as signals to white blood cells, but also help the degradation of damaged tissue. This stage is also called the stage of inflammatory response. It begins when injury occurs, lasts for 48 h, and is important because of the arrival of white blood cells.

Ground substance proliferation does not take place until Day 3 or 4. The existence of an adequate amount of ground substance (which is a gel-like matrix composed of proteins, carbohydrates, and water) is necessary for the aggregation of collagenous proteins into the shape of fibrils.

The stage of collagen protein formation begins at Day 5 following the injury, and is characterized by the transformation of the immature (soluble) collagen into the mature form of the molecule. Collagen transforms as a result of cross-links forming between the tropocollagen molecules. From Day 6 to Day 14, the proportion of cross-linked collagen increases. It is of crucial importance to stop the inflammation before Day 5 because the enzymes prevent formation of cross-links and degrade newly synthesized soluble collagen.

In the final stage, from Day 14 onward, collagen continues to increase and begins to organize into fibrils that reorient themselves in line with the tensile force applied to the tissue. It is very important to contract the adjacent muscles because the contraction causes the stress of collagen fibrils and generates electric potential due to the piezoelectric effect. The potential itself orients collagen fibrils in line with the tensile force of the muscle contraction. With this event, the process of healing is terminated, and the tendon is capable of withstanding further mechanical loads.

Arnoczky et al.[9] studied activation of stress-activated protein kinases in tendon cells following cyclic strain. Cyclic strain has been shown to benefit tendon health. However, repetitive loading has also been implicated in the etiology of tendon overuse injuries. Recent studies demonstrated that in several cell lines cyclic strain was associated with an activation of stress-activated protein kinases (SAPKs). These SAPKs, in turn, were shown to be important upstream regulators of a variety of cell processes including apoptosis. A similar mechanism could be responsible for initiating the pathological events (localized cell death) seen in tendon overuse injury. According to Kjaer,[40] we are only just beginning to master methodologies to evaluate tissue changes in tendon and muscle that will allow for better understanding of adaptation to mechanical loading in sports activities. Such knowledge of muscle–tendon force development and tissue reaction to movement will be important for understanding the etiology and pathogenesis of overuse injuries, and will provide the basis for better diagnostic approaches and better treatment modalities. Herein lies a major scientific challenge.

Although conditions related to tendons and tendon insertions are primarily considered overuse injuries of the musculoskeletal system, some such injuries involve bones,[29,58] muscles,[79] joint cartilage,[1] bursae,[59] and peripheral nerves.[68,69] One joint that appears to be particularly susceptible to overuse conditions is the patellofemoral joint, where abnormal wear of hyaline cartilage on the retropatellar surface may occur, resulting in anterior knee pain. This condition is further explored in Chapter 8. Chapter 11 is dedicated to the inflammation of the bursae (bursitis), stressing the problem of the chronic bursitis caused by repetitive trauma from either friction of the overlying tendon or external pressure applied above the bursae. Nerve tissue is also subject to overuse injury. Sensory, motor, or mixed sensory-motor peripheral nerves may be affected by constant and/or repetitive loading and pressure on nerves, as well as by the pathomechanics of the special anatomic area such as carpal tunnel, tarsal tunnel, etc.[69] These nerve entrapment disorders of the sports participant are discussed in Chapter 13.

Pathoanatomical changes that can be seen in overuse injuries of the musculoskeletal system depend on the type of tissue affected and on the localization and clinical stage of the injury. There is a large pathohistological scale from inflammatory response to degenerative changes reported by many authors[19,28,70] and confirmed by intraoperative examination in our own patients. We briefly describe pathohistological findings concerning different localizations of overuse injuries in our operated patients. The tissue sections were obtained and histologically analyzed courtesy of Nikola Sipus, from the Institute for Chemical Pathology, University of Zagreb. Tissue samples were obtained from all of the patients who underwent surgery. The samples were taken from the tendon insertion site and from sites of the macroscopic changes in the tendon and its sheath. The tissue samples were fixed in formalin, embedded in paraffin, and stained with hemalaun-eosin. Histological changes of the tendon tissue, the bone–tendon interface, and the tendon sheath, as well as the blood vessels and nerves in the tendon and its sheath, have been analyzed.

The pathohistological sections shown here relate to Achilles tendinitis or patellar tendinitis, which is understandable as these localizations are the most common to incite surgical treatment.

The formation of edema and tissue necrosis on certain parts of the tendon is the first noticeable change (Figure 1.2 and Figure 1.3). After a short period of time, inflammatory cells migrate to the damaged area. The most abundant among them are mononuclears (Figure 1.4). Because infection is not the issue in this case, there are very few granulocytes among the inflammatory cells. The

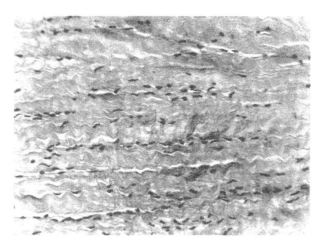

FIGURE 1.2 Normal tendon (original magnification × 200).

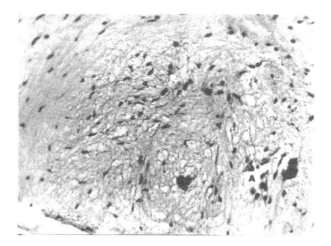

FIGURE 1.3 Necrotic focus in tendon accompanied by severe edema of the surrounding tissue and initial accumulation of mononuclears (A) (original magnification × 200).

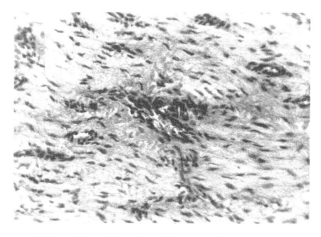

FIGURE 1.4 Tendon remodeling with proliferation with connecting tissue strongly interspersed with blood capillaries. Inflammatory infiltrates of mononuclears are sparse (original magnification × 200).

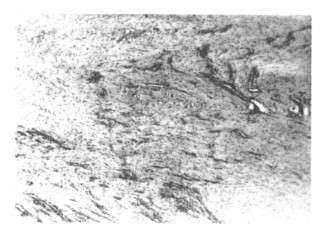

FIGURE 1.5 Remodeled tendon has irregular structure and contains a greater number of blood capillaries (original magnification × 60).

first stage of tissue healing, the inflammatory response, is followed by remodeling of the damaged tendon. The remodeling occurs through connective tissue proliferation and formation. Proliferation of collagen molecules continues from within the cells of the damaged tendon but soon organizes into collagen fibrils.

The number of blood capillaries also increases, but as the process develops, the number decreases back to normal. The scar formed after the tendon is remodeled differs from the normal uninjured tendon in random organization of collagen fibers and greater number of blood capillaries (Figure 1.5). Changes that affect the bone–tendon interface are characterized by edema development and bleeding and sometimes even by disjunction of the tendon fibers from the bone. Lesser damage of the bone–tendon interface causes edema of all tissue structures, which is then followed by inflammation. The cells most commonly involved in the inflammatory process are mononuclears and lymphocytes (Figure 1.6). The connective tissue scar usually degenerates, and the largest part of the tendon (sometimes even the periost) becomes acellular and full of homogeneous hyaline matrix (Figure 1.7). Those scars are very often spread over surrounding tissue structures, changing the appearance of the surrounding tissue. The first sign of the changes of the tendon sheath is bleeding in the early stages of the injury. Bleeding is soon followed by a secondary inflammation. Because

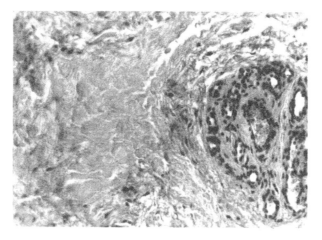

FIGURE 1.6 Damage of the tendon–bone insertion. Connective tissue edema. Blood capillaries are dilated and surrounded by inflammatory cells: lymphocytes and mononuclears (original magnification × 200).

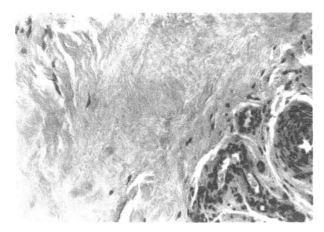

FIGURE 1.7 Scars on the Achilles tendon insertion site. Strong hyaline degeneration of the tendon's connective tissue makes the connective tissue practically acellular. Mononuclears are rare (original magnification × 200).

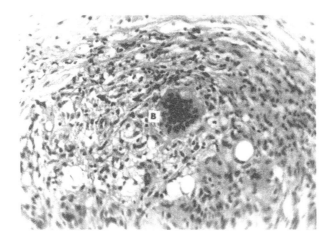

FIGURE 1.8 Tendon sheath inflammation accompanied by multiplication of the granulation tissue-rich macrophages. Rare giant cells of the foreign body are also present, and their cytoplasm contains phagocytic necrotic material (B) (original magnification × 200).

the tendon is poorly provided with blood and lymph, the tendon sheath plays an active role in tissue remodeling. This process is accompanied by a proliferation of macrophages and quite often gigantic cells of the foreign body, which fagocite larger particles of the necrotic tendon (Figure 1.8).

Changes in blood vessels can be divided into changes in the arteries, capillaries, and veins. Inflammatory cells leave the arteries, and capillaries during the inflammatory infiltrates are frequently seen. Although generally younger individuals are involved, the later stages are characterized by a proliferation of endotel accompanied by endarteritic changes, which significantly decrease the breadth of the blood vessel. In some cases, this leads to an obliteration of the artery (an example is shown in Figure 1.9, depicting the area of insertion of the Achilles tendon into the calcaneus). Smaller veins frequently have thrombocytes. In later stages, these thrombocytes are organized (Figure 1.10) and in some cases recanalized (Figure 1.11).

Changes in nerves of overuse injuries, until now, have not been specifically analyzed. However, we have found significant changes in the nervous tissue in the area of the injured tendon or in the area of its insertion. To better explain the changes affecting nerves, Figure 1.12 is a photograph of a normal nerve with a sheath of normal breadth. (In our opinion, intense pain in the area of the

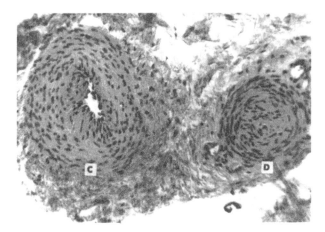

FIGURE 1.9 Changes affecting arteries close to the scarred tendon insertion site. Severe endarteritis with constriction of the arterial lumen (C), resulting in total obliteration of the artery (D) (original magnification × 200).

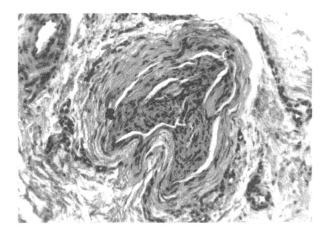

FIGURE 1.10 Changes in the vein close to the tendon scar. Chronic thrombosis of the vein with thromb organization (original magnification × 200).

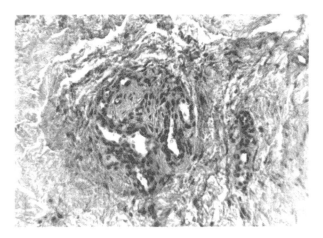

FIGURE 1.11 Recanalized thromb of a smaller vein localized in the scar on the tendon insertion site (original magnification × 200).

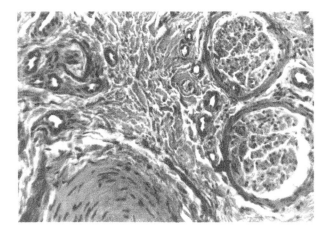

FIGURE 1.12 Normal nerve with unaffected sheath.

injured tendon, or in the area of its insertion, with frequent morphologically insignificant changes is caused by changes on the ends of peripheral nerves.) Our pathohistological analysis has shown the presence of perineuritis accompanied by an increase of breadth of the nerve sheath, which later compresses the nerve. These changes are frequently very noticeable (as shown in Figure 1.13).

Recently, the term *tendinosis* (tendon degeneration), instead of "tendinitis," is used more and more. The pathways and cellular mechanisms that lead to tendinosis are not well understood.[37] Frequently, tendinosis can be found in conjunction with the chronic forms of peritendinitis and tendinitis, although this does not indicate a causal relationship, in either direction.[32] A popular theory in the medical literature suggests that tendon degeneration passes through acute, recurrent, subacute, subchronic, and chronic phases of tendinitis before actual degeneration develops.[25,70,71] Clinically, the term tendinosis can be described as a focal area of intratendinous degeneration that may by initially asymptomatic.[50] Clancy and Leadbetter[50] note that no signs of intratendinous inflammation are present in tendinosis. If intratendinous inflammation is combined with tendinosis (symptomatic degeneration), they called it tendinitis. Jozsa and Kannus,[32] in turn, prefer to keep "tendinosis" and "tendinitis" separate entities so that both may occur independently or together, as is the case with tendinosis and peritendinitis. Thus, Jozsa and Kannus[32] do not exclude the possibility of pure tendinitis.

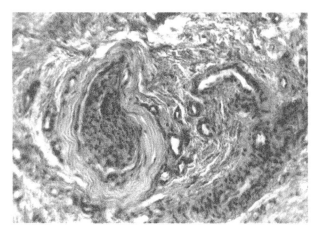

FIGURE 1.13 Changes in the nerve situated in the scar on the Achilles tendon insertion site. The nerve sheath is thickened and compresses the nerve (original magnification × 200).

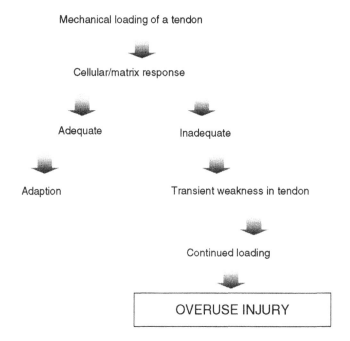

Mechanical loading of a tendon

Cellular/matrix response

Adequate   Inadequate

Adaption   Transient weakness in tendon

Continued loading

OVERUSE INJURY

SCHEME 1.2 Tendon response to a mechanical loading.

Without a complete understanding of the etiopathogenesis of overuse injuries of the musculoskeletal system, there can be no early diagnosis or adequate therapy prescribed. According to Leadbetter,[50] the microtraumatic response to load and use is best understood within the context of a failed adaptation to physical load and use (Scheme 1.2). The etiology of these syndromes is multifactorial. In other words, numerous factors contribute to the development of overuse injuries (Table 1.1). A combination of extrinsic factors, such as training errors and environmental factors, and intrinsic or anatomical factors, such as bony alignment of the extremities, flexibility deficits, and ligamentous laxity, predisposes athletes to develop overuse injuries.[44]

Awareness of anatomical factors that may predispose individuals to overuse injuries allows the clinician to develop individual prehabilitation programs designed to decrease the risk of overuse injury. The purpose of the prospective study of Kaufman et al.[35] was to determine whether an association exists between foot structure and the development of musculoskeletal overuse injuries. The study group was a well-defined cohort of 449 trainees at the Naval Special Warfare Training Center in Coronado, CA. Before beginning training, measurements were made of ankle motion, subtalar motion, and the static (standing) and dynamic (walking) characteristics of the foot arch. The subjects were followed prospectively for injuries throughout training. The authors of the study identified risk factors that predispose people to lower extremity overuse injuries. These risk factors include dynamic pes planus, pes cavus, restricted ankle dorsiflexion, and increased hindfoot inversion, all of which are subject to intervention and possible correction. Hintermann and Nigg[27] consider that the individual transfer mechanism of foot eversion into internal tibial rotation may be of some predictable value for lower extremity overloading and related overuse injuries.

II. CLINICAL PICTURE AND DIAGNOSTICS

The clinical picture in the early stages of overuse injuries is characterized by a feeling of tightness. This is generally followed by pain in one part or in the whole musculotendinous unit during passive or active stretching, during contraction of the affected muscle against resistance, and in lateral stages during normal contraction of the muscle. These symptoms are followed by

TABLE 1.1
Predisposing Factors Leading to Overuse Injuries of the Musculoskeletal System

Internal (Intrinsic)	External (Extrinsic)
Anatomical malalignment	Training errors
Leg length discrepancy	Abrupt changes in intensity, duration, and/or frequency
Excessive femoral anteversion	of training
Knee alignment abnormalities (genu valgum, varum, or	Poorly trained and unskilled athlete
recurvatum)	Surface
Position of the patella (patella infera or alta)	Hard
Excessive Q-angle	Uneven
Excessive external tibial rotation	Footwear
Flat foot	Inappropriate running shoes
Cavus foot	Worn-out running shoes
Muscle-tendon imbalance of	
Flexibility	
Strength	
Other	
Growth	
Disturbances of menstrual cycle	

TABLE 1.2
Classification System for the Effect of Pain on Athletic Performance[19]

Level	Description of Pain	Level of Sports Performance
1	No pain	Normal
2	Pain only with extreme exertion	Normal
3	Pain with extreme exertion, 1 to 2 h afterward	Normal or slightly decreased
4	Pain during and after any vigorous activities	Somewhat decreased
5	Pain during activity, forcing termination	Markedly decreased
6	Pain during daily activities	Unable to perform

pain felt during palpation, and sometimes by the presence of swelling in the affected area. The final symptoms include spontaneous pain felt during complete rest, which can in some cases radiate along the length of the whole affected muscle. With regard to the time that the pain appears during athletic activities and to the intensity of the pain, several stages of development are recognized. Based on the correlation between the intensity of the pain, or in other words, the stage of the disease and the remaining athletic capacity, Curwin and Stanish[19] differentiate six stages of development in overuse injuries (Table 1.2).

The diagnosis of overuse injuries must stem from a careful history as well as a thorough physical examination. To identify the injured structure, it is essential to characterize the pain (e.g., where, when, and how long it lasts) and to ask questions establishing the etiological factors that lay the groundwork for the affliction. However, exclusion of macrotrauma is key to proper categorization of the injury as one of overuse. Diagnostic tools include the following:

Physical examination is the basic and most important diagnostic method, whereas all other methods can be regarded as auxiliary methods that are useful only in concert with a detailed physical examination. The characteristics of physical examination with regard to various overuse injuries are discussed in Chapters 3 through 15.

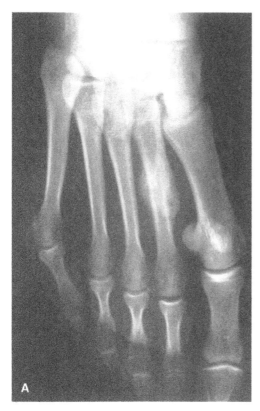 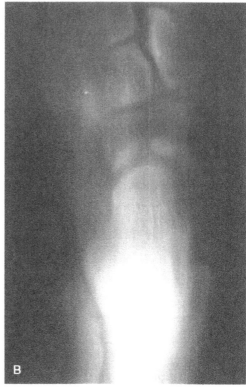

FIGURE 1.14 Stress fracture of the second metatarsal bone (A) and of the tarsal navicular bone (B).

Radiographic examination is rarely of value in establishing a diagnosis of overuse injuries, with the exception of stress fractures (Figure 1.14). Radiographic examination can be used to detect causative factors that lead to development of overuse injuries such as malalignment of the extensor system of the knee, static deformation of the lower extremity, and others.

Computerized tomography (CT) is a useful method when diagnosing the presence of an overuse injury and has the added advantage of being able to diagnose changes in muscles and tendons (e.g., in patients with ruptured tendons), as well as those in bone.

Bone scan with technetium-99m diphosphonate is of great help in early diagnosis of stress fractures. In recent times, its diagnostic capabilities have been significantly increased especially with regard to diagnosing changes in tendons and muscles in overuse injuries (Figure 1.15).[21,34]

Sonographic examination is, without doubt, the most useful auxiliary method used today in diagnosis of overuse injuries. In fact, we could almost say it is an unavoidable method when diagnosing overuse injuries.[22,33,57,74] Ultrasonography is very helpful when diagnosing tendinitis/tendinosis (Figure 1.16), peritendinitis, enthesitis, tendon (Figure 1.17) and muscle rupture (Figure 1.18), bursitis, and even stress fractures. The importance of sonographic examination is enhanced by its ability to perform dynamic investigations (e.g., investigation of the muscle during contraction and relaxation, investigation of the tendon during passive and active stretching, etc.).

Thermography is an auxiliary method that in recent times has been successfully applied in diagnosing overuse injuries. However, its greatest value is its ability to monitor the course of the disorder objectively, both when monitoring the development of overuse injury *sua sponte* and when evaluating the effect of prescribed therapy (Figure 1.19).

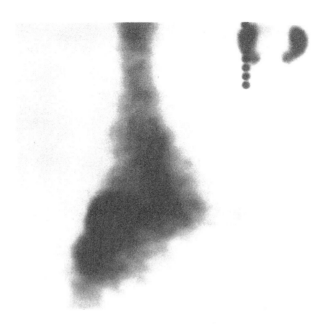

FIGURE 1.15 Bone scan demonstrating tarsal navicular stress fracture.

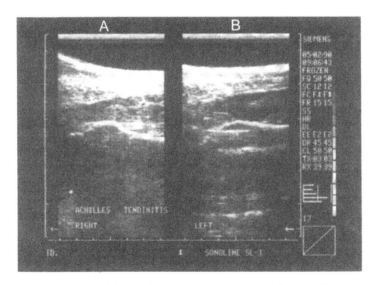

FIGURE 1.16 Sonogram of the Achilles tendon. (A) Achilles tendonitis/tendinosis; (B) normal tendon.

Arthroscopy is of significant value in the detection and treatment of injuries to the joint cartilage.[31] It is most commonly applied to the knee joint, but is also applied to other larger and smaller joints.

Magnetic resonance imaging (MRI) is the diagnostic method of choice in all pathological changes of the musculoskeletal system and thus is eminently applicable when diagnosing overuse injuries. MRI is able to investigate all of the tissues present in the musculoskeletal system and diagnose any pathological changes in them.[8,13,43,73,78]

Pedobarographic analysis with gait analysis reveals possible etiological factors of the over-use injuries of the lower extremities. Pedobarogram of a basketball player (Figure 1.20) shows varo-excavatus deformity of the foot, causing plantar fasciitis in this athlete, cured by adequate insole.

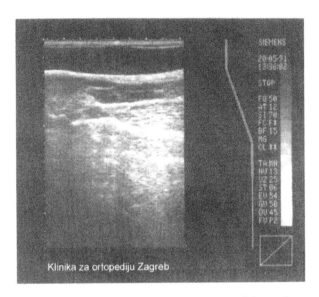

FIGURE 1.17 Sonogram of the Achilles tendon shows acute rupture of the tendon.

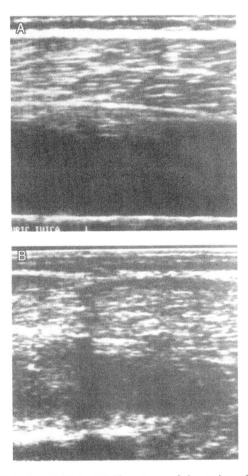

FIGURE 1.18 Sonogram of the lateral thigh. (A) Hematoma of the region of the vastus lateralis muscle; (B) sonographically controlled puncture.

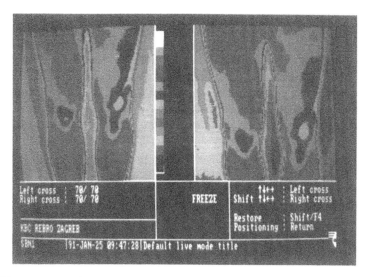

FIGURE 1.19 Thermography of both knees showing hypothermy in the patellar area of the afflicted knee.

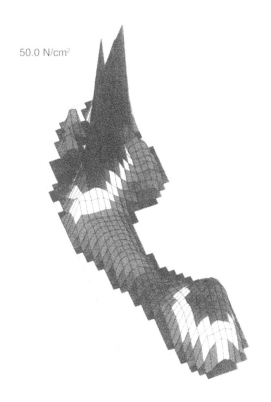

FIGURE 1.20 Pedobarographic analysis in a basketball player with plantar fasciitis.

III. TREATMENT

Treatment of overuse injuries of the musculoskeletal system in the vast majority of cases is non-operative. Surgical treatment is indicated only after failure to respond to a rigorous non-operative program. The patients must qualify for surgery. Lack of compliance and inadequate rehabilitation most often lead to inappropriate surgery and poor results. The basic principle of non-operative treatment is that it should begin as early as possible — in other words, as soon as the first symptoms appear. The most common error is that patients do not pay sufficient attention to the early symptoms and proceed with their everyday athletic or nonathletic activities with unchanged intensity. The basic postulates of non-operative treatment for overuse injuries are based on the following principles: reducing the pain, controlling the inflammation, facilitating tissue healing, and monitoring further activities.[6,10,36,60,61,63]

Any non-operative treatment program must be individually adapted to every patient with regard both to the localization of the pain and to the stage of the disease.[14,18,47,53] The program should consist of the following: a short-term cessation or modification of athletic activities, icing applied to the tender area, application of NSAIDs, stretching exercises for the affected muscles, strengthening exercises for the affected muscle group,[80] correction of the predisposing causative factors[39,40] (training errors, anatomical deviations that impede the normal biomechanics of the activity, inadequate athletic footwear, and even the surface on which the athlete habitually trains).

Physical modalities (cryotherapy, thermotherapy, therapeutic ultrasound, high-voltage pulse galvanic stimulation, electrical stimulation, laser stimulation, extracorporeal shock-wave therapy,[81] etc.) are frequently prescribed to promote healing and recovery after injury. Icing effectively relieves pain and muscle spasm; it lessens the inflammatory reaction by lowering the level of chemical activity and by vasoconstriction. There is much claimed and much more unknown about the various physical techniques, their indications, efficacy, and potential to modify the inflammation repair cycle, such that it is safe to say that the role of physical modalities remains largely experiential and theoretical.[52] Although some authors recommend a total cessation of athletic activities, we believe that in the early stages of disease complete cessation is not mandatory. The patient, aside from submitting to all other non-operative methods of treatment, should be encouraged simply to reduce the intensity of the training program, especially those activities that cause pain. In later stages of disease, a complete cessation of athletic activities is mandatory for a period of no less than 3 to 4 weeks. The functional capabilities of the athlete can be maintained during this time by alternative training programs such as swimming or bicycling.[60,61]

The principal purpose in applying NSAIDs is to control and regulate the inflammatory process and to monitor its duration such that it does not last longer than its primary phase, which has a positive effect on tissue healing. Almekinders et al.[3] observed in an *in vitro* investigation that NSAIDs may have potentially negative effects on tendon fibroblasts during the proliferative phase of healing, as the medication has been associated with decreased DNA synthesis, but may have positive effects in the maturation and remodeling phase, as they stimulate protein synthesis. It is difficult to combine the experimental and clinical data on NSAIDs into a simple clinical recommendation but Jozsa and Kannus[32] recommend that NSAIDs be administered during the first 3 weeks of tendon healing (i.e., during the inflammatory and proliferative phases).

Corticosteroid injection therapy continues to be widely employed, although the mechanism of its alleged therapeutic effect has not been documented in humans. The best indication for steroid injection remains a localized inflammatory site such as synovial cavity, bursa, or tendon synovial sheath. Side effects observed after corticosteroid injection can be problematic, and the patient should be warned of the risk of local corticosteroid injection. Sports participation after injection adjacent to a major tendon should be delayed for a minimum of 2 to 3 weeks. According to Leadbetter,[51,52] improper use and abuse of corticosteroid injection consists of the following: acute trauma, intratendinous injection, infection, multiple injections (more than three), injection immediately before competition, and frequent intra-articular injections.

In the treatment of overuse injuries, stretching exercises are also prescribed — principally, so-called passive stretching exercises.[4,5,80] The basic principles of these exercises consist of a precisely defined stance to which patients must adhere while performing the exercise. They should carry out slow and gradual movements until they feel a stretching sensation; then they should hold that position for a certain period of time.[67] During the performance of passive stretching exercises, the often-quoted principle, "no pain, no gain," should be forgotten. The reason is that staying in a stretched position that causes pain decreases the length of time the patient can stay in that particular position. It increases the possibility of a reflex muscle contraction and can lead to muscle damage.[41] On the other hand, remaining in the point of "primary" stretching enables the complete relaxation of the targeted muscles, and likewise enables the patient to hold that position for a relatively longer period of time. The athlete who performs stretching exercises for the first time is advised to hold the position of primary stretching for 15 s. This period of time is gradually increased but should not exceed 30 s. The principal effects of stretching exercises — a decrease of muscle–tendon tension, improvement of vascularization in the musculotendinous functional unit, and an increase in the breadth of movements — reduce the possibility of injury development. Increase of flexibility, which also reduces injury development risk, is another long-term benefit of stretching exercises.

Surgical treatment of overuse injuries of the musculoskeletal system is the final option. In other words, surgical treatment is recommended only after all non-operative methods of treatment have failed.[11,15] During surgical procedure, diseased, scarred, and degenerated tissue, calcificates, chronically changed bursae, and other tissue are excised.[66,70] Whenever possible, the surgical treatment should target the causative factors that led to the development of the overuse injury, e.g., removing the tuber of the calcaneus, which causes retrocalcanear bursitis, or correctly orienting the extensor system of the knee (realignment). In some cases, the aim of the surgical procedure is to increase the vascularization of the injured area. This can be achieved by drilling the bone, by adhesiolysis of the tendon, or by other means. In some cases, surgical treatment is unavoidable, i.e., ruptured tendons, muscle rupture, and depending on the localization, stress fracture. Indications for surgical treatment of various overuse injuries of the musculoskeletal system are discussed in detail in Chapters 3 through 15. However, we would stress at this time the importance of postoperative rehabilitation because, without an adequately carried out postoperative program of treatment, no surgical intervention, however well performed, can achieve good results.

According to Curwin and Stanish,[19] both the surgical and non-operative treatment methods should be chosen depending on the stage of healing of the damaged tissue of the musculoskeletal system (Table 1.3). Whatever the treatment program selected, it must adhere to the following principles: (1) protection of the early phases of tissue healing, (2) avoidance of excessive immobilization, (3) restoration of total limb function, (4) safe progressive return to competition or work activity, and (5) elimination of faulty or abusive technique.

Unfortunately, at present, no single method, either surgical or non-operative, for any localization of overuse injury exists that can guarantee 100% good results. Thus, prevention is of utmost importance. To prevent overuse injury successfully or, in other words, to reduce as much as possible the risk of developing overuse injuries, we should be well acquainted with the predisposing factors leading to the development of these overuse syndromes and should attempt to assert some influence over the factors. In prevention, as in the treatment of overuse injuries, the physician should take into account the individual needs of each patient as it is incorrect to treat, for example, a recreational runner with the same therapy that would be prescribed for a top-level, professional athlete.[25] Stretching exercises play an important role in the *prevention* of overuse injuries as well. It is also important to note that prevention of overuse injuries of the musculoskeletal system has been greatly enhanced by numerous investigations carried out during the past 20 years. This research has described many predisposing causative factors of these injuries and has suggested ways of both treating and preventing them.[25,66,77] Perhaps one of the best examples of how these investigations have contributed not only to therapy, but also to decreasing the frequency of some overuse injuries, is Achilles tendinitis. As a result of adequate and correct prevention regarding training (monitoring

TABLE 1.3
Forms of Treatment for Overuse Injuries[19]

Treatment	Used in This Stage of Healing[a]
Rest	1,2,3
Stop activity	
Cast immobilization	
Taping/support	1,2,3,4
Physical modalities	1,2,3
Ice	
Electric stimulation	
"Deep heat"	
Ultrasound	
Drugs	
Anti-inflammatory drugs (oral)	1,2,3
Steroids (injections)	
Exercise	3,4
Stretching	
Strengthening	
Surgery	1 (rupture) or 4 (chronic)

[a] 1 = cell mobilization (inflammatory response); 2 = ground substance proliferation; 3 = collagen protein formation; 4 = final organization.

the training process so that there are no sudden increases in the intensity of training), prevention regarding the surface (avoiding running on steep inclines and on uneven, rough, and hard surfaces) and prevention regarding footwear (wearing adequate athletic footwear), as well as prevention regarding orthotic correction of biomechanical irregularities that cause excessive pronation of the foot during running (pes planovalgus, pes cavus, and others), the incidence of Achilles tendinitis has dropped by more than 50% during the time. In addition to education (to which we hope to contribute with this book), prevention, as well as treatment of overuse injuries of the musculoskeletal system, depends on the close collaboration among athlete, coach, and physician.

Hippocrates noted: "Healing is a matter of time but is sometimes also a matter of opportunity." Leadbetter[52] added:

In this age, when sports medicine has been an art earnestly seeking its science, the modern sports medicine clinician must be increasingly aware of the biologic events and reparative capabilities of human tissues. For while the art of sports medicine may be extended through experience, the future therapeutic opportunities of sports medicine will be extended only by its scientific basis.

IV. NOMENCLATURE

The various terms applied to different overuse injuries have not been recognized by all authors as yet. All connective tissues are not the same. Intrinsic differences in the biologic nature of connective tissues have yet to be fully understood in regard to their impact on the quality of healing.[52] Classifications and terminology of the clinicopathological entities of overuse injuries are not clear and definitive.[32,45,52,71] The reasons for this confusion are that symptoms, clinical signs, and histological findings of each entity overlap with those of other entities, conditions can coexist, and true knowledge on the etiology, pathogenesis, and histopathology of overuse injury problems is still rather scarce.[32] Sports physicians in the U.S. have tried to create a new classification of tendon disorders and injuries.[50] They describe four pathologic conditions: (1) paratenonitis, a class including "tenosynovitis," "tenovaginitis," and "peritendinitis"; (2) paratenonitis with tendinosis, a class replacing "tendinitis"; (3) tendinosis, a class also replacing "tendinitis"; and (4) tendinitis, a class replacing acute (less than 2 weeks), subacute (4 to 6 weeks), and chronic (more than 6 weeks) "tendon strain and tear." However, although this classification is systematic and in many respects an improvement, it has problems similar to the other classification systems.[32] Kvist[45,46] believes that, as long as there is little knowledge in this area, we must accept overlapping terms to describe the clinicopathological entities of tendon disorders and tendon injuries. With regard to the basic pathohistological substrate of overuse injury, whether it is inflammation or a degenerative process, the question arises whether one should use the term tendinitis or tendinopathic change (tendinosis). Maffulli et al.[56] consider that the terms such as tendinosis, paratendinitis, and tendinitis imply specific, histopathologically proven conditions, and should be used only after an excision biopsy has been examined by a pathologist. None of the above terms should be used in clinical practice when talking of overuse tendon injuries. The clinical syndrome characterized by a combination of pain, swelling (diffuse or localized), and impaired performance should be labeled tendinopathy. Depending on the tissues affected, the terms tendinopathy, paratendinopathy, or pantendinopathy should be used. The term tendinosis was first used in this context by Puddu et al.[71] implying tendon degeneration without clinical or histological signs of intratendinous inflammation. The finding that the pathological bases of the overuse tendon condition in athletes are due to tendinosis is not new. In 1986, Perugia et al.[70] noted the "remarkable discrepancy between the terminology generally adopted for these conditions (which are obviously inflammatory since the ending -itis is used) and their histopathological substratum, which is largely degenerative."

We believe that the primary cause lies in the inflammation process, which during the course of its chronic stage leads to degenerative changes. For this reason, we use terms ending with "itis," or "osis" individually according to the stage of overuse injury. When naming various individual syndromes, we also place full attention on the precise localization of the injury. For this reason, we use the term *tendinitis* when the injury is located on the tendon, *peritendinitis,* when the injury is located on the tendon sheath, *miotendinitis,* when the injury is located in the area where the muscle connects with the tendon, and *enthesitis,* when the injury is located in the area of insertion of the tendon to the bone. In the medical literature there are many synonyms for the term enthesitis: insertitis, insertion tendinopathy, insertional tendinitis, insertion tendinitis, insertion tendinosis, insertiopathy, insertionitis, enthesopathy, tenoperiostitis, tendoperiostitis, tenoperiostosis, and tendoperiostosis.

In most cases, however, we use the term based on the pathoanatomical localization of the injury, or in other words the term that is most commonly known and that is generally used in the medical literature. In general terms, overuse injuries have acquired their terms according to the following:

- Affected anatomical structure (i.e., epicondylitis humeri radialis, hip external rotator syndrome, bicipital tendinitis, plantar fasciitis, patellar tendinitis/tendinosis, and others)
- Athletic activity in which it most frequently occurs (jumper's knee, rower's forehand, pitcher's elbow, swimmer's knee, runner's knee, etc.)
- Cause of development (impingement shoulder syndrome, impingement in the wrist or ankle joint, etc.)
- Characteristic symptom or clinical picture (trigger finger, low back pain, groin pain, snapping hip syndrome, anterior knee pain, etc.)
- Author who first or most precisely described the syndrome (de Quervain disease, Hoffa disease, Osgood-Schlatter disease, Haglund disease, Sever disease, etc.)

Whatever the term applied, the basic characteristic of all these syndromes is chronic, cumulating microtraumatic injury. Because of this, the most accurate term is the general term, overuse injuries.

REFERENCES

1. **Allan, D.A.** Structure and physiology of joints and their relationship to repetitive strain injuries. *Clin. Orthop.*, 1998; 351: 32–38.
2. **Almeida, S.A., Williams, K.M., Shaffer, R.A., and Brodine, S.K.** Epidemiological patterns of musculoskeletal injuries and physical training. *Med. Sci. Sports Exerc.*, 1999; 31: 1176–1182.
3. **Almekinders, L.C., Baynes, A.J., and Bracey, L.W.** An *in vitro* investigation into the effects of repetitive motion and nonsteroidal antiinflammatory medications on human tendon fibroblasts. *Am. J. Sports Med.*, 1995; 23: 119–123.
4. **Alter, M.J.** *Science of Stretching.* Champaign, IL: Leisure Press, 1990.
5. **Anderson, B.** *Stretching,* 20th ed. Bolinas, CA: Shelter Publications, 1987.
6. **Andrews, J.R.** Overuse syndromes of the lower extremity. *Clin. Sports Med.*, 1983; 2:137–148.
7. **Archambault, J.M., Wiley, J.P., and Bray, R.C.** Exercise loading of tendons and the development of overuse injuries. *Sports Med.*, 1995; 20: 77–89.
8. **Arendt, E.A. and Griffiths, H.J.** The use of MR imaging in the assessment and clinical management of stress reactions of bone in high-performance athletes. *Clin. Sports Med.*, 1997; 16: 291–306.
9. **Arnoczky, S.P., Tian, T., Lavagnino, M. et al.** Activation of stress-activated protein kinases (SAPK) in tendon cells following cyclic strain: the effects of strain frequency, strain magnitude, and cytosolic calcium. *J. Orthop. Res.*, 2002; 20: 947–952.
10. **Barry, N.N. and McGuire, J.L.** Overuse syndromes in adult athletes. *Rheum. Dis. Clin. North Am.*, 1996; 22: 515–530.
11. **Benezis, C., Simeray, J., and Simon, L., Eds.** *Muscles, Tendons et Sport.* Paris: Masson, 1990.
12. **Bennell, K.L., Malcolm, S.A., Wark, J.D., and Brukner, P.D.** Models for the pathogenesis of stress fractures in athletes. *Br. J. Sports Med.*, 1996; 30: 200–204.
13. **Bohndorf, K., Imhof H., and Pope, T.L., Jr., Eds.** *Musculoskeletal Imaging. A Concise Multimodality Approach.* New York: G. Thieme, 2001.
14. **Brody, D.M.** Running injuries. *Clin. Symp.*, 1987; 39:1–36.
15. **Catonne, Y. and Saillant, G.** *Lesions Traumatiques des Tendons chez le Sportif.* Paris: Masson, 1992.
16. **Ciullo, J.V. and Zarins, B.** Biomechanics of the musculotendinous unit: relation to athletic performance and injury. *Clin. Sports Med.*, 1983; 2:71–86.
17. **Clain, M.R. and Hershman, E.B.** Overuse injuries in children and adolescents. *Phys. Sportsmed.*, 1989; 17: 111–123.
18. **Clement, D.B., Taunton, J.E., Smart, G.W.** et al. A survey of overuse running injuries. *Phys. Sportsmed.*, 1981; 9:47–58.
19. **Curwin, S. and Stanish, W.D.** *Tendinitis: Its Etiology and Treatment.* Lexington, KY: Collamore Press, 1984; 1–67.
20. **Dalton, S.E.** Overuse injuries in adolescent athletes. *Sports Med.*, 1992; 13:58–70.
21. **Drubach, L.A., Connolly, L.P., D'Hemecourt, P.A., and Treves, S.T.** Assessment of the clinical significance of asymptomatic lower extremity uptake abnormality in young athletes. *J. Nucl. Med.*, 2001; 42: 209–212.
22. **Fornage, B.D.** *Ultrasonography of Muscles and Tendons.* New York: Springer-Verlag, 1988.
23. **Grieco, A., Molteni, G., De Vito, G., and Sias, N.** Epidemiology of musculoskeletal disorders due to biomechanical overload. *Ergonomics,* 1998; 41: 1253–1260.
24. **Hart, D.A., Archambault, J.M., Kydd, A. et al.** Gender and neurogenic variables in tendon biology and repetitive motion disorders. *Clin. Orthop.*, 1998; 351: 44–56.
25. **Hess, G.P., Cappiello, W.L., Poole, R.M. et al.** Prevention and treatment of overuse tendon injuries. *Sports Med.*, 1989; 8: 371–384.
26. **Higgs, P.E. and Young, V.L.** Cumulative trauma disorders. *Clin. Plast. Surg.*, 1996; 23: 421–433.
27. **Hintermann, B. and Nigg, B.M.** Pronation in runners. Implications for injuries. *Sports Med.*, 1998; 26: 169–176.
28. **Hunter-Griffin, L.Y.** Overuse injuries. *Clin. Sports Med.*, 1987; 6: 225–466.
29. **Hulkko, A. and Orava, S.** Stress fractures in athletes. *Int. J. Sports Med.*, 1987; 8: 221–226.
30. **Hunter, S.C. and Poole, R.M.** The chronically inflamed tendon. *Clin. Sports Med.*, 1987; 6: 371–388.
31. **Johnson, L.L.** *Arthroscopic Surgery: Principles and Practice,* 3rd ed. St. Louis: C.V. Mosby, 1986.

32. **Jozsa, L. and Kannus, P.** *Human Tendons. Anatomy, Physiology, and Pathology.* Champaign, IL: Human Kinetics, 1997.
33. **Kainberger, F., Ulreich, N., Huber, W. et al.** Tendon overuse syndrome: imaging diagnosis. *Wien. Med. Wochenschr.*, 2001; 151: 509–512.
34. **Kannangara, S., Bruce, W., Hutabarat, S.R., Magee, M., and Van der Wall, B.** Scintigraphy in severe tenosynovitis of the tibialis posterior tendon. *Clin. Nucl. Med.*, 1999; 24: 694–695.
35. **Kaufman, K.R., Brodine, S.K., Shaffer, R.A., Johnson, C.W., and Cullison, T.R.** The effect of foot structure and range of motion on musculoskeletal overuse injuries. *Am. J. Sports Med.*, 1999; 27: 585–593.
36. **Kannus, P., Jarinen, M., and Niittymaki, S.** Long- or short-acting anesthetic with corticosteroid in local injections of overuse injuries? A prospective, randomized, double blind study. *Int. J. Sports Med.*, 1990; 11: 397–400.
37. **Kannus, P. and Jozsa, L.** Histopathological changes preceding spontaneous rupture of the tendon. A controlled study of 891 patients. *J. Bone Joint Surg. Am.*, 1991; 73: 1507–1525.
38. **Keller, K., Corbett, J., and Nichols, D.** Repetitive strain injury in computer keyboard users: pathomechanics and treatment principles in individual and group intervention. *J. Hand Ther.*, 1998; 11: 9–26.
39. **Kilmartin, T.E. and Walace, W.A.** The scientific basis for the use of biomechanical foot orthoses in the treatment of lower limb sports injuries — a review of the literature. *Br. J. Sports Med.*, 1994; 28: 180–184.
40. **Kjaer, M.** The treatment of overuse injuries in sports. *Scand. J. Med. Sci. Sports*, 2001; 11: 195–196.
41. **Komi, V.P., Ed.** *Strength and Power in Sport.* London: Blackwell Scientific Publications, 1992.
42. **Korkia, P.K., Taustall-Pedoe, D.S., and Maffuli, N.** An epidemiological investigation of training and injury patterns in British triathletes. *Br. J. Sports Med.*, 1994; 28: 191–196.
43. **Krampla, W., Mayrhofer, R., Malcher, J. et al.** MR imaging of the knee in marathon runners before and after competition. *Skel. Radiol.*, 2001; 30: 72–76.
44. **Krivickas, L.S.** Anatomical factors associated with overuse sports injuries. *Sports Med.*, 1997; 24: 132–146.
45. **Kvist, M.** Achilles Tendon Overuse Injuries, dissertation, 1991; University of Turku, Turku, Finland.
46. **Kvist, M.** Achilles tendon injuries in athletes. *Sports Med.*, 1994; 18: 173–201.
47. **La Cava, G.** L'enthesite ou maladie des insertions. *Press Med.*, 1959; 67: 9.
48. **Laursen, B., Jensen, B.R., Garde, A.H., and Jorgensen, A.H.** Effect of mental and physical demands on muscular activity during the use of computer mouse and a keyboard. *Scand. J. Work Environ. Health*, 2002; 28: 215–221.
49. **Leadbetter, W.B., Buckwalter, J.A., and Gordon, S.L., Eds.** Sports-induced inflammation: clinical and basic science concepts. Park Ridge, IL: American Academy of Orthopaedic Surgeons, 1990.
50. **Leadbetter, W.B.** Cell-matrix response in tendon injury. *Clin. Sports Med.*, 1992; 11: 533–578.
51. **Leadbetter, W.B.** Anti-inflammatory therapy and sport injury: the role of non-steroidal drugs and corticosteroid injections. *Clin. Sports Med.*, 1995; 14: 353–410.
52. **Leadbetter, W.B.** Soft tissue athletic injury, in Fu, H.F. and Stone, D.A., Eds. *Sports Injuries, Mechanisms-Prevention-Treatment*, 2nd ed. Philadelphia: Lippincott/Williams & Wilkins, 2001, 839–888.
53. **Lehman, W.L., Jr.** Overuse syndromes in runners. *AFP*, 1984; 29: 157–161.
54. **Litchfield, R., Hawkins, R., Dillman, C.J., Atkins, J., and Hagerman, G.** Rehabilitation for the overhead athletes. *J. Orthop. Sports Phys. Ther.*, 1993; 18: 433–441.
55. **Lysholm, J. and Wiklaner, J.** Injuries in runners. *Am. J. Sports Med.*, 1987; 15: 168–171.
56. **Maffulli, N., Khan, K.M., and Puddu, G.** Overuse tendon conditions: time to change a confusing terminology. *Arthroscopy*, 1998; 14: 840–843.
57. **Matasovic, T., Ed.** *Diagnostic Ultrasound of the Locomotor System.* Zagreb: Skolska Knjiga, 1990.
58. **Matheson, G.O., Clement, D.B., McKenzie, D.C. et al.** Stress fractures in athletes. *Am. J. Sports Med.*, 1987; 15: 46–57.
59. **McCarthy, P.** Managing bursitis in the athlete: an overview. *Phys. Sportsmed.*, 1989; 17: 115–125.
60. **McKeag, D.B. and Dolan, C.** Overuse syndrome of the lower extremity. *Phys. Sportsmed.*, 1989; 17: 108–123.
61. **Micheli, L.J.** Lower extremity overuse injuries. *Acta Med. Scand.* (Suppl.), 1986; 711: 171–177.

62. **Molteni, G., De Vito, G., Sias, N., and Grieco, A.** Epidemiology of musculoskeletal disorders caused by biomechanical overload. *Med. Lav.,* 1996; 87: 469–481.
63. **O'Connor, F.G., Sobel, J.R., and Nirschl, R.P.** Five-step treatment for overuse injuries. *Phys. Sportsmed.,* 1992; 20: 128–142.
64. **O'Neill, D.B. and Micheli, L.J.** Overuse injuries in the young athletes. *Clin. Sports Med.,* 1988; 7: 591–610.
65. **Pascarelli, E.F. and Hsu, Y.P.** Understanding work-related upper extremity disorders: clinical findings in 485 computer users, musicians, and others. *J. Occup. Rehabil.,* 2001; 11: 1–21.
66. **Pećina, M.** *Overuse Injuries of the Musculoskeletal System.* Zagreb: Globus, 1992.
67. **Pećina, M.** *Stretching.* Zagreb: Globus, 1992.
68. **Pećina, M., Bojanić, I., and Markiewitz, A.D.** Nerve entrapment syndromes in athletes. *Clin. J. Sports Med.,* 1993; 3: 36–43.
69. **Pećina, M.M, Krmpotic-Nemanic, J., and Markiewitz, A.D.** *Tunnel Syndromes. Peripheral Nerve Compression Syndromes,* 3rd ed. Boca Raton, FL: CRC Press, 2001.
70. **Perugia, L., Postacchini, F., and Ippolito, E.** *The Tendons: Biology–Pathology–Clinical Aspects.* Milan: Editrice Kurtis, 1986.
71. **Puddu, G., Ippolito, E., and Postacchini, F.A.** A classification of Achilles tendon disease. *Am. J. Sports Med.,* 1976; 4: 145–150.
72. **Renstroem, P. and Johnson, R.J.** Overuse injuries in sports: a review. *Sports Med.,* 1985; 2: 316–333.
73. **Resnick, D., Ed.** *Diagnosis of Bone and Joint Disorders.* Philadelphia: W.B. Saunders, 1996.
74. **Ribarić, G., Pećina, H.I., and Pećina, M.** Jumper's knee — comparison of clinical, radiological and sonographic findings. *Croat. J. Sports Med.,* 1996; 11: 67–75.
75. **Rodineau, J. and Simon, L., Eds.** *Microtraumatologie du Sport.* Paris: Masson, 1990.
76. **Ross, J.** A review of lower limb overuse injuries during basic military training. Part 1: Types of overuse injuries. *Mil. Med.,* 1993; 158: 410–415.
77. **Schwellnus, M.P., Jordaan, G., and Noakes, T.D.** Prevention of common overuse injuries by the use of shock absorbing insoles. *Am. J. Sports Med.,* 1990; 18: 636–641.
78. **Shin, A.Y., Morin, W.D., Gorman, J.D., Jones, S.B., and Lapinsky, A.S.** The superiority of magnetic resonance imaging in differentiating the cause of hip pain in endurance athletes. *Am. J. Sports Med.,* 1996; 24: 168–176.
79. **Sjogaard, G. and Sjogaard, K.** Muscle injury in repetitive motion disorders. *Clin. Orthop.,* 1998; 351: 21–31.
80. **Stanish, W.D., Rubinovich, R.M., and Curwin, S.** Eccentric exercise in chronic tendinitis. *Clin. Orthop.,* 1986; 208: 65–68.
81. **Steinacker, T. and Steuer, M.** Use of extracorporeal shockwave therapy (ESWT) in sports orthopedics. *Sportverletz. Sportschaden,* 2001; 15: 45–49.
82. **Taunton, J.E., McKenzie, D.C., and Clement, D.B.** The role of biomechanics in the epidemiology of injuries. *Sports Med.,* 1988; 6: 107–120.
83. **Zecevic, A., Miller, D.I., and Harburn, K.** An evaluation of the ergonomics of three computer keyboards. *Ergonomics,* 2000; 43: 55–72.

2 MR Imaging in Diagnosis of Overuse Injuries*

A number of overuse syndromes are poorly understood because of the traditional lack of objective tests to confirm the presence of tissue abnormality. Magnetic resonance imaging (MRI), a noninvasive diagnostic tool, objectively confirms the presence of the exact tissue abnormality, demonstrates the location and degree of involvement, and helps clarify complex pathomorphological and pathophysiological conditions. It can also predict the length of time the patient will be disabled and helps in monitoring patients' response to treatment, which may help return the patients/athletes to their former activities. MRI findings in overuse injuries are based on morphological changes and signal intensity alterations of involved muscles and their tendons, cartilage, bones, and surrounding soft tissues.

I. MUSCLES AND TENDONS

MRI alteration in muscle can be seen in some occupational or sport and recreational overuse syndromes. In those cases, MRI may be used to determine the muscle or muscles involved, to localize and grade the edema-like process within involved muscle, and to assess associated soft-tissue abnormalities. Findings on MRI may include hyperintense signal intensity in the region of the injury, near the myotendinous junction on T2-weighted or short tau inversion recovery (STIR) images. The area of signal abnormality may also surround a previously formed fibrous scar.[93] Muscle pain secondary to overuse is the result of various types of injury: muscle strain, tendinitis, tendinosis, bursitis.[99]

Muscle Strain. Muscle strain can be graded from muscle spasm or cramp to true muscle tear that occurs within the muscle, at the muscle–tendon junction, or at the origin or insertion of the muscle. Commonly strained muscles include the hamstrings, rectus femoris, hip adductors, hip flexors, and medial gastrocnemius. Paraspinal musculature can also be subject to strain, particularly in the lumbar and cervical region. First-degree strain produces minimal disruption of the tissue and the appearance on MR images is similar to that of a contusion. A diffuse, infiltrative pattern of edema and hemorrhage is found without evidence of architectural disturbance. There may be an associated band of perifascial fluid, typically seen approximately 3 days after injury.[93] MR images of second-degree strain, which corresponds with a variable degree of muscle separation from tendon and fascia, demonstrate focal areas of muscle fiber disruption. In third-degree strain, muscle paresis occurs with complete disruption of the myotendinous junction or tendo-osseous avulsion. MR images usually show complete discontinuity of the muscle, usually at the musculotendinous junction, as high-signal-intensity disruption on T2-weighted and STIR images, and the ends of injured muscle may appear wavy or lobulated (Figure 2.1 and Figure 2.2). When muscle pain or soreness occurs in an otherwise healthy individual several hours or days following exercise, it is termed *delayed-onset muscle soreness* (DOMS). The pathomorphology of DOMS seems to involve increased intramuscular fluid pressure, inflammation, and perhaps damage to corresponding connective tissue. The appearance of DOMS on MR images is similar to a first-degree strain.[89,93,99]

---

* Contributed by Igor Borić.

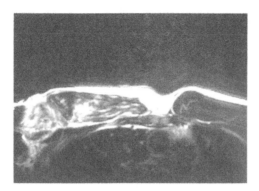

FIGURE 2.1 Axial STIR image shows partial rupture of clavicular part of the pectoralis major muscle.

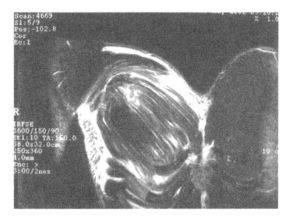

FIGURE 2.2 Coronal STIR image shows partial rupture of the clavicular part of the pectoralis major muscle.

Axial plane imaging of muscle strain is useful to demonstrate associated muscle retraction and atrophy, which are seen as high signal intensity on T1-weighted images. Coronal and sagittal images provide a longitudinal display of the entire muscle group on a single image. A comparison with the contralateral extremity is important in evaluating the symmetry of each muscle group.[99] Follow-up MRI studies can clearly demonstrate atrophy, fibrosis, and calcium deposition.[93]

Tendinitis/Tendinosis. Its exquisite soft-tissue contrast resolution, noninvasive nature, and multiplanar capabilities make MRI an invaluable tool for the detection and assessment of a variety of tendon disorders. Tendinosis, a focal area of degeneration, is seen on MRI as an area of increased signal intensity on T1- and T2-weighted images within normal-thickness or thickened tendon.[89] The MRI findings in tendinitis include mildly to moderately increased signal on T1- and T2-weighted or STIR images within thickened, poorly shaped tendon (Figure 2.3 and Figure 2.4). Tendinitis usually occurs at the level of tendon insertion.[15] Peritendinitis, inflammation of peritendinous soft-tissue, is seen as high signal intensity on fat-suppressed sequences (Figure 2.5). Partial tear is seen as an area of discrete, hyperintense signal intensity within the tendon, whereas intratendon hyperintensity with discontinuity in tendon fibers indicates a full-thickness tear. Dynamic contrast-enhancement MRI shows early contrast enhancement at tendon lesions, and increased severity of tendon pathology correlates with signal enhancement.[54] MRI is not able to distinguish age-related tendon degeneration from acute tendinosis. It may also be difficult to distinguish areas of chronic tendinitis from intrasubstance tendon tears. Each of the above-mentioned entities is distinct, although they often occur in combination.[99]

Bursitis. There are many bursae in the body located between tendons or muscles and over bony prominences.[99] Bursal inflammation may be caused by a variety of conditions, including

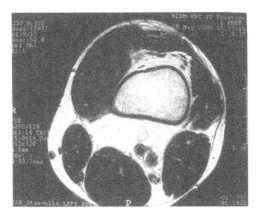

FIGURE 2.3 Axial fat-suppressed T2-weighted fast spin-echo image shows focal enlargement of quadriceps muscle — chronic tendinitis.

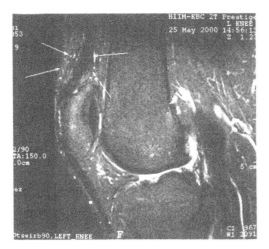

FIGURE 2.4 Sagittal STIR image shows focal enlargement of quadriceps muscle with intratendinous foci of increased signal — chronic tendinitis.

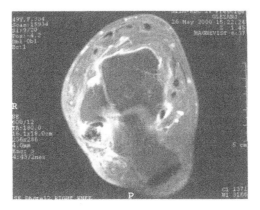

FIGURE 2.5 Axial fat-suppressed T1-weighted spin-echo image shows increased thickness of the peroneus brevis tendon and muscle with increased signal intensity within the tendon and peritendinous fluid — chronic tendinitis.

repetitive irritation or direct trauma with hemorrhage. Bursitis is well demonstrated on MRI as bursal distension with abnormal high signal intensity of bursal fluid collection on coronal or axial T2-weighted and fat-suppressed sequences. Those pulse sequences are also most useful for detecting accompanying musculotendinous injury or stress lesion in the bone marrow, conditions that may be clinically confused with bursitis. Knowledge of normal bursal anatomy and tissue MR signal characteristics helps in differentiation of a fluid-filled bursa from a soft-tissue tumor.[1,49,82]

A. SHOULDER IMPINGEMENT SYNDROME

Overuse injuries of the shoulder are common in the athletic population as well as in people performing certain occupations or recreational activities. Although imaging evaluation of shoulder injuries usually starts with conventional radiographs and ultrasound examination, additional studies should include MRI. With MRI the status and integrity of muscles, tendons, ligaments, labrocapsular complex, and cartilage can be easily evaluated.[28] Although routine imaging protocols vary widely, complete examination of the shoulder usually can be accomplished with coronal oblique T1- and T2-weighted images with fat suppression or STIR images, sagittal oblique T2-weighted images, and axial gradient echo scans (usually GRE T2*). MR resonance arthrography is useful, especially if the labrum is at issue.[17] Shoulder impingement lesions are evaluated on the basis of tendon morphology and changes in signal intensity within the specific rotator cuff tendon. Additionally, pathomorphological changes in the coracoacromial arch, the acromioclavicular joint, and the subacromial-subdeltoid bursa may be identified in a spectrum of findings in impingement lesions.[17,28,39,74]

1. Rotator Cuff Impingement

Based on the theory that impingement is caused by mechanical wear and repetitive microtrauma from overuse, Neer[71] has developed a three-stage classification for tendon impingement: in stage 1 tendon, edema and hemorrhage are present; stage 2 is characterized by fibrosis and tendinitis, and in stage 3 partial or complete tear of the tendon is present.[71] As seen on MRI, according to Neer's classification[71] stage 1 tendon is thickened or normal in shape with foci of increased signal intensity on T2-weighted or STIR images, which represent focal edema or hemorrhage. Tendinosis/fibrosis in stage 2 shows intratendinous mildly increased signal intensity on T1- and T2-weighted images with widening of the tendon shape, which may be irregular. Occasionally in stage 2, tendinitis is present as increased signal intensity on T2-weighted or STIR images within the tendon or in peritendinous tissue, including bony edema at the insertional area of the humerus.

Partial cuff tear is seen as discrete hyperintense signal intensity within the tendon. Sometimes a tear will not appear as fluid intensity but its signal will almost always be greater than the signal from muscles. Similar signal intensity is found in tendinitis and acute cuff contusion. However, tears will be oriented to the long tendon axis, will be seen on both fat-suppressed and non-fat-suppressed images, and will have ill-defined margins. The majority of partial tears communicate with the articular surface of the tendon, and some authors suggest using intra-articular gadolinium (MR arthrography) for their detection. This procedure will identify only tears that communicate with the articular surface of the tendon, but not partial tears located within the tendon. Discontinuity in tendon fibers with intratendon hyperintensity of fluid represents full-thickness cuff tear (Figure 2.6). The fluid collection is usually well demarcated, but in the case of a chronic tear, hypertrophic synovium or granulation tissue may partially fill the defect and modify the signal intensity. In the case of complete cuff tears, fluid in the subacromial bursa is often present, especially if the tear is relatively acute or if the impingement is exacerbated. Musculotendinous junction retraction implies a relatively large tear. Retraction is best seen on coronal oblique and axial images. The presence of fatty atrophy of the retracted muscle belly indicates a chronic tear. The supraspinatus tendon is the only tendon in the body that must function in a space delineated by two bony structures: the

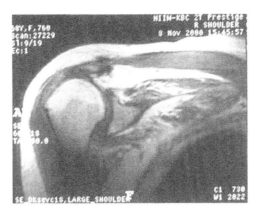

FIGURE 2.6 Coronal oblique T2-weighted fast spin-echo image shows full-thickness supraspinatus tear with proximal retraction.

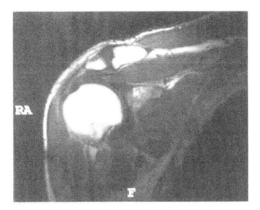

FIGURE 2.7 Coronal oblique T1-weighted image: degenerative acromioclavicular joint disease.

coracoacromial arch (acromion, acromioclavicular joint, distal clavicle, coracoacromial and cora-cohumeral ligament) superiorly and the humeral head inferiorly.

The factors that contribute to bony supraspinatus impingement include anterior acromial spurs, the shape of acromion (curved or overhanging edge), the slope of the acromion (flat or decreased angle), and the changes of the acromioclavicular joint (callus formation, hypertrophic osteoarthrosis) (Figure 2.7). The shape of the acromion as seen on sagittal oblique MR images has been classified into three types by Bigliani: type 1 has a flat undersurface; type 2 acromion has a smooth, curved, inferior surface (Figure 2.8); and type 3 acromion has an anterior hook or break (Figure 2.9).[17] Less frequent mechanisms of supraspinatus impingement include bony abnormalities that are unrelated to the coracoacromial arch — not "outlet impingement" (prominence of the greater tuberosity as fracture, malunion or nonunion, subluxation or luxation of the glenohumeral joint).[10]

2. SLAP Lesion

MRI has proved to be a sensitive, specific, and accurate modality for evaluating glenoid labrum with sensitivity to 88% and specificity to 95%.[21,28] Routinely, axial images are obtained using T1-weighting, T2*-weighting sequences and fat-suppressed T2-weighted fast spin-echo sequences. When MR arthrography with a paramagnetic contrast agent is used, precontrast T1-weighted images, postcontrast T2*-weighted axial images, and postcontrast T1-weighted fat-suppressed axial, sagittal, and coronal oblique images are obtained. The intact fibrous labrum demonstrates low signal intensity on all pulse sequences. Zlatkin and colleagues[114] have devised a four-category system of

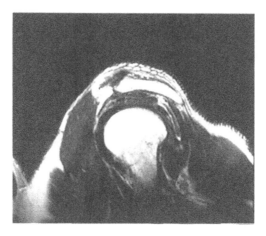

FIGURE 2.8 Sagittal oblique T1-weighted image: type 2 acromion is concave inferiorly.

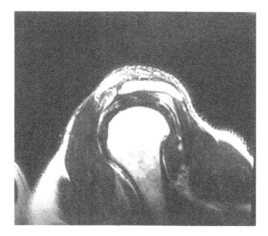

FIGURE 2.9 Sagittal oblique T1-weighted image shows type 3 acromion: prominent anterior hook decreases the acromiohumeral distance with a significant risk of rotator cuff impingement.

classification for abnormal labral signal intensity. In type 1, there is increased signal intensity within the labrum, but there is no surface extension. Type 1 corresponds to internal labral degeneration without tear. In type 2, the blunted or frayed labrum demonstrates normal dark signal intensity. In type 3, T1-weighted or T2*-weighted images demonstrate increased signal intensity that extends to the surface, indicating a labral tear. In type 4, a labral tear is depicted by a combination of abnormal morphology with type 2 features and increased signal intensity extending to the surface of the labrum with type 3 features. Large tears and detachments may demonstrate a more diffuse increase in signal intensity, whereas discrete tears maintain linear morphology.[114]

3. Subacromial Bursitis

Usually, the normal subacromial–subdeltoid bursal complex appears on MRI as a thin line of fat. Subacromial bursitis as hypertrophic synovitis results with thickening of the fat line. Bursal distension on MRI is seen as decreased signal intensity or loss of peribursal fat on T1-weighted images and abnormal increased signal intensity of bursal fluid collection on coronal oblique or axial T2-weighted and fat-suppressed sequences. Fat-suppressed T2-weighted images are more sensitive than non-fat-suppressed T2-weighted images in identifying small amounts of subarachnoidal bursal fluid on coronal oblique or axial images.[9,20] Low signal intensity within a thickened subacromial bursa on T1- and T2-weighted images indicates a proliferative process in chronic bursitis. It is unusual to see a fluid-filled bursa in the presence of normal cuff.[20,109]

B. HUMERAL EPICONDYLITIS

Lateral epicondylitis, also known as tennis elbow, is caused by degeneration and tearing of the common extensor tendon. Tendinosis and tearing usually involve the extensor carpi radialis brevis portion of the common extensor tendon anteriorly.[31] Medial epicondylitis, also known as golfer's elbow, pitcher's elbow, or medial tennis elbow, is caused by degeneration of the common flexor tendon secondary to overload of the flexor/pronator muscle group that arises from the medial epicondyle.[30,31] MRI can clearly determine if there is tendinosis vs. partial tear or complete rupture. In the case of degenerative tendinosis, tendon fibers are normal or thickened, thin in the case of a partial tear, or absent in the case of a complete tear. On MRI tendinosis appears as focal areas of increased signal intensity on T1- and T2-weighted images within the tendon, which represents focal fibrous or fibrosclerotic degeneration of the tendon tissue.[78,94] In a partial or complete tear of the tendon, an edema or hemorrhage pattern and various amounts of peritendinous fluid are found, best seen on T2-weighted or fat-suppressed images.[30,31,78,94] Increased marrow T2 signal within involved epicondyle is occasionally seen. Musculus anconeus edema and radial head bursitis are very rarely found.[19,63] Ulnar neuritis commonly accompanies common flexor tendinosis. In those cases, MRI detects various amounts of perineural fluid, swelling, and enlargement of the nerve.[90] MR sequences in all three planes (sagittal, coronal, and axial) are useful for assessment of the degree of tendon injury.[16] In addition to localization and characterization of injury, MRI also helps to follow possible lack of response to treatment.[78]

C. GROIN PAIN

Many muscles have their origin in the pubic symphysis: ramus superior or inferior of pubic bone, inguinal ligament, trochanter minor, or spina illiaca. All these muscles may suffer during repetitive overload or overuse. If pathomorphological changes occur at their origin, the clinical sign is unique — groin pain. The role of MRI in evaluation of groin pain is in distinguishing musculotendinous injuries from bony injuries or other pathological conditions.[99] Axial MR images are very useful in evaluation of muscle and tendon morphology as well as signal intensity. Tendinopathy of the hip adductors, gluteal muscles, abdominal wall muscles, and of their proximal tendons is a common finding on MRI.[49,52] T1- and T2-weighted images may demonstrate mildly to moderately increased intrasubstance signal on T1-weighted images of normal or thickened tendon with various intensities of muscle edema depending on the duration of the symptoms.[56] In the acute phase, bone marrow edema appears as hyperintensity on T2-weighted or STIR images in the region of tendon insertion (ramus inferior and ramus superior of pubic bone, ramus and tuber of ishial bone), but in the chronic phase decreased signal intensity on all pulse sequences is present due to sclerotic degenerative changes of the bone. The GRE T2* sequence is very useful for demonstrating bony changes.[5,12,99] It is very important to evaluate bony structures and articular cartilage of hip, pelvis, and sacrum including sacroiliac joint to exclude arthrotic changes as the cause of the groin pain.[73] Osteohondral lesions of the femoral head appear as focal areas of high T2-weighted and low T1-weighted signals on MR images. Labral lesions could be the cause of persistent groin pain, especially in young athletes.[107] MR arthrography, as a minimally invasive diagnostic technique, has shown an excellent accuracy of over 90% in detecting those lesions.[61]

D. SNAPPING HIP

Based on etiology, the snapping hip syndrome can be divided into three types: external, internal, and intra-articular. The external type is due to a sudden displacement of the iliotibial band or gluteus maximus over the greater trochanter with irritation of the greater trochanteric bursa. The internal variant is caused by the psoas tendon passing over the iliopectineal eminence on the pubis, femoral head, or anterior hip capsule with a palpable and audible snapping.[45,99,110] The intra-articular snapping hip type is due to a lesion in the joint itself.[2] Optimal visualization of pathomorphological changes and signal abnormalities by MRI is on axial and coronal images. Additional sagittal plane images can help, especially in planning surgical treatment.[2] In the external type of snapping hip, coronal and axial T2-weighted or STIR images can demonstrate a thickened area of the posterior iliotibial band or anterior edge of the gluteus maximus muscle and iliotibial bursitis as a bursal collection in the greater trochanter bursa. MR findings in the internal type of snapping hip include iliopsoas bursitis as a bursal collection adjacent to the iliopsoas tendon, which correlates with snapping or clicking of the hip during external and internal rotation.[40,43] Intra-articular loose bodies or labral tears are unusual, but should be considered in the differential diagnosis of snapping hip syndrome. In those conditions, GRE echo T2* sequence and MR arthrography will be helpful as well for assessment of articular cartilage.[21]

E. Hamstring Syndrome

Hamstring muscle injuries (semimembranosus, semitendinosus, and biceps femoris) present a variable appearance over time that can be characterized by MRI.[15] Distinctive findings are seen in acute or chronic injury. The injuries occur in diverse locations within the muscles: at proximal and distal musculotendinous junctions, within the muscle belly, or at the ends of the muscle with a characteristic featherlike edema pattern on MRI.[15,20,54,55,85] The biceps femoris is the most commonly injured hamstring muscle, followed by the semitendinosus and semimembranosus muscles. Although hamstring injuries often involve one muscle injured proximally, De Smet[22] has found that multiple muscle injuries were involved in 33% and the injuries were distal in 40%. Intermediate signal intensity on T1-weighted images within thickened conjoined hamstring tendon (the hamstring muscle originates in a conjoined tendon from the posterolateral aspect of the ischial tuberosity) indicating tendinopathy, or soft-tissue edema within tendon and in its surroundings indicating tendinitis, can be found. Internal derangement of muscle fibers leading to edema or hemorrhage and typically partial tearing[54] is also seen as high signal intensity within the muscle or the musculotendinous junction on T2-weighted or STIR images (Figure 2.1 and Figure 2.2).[20] Localized organization of hemorrhage leading to a hematoma has a variable appearance on MRI, depending both on the oxidation state of hemoglobin and the temporal dissolution of the clot, but is distinguished by its focal appearance and relatively high signal intensity on fat-suppressed sequences. Myositis ossificans, a chronic complication of hematoma, is best seen, using a GRE T2* sequence, as peripheral pattern of low signal intensity of calcification around the mass. Chronic inflammation and fibrosis may involve the sciatic nerve coursing near the injured muscles.[15,99] MRI findings, which determine the severity of the injury, can be also predictive factors in prognosis of convalescence interval,[79] and can show risk factors for hamstring muscle injury, such as a previous posterior thigh injury.[105]

F. Iliotibial Band Friction Syndrome

The iliotibial band is seen on MR images as a thin band of low signal intensity, parallel to the femur, with an anterolateral tibial insertion. The iliotibial band friction syndrome is caused by abnormal contact of the iliotibial band and the lateral femoral condyle, which leads to friction and inflammation between the iliotibial tract and the anterolateral femoral condyle. T2-weighted or STIR coronal images show an ill-defined high-signal-intensity area deep to the iliotibial band, lateral to the lateral femoral condyle. The signal alteration is seen predominantly in the region beneath the posterior fibers of the iliotibial band. The iliotibial band itself does not show any signal alteration or increased thickness.[69,72]

G. PATELLAR TENDINITIS/TENDINOSIS

Patellar tendinitis, also called as jumper's knee, usually affects the patellar tendon at its proximal insertion at apex patellae. Tendinitis usually occurs in adults, and findings include microtears of the tendon tissue with reactive inflammation, devitalization, and areas of focal degeneration mostly in the region of the proximal patellar tendon junction.[27,46,81] The medial portion of the tendon is most commonly involved and the posterior margin of the tendon is usually poorly defined.[27,86,111] Acute patellar tendinitis (symptoms for less than 2 weeks) may demonstrate greater signal intensity abnormalities in the peritendon region, without intrasubstance tendon changes.[24,96] In chronic patellar tendinitis (symptoms more than 6 weeks) enlargement in the proximal third of the tendon and a focal area of low signal intensity on T1-weighted images with increased signal intensity on T2-weighted or STIR images may be seen before development of late phase, which includes chronic tears within the tendon.[12,24,27,68,87,96] In this phase MR findings are similar to acute partial intrasubstance patellar tendon tears, except for the presence of subcutaneous edema, which is a sign of acute partial tears. The asymptomatic patellar tendon may contain foci of increased signal intensity at either or both ends when imaged on gradient-echo sequences, but the tendon shows uniform thickness throughout most of its length.[83] Axial and sagittal MR images are most appropriate to demonstrate changes of the tendon.[27]

H. ACHILLES TENDINITIS/TENDINOSIS

The Achilles tendon does not possess a true tendon synovial sheath, so inflammatory conditions of the tendon are classified as tendinitis (intrasubstance inflammation within the Achilles tendon), paratendinitis (inflammatory changes around the Achilles tendon), and peritendinitis, which represents inflammation of the peritenon. Based on MR findings, it is possible to distinguish those three conditions.[37,44] There are two distinct sites of tendon injury: intrasubstance tendinitis occurs about 2 to 6 cm proximal to the tendon insertion on the calcaneus; insertional tendinitis occurs at the tendon–bone junction and may be associated with a bony protuberance of the calcaneus.[44] MR images in Achilles tendinitis show focal or fusiform thickening of the tendon with diffuse or linear low to intermediate signal intensity on T1-weighted, T2-weighted, or STIR images, which represent tendon mucinous or mixoid degeneration (Figure 2.10 through Figure 2.12). Inflammatory changes may coexist with degeneration and demonstrate increased signal intensity on T2-weighted and STIR images. Axial and sagittal images can be used to differentiate peritendinitis — edema (increased signal on T2-weighted and STIR images) along the Achilles tendon without thickening and intrasubstance signal abnormalities of the tendon — from intratendinous degeneration and partial/full-thickness tears. A partial tear is seen as discrete hyperintense signal intensity within the tendon, but intratendon hyperintensity with discontinuity in tendon fibers represents full-thickness

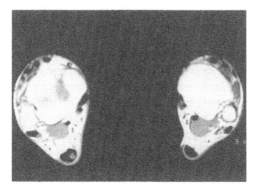

FIGURE 2.10 Axial T1-weighted chronic Achilles tendinitis with focal tendon thickening.

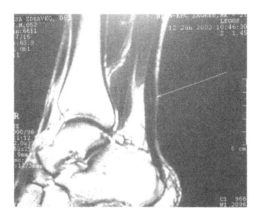

FIGURE 2.11 Sagittal T2-weighted image shows focal Achilles tendon thickening with intratendinous increased signal intensity.

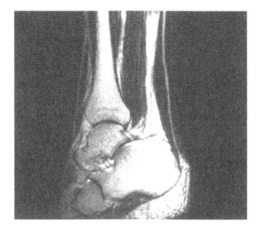

FIGURE 2.12 Sagittal T1-weighted chronic Achilles tendinitis with focal thickening and anterior tendon convexity.

tears.[8,37,44] Chronic Achilles tendinitis seen as focal or diffuse widening of the tendon diameter; intrasubstance increased signal intensity may not be evident in uncomplicated chronic conditions, the same are MR findings in healed Achilles tendon tear.[66] It may be difficult to distinguish areas of chronic tendinitis from acute intrasubstance tendon tears.[32]

I. PLANTAR FASCIITIS

Plantar fasciitis is an overuse injury common in runners, dancers, and other athletes. Microtears of the plantar fascia occur with overuse, leading to attempted repair and chronic inflammation.[37,97] In the acute phase, plantar fasciitis presents as inflammation of the plantar fascia, commonly near its calcaneal origin.[67] Chronic changes progress to collagen necrosis, angiofibroblastic hyperplasia, and matrix calcification.[47] With its superior soft-tissue contrast resolution and multiplanar capability, MRI delineates the anatomy of plantar aponeurosis and perifascial soft tissues and may allow precise location and definition of the extent of involvement in the disease process.[70,84,101] Normal plantar fascia is best seen on coronal and sagittal MR images as a fusiform and sharply shaped band of homogeneous low signal intensity on all pulse sequences that arises from the medial calcaneal tuberosity, spans the bottom of the foot, and inserts onto the base of each proximal phalanx.[97,112] Normally, the plantar fascia should be no greater than 3 mm in thickness on coronal

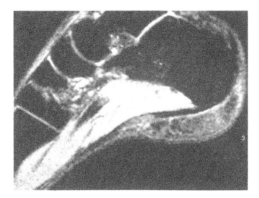

FIGURE 2.13 Sagittal T1-weighted image shows a focal area of plantar aponeurosis thickening in plantar fasciitis.

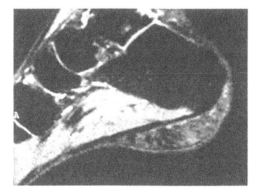

FIGURE 2.14 Hyperintensity involving the calcaneal attachment of the plantar aponeurosis and adjacent plantar soft tissue on sagittal fat-suppressed T2-weighted fast spin-echo image with focal area of plantar aponeurosis thickening.

and sagittal images.[7,48] In plantar fasciitis, coronal and sagittal MR images demonstrate hyperintense signal intensity of edema around the plantar fascia on T2-weighted, T2*-weighted, STIR, and fat-suppressed T2-weighted images. T1-weighted sagittal images display the low signal intensity fascia with a focal area of thickening, usually at the calcaneal insertion, and the fascia layer often measures 6 to 10 mm (Figure 2.13 and Figure 2.14).[7,94,101] Subtle bone marrow edema also may be found near the calcaneal insertion of the fascia.[33,36,67,84] Increased signal intensity within the fascia on T2-weighted images indicates a plantar fascia tear.[7,33]

II. BONES

A. STRESS FRACTURES

The radiographic findings of stress fracture are often subtle. Radiographs may be negative for several weeks after the onset of symptoms. In those cases, bone scan or MRI may be used to confirm the clinical diagnoses.[96] In case of stress fracture, MRI shows an abnormal signal, which represents edema or hemorrhage related to accumulated tissue microdamage — bone marrow edema as well as periosteal edema, edema in adjacent muscle, and sometimes a fracture line. On MR images a stress fracture demonstrates a diffuse pattern of decreased signal intensity on T1-weighted images and increased signal intensity on fat-saturated T2-weighted or STIR images, with variable presence of a low signal intensity fracture line. Increases in the signal on edema-sensitive sequences

TABLE 2.1
Grading System of Stress Fracture According to MRI Appearance

Grade of Injury	MRI Appearance
Grade I	Periosteal edema: mild to moderate on T2-weighted images
	Marrow edema: normal signal intensity on T1- and T2-weighted images
Grade II	Periosteal edema: moderate to severe on T2-weighted images
	Marrow edema: only on T2-weighted images
Grade III	Periosteal edema: moderate to severe on T2-weighted images
	Marrow edema on T1 and T2-weighted images
Grade IV	Periosteal edema: mild to moderate on T2-weighted images
	Marrow edema on T1 and T2-weighted images
	Fracture line clearly visible

Source: Modified from Fredericson et al.[29]

become less prominent with increasing duration of symptoms. High signal intensity representing bone marrow edema may not be present if the patient is imaged more than 4 weeks after the onset of symptoms.[50,58,88,90,96] The fracture line is seen as a low signal line on all pulse sequences and often is best seen on T2-weighted images, outlined by the high signal of the bone marrow edema.[6] It is continuous with the cortex and extends into the intramedullary space, oriented perpendicular to the cortex and the major weight-bearing trabecula. On T1-weighted images the fracture line may be obscured by the surrounding low signal edema. If a discrete fracture line is invisible on MR images, the lesion should be categorized as bony stress reaction. These areas of edema have a similar appearance to bone contusional injuries (bone bruises) as well as other less common conditions such as transient bone marrow edema syndrome, very early avascular osteonecrosis, osteomyelitis, and infiltrative neoplasm. The findings must be carefully correlated with the clinical symptoms and signs to differentiate between the various diagnoses.[6,24,29,60,64,104]

According to MRI findings, stress fractures have been classified into four different grades (Table 2.1; this grading system is a modification of the grading system by Fredericson et al.[29]): a grade I injury indicates mild to moderate periosteal edema only on the fat-suppressed T2-weighted image without bone marrow changes; grade II shows abnormal increased signal both at the periosteum and bone marrow on fat-suppressed T2-weighted images; grade III injuries show marrow edema on T1-weighted imaging as well; and grade IV shows the presence of a fracture line. Grade IV may also show moderate muscle edema.[29] Gadolinium administration may produce enhancement of bone contusion and in this setting enhancement is most conspicuous when fat-suppressed T1-weighted images are obtained.

Thin-section computerized tomography (CT) may also be helpful in the follow-up of these injuries, to detect subtle, early fragmentation of the bone.[6,96]

MRI is used to differentiate stress fractures from other pathological processes, especially from neoplastic processes. The linear segment of the stress fracture (decreased signal intensity on T1-weighted image) is usually accompanied by marrow edema. The lack of a soft-tissue mass, cortical destruction, and characteristic marrow extension effectively excludes a neoplasm from the differential diagnoses.[75] The sensitivity of MRI for stress fractures is 95 to 100%, specificity 80 to 86%, and accuracy 91 to 95%.[6,23,50,60,64,88,90]

During MR examination, a marker for planing should be placed over the region of interest (or pain) and the images in different plane (axial, coronal, or sagittal) should be performed depending on involved bone.[80]

Stress fractures of the inferior pubic ramus are fairly uncommon and occur primarily in long-distance runners and joggers. On MRI, the bony pelvis is best evaluated by imaging in the axial and

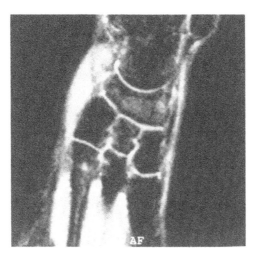

FIGURE 2.15 Axial STIR image shows increased signal intensity of bone marrow edema of the tarsal navicular bone in stress fracture.

coronal planes. A stress fracture demonstrates a characteristic pattern: decreased signal intensity on T1-weighted images and increased signal intensity on fat-saturated T2-weighted or STIR images with or without the presence of a visible fracture line. In the absence of a fracture line, it may be difficult on MRI to distinguish between the lesion and unilateral osteitis pubis or the gracilis syndrome.[42,51]

Stress fractures of the femoral neck are most frequently seen in military recruits, long-distance runners, ballet dancers, and elderly people. On MRI, stress fracture often presents as a serpinginous, low signal intensity line on T1-weighted images, which is variably evident on T2-weighted or STIR images. This line extends to the endosteal cortex, represents impaction of trabecular bone, and is usually surrounded by a zone of edema, inflammation, intraosseous hemorrhage, and/or granulating tissue. The fracture line does not traverse the entire femoral neck as do most other fracture lines associated with stress fractures.[11,25,42,76]

Stress fractures that involve the *femoral diaphysis* cause poorly localized thigh pain. MRI shows periosteal edema as well as bone marrow edema that involves the posteromedial aspect of the femur near the junction of the proximal and middle thirds of the femoral diaphysis. Axial plane T2-weighted imaging usually demonstrates the pathomorphology best.[11,25,42,76]

Distinguishing a *tibial stress reaction or fracture* from the shin splint syndrome is often very difficult without MRI. MRI can clearly demonstrate a pattern of tibial stress fracture as well as periostitis, posterior tibial muscle tendinitis, or compartment syndrome.[3,6,57]

MRI is sensitive to the hyperemia, morphology, and location of *calcaneal stress fracture,* intra-articular or extra-articular. STIR and fat-suppressed T2-weighted images are used to identify these areas of hyperintensity. T1-weighted images may be unremarkable or may demonstrate a fracture line.[37]

In addition to demonstrating *talar stress fractures* in the classical location (paralleling the talonavicular articulation at the level of the talar neck), MRI depicts other fracture locations. Those fractures involve vertically and horizontally oriented fractures of the medial aspect of the poster-oinferior talus, and transverse or horizontal fractures of the talar body parallel to the tibiotalar joint.[65,108]

Most *stress fractures of the tarsal navicular bone* are characterized as partial and linear. Sagittal plane MR images are useful for identification of fractures involving one or both cortices. Axial images may be used to show fracture lines that are parallel with the sagittal plane (Figure 2.15). MRI is also helpful in differentiating tarsal navicular stress fracture from symptomatic accessory tarsal navicular bone.[4,13]

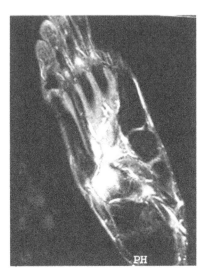

FIGURE 2.16 Axial STIR image demonstrates high signal intensity representing bone marrow edema in stress fracture of cuboid and fourth metatarsal bone.

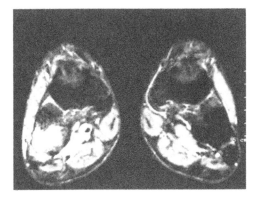

FIGURE 2.17 Coronal STIR image shows high signal intensity representing bone marrow edema of the cuboid bone.

MRI is especially useful for distinguishing *metatarsal stress fractures* from other pathological conditions in this area, as well as from synovitis of the Lisfranc joint, degenerative joint changes with negative conventional radiographs, or arthrosis. To see the full extent of each metatarsal bone on one image, the axial image of the foot should be obliqued into the plane of the metatarsal bone (Figure 2.16 and Figure 2.17).[34–36,59,95]

B. OSTEITIS PUBIS

Osteitis pubis, pain in the pubic region or groin that may radiate into the perineum, lower abdomen, or medial thigh, has been reported in association with long-distance running, soccer, rugby, football, ice hockey, and weight lifting. The etiological factor most often found is repetitive overuse of the adductor muscles. Sacral stress fracture or sacroiliac joint degeneration due to transmission of abnormal stresses across the pelvic ring structure can be seen in association with sports-related osteitis pubis.[5,103,106] Radiographic changes in osteitis pubis are usually absent during the first weeks of symptoms and may be absent months after the onset of symptoms. In the acute phase, MRI reveals a pattern of bone marrow edema as high signal intensity on T2-weighted or STIR images within the pubic bone with an associated symphysis pubis joint effusion.[5,103] The bone marrow edema may extend into the pubic rami. In the later phase of fibrosis and sclerosis, low signal intensity on T1- and T2-weighted images is found.[26,62] Those changes are always well depicted on the axial plane.[5]

C. SPONDYLOLYSIS

Isthmic spondylolysis with a lesion in the pars interarticularis may be a significant cause of pain in a given individual, particularly in adolescent athletes involved in sports with repetitive spinal motions. The pars lesion likely represents a stress fracture of the bone caused by the cumulative effects of repetitive stress imposed by physical activity.[92] Early diagnosis of isthmic, usually lumbar, spondylolysis cannot always be established on plain radiographs and CT scans. MRI shows typical bone marrow changes, even at an early stage.[98] Locally ill-defined bone marrow edema in pars interarticularis and the pedicle is seen as high signal intensity on fat-suppressed T2-weighted or STIR images, which is an early MR sign of isthmic spondylolysis before evidence of the fracture line.[98] Axial MR images at the level of the spondylolytic defect demonstrate low signal intensity sclerosis, fragmentation, or a discontinuity in the region of the pars defect. Latter hypertrophic bone and fibrocartilaginous overgrowth at the pars defect often produce a lateral recess or central canal stenosis that may result in nerve root impingement.[91] Spondylolysis may result in lytic spondylolisthesis, when anterior displacement of one vertebra on to another occurs secondary to bilateral fractures or defects in the pars interarticularis. Peripheral parasagittal images, in the sagittal plane, particularly T2*-weighted or T1-weighted images, demonstrate the defect or fracture line in pars interarticularis of the vertebra with perifocal bone marrow edema seen as high signal intensity on fat-suppressed T2-weighted or STIR images. The anteroposterior diameter of the spinal canal is increased in the presence of spondylolytic spondylolisthesis. The posterior aspects of the two involved vertebrae may be seen in the same axial image. MRI should be the first and only imaging modality in young patients with low back pain during and after exercise and pain with hyperextension of the spine.[91]

III. CARTILAGE

Overuse injuries as well as other sports-related injuries involve different parts of the body and different tissues. Those injuries often involve joint structures including articular cartilage. Overuse injuries may involve articular cartilage alone or result in osteohondral lesions, which may impair the mechanical properties of the cartilage.[102] Articular cartilage lesions or damage lead to partial breakdown in the proteoglycan matrix with a small increase in total water content and in changes in the size and arrangement of collagen fibers. All these changes in the macromolecular matrix lead to an alteration in the mechanical and chemical properties of the cartilage, as well as changes in normal signal intensity of articular cartilage on MRI. That is the reason MRI is the diagnostic method of choice in evaluation of articular cartilage. MRI is also the only diagnostic modality for direct non-invasive visualization of the articular cartilage.[38,53]

Different articular cartilage changes can be seen using MRI, including softening, edema, and fissuring. Arthroscopic grades of cartilage lesions have been correlated with findings on MRI and often have been compared with the stages of chondromalacia. In arthroscopic grade 1 chondral lesion, T1-weighted images show focal areas of decreased signal intensity without cartilage surface or subchondral bone extension. Fat-suppressed T2-weighted fast spin-echo images show focal areas of hyperintensity in the absence of any change in the smooth cartilage surface. Small irregularities of the articular cartilage, less than 1 mm, also seen using a fat-suppressed T2-weighted fast spin-echo sequence, represent the earliest changes of softening and swelling of the cartilage. Focal basal or deep layer hyperintensity is also seen in this early stage (Figure 2.18). In grade 2, indicated by blisterlike swelling, T1-weighted images show areas of decreased signal intensity extending to the articular cartilage surface with sharp cartilage margin. Fat-suppressed T2-weighted fast

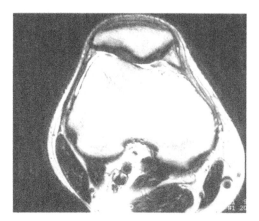

FIGURE 2.18 Axial fat-suppressed T2-weighted fast spin-echo image shows hyperintensity within normal articular cartilage thickness of medial and lateral patellar facets as sign of early softening and swelling — corresponding to findings in arthroscopic grade 1 chondromalacia.

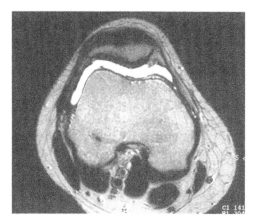

FIGURE 2.19 Axial fat-suppressed T2-weighted fast spin-echo image demonstrates focal ulceration and irregularity of cartilage surface on lateral patellar facet — grade 3 chondromalacia patellae.

spin-echo images demonstrate the blister lesion, which may or may not be associated with underlying articular cartilage signal inhomogeneity. This finding represents a focal separation of the superficial and deep layers of articular cartilage. Focal areas of decreased signal intensity associated with loss of the sharp articular margin between the two articular cartilage surfaces present the grade 3 articular cartilage lesion (Figure 2.19 and Figure 2.20). Fat-suppressed T2-weighted fast spin-echo images show fluid collection in surface articular cartilage defects as high-signal-intensity sites. In grade 4 chondral lesions, the ulceration and subchondral bone changes are represented on MRI by articular cartilage defects, exposed subchondral bone, and underlying fluid in subchondral bone (Figure 2.21 and Figure 2.22). On T1-weighted images there are low signal intensity changes in the subchondral bone, which may be hyperintense on fat-suppressed T2-weighted fast spin-echo images or STIR images.

MRI can reliably detect and stage osteochondral lesions.[38,53] The accuracy of staging is improved by performing MR arthrography using dilute gadolinium. On MRI, the focus of osteochondral lesion demonstrates low signal intensity on T1- and T2-weighted images.[107] A staging system for osteochondral lesions was developed based on arthroscopic findings. In stage 1, the articular cartilage is intact. In stage 2, an articular cartilage defect is present but without a loose body. On fat-suppressed T2-weighted fast spin-echo images high signal intensity articular fluid implies

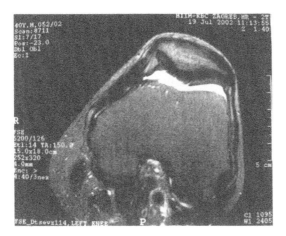

FIGURE 2.20 Axial fat-suppressed T2-weighted fast spin-echo image shows deep fissures of the patellar articular facet.

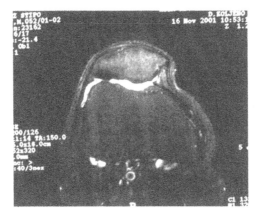

FIGURE 2.21 Axial fat-suppressed T2-weighted fast spin-echo image shows partial articular cartilage loss of the patellar facet.

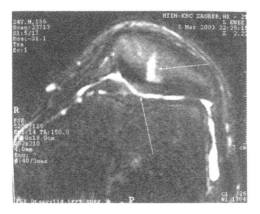

FIGURE 2.22 Axial fat-suppressed T2-weighted fast spin-echo image demonstrates focal hyperintensity within patellar articular cartilage with sclerotic subchondral bone and reactive bone marrow edema.

fissuring and irregularity of the articular cartilage surface. In stage 3, a partially detached osteo-chondral fragment is found. When the subchondral fluid collection circles the entire fragment of osteochondral lesion in its circumference, it is a MR sign of lesion instability. Hyperintensity between the lesion and adjacent bone visualized on T2-weighted or fat-suppressed T2-weighted fast spin-echo or STIR images represents either fluid or granulation tissue. Focal cystic regions deep to the lesion are also signs of instability of the fragment. Stage 4 is characterized by a loose body with a crater filled with fibrous tissue.[38,102] MR arthrography with intra-articular gadolinium contrast may improve visualization of fluid across the articular cartilage surface.

There is no consensus about the best sequence for the articular cartilage evaluation. Three-dimensional T-1 weighted gradient-echo sequences with fat suppression provide high accuracy in the detection of cartilage surface defects. Fast spin-echo imaging with heavy T2-weighting demonstrates cartilage defects in the presence of joint effusion accurately too, but minimal slice thickness in two-dimensional imaging is limiting. Fat-suppressed sequences and MR arthrography are especially useful in demonstrating the chondral surfaces. Fat-suppressed T2-weighted fast spin-echo may be more sensitive to basal articular cartilage changes than MR arthrography, which is better for the detection of articular cartilage surface irregularity. Those sequences provide excellent contrast between the low-signal cartilage and a high-signal joint fluid and the frequently present high signal in the underlying bone often serves as a useful indicator of injury to the overlying cartilage.[53] Conventional T2-weighted images may be associated with false-positive diagnoses, because this sequence does not provide enough contrast differentiation between articular cartilage and cortical bone. T2* gradient-echo images are no longer used to evaluate cartilage lesions, because the high signal intensity of the articular cartilage does not allow enough contrast resolution to successfully detect areas of articular cartilage softening and inhomogeneity. High-energy joint loading can cause cartilage damage without visible tissue disruption. To demonstrate this early stage of chondral injury, special techniques are necessary. These include diffusion-weighted imaging, measurements of magnetization transfer as a function of collagen concentration, proton density mapping to plot distribution of water in hyaline cartilage, and sodium imaging to visualize ions bound to proteoglycans. Although promising techniques, they are still experimental. It is important to remember potential pitfalls such as focal signal abnormalities in the patellar cartilage caused by pulsation artifacts from the popliteal artery. Fat signal intensity anterior to the trochlear groove may produce false-positive interpretations of articular cartilage irregularities when using fat-suppressed axial images or STIR images.[38,53,102]

IV. NERVE

Long-term repetitive microtrauma can lead to nerve entrapment syndromes. MRI of the nerves is still in a relatively early stage of development.[41]

According to Christine B. Chung,[18] MRI with its excellent soft-tissue contrast and multiplanar imaging capabilities is the diagnostic imaging method of choice for compressive or entrapment neuropathies. I agree with Christine B. Chung and as confirmation I present a few of my own cases:[14,77]

Piriformis muscle syndrome (Figure 2.23 and Figure 2.24)
Peroneus tunnel syndrome (Figure 2.25 and Figure 2.26)
Supracondylar process syndrome (Figure 2.27 and Figure 2.28)

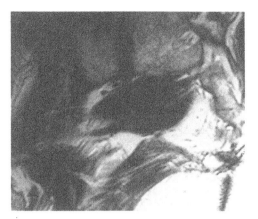

FIGURE 2.23 Coronal oblique T2-weighted image shows two heads of the divided right piriformis muscle, tendinous portion between the muscle heads and course of the common peroneal nerve through the piriformis muscle between the tendinous portion of the muscle.

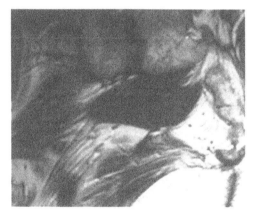

FIGURE 2.24 Coronal oblique T2-weighted image shows the course of the common peroneal nerve through the piriformis muscle.

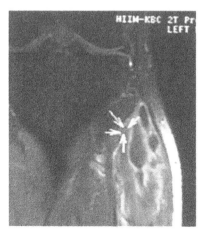

FIGURE 2.25 Contrast-enhanced coronal T1-weighted image with fat suppression shows multilobulated, septed ganglion with peripheral rim enhancement and compression of the common peroneal nerve at the level of below the fibular head.

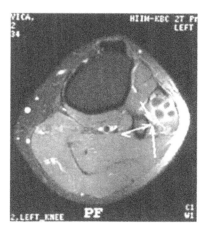

FIGURE 2.26 Contrast-enhanced axial T1-weighted image with fat suppression shows multilobulated, septed ganglion with peripheral rim enhancement and compression of the common peroneal nerve at the level of below the fibular head.

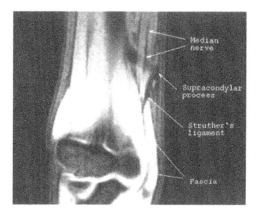

FIGURE 2.27 Coronal T2*-weighted image shows relationship of the supracondylar process, Struther's ligament, and median nerve proximal to the elbow.

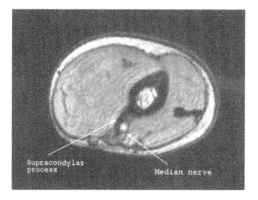

FIGURE 2.28 Axial three-dimensional GRE T1-weighted image shows position of the median nerve according to supracondylar process.

REFERENCES

1. **Al-Khodairy, A.T., Gobelet, C., Nancoz, R., and De Preux, J.** Iliopsoas bursitis and pseudogout of the knee mimicking L2-L3 radiculopathy: case report and review of the literature. *Eur. Spine J.*, 1997; 6: 336–341.

2. **Allen, W.C. and Cope, R.** Coxa saltans: the snapping hip revisited. *J. Am. Acad. Orthop. Surg.*, 1995; 3: 303–308.

3. **Anderson, M.W., Ugalde, V., Batt, M., and Gacayan, J.** Shin splints: MR appearance in a preliminary study. *Radiology*, 1997; 204(1): 177–180.

4. **Ariyoshi, M., Nagata, K., Kubo, M. et al.** MRI monitoring of tarsal navicular stress fracture healing — a case report. *Med. J.*, 1998; 45: 223–225.

5. **Barile, A., Erriquez, D., and Cacchio, A. et al.** Groin pain in athletes: role of magnetic resonance. *Radiol. Med.* (Torino), 2000; 100: 216–222.

6. **Bergman, G. and Fredericson, M.** MR finds runners' overuse injuries. *Diagn. Imaging Sports Imaging Suppl.*, 2000; 16: 12–16.

7. **Berkowitz, J.F., Kier, R., and Rudicel, S.** Plantar fasciitis: MR imaging. *Radiology*, 1991; 179: 665–667.

8. **Berthoty, D., Sartoris, D.J., and Resnick, D.** Fast scan magnetic resonance of Achilles tendonitis. *J. Foot Surg.*, 1989; 28: 171–173.

9. **Blevins, F.T.** Rotator cuff pathology in athletes. *Sports Med.*, 1997; 24: 205–220.

10. **Bigliani, L.U.** The morphology of the acromion and its relationship to rotator cuff tears. *Orthop. Trans.*, 1986; 10: 216.

11. **Boden, B.P. and Speer, K.P.** Femoral stress fractures. *Clin. Sports Med.*, 1997; 16: 307–317.

12. **Bodne, D., Quinn, S.F., Murray, W.T. et al.** Magnetic resonance images of chronic patellar tendinitis. *Skel. Radiol.*, 1988; 17: 24–28.

13. **Bojanić, I., Pećina, H.I., and Pećina, M.** Stress fractures. *Arh. Hig. Rada Toksikol.*, 2001; 52: 471–82.

14. **Borić, I., Pećina, H.I., and Pećina, M.** MRI of tunnel syndromes. European Congress of Radiology, Vienna, 2002. *Eur. Radiol.*, 2002; 12(Suppl. 1): 446.

15. **Brandser, E.A., el-Khoury, G.Y., Kathol, M.H. et al.** Hamstring injuries: radiographic, conventional tomographic, CT, and MR imaging characteristics. *Radiology*, 1995; 197: 257–262.

16. **Bredella, M.A., Tirman, P.F., Fritz, R.C. et al.** MR imaging findings of lateral ulnar collateral ligament abnormalities in patients with lateral epicondylitis. *Am. J. Roentgenol.*, 1999; 173: 1379–1382.

17. **Chung, C.B., Lektrakul, N., Gigena, L. et al.** Magnetic resonance imaging of the upper extremity: advances in technique and application. *Clin. Orthop.*, 2001; 383: 162–174.

18. **Chung, C.B.** Personal communications.

19. **Coel, M., Yamada, C.Y., and Ko, J.** MR imaging of patients with lateral epicondylitis of the elbow: importance of increased signal of the anconeus muscle. *Am. J. Roentgenol.*, 1993; 161: 1019–1021.

20. **Cohen, R.B. and Williams, G.R., Jr.** Impingement syndrome and rotator cuff disease as repetitive motion disorders. *Clin. Orthop.*, 1998; 351: 95–101.

21. **De Paulis, F., Cacchio, A., Michelini, O. et al.** Sports injuries in the pelvis and hip: diagnostic imaging. *Eur. J. Radiol.*, 1998; 27(Suppl. 1): 49–59.

22. **De Smet, A.A. and Best, T.M.** imaging of the distribution and location of acute hamstring injuries in athletes. *Am. J. Roentgenol.*, 2000; 174: 393–399.

23. **Deutsch, A.L., Coel, M.N., and Mink, J.H.** Imaging of stress injuries to bone. Radiography, scintigraphy, and MR imaging. *Clin. Sports Med.*, 1997; 16: 275–290.

24. **Duri, Z.A., Aichroth, P.M., Wilkins, R. et al.** Patellar tendonitis and anterior knee pain. *Am. J. Knee Surg.*, 1999; 12: 99–106.

25. **Egol, K.A., Koval, K.J., Kummer, F. et al.** Stress fractures of the femoral neck. *Clin. Orthop.*, 1998; 348: 72–78.

26. **Ekberg, O., Sjoberg, S., and Westlin, N.** Sports-related groin pain: evaluation with MR imaging. *Eur. Radiol.*, 1996; 6: 52–55.

27. **El-Khoury, G.Y., Wira, R.L., Berbaum, K.S. et al.** MR imaging of patellar tendinitis. *Radiology*, 1992; 184: 849–854.

28. **Farooki, S. and Seeger, L.L.** MR imaging of sports injuries of the shoulder. *Semin. Musculoskel. Radiol.,* 1997; 1: 61–63.
29. **Fredericson, M., Bergman, G., Hoffman, K.L. et al.** Tibial stress reaction in runners: correlation of clinical symptoms and scintigraphy with a new MRI grading system. *Am. J. Sports Med.,* 1995; 23: 472–481.
30. **Fritz, R.C.** MR imaging in sports medicine: the elbow. *Semin. Musculoskel. Radiol.,* 1997; 1: 29–49.
31. **Fritz, R.C. and Stoller, D.W.** Elbow, in *Magnetic Resonance Imaging in Orthopaedics and Sports Medicine,* 2nd ed., Stoller, D.W., Ed. Philadelphia: Lippincott-Raven, 1997; 779–788.
32. **Gillet, P., Blum, A., Hestin, D. et al.** Magnetic resonance imaging may be an asset to diagnose and classify fluoroquinolone-associated Achilles tendinitis. *Fundam. Clin. Pharmacol.,* 1995; 9: 52–56.
33. **Grasel, R.P., Schweitzer, M.E., Kovalovich, A.M. et al.** MR imaging of plantar fasciitis: edema, tears, and occult marrow abnormalities correlated with outcome. *Am. J. Roentgenol.,* 1999; 173: 699–701.
34. **Harmath, C., Demos, T.C., Lomasney, L. et al.** Stress fracture of the fifth metatarsal. *Orthopedics,* 2001; 24: 204–208.
35. **Harrington, T., Crichton, K.J., and Anderson, I.F.** Overuse ballet injury of the base of the second metatarsal. A diagnostic problem. *Am. J. Sports Med.,* 1993; 21: 591–598.
36. **Hodler, J., Steinert, H., Zanetti, M. et al.** Radiographically negative stress related bone injury. MR imaging versus two-phase bone scintigraphy. *Acta Radiol.,* 1998; 39: 416–420.
37. **Hollister, M.C. and De Smet, A.A.** MR imaging of the foot and ankle in sports injuries. *Semin. Musculoskel. Radiol.,* 1997; 1: 105–126.
38. **Imhof, H., Nöbauer-Huhmann, I.M., Krestan, C. et al.** MRI of cartilage. *Eur. Radiol.,* 2002; 12: 2781–2793.
39. **Jacobson, J.A.** Musculoskeletal sonography and MR imaging. A role for both imaging methods. *Radiol. Clin. North Am.,* 1999; 37: 713–735.
40. **Janzen, D.L., Partridge, E., Logan, P.M. et al.** The snapping hip: clinical and imaging findings in transient subluxation of the iliopsoas tendon. *Can. Assoc. Radiol. J.,* 1996; 47: 202–208.
41. **Jarvik, J.G., Yuen, E., Haynor, D.R. et al.** MR nerve imaging in a prospective cohort of patients with suspected carpal tunnel syndrome. *Neurology,* 2002; 58: 1597–1602.
42. **Jean, J.L., Lee, G.H., Tang, H.L. et al.** Stress fracture of the femoral neck in young adult: report of four cases. *Chang Gung Med. J.,* 2001; 24: 188–195.
43. **Johnston, C.A., Wiley, J.P., Lindsay, D.M. et al.** Iliopsoas bursitis and tendinitis. A review. *Sports Med.,* 1998; 25: 271–283.
44. **Keene, J.S., Lash, E.G., Fisher, D.R. et al.** Magnetic resonance imaging of Achilles tendon ruptures. *Am. J. Sports Med.,* 1989; 17: 333–337.
45. **Kerr, R.** MR imaging of sports injuries of the hip and pelvis. *Semin. Musculoskel. Radiol.,* 1997; 1: 65–82.
46. **Khan, K.M., Bonar, F., Desmond, P.M. et al.** Patellar tendinosis (jumper's knee): findings at histopathologic examination, US, and MR imaging. Victorian Institute of Sport Tendon Study Group. *Radiology,* 1996; 200: 821–827.
47. **Kier, R.** Magnetic resonance imaging of plantar fasciitis and other causes of heel pain. *Magn. Reson. Imaging Clin. North Am.,* 1994; 2: 97–107.
48. **Kier, R.** Imaging of foot and ankle tumors. *Magn. Reson. Imaging,* 1993; 11: 149–162.
49. **Kingzett-Taylor, A., Tirman, P.F., Feller, J. et al.** Tendinosis and tears of gluteus medius and minimus muscles as a cause of hip pain: MR imaging findings. *Am. J. Roentgenol.,* 1999; 173: 1123–1126.
50. **Kiuru, M.J., Pihlajamaki, H.K., Hietanen, H.J. et al.** MR imaging, bone scintigraphy, and radiography in bone stress injuries of the pelvis and the lower extremity. *Acta Radiol.,* 2002; 43: 207–212.
51. **Kiuru, M.J., Pihlajamaki, H.K., Perkio, J.P. et al.** Dynamic contrast-enhanced MR imaging in symptomatic bone stress of the pelvis and the lower extremity. *Acta Radiol.,* 2001; 42: 277–285.
52. **Klinkert, P., Jr., Porte, R.J., de Rooij, T.P. et al.** Quadratus femoris tendinitis as a cause of groin pain. *Br. J. Sports Med.,* 1997; 31: 348–349.
53. **Kneeland, J.B.** MR imaging of articular cartilage and of cartilage degeneration, in *Magnetic Resonance Imaging in Orthopaedics and Sports Medicine,* 2nd ed., Stoller, D.W., Ed. Philadelphia: Lippincott-Raven, 1997; 83–91.

54. **Kujala, U.M., Orava, S., and Jarvinen, M.** Hamstring injuries. Current trends in treatment and prevention. *Sports Med.*, 1997; 23: 397–404.

55. **Kurosawa, H., Nakasita, K., Nakasita, H. et al.** Complete avulsion of the hamstring tendons from the ischial tuberosity. A report of two cases sustained in judo. *Br. J. Sports Med.*, 1996; 30: 72–74.

56. **Lacroix, V.J., Kinnear, D.G., Mulder, D.S. et al.** Lower abdominal pain syndrome in national hockey league players: a report of 11 cases. *Clin. J. Sport Med.*, 1998; 8: 5–9.

57. **Lambros, G. and Alder, D.** Multiple stress fractures of the tibia in a healthy adult. *Am. J. Orthop.*, 1997; 26: 687–688.

58. **Lassus, J., Tulikoura, I., Konttinen, Y.T. et al.** Bone stress injuries of the lower extremity: a review. *Acta Orthop Scand.*, 2002; 73: 359–368.

59. **Lechevalier, D., Fournier, B., Leleu, T. et al.** Stress fractures of the heads of the metatarsals. A new cause of metatarsal pain. *Rev. Rhum. Engl. Ed.*, 1995; 62: 255–259.

60. **Lee, J.K. and Yao, L.** Stress fractures: MR imaging. *Radiology,* 1988; 169: 217–220.

61. **Leunig, M., Werlen, S., Ungersbock, A. et al.** Evaluation of the acetabular labrum by MR arthrography. *J. Bone Joint Surg. Br.*, 1997; 79: 230–234.

62. **Major, N.M. and Helms, C.A.** Pelvic stress injuries: the relationship between osteitis pubis (symphysis pubis stress injury) and sacroiliac abnormalities in athletes. *Skel. Radiol.*, 1997; 26: 711–717.

63. **Martin, C.E. and Schweitzer, M.E.** MR imaging of epicondylitis. *Skel. Radiol.*, 1998; 27: 133–138.

64. **Martin, S.D., Healey, J.H., and Horowitz, S.** Stress fracture MRI. *Orthopedics,* 1993; 16: 75–78.

65. **Masciocchi, C., Maffey, M.V., and Mastri, F.** Overload syndromes of the peritalar region. *Eur. J. Radiol.*, 1997; 26: 46–53.

66. **McGarvey, W.C., Singh, D., and Trevino, S.G.** Partial Achilles tendon ruptures associated with fluoroquinolone antibiotics: a case report and literature review. *Foot Ankle Int.*, 1996; 17: 496–498.

67. **McGonagle, D., Marzo-Ortega, H., and O'Connor, P. et al.** The role of biomechanical factors and HLA-B27 in magnetic resonance imaging-determined bone changes in plantar fascia enthesopathy. *Arthritis Rheum.*, 2002; 46: 489–493.

68. **McLoughlin, R.F., Raber, E.L., Vellet, A.D. et al.** Patellar tendinitis: MR imaging features, with suggested pathogenesis and proposed classification. *Radiology,* 1995; 197: 843–848.

69. **Muhle, C., Ahn, J.M., Yeh, L. et al.** Iliotibial band friction syndrome: MR imaging findings in 16 patients and MR arthrographic study of six cadaveric knees. *Radiology,* 1999; 212: 103–110.

70. **Narvaez, J.A., Narvaez, J., Ortega, R. et al.** Painful heel: MR imaging findings. *Radiographics,* 2000; 20: 333–352.

71. **Neer, C.S.** Anterior acromioplasty for the chronic impingement syndrome: a preliminary report. *J. Bone Joint Surg. Am.*, 1972; 54: 41.

72. **Nishmura, G., Yamato, M., Tamai, K. et al.** MR findings in iliotibial band syndrome. *Skel. Radiol.*, 1997; 26: 533–537.

73. **Notzli, H.P., Wyss, T.F., Stoecklin, C.H. et al.** The contour of the femoral head-neck junction as a predictor for the risk of anterior impingement. *J. Bone Joint Surg. Br.*, 2002; 84: 556–560.

74. **O'Neil, B.A., Forsythe, M.E., and Stanish, W.D.** Chronic occupational repetitive strain injury. *Can. Fam. Physician,* 2001; 47: 311–316.

75. **Pauleit, D., Sommer, T., Textor, J. et al.** MRI diagnosis in longitudinal stress fractures: differential diagnosis of Ewing sarcoma. *Rofo,* 1999; 170: 28–34.

76. **Pearce, D.H., White, L.M., and Bell, R.S.** Musculoskeletal images. Bilateral insufficiency fracture of the femoral neck. *Can. J. Surg.*, 2001; 44: 11–12.

77. **Pećina, M., Borić, I., and Antićević, D.** Intraoperatively proven anomalous Struthers' ligament diagnosed by MRI. *Skel. Radiol.*, 2002; 31: 532–535.

78. **Pfahler, M., Jessel, C., Steinborn, M. et al.** Magnetic resonance imaging in lateral epicondylitis of the elbow. *Arch. Orthop. Trauma Surg.*, 1998; 118: 121–125.

79. **Pomeranz, S.J. and Heidt, R.S., Jr.** MR imaging in the prognostication of hamstring injury. Work in progress. *Radiology,* 1993; 18: 897–900.

80. **Popovic, N., Ferrara, M.A., Daenen, B. et al.** Imaging overuse injury of the elbow in professional team handball players: a bilateral comparison using plain films, stress radiography, ultrasound, and magnetic resonance imaging. *Int. J. Sports Med.*, 2001; 22: 60–67.

81. **Popp, J.E., Yu, J.S., and Kaeding, C.C.** Recalcitrant patellar tendinitis. Magnetic resonance imaging, histologic evaluation, and surgical treatment. *Am. J. Sports Med.*, 1997; 25: 218–222.

82. **Potter, H.G., Sharon, S., and Adler, R.S.** Imaging of the hip in athletes. *Sports Med. Arthrosc. Rev.,* 2002; 10: 115–122.
83. **Reiff, D.B., Heenan, S.D., and Heron, C.W.** MRI appearances of the asymptomatic patellar tendon on gradient echo imaging. *Skel. Radiol.,* 1995; 24: 123–126.
84. **Roger, B. and Grenier, P.** MRI of plantar fasciitis. *Eur. Radiol.,* 1997; 7: 1430–1435.
85. **Sallay, P.I., Friedman, R.L., Coogan, P.G. et al.** Hamstring muscle injuries among water skiers. Functional outcome and prevention. *Am. J. Sports Med.,* 1996; 24: 130–136.
86. **Schmid, M.R., Hodler, J., and Cathrein, P. et al.** Is impingement the cause of jumper's knee? Dynamic and static magnetic resonance imaging of patellar tendinitis in an open-configuration system. *Am. J. Sports Med.,* 2002; 30: 388–395.
87. **Shalby, M. and Almekinders, L.C.** Patellar tendinitis: the significance of magnetic resonance imaging findings. *Am. J. Sports Med.,* 1999; 27: 345–349.
88. **Sijbrandij, E.S., van Gils, A.P., and de Lange, E.E.** Overuse and sports-related injuries of the ankle and hind foot: MR imaging findings. *Eur. J. Radiol.,* 2002; 43: 45–56.
89. **Speer, K.P., Lohnes, J., and Garrett, W.E., Jr.** Radiographic imaging of muscle strain injury. *Am. J. Sports Med.,* 1993; 21: 89–95.
90. **Spitz, D.J. and Newberg, A.H.** Imaging of stress fractures in the athlete. *Radiol. Clin. North Am.,* 2002; 40: 313–331.
91. **Staebler, A., Paulus, R., Steinborn, M. et al.** Spondylolysis in the developmental stage: diagnostic contribution of MRI. *Rofo,* 2000; 172: 33–37.
92. **Standaert, C.J., Herring, S.A., Halpern, B. et al.** Spondylolysis. *Phys. Med. Rehabil. Clin. North Am.,* 2000; 11: 785–803.
93. **Steinbach, L.S., Fleckenstein, J.L., and Mink, J.H.** MR imaging of muscle injuries. *Semin. Musculoskel. Radiol.,* 1997; 1: 127–141.
94. **Steinborn, M., Heuck, A., Maier, M. et al.** MRI of plantar fasciitis. *Rofo,* 1999; 170: 41–46.
95. **Steinbronn, D.J., Bennett, G.L., and Kay, D.B.** The use of magnetic resonance imaging in the diagnosis of stress fractures of the foot and ankle: four case reports. *Foot Ankle Int.,* 1994; 15: 80–83.
96. **Stoller, D.W., Dilworth Cannon, W., and Anderson, L.J.** Fractures, in *Magnetic Resonance Imaging in Orthopaedics and Sports Medicine,* 2nd ed., Stoller, D.W., Ed. Philadelphia: Lippincott-Raven, 1997; 417–432.
97. **Stoller, D.W. and Ferkel, R.D.** Plantar fasciitis, in *Magnetic Resonance Imaging in Orthopaedics and Sports Medicine,* 2nd ed., Stoller, D.W., Ed. Philadelphia: Lippincott-Raven, 1997; 587.
98. **Stoller, D.W., Hu, S.S., and Kaisser, J.A.** Spondylolisthesis. in *Magnetic Resonance Imaging in Orthopaedics and Sports Medicine,* 2nd ed., Stoller, D.W., Ed. Philadelphia: Lippincott-Raven, 1997; 1075–1084.
99. **Stoller, D.W., Maloney, W.J., and Glick, J.M.** Hip pain in the athlete, in *Magnetic Resonance Imaging in Orthopaedics and Sports Medicine,* 2nd ed., Stoller, D.W., Ed. Philadelphia: Lippincott-Raven, 1997; 156–167.
100. **Theodorou, D.J., Theodorou, S.J., Farooki, S. et al.** Disorders of the plantar aponeurosis: a spectrum of MR imaging findings. *Am. J. Roentgenol.,* 2001; 176: 97–104.
101. **Theodorou, D.J., Theodorou, S.J., Kakitsubata, Y. et al.** Plantar fasciitis and fascial rupture: MR imaging findings in 26 patients supplemented with anatomic data in cadavers. *Radiographics,* 2000; 20(Suppl.): S181–S197.
102. **Tratting, S.** Overuse of hyaline cartilage and imaging. *Eur. J. Radiol.,* 1997; 25: 188–198.
103. **Tuite, M.J. and De Smet, A.A.** MRI of selected sports injuries: muscle tears, groin pain, and osteochondritis dissecans. *Semin. Ultrasound CT MR,* 1994; 15: 318–340.
104. **Tyrrell, P.N. and Davies, A.M.** Magnetic resonance imaging appearances of fatigue fractures of the long bones of the lower limb. *Br. J. Radiol.,* 1994; 67: 332–338.
105. **Verrall, G.M., Slavotinek, J.P., Barnes, P.G. et al.** Clinical risk factors for hamstring muscle strain injury: a prospective study with correlation of injury by magnetic resonance imaging. *Br. J. Sports Med.,* 2001; 35: 435–439.
106. **Verrall, G.M., Slavotinek, J.P., and Fon, G.T.** Incidence of pubic bone marrow oedema in Australian rules football players: relation to groin pain. *Br. J. Sports Med.,* 2001; 35: 28–33.
107. **Weaver, C.J., Major, N.M., Garrett, W.E. et al.** Femoral head osteochondral lesions in painful hips of athletes: MR imaging findings. *Am. J. Roentgenol.,* 2002; 178: 973–977.

108. **Weishaupt, D. and Schweitzer, M.E.** MR imaging of the foot and ankle: patterns of bone marrow signal abnormalities. *Eur. Radiol.*, 2002; 12: 416–426.

109. **Wright, T., Yoon, C., and Schmit, B.P.** Shoulder MRI refinements: differentiation of rotator cuff tear from artifacts and tendonosis, and reassessment of normal findings. *Semin. Ultrasound CT MR*, 2001; 22: 383–395.

110. **Wunderbaldinger, P., Bremer, C., Matuszewski, L. et al.** Efficient radiological assessment of the internal snapping hip syndrome. *Eur. Radiol.*, 2001; 11: 1743–1747.

111. **Yu, J.S., Popp, J.E., Kaeding, C.C. et al.** Correlation of MR imaging and pathologic findings in athletes undergoing surgery for chronic patellar tendinitis. *Am. J. Roentgenol.*, 1995; 165: 115–118.

112. **Yu, J.S., Smith, G., Ashman, C. et al.** The plantar fasciotomy: MR imaging findings in asymptomatic volunteers. *Skel. Radiol.*, 1999; 28: 447–452.

113. **Yu, J.S., Spigos, D., and Tomczak, R.** Foot pain after a plantar fasciotomy: an MR analysis to determine potential causes. *J. Comput. Assist. Tomogr.*, 1999; 23: 707–712.

114. **Zlatkin, M.B.** Evaluation of rotator cuff disease and glenohumeral instability with MR imaging: correlation with arthroscopy and arthrotomy in a large population of patients. *Magn. Reson. Imaging*, 1990; 8(Suppl. 1): 78.

Part II

Upper Extremities

3 Shoulder

The glenohumeral joint has the greatest range of movement of any joint in the human body. The joint is able to rotate in every direction to reach every part of the body. Further, all the movements performed by the shoulder joint are within eyesight range, i.e., within the area supervised by our sight, which is very important during work and exercise.

On the one hand, the mobility of the shoulder joint is enabled by the disproportional concave and convex joint bodies and the large volume of the joint capsule. On the other hand, the stability of the joint is ensured by the action of many muscles whose tendons are contained in the joint capsule itself. The importance of the arm in human activities is beyond question, especially during work activities and sports involving the arm in an overhead position (racket sports, volleyball, water polo, swimming, etc.). Because of the numerous tendons and bursae in the glenohumeral area, the high incidence of overuse syndromes in such an area is expected.

We illustrate the point with the words of Uhthoff and Sarkar:[167] "We were aware of this problem when we formulated the following classification, which is based on where the lesion originates. If the lesion arises in the substance of the tendon, the category has been designated intrinsic or primary. On the other hand, if the involvement of the tendon is apparently related to lesion in an adjacent or remote structure, or to systemic diseases, the category is extrinsic or secondary" (Table 3.1 and Table 3.2).

I. IMPINGEMENT SYNDROME OF THE SHOULDER

Impingement syndrome is an entity[48,65,114,115] that includes a series of damages resulting from the clash of the rotator cuff of the glenohumeral joint (m. supraspinatus, m. infraspinatus, m. subscapularis, m. teres minor), subacromial bursa, and sometimes the long head of the biceps brachii muscle tendon against the frontal part of the acromion, acromioclavicular ligament, coracoid processus, and acromioclavicular joint (Figure 3.1). The clash occurs when the arm is lifted high above the head in an overhead position (Figure 3.2). The rotator cuff of the shoulder and especially the supraspinatus muscle suffer the most damage during this clash. There are other terms found in literature denoting this entity, e.g., rotator cuff tendinitis, supraspinatus syndrome, subacromial compressive syndrome, pitcher's shoulder, and, in our experience, volleyball shoulder.

Gerber et al.[50] stressed the role of the coracoid process in chronic impingement syndrome. The pain appears in abduction and internal rotation of the arm, and according to them this is "subcoracoid impingement" of the shoulder. According to Paulson et al.[125] anterior shoulder problems including coracoid impingement syndrome are extremely common in athletes engaged in throwing activities.

Impingement of the deep surface of the supraspinatus tendon on the posterosuperior glenoid rim was described by Walch et al.[172] in 1992 and termed "glenoidal or internal impingement of the shoulder." In the position of the arm at 90° of abduction and maximal external rotation the supraspinatus tendon comes in contact with the posterosuperior glenoid rim (Figure 3.3). Walch et al.[172] were the first to describe glenoidal impingement in athletes participating in throwing activities. In the final stage of the syndrome, rupture of the supraspinatus tendon may occur. Meister[109] considers that the articular surface of the rotator cuff can become diseased secondary to direct abutment against the glenoid rim and labrum. Damage to the undersurface of the rotator cuff can occur from contact at the extremes of shoulder motion and can increase secondary to adaptive changes in bone and soft tissue. According to McFarland et al.[107] the finding of contact of the rotator

TABLE 3.1
Primary (Intrinsic Origin) Tendinopathies of Rotator
Cuff, Bicipital Tendon, or Both

Apparent Causative Factor(s)	Clinical Syndrome
Trauma	Tendinitis
	Impingement
	Rupture
	Instability
Reactive	Calcifying tendinitis with or without impingement
Degeneration	Instability
	Impingement
	Rupture
Hyperelasticity (Ehlers-Danlos syndrome)	Instability
Idiopathic	Frozen shoulder

TABLE 3.2
Secondary (Extrinsic Origin) Tendinopathies of
Rotator Cuff, Bicipital Tendon, or Both

Apparent Causative Factor(s)	Clinical Syndrome
Anatomic variations of bony tissue	Tendinitis
Large coracoid process	Impingement
"Beaking" of the acromion	Rupture
Supratubercular ridge	
Pathologic changes in the bony tissue	Tendinitis
Acromial spur	Impingement
Osteophytes of the acromioclavicular (a-c) joint	Rupture
Systemic diseases	Tendinitis
Metabolic	Frozen shoulder
Endocrine	
Rheumatic	
Remote causes	Tendinitis
Cervical disc	Frozen shoulder
Intrathoracic/intra-abdominal disorders	

cuff to the posterosuperior glenoid with the arm in abduction and external rotation can occur in a wide spectrum of shoulder diseases and is not limited to the throwing athlete. Halbrecht et al.[63] evaluated and compared the findings of gadolinium-enhanced magnetic resonance imaging (MRI) studies of throwing and nonthrowing shoulders in college baseball athletes. Abnormalities of the rotator cuff and superior labrum are seen in asymptomatic throwing shoulders but not nonthrowing shoulders. From examination of a large number of skeletal specimens (1232 shoulders) Edelson and Teitz[43] conclude that internal impingement of the shoulder may also be a significant mechanism in the development of rotator cuff pathosis. Giombini et al.[52] reported that posterosuperior glenoid rim impingement is a cause of shoulder pain in top-level water polo players. The study of Paley et al.[122] supports the concept of impingement of the posterior cuff undersurface with the posterosuperior glenoid rim in the overhead throwing athlete with shoulder pain. According to Sonnery-Cottet et al.[152] the results of arthroscopic treatment of posterosuperior glenoid impingement in tennis

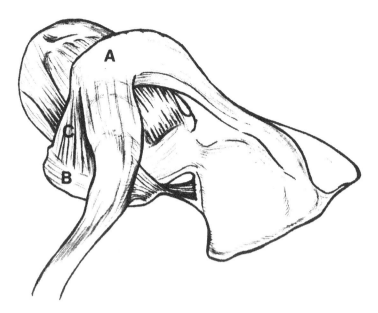

FIGURE 3.1 The shoulder joint roof is composed of the acromion (A), coracoid process (B), and coracoacromial ligament (C).

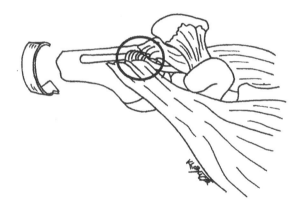

FIGURE 3.2 Mechanism of the clash development in subacromial area of the shoulder joint.

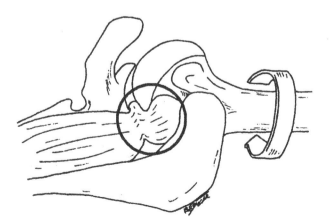

FIGURE 3.3 Mechanism of the glenoidal or internal impingement of the shoulder joint.

players are encouraging in terms of the high number of patients returning to tennis. Thermal capsular shrinkage can also be safely used to treat internal impingement in the throwing athlete. Jobe[82,83] describes superior glenoid impingement as a special diagnostic entity. Superior glenoid impingement places five structures at risk: the rotator cuff, the superior labrum, the greater tuberosity, the superior glenoid, and the inferior glenohumeral ligament. Struhl[158] introduces the concept of anterior internal impingement in patients with signs and symptoms of classic impingement syndrome and arthroscopic evidence of articular-side partial rotator cuff tear. Gerber and Sebesta[51] suggest that in addition to the posterosuperior impingement of the supraspinatus tendon originally described by Walch, anterosuperior impingement of the deep surface of the subscapularis is a form of intra-articular impingement responsible for painful structural disease of the shoulder. If the internal impingement of the shoulder is recognized early, non-operative intervention may be successful. When non-operative treatment fails, the use of arthroscopy to treat torn rotator cuff and labral tissue and capsular laxity may be indicated to resolve symptoms and restore the premorbid level of function.[109]

Ellenbecker and Derscheid[44] reported that impingement syndrome most often occurs in athletes as a consequence of shoulder area overuse, that is, as repetitive motion disorder.[37] Jobe and Bradley[85] describe an increased incidence of the syndrome in baseball, volleyball, tennis, rugby, athletics, water polo, and swimming, i.e., all sports that require an extended use of the arm in an overhead position, including elite rock climbing.[19,156,173,178] An epidemiological survey was conducted by Lo et al.[99] to collect data relating to the prevalence and frequency of shoulder pain and other related problems among different athletic groups who use vigorous upper arm activities. A questionnaire was administered on site, thus ensuring that the response rate was 100%. Analysis of the results revealed that, of the 372 respondents, a total of 163 athletes (43.8%) indicated that they had shoulder problems and 109 (29%) were suffering pain as well. Diffuse pain was indicated by 20 respondents (5.4%), and localized pain during movement was reported in 89 respondents (23.9%). The prevalence of shoulder pain ranked highest among volleyball players ($N = 28$), followed by swimmers ($N = 22$), then badminton, basketball, and tennis participants, who were equally affected ($N = 10$ for each). Neviaser[119] defines impingement syndrome on rotator cuff muscle as tendinitis caused by prolonged tendon pressure on the coracoacromial arch and the acromioclavicular joint. Butters and Rockwood[27] and Neviaser[119] reported that the impingement syndrome is regularly characterized by subacromial (subdeltoid) bursa damage and damage to the long head of biceps brachii tendon because these structures are connected by the synovial sheath of the shoulder joint.

The shoulder joint is an example of a spheric joint, granted, with exceptional mobility and dynamic stability.[44,140,143] The joint consists of a spacious joint capsule, enforced with the glenohumeral ligament and the labrum glenoidale on the front aspect. The shoulder joint roof is composed of the coracoacromial arch, which consists of the coracoid processus and the acromion of the scapula connected by the broad coracoacromial ligament (Figure 3.1). The subacromial (subdeltoid) bursa is situated beneath the coracoacromial arch. It is one of eight synovial bursae that can be found in this area. Dynamic stability of the joint is determined by the synchronous action of the shoulder muscle. The muscles are divided into three major groups: (1) the costohumeral group (pectoralis major muscle and latissimus dorsi muscle), (2) the spinoscapular group (trapezius muscle, rhomboideus muscle, serratus anterior muscle, and levator scapulae muscle), and (3) the scapulohumeral group (rotator cuff and coracobrachialis muscle).

The rotator cuff of the shoulder joint is constructed of short muscles: the supraspinatus muscle, infraspinatus muscle, teres minor muscle, and subscapularis muscle. These four muscles originate in the scapula and attach to both tubercules of the humerus. The supraspinatus, infraspinatus, and teres minor muscles attach downward on the tubercul major, while subscapularis muscle attaches to the tubercul minor. The supraspinatus muscle traverses through the so-called supraspinatus tunnel rimmed with the coracoid processus on the front, with the acromion and the spina scapulae on the back, and with the coracoacromial ligament from above. Because of its special anatomic determination, the supraspinatus muscle plays an important role in the rotator cuff. It represents the locus minoris resistentiae in the mechanical sense of the rotator cuff.[97,98] It is well known that the musculotendinous units of the rotator cuff act as dynamic stabilizers of the glenohumeral joint, but at the same time prevent the joint capsule from excessive anterior or posterior shift (especially the supraspinatus muscle since it is encompassed in the joint capsule from the upper side).

Biomechanical and electromyographic investigations have shown the importance of the supraspinatus muscle's preventive role in upper and lower instability.[143] In addition, between one third and one half of shoulder joint strength during external rotation (infraspinatus muscle, teres minor muscle) is due to the rotator cuff muscles, whereas the subscapularis muscle acts as a strong internal rotator. External rotation plays an important role in abduction of the arm because it prevents the tubercul major from hitting the glenoid and enables arm abduction greater than 90°.[140] Internal rotation of the shoulder joint is important in anteflexion of the arm because of the similar mechanism of avoiding the clash between the humerus head and the coracoacromial ligament. The synchronous action of the teres minor and subscapularis muscles strongly contributes to the fixation of the humerus head (depression action) to the glenoid in any position of arm elevation. The supraspinatus muscle is the fixator of the humeral head in initial abduction that, according to recent findings, does not necessarily start with supraspinatus muscle contraction alone. The deltoideus muscle plays an equal role in abduction initiation.[74] The role of the long head of the biceps brachii is characterized by assisting the depression and fixation of the humeral head to the glenoid. Its role is stressed in cases of weakness of the first three muscles (infraspinatus muscle, subscapularis muscle, and teres minor muscle).

Recent investigations point to the nutritive role of the rotator cuff. Muscle tension of the rotator cuff of the shoulder mechanically assists synovial fluid flow through the joint. In this way, the cartilage of the joint surfaces are equally provided with synovial fluid. Finally, the rotator cuff muscles represent a liquid-proof coating of the joint capsule, enabling the loss of synovial fluid due to minor tears of the joint capsule.

A. ETIOPATHOGENESIS

The clash of the humerus head against the coracoacromial arch and the pressure on the surrounding soft tissues result in damage to the rotator cuff tendons; this also leads to an inflammatory reaction characteristic of impingement syndrome. There is an area of relative avascularity on the supraspinatus muscle tendon near its insertion on the tubercul major of the humerus (Figure 3.4).[23,31,136] A similar region is present on the upper part of the tendon of the long head of biceps brachii. This region is called the *critical zone of the rotator cuff.* Rathburn and McNab[136] suggest that the anatomical position of the rotator cuff tendons plays an important role in the development of the critical zone because it exposes the tendons to constant pressure from the humeral head, squeezing the blood out of the surrounding blood vessels even when the arm is stationary in a position of abduction or neutral rotation.

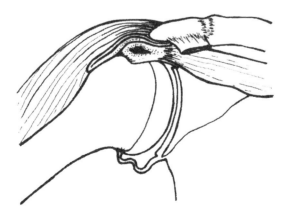

FIGURE 3.4 Degenerative changes in the "critical zone" area of the supraspinatus muscle tendon.

Investigations carried out on numerous anatomical specimens of the scapula have shown that the development of impingement syndrome is both correlated and enhanced by an acromion with a lesser inclination and an acromion with a slightly pushed out anterior part or lower area, or by the presence of anterior acromial spurs and inferior acromioclavicular osteophytes.[13,61] Results obtained by Neer[114,115] indicate that in 95% of the patients suffering from impingement syndrome, damage to the rotator cuff occurs as a consequence of a similarly or identically developed acromion. In some cases, impingement syndrome can develop as a consequence of the existence of the os acromiale, a special part of the acromion believed to be an ununited ossification center of that acromion. Contrary to the opinion expressed by Neer, Post et al.[131,132] believe that the cause of the impingement syndrome is not necessarily and exclusively related to anatomical deviations. The results of their investigations indicate that the development of the impingement syndrome can also be initiated by weak external rotators of the shoulder joint infraspinatus and teres minor muscles. An existing weakness of the external rotators of the shoulder joint results in inadequate fixation of the humeral head in the glenoid fossa in the superior direction. This significantly increases the pressure of the humeral head on the tendon blood vessels of the shoulder joint's rotator cuff, which leads to an increasingly greater degeneration of the so-called critical zone accompanied by progressive development of the impingement syndrome.

The development and treatment of impingement syndrome in athletes was described by Jobe et al.[84–87] and Tibone et al.[163] Their results indicate that acute trauma to the shoulder and repeated overhead arm movements, characteristically performed in numerous sports and intensive work, can increase the speed of progression of the impingement syndrome.[5,46,90] Ellenbecker and Derscheid[44] note that concomitant, but unsynchronized, actions of the rotator muscles cause abnormal movements of the upper extremity allowing the humeral head to clash against the coracoacromial arch. Jobe and Bradley[85] and Scheib[145] opine that impingement syndrome develops as a result of instability of the shoulder joint. According to their opinion, the pathogenetic course of injury to the rotator cuff comprises instability of the shoulder joint, subluxation, impingement, and destruction of the rotator cuff. Jobe and Bradley[85] term the preceding course of events the *shoulder instability complex.* Pieper et al.[127,128] describe *secondary impingement* of the rotator cuff, encountered typically in athletes who participate in "overhead" sports, as caused by the instability of the shoulder joint.[54] Impingement of the rotator cuff can be caused by chronic anterior instability of the shoulder joint. This particular injury is frequently found in athletes who repeatedly engage in overhead arm motions in abduction/external rotation of the arm, i.e., such sports as volleyball, European handball, tennis, badminton, and swimming.[6,7,18,89,105,108,130,164,178]

Shoulder dysfunction in overhead athletes may be caused by shoulder instability. However, a possible instability in the shoulder is often silent and difficult to demonstrate by ordinary tests and has therefore been termed by some investigators "functional instability." This functional instability in the shoulder may lead to a vicious cycle involving microtrauma and attenuation of the capsular complex, and may eventually lead to shoulder impingement syndrome and to shoulder pain.[11] Patients who do not respond to conservative treatment such as muscular stabilization are treated surgically.

In brief, we can conclude that there are two principal theories regarding the development of impingement syndrome: the anatomic theory and the dynamic theory. Proponents of the anatomic theory believe that impingement syndrome is caused principally by decreased vascularization of some of the tendons of the rotator cuff, whereas proponents of the dynamic theory emphasize the relative weakness of those muscles. At the same time it is quite clear that some causative factors can synergistically combine to produce impingement syndrome of the shoulder joint. These include the os acromiale, acute trauma to the shoulder, and excessive repeated strain placed on the upper extremity during some athletic activities. A possible mechanism leading to the development of impingement syndrome of the shoulder is stated as follows: Clash of the humeral head against the acromion causes injury to the surrounding soft tissue, the tendon of the supraspinatus muscle, the long head of the biceps brachii muscle, and the subacromial bursa, which results in inflammatory processes and scarred healing. After a certain period of time, the scar degenerates, frequently resulting in partial or total rupture of the tendon. Depending on the degree of change in the tendons of the shoulder joint rotator cuff, various functions of the rotator cuff are affected.[1] The humeral head is not firmly fixed in the glenoid fossa during arm motions and has a tendency to translate in the superior direction. Such an unstable humeral head causes pain, decreases the range of movements possible in the shoulder joint, causes instability of the shoulder joint, and disrupts the normal flow of the synovial liquid that nourishes the joint cartilage; all this leads to further progression of the injury. The final stages of impingement syndrome are characterized by destruction of the rotator cuff, primarily the supraspinatus muscle and the long head of the biceps brachii muscle (and, in some cases, morphological changes of the humeral head, also known as arthropathy, caused by injury to the rotators of the shoulder joint).

Vascular endothelial growth factor expression in the subacromial bursa is increased in patients with impingement syndrome[179] and the differential regulation of the two forms of interleukin-1β mRNA may play an important role in shoulder pain in rotator cuff disease, regulating interleukin-1β-induced subacromial synovitis.[56]

The synovial osteochondromatosis of the shoulder joint presenting as chronic impingement syndrome in a 44-year-old tennis player was reported by Baums et al.,[10] and Demirhan et al.[42] reported a case of synovial chondromatosis of the subcoracoid bursa, which resulted in impingement symptoms.

B. CLINICAL PICTURE AND DIAGNOSTICS

Impingement syndrome is an injury that is characterized by a chronic course. Patients frequently correlate the symptoms of the injury with some acute trauma to the shoulder, but detailed anamnesis usually results in the patient remembering earlier painful sensations in the shoulder joint.

The dominant symptoms of impingement syndrome are tenderness in the shoulder area, crepitations, decreased range of movements in the shoulder joint,[166,176] and varying loss of strength in the surrounding musculature. The pain may be categorized in intensity depending on arm activities: pain caused while performing strenuous activities of the arm, pain caused by moderate or strong activities, and pain when the arm is stationary.[53,70,71]

The condition may appear at any age. Athletes and people with physically difficult occupations are at a greater risk to develop these injuries. Neer[114] has developed an elaborate hypothesis on the progression of the impingement syndrome in three stages based on pathoanatomical examinations (Table 3.3). In Stage 1, edema and inflammation occur. In the beginning of this stage, excessive bowing of the shoulder rotator tendon is noticeable; there is microscopic or partial damage to some of the tendon fibers. Bleeding is sometimes present but usually not to a large degree. The age of the patients in this group is usually less than 25 years. The main characteristic of Stage 1 is good prognosis in the sense of reversibility of pathological changes.

Stage 2 lesions are characterized by fibrosis and tendinitis and clearly indicate chronicity. Repetitive episodes of mechanical inflammation of the shoulder rotator tendon, edema, cellular infiltration, and vascular invasion of the tendon are followed by connective tissue reparation and fibrosis of different stages. Nirschl[120] refers to this stage as *angiofibroblastic hyperplasia of the tendons*. The subacromial bursa is also thickened and fibrous. Lesions of this stage are characteristically found in patients between 25 and 40 years of age. The shoulder functions satisfactorily during "easy" activities. However, when performing stronger repetitive movements in an overhead position, such as in throwing sports, the rotator cuff becomes insufficient.

Tears in the tendons of the rotator cuff, tears in the tendon of the long head of the biceps brachii muscle, and changes in the bone represent the main characteristics of Stage 3. Progression of the impingement syndrome is characterized by the appearance of complete, incomplete, or superficial/roughened areas located on the surface of the tendon, which cause bursitis and tears in the tendons of the rotator cuff of the shoulder.[117] Measured at their largest diameter, tears in the tendons of the rotator cuff can be small (less than 1 cm in diameter), average (from 1 to 3 cm in diameter),

TABLE 3.3
Classification of Impingement Syndrome
According to Neer[133]

Stage 1: Edema and Hemorrhage

Typical age	<25
Differential diagnosis	Subluxation
	A/C arthritis
Clinical course	Reversible
Treatment	Conservative

Stage 2: Fibrosis and Tendinitis

Typical age	25–40
Differential diagnosis	Frozen shoulder
	Calcium deposits
Clinical course	Recurrent pain with activity
Treatment	Consider bursectomy
	C/A ligament division

Stage 3: Bone Spurs and Tendon Rupture

Typical age	>40
Differential diagnosis	Cervical radiculitis
	neoplasm
Clinical course	Progressive disability
Treatment	Anterior acromioplasty
	Rotator cuff repair

large (from 3 to 5 cm in diameter), and massive (larger than 5 cm in diameter). Stage 3 is usually found in patients older than 40 years of age. Surgical treatment is the only form of therapy for this stage of impingement syndrome.

Lesions in the tendon of the long head of the biceps brachii muscle appear on average in a 1:7 ratio in comparison to lesions in the tendons of the rotator cuff. Lesions in the tendon of the biceps brachii muscle can, however, sometimes represent the first sign of a developing impingement syndrome.[51] Pathological changes in bone tissue, i.e., the collapse of the humeral head, represent the final stage of impingement syndrome. They develop typically only after the presence of long-term destruction of the shoulder rotator tendons and a complete insufficiency of the rotator net. This stage is followed by pathological changes in the whole shoulder joint-cuff tear arthropathy.[84,112,115] Partial or complete destruction of the tendons of the shoulder rotators is sometimes accompanied by nutritive changes in the joint cartilage, which is characterized by development of hydroxyapatites, active collagenasis, and neutral proteases. This clinical entity is known as *Milwaukee shoulder*.[9]

Clinical signs characteristic of impingement syndrome include general tenderness in the anterior part of the acromion or in the humeral greater tubercule area, a painful arch during abduction of the upper extremity more than 90°, and a positive impingement sign and hypotrophy of the rotator cuff muscles. The impingement test and the presence of the impingement sign are used in differential diagnosis to ascertain if the painful symptoms are the result of impingement of the shoulder joint and not the result of other changes in the shoulder (Figure 3.5 and Figure 3.6).

A positive impingement sign, according to Neer, is the presence of tenderness in the shoulder area when the physician performs anteflexion on the patient's injured shoulder simultaneously with internal rotation of the upper arm. According to Hawkins and Kennedy,[65] a positive impingement sign consists of pain in the shoulder area when the physician performs a strong internal rotation of the patient's arm in a 90° anteflexion position. The impingement test (Figure 3.6) is used in

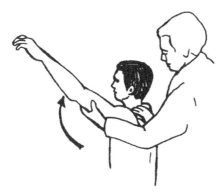

FIGURE 3.5 Impingement sign performance.

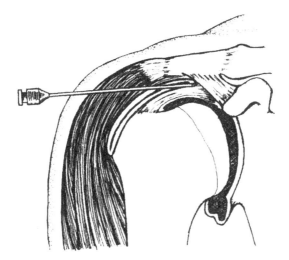

FIGURE 3.6 Impingement test.

clinical diagnostics when making differential diagnoses to rule out the possibility of the painful sensations resulting from anterior subluxation of the shoulder joint, acromioclavicular arthritis, cervical radiculitis, "frozen shoulder," traumatic bursitis, calcifying tendinitis, or neoplasmas. A diagnosis of impingement syndrome is confirmed, if after injection of 10 cc of 1.0% xylocain below the anterior edge of the acromion the patient is able to perform the impingement sign without any pain. A study by Calis et al.[28] found that the most sensitive clinical diagnostic test was Hawkins test. MacDonald et al.[101] conclude that the Neer and Hawkins impingement signs are sensitive for appearances suggestive of subacromial bursitis and rotator cuff partial or complete tearing with a high negative predictive value. However, the tests lack specificity in comparison with arthroscopic findings. Buchberger[25] introduces a new physical examination procedure for the differentiation of acromioclavicular joint lesions and subacromial impingement by applying downward pressure over the lateral one third of the clavicle while passively inducing slight adduction, external rotation, and forced forward flexion to the humerus with the patient in the seated position.

Jobe et al.[84,85] have described a test for the supraspinatus muscle used in differentiating tendon injuries between the supraspinatus muscle and other rotators of the shoulder joint. The test is performed by having the patient stand with the arms held in a position of 90° abduction and horizontal abduction of 30° with full internal rotation. The physician holds the patient's upper arms and resists the patient's efforts to lift the arms in an upward direction (Figure 3.7). If weakness or pain in the shoulder joint appears, the supraspinatus muscle test is considered positive, and the

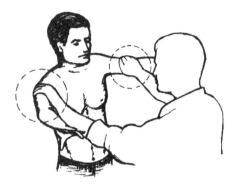

FIGURE 3.7 Supraspinatus test.

probable localization of the injury to the rotator cuff is the supraspinatus muscle tendon. During performance of this maneuver, the infraspinatus, subscapularis, and teres minor muscles are completely inactive, which can be verified by determining the electrical activity in them.

Lyons and Tomlinson[100] have studied the reported clinical assessment of the presence and extent of a rotator cuff tear in 42 patients in a special shoulder clinic. The preoperative diagnosis was compared with the findings at operation. The clinical tests had a sensitivity of 91% and a specificity of 75%. It is important to exploit clinical examination before resorting to costly and sometimes harmful special investigations.

Radiographic analysis of the shoulder joint includes transaxillar lateral and anteroposterior radiographs during both the internal and external rotation of the humerus. Although not a particularly precise diagnostic method, radiographic analysis sometimes enables the examining physician to confirm the presence of calcium deposits in the tendons of the rotator cuff, sclerotic changes in the greater tubercule of the humerus, a decrease of the subacromial area to less than 6 mm, eburnation of the anterior part of the acromion (Figure 3.8), and degenerative changes in the acromioclavicular joint.[39,48] On the modified Stryker view it is possible to see a bony exostosis of the posterior inferior glenoid, so-called thrower's exostosis, or Bennett's lesion of the shoulder. The lesion is characteristic in professional baseball players. In the past, fluoroscopy, shoulder arthrography, subacromial bursography, and bursotomography were fundamental diagnostic

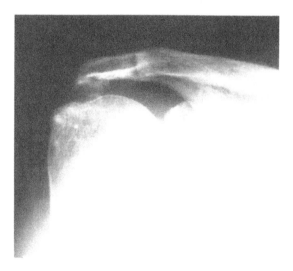

FIGURE 3.8 Roentgenogram demonstrating subacromial sclerosis, acromial spurs, and cystic changes of the greater tuberosity of the humerus as a result of the impingement process.

imaging modalities in shoulder impingement syndrome.[39] Roentgenographic assessment of acromial morphologic condition in shoulder impingement syndrome has been presented by many authors.[75,91,123,126,141] According to Kitay et al.[91] the supraspinatus and caudal tilt views correlate significantly with distinct intraoperative measurements of acromial spur size. Hyvonen et al.[75] consider that the supraspinatus outlet view in the diagnosis of Stages 2 and 3 impingement syndrome can be used as an adjunctive to other diagnostic modalities. Petje et al.[126] conclude that anteroposterior view radiographs with an individual caudally tilted beam, depending on the acromion slope, can show the whole spur and/or size of the osteophyte on the anterior margin of the acromion. In our department on the basis of clinical diagnosis we perform anteroposterior, axillary, 30° caudal tilt, and supraspinatus outlet views roentgenograms.

Contrasting arthrography is sometimes employed to analyze the continuity of the tendons as well as to verify diagnoses of complete tendon rupture.[96] Subacromial bursography and bursotomography are auxiliary methods used to confirm injury to the joint bursae. Cone et al.[39] consider these methods, as well as fluoroscopy and arthrography, to be useful diagnostic methods for detecting the beginning stages of impingement syndrome, and Cicak et al.[41] described ultrasound guidance of needle placement for shoulder arthrography. Computerized tomography (CT) is used when analyzing bone pathology of the humeral head and the glenohumeral joint. Advanced arthrography of the shoulder with CT and MR imaging is also recommended.[134]

Numerous authors[22,38,62,72,85,92,93,104,110,112,137,160] have recently expressed their belief that ultrasound examination of the rotator cuff is an unavoidable diagnostic method when attempting to determine the presence of partial or total tendon ruptures (Figure 3.9 and Figure 3.10) and inflammatory changes in the tendon and tendon sheath. Hedtmann and Fett[72] consider that the limits of ultrasonography lie in estimation of tear size in global tears, because retraction of tendon stumps under acromion cannot be visualized, and in evaluation of the status of rotator cuff muscles, because whereas volumetric information about atrophy can be gained by ultrasonography, differentiation between simple atrophy and fatty degeneration is not possible. Martin-Hervas et al.[104] compared the accuracy of ultrasonography and MR imaging in the diagnosis of rotator cuff injuries using arthroscopy or open surgery findings. The diagnosis of full-thickness rotator cuff tear was highly specific in both imaging techniques, but was not as sensitive in ultrasonography (57.7%) as on MR (80.8%). Read and Perko[137] report that ultrasonography is a sensitive and accurate method of identifying patients with full-thickness tears of the rotator cuff, extracapsular biceps tendon pathology, or both. According to Swen et al.[160] ultrasonography and MR imaging are equally valuable in the assessment of full-thickness rotator cuff tears.

Although recognized as useful in detecting soft-tissue inflammation and infection, technetium-99m human immunoglobulin has been studied in evaluating regional inflammatory shoulder conditions,[34] either subacromial impingement or adhesive capsulitis. Gratz et al.[59] recommend arthroscintigraphy as a sensitive technique for detection of rotator cuff ruptures.

Wilbourn[177] recommends the use of electromyographic analysis of the muscles of the rotator cuff with the aim of ruling out the possibility of radiculopathy when diagnosing impingement syndrome. Electromyographic analysis performed by Reddy et al.[138] showed that in the impingement group, the supraspinatus and teres minor revealed a diminution of muscle function in comparison with shoulders in the normal group. This study demonstrates that muscle activity in subjects with impingement is most notably decreased in the first arc of motion. Hancock and Hawkins[64] applied electromyographic analysis in the throwing shoulder.

Neviaser,[118] on the other hand, indicates the exceptional contribution of arthroscopy to both the diagnostics and the treatment of impingement syndrome. Arthroscopy enables a direct view of the current state of the internal structures of the shoulder joint, tendons, bursae, cartilage, and tendon and synovial sheaths; at the same time it offers the possibility of therapeutic intervention.[118,121,149]

MR imaging is a very useful diagnostic method, which enables the detection of even very small lesions in the soft tissues and the neurovascular structures.[3,16,40,45,57,58,73,81,102,165,168] Complete and partial tears of the rotator cuff, as well as factors contributing to impingement, can be detected and

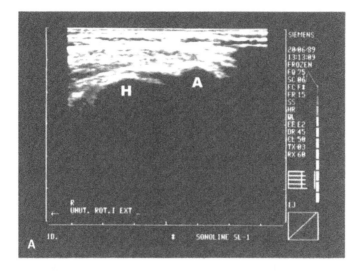

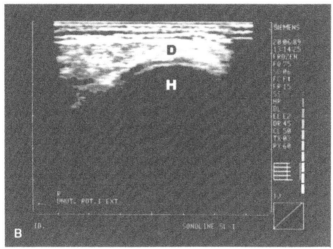

FIGURE 3.9 Longitudinal (A) and transversal (B) sonogram show a complete tear of the rotator cuff. The cuff lacks apposition of the deltoid muscle (D) to the humeral head (H). A = acromion.

characterized with MR imaging.[45] Graichen et al.[57,58] describe a technique for determining the spatial relationship between the rotator cuff and the subacromial space in arm abduction using MR imaging and three-dimensional image processing. MacGillivray et al.[102] performed three-dimensional MR imaging or CT on 132 symptomatic shoulders to more completely describe acromion morphology and its relationship to impingement syndrome. Age distribution from the second to eighth decade demonstrated a consistent and gradual transition from a flat acromion in the younger decades to a more hooked acromion in the older decades that was significant in both the midsagittal and lateral sagittal planes. MR imaging provides a comprehensive evaluation of a wide spectrum of both intra-articular and extra-articular pathology of the shoulder. MR imaging enables the detection or exclusion of degenerative and post-traumatic diseases of the shoulder with reasonable accuracy. MR arthrography is useful in the visualization of subtle anatomic details and further improves the differentiation.[94,133,139,161] Bergman and Fredericson[12] investigated how long injected fluid from an impingement test remains in the bursa or adjacent soft tissue after an injection. By 3 days after the injection, the soft tissue fluid had returned to preinjection levels and no patients showed rotator cuff signal abnormalities related to the impingement test injection.

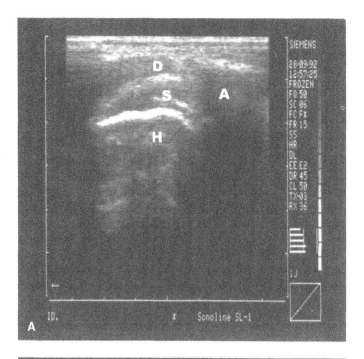

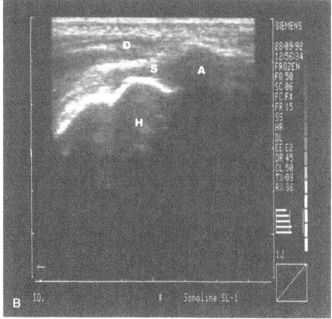

FIGURE 3.10 (A) Longitudinal sonogram shows focal thinning of the supraspinatus tendon (S). (B) Normal supraspinatus tendon; H = humeral head; A = acromion; D = deltoid muscle.

According to Godefroy et al.[55] the choice of imaging modality depends on the information expected from each technique. In the case of instability, plain films demonstrate bone abnormalities such as Hill Sachs and/or Bankart lesions. Arthro-CT or arthro-MR imaging need not be performed in all cases but can provide additional information about the intra-articular structures and the glenoid labrum. The rotator cuff is initially evaluated by plain films, which demonstrate anatomical conditions resulting in impingement syndrome as well as indirect signs of tendinopathy. Direct visualization of tendons may be achieved by ultrasonography, arthro-CT, and arthro-MR imaging. Ultrasonography is a dynamic, non-invasive, and accurate technique for evaluation of rotator cuff tear but is very operator dependent. Arthro-CT is more reproducible and reveals accurately partial tear as well as anterior tears involving biceps or subscapularis tendons. MR imaging is very useful in visualizing the rotator cuff and adjacent anatomical structures.

C. TREATMENT

Treatment for impingement syndrome, in the most general terms, can be divided into non-operative and operative treatment. Non-operative treatment is indicated for the first stage of the disease. Lasting at least several months, non-operative treatment is also indicated for patients suffering from Stage 2 of the disease, whereas surgical treatment is indicated only when, and if, conservative treatment fails to produce any significant results for patients with Stage 2 disease. Patients suffering from Stage 3 of the disease must always be treated surgically.

Thus, non-operative treatment is recommended for patients suffering from Stage 1 and 2 impingement syndrome. Treatment during the acute, painful stage of the injury consists of rest, physical therapy, electrotherapy, cryotherapy, and application of oral nonsteroidal anti-inflammatory drugs.[48,62,65,67,106,111,140] Local application of corticosteroids is also described as part of non-operative treatment for impingement syndrome. The corticosteroids are applied onto the inflamed area and not directly on the tissue. The principal effects of corticosteroid therapy include reduction of the edema and the inflammatory reaction. However, repeatedly applying corticosteroids into the same area, carries a certain risk; thus, their use and application must be tempered with necessary prudence.[129] Friction massage, stretching exercises (Figure 3.11 through Figure 3.13), and strengthening exercises for the rotator musculature of the shoulder joint (Figure 3.14 through Figure 3.16) are recommended, both as prevention and as part of treatment, for patients who are not suffering from the acute stage of impingement syndrome.[8,24,26,29,44,79,85,135]

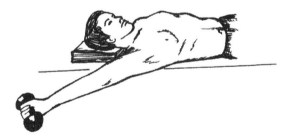

FIGURE 3.11 Rotator cuff extension. The patient lies on his back with the shoulder in a position of 135° and the elbow in a position of 45°. The weight passively stretches the rotator cuff in the direction of the external rotation.

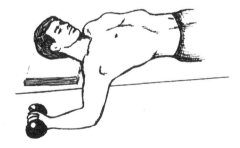

FIGURE 3.12 Rotator cuff extension. The patient lies on his back with his shoulder and elbow in a position of 90°. The weight passively stretches the rotator cuff in the direction of the external rotation.

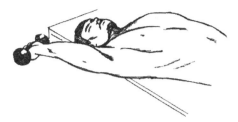

FIGURE 3.13 Rotator cuff extension. The patient lies on his back with his shoulder in a position of 170° and his elbow at 45°. The weight passively stretches the rotator cuff in the direction of the external rotation.

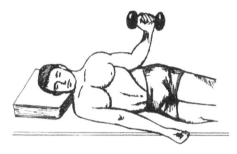

FIGURE 3.14 Strengthening of the infraspinatus and teres minor muscle. The patient lies on one side with his elbow on his thorax in a position of 90°. The weight is slowly lifted in the external rotation direction and slowly lowered in the internal rotation direction.

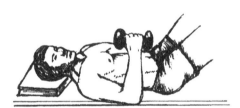

FIGURE 3.15 Strengthening of the subscapularis muscle. The patient lies on his back, with his elbow along his thorax in a position of 90°. The weight is lowered in an external rotation direction and then lifted in the internal rotation direction.

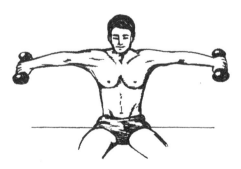

FIGURE 3.16 Strengthening of the supraspinatus muscle. The patient sits erect, with his shoulder in 90° abduction, 30° horizontal abduction, and total interior rotation. The weight is slowly lowered in a 45° arch and then lifted to the starting position.

Extracorporeal shock wave therapy is a new therapeutic procedure for chronically painful tendinitis of the rotator cuff.[148] Treatment at high dose or low dose could be effective if the total cumulative amount of applied energy is similar.[148]

Operative treatment is indicated for patients suffering from Stage 3 of the disease.[14,15,35,36,49,66,116,169] Neer[113-115] describes an operative technique called *anterior acromioplasty*. The main principle of the procedure consists of remodeling excessively protuburant, large, and downward-slanting acromions. In addition, the tendons of the shoulder rotators, the tendon of the long head of the biceps brachii muscle, the subacromial bursa, and the acromioclavicular joint is also inspected during the operation. This is done because it is quite possible for two or more structures of the shoulder to be damaged or injured at the same time. Osteophytes on the acromioclavicular joint and calcificates on the coracoacromial ligament are always removed. Resection of either the acromioclavicular joint or the coracoacromial ligament is performed if it is judged that these structures represent the immediate cause for the development of impingement syndrome. An inflammatorily altered, fibrous subacromial bursa is always excised. Tenodesis is performed when damage to the long head of the biceps brachii muscle is evident. Acromioplasty is an effective procedure in the treatment of shoulder impingement syndrome, and the type of bone resection does not influence the clinical outcome.[20,78,159]

Anterior acromioplasty, subacromial decompression, shaving of incomplete ruptures in rotator cuff tendons, and refixation of the origins of the rotator muscles in cases of complete rupture are frequently performed arthroscopically.[69,95,118,121,124,142,146,149,154,155,157,174,175] Checroun et al.[32] consider that the outcome from arthroscopic subacromial decompression is similar to open decompression. Arthroscopic procedure allows earlier rehabilitation than open decompression because complete detachment of the deltoid is not performed. Regarding arthroscopic vs. open acromioplasty, Spangehl et al.[153] found that for pain and function both procedures led to significant improvement, but the open technique may be superior. Schroder et al.[147] report the results of 238 consecutive patients who underwent a total of 261 acromioplasties either in conventional open technique or arthroscopically. Compared to the open technique, the arthroscopic procedure had a statistically significant superior result concerning outcome, operating time, and hospital stay. Arthroscopic procedures performed by less-experienced surgeons had inferior results. Arthroscopic subacromial decompression with a holmium:YAG laser[21,76] has been performed, but it is recommended that further research be conducted to establish the safety and efficacy of the technique.

Technical falls are the most common cause for revision operation after subacromial arthroscopic decompression.[4,103] This demonstrates the demanding nature of this kind of operative procedure. When a revision procedure is necessary, individual strategies should be developed; the decision whether to perform arthroscopic or open revision is especially important.

All authors agree that anterior acromioplasty and revision of the surrounding tissue generally produce satisfying results, which are evident during the short time that the patient is monitored after the operation.[17,48,62,68,144,162,163] However, recidives of impingement syndrome after surgical treatment have been described in patients who have previously participated at the highest level in various sports.[68] The long-term success of anterior acromioplasty in athletes significantly depends on scrupulously following the postoperative rehabilitation program. For precisely this reason, Post and Cohen[132] recommend a combination of anterior acromioplasty and stretching and strengthening exercises for the rotator cuff of the shoulder joint. Ellenbecker and Derscheid[44] describe the importance of strengthening the complete musculature of the shoulder joint.

In cases of secondary impingement that has developed as a consequence of instability of the shoulder joint, the primary causative factor must be treated. According to Pieper et al.,[127,128] and numerous other authors,[47,80,87,171] surgical treatment is indicated for these cases. The treatment consists of anterior reconstruction of the capsule and/or the glenoid labrum, and in addition, if necessary, subacromial decompression and revision of the rotator cuff. Between October 1988 and April 1992, Pieper et al.[127,128] operated on 66 shoulders in 64 top athletes suffering from chronic anterior or multidirectional instability of the shoulder joint that had led to the development of impingement syndrome of the rotator cuff. In all cases, the athletes themselves were not aware of the instability. Conservative treatment failed to produce significant results. The success ratio for surgical treatment of the athletes was close to 90%.

II. BICIPITAL TENDINITIS

Bicipital tendinitis is a term used to define overuse of the long head of the biceps brachii muscle. The biceps brachii muscle belongs to the group of anterior, upper arm muscles and is characterized by having two heads — caput longum (long head) and caput breve (short head). The long head of the biceps originates from the supraglenoid tubercle of the scapula, passes over the top of the humeral head, and courses distally, passing through the intertubercular sulcus. The tendon is contained within an invaginated envelope of synovial membrane as it passes through the shoulder joint. The short head originates from the coracoid process of the scapula. The two heads unite approximately in the middle of the upper arm, in the region of the deltoid tuberosity (Figure 3.17). The biceps brachii muscle ends with two tendons, the stronger and shorter of which attaches to the radial tuberosity and, in effect, represents an extension of the caput longum. One tendon plate, the musculus bicipitis brachii aponeurosis, with fibers consisting of extensions from the short head of the biceps brachii, departs from the medial edge of the stronger tendon and proceeds medially into the forearm fascia, which it strengthens. The biceps brachii muscle is a two-joint muscle. The long head of the muscle moves the arm away from the body and rotates it inwardly, whereas the short head moves the arm toward the body. Synergistic deployment of both heads produces ante-flexion of the arm in the shoulder. In the elbow joint, the muscle acts as both a flexor and a strong supinator of the forearm. The biceps brachii muscle is innervated by the musculocutaneous nerve.

A. ETIOPATHOGENESIS

Bicipital tendinitis is a condition that may occur as an isolated entity, primary tendinitis, or, more frequently, may be seen in conjunction with significant pathology elsewhere in the shoulder, such as impingement syndrome and frontal instability of the shoulder (secondary tendinitis).[192,196,199,206] The long head of the biceps tendon can be affected at two district sites: inside the joint and inside the bicipital (intertubercular) groove.

In cases of primary tendinitis, the damage to the tendon is localized within the intertubercular groove, characterizing it as a tenosynovitis, an inflammatory process involving the tendon and its sheath. Besides external factors, such as direct trauma or overuse of the arm in an overhead position (smash in volleyball, serve in tennis, or pitch in baseball), development of primary tendinitis may also be due to abnormalities in the soft-tissue parts that surround the tendon (e.g., coracohumeral ligament) and to abnormalities in the intertubercular groove (e.g., in cases with abnormally shallow intertubercular grooves that lead to subluxation of the tendon).

The causes of bicipital tendinitis are definitely age related. Anomalies of the groove and repeated traumas are the most common causes in young individuals, whereas degenerative tendon changes predominate in the older population. Radiologic signs of groove degeneration correlated in 43.6% with biceps tendon disease on the sonogram.[202] Pfahler et al.[202] revealed statistically significant correlations between groove anatomy and long biceps tendon disease, which should be considered more when shoulder problems are evaluated. In a prospective study, 200 consecutive shoulders underwent arthroscopic subacromial decompression for impingement syndrome, Murthi et al.[198] concluded that the high incidence of chronic inflammation of the long head of the biceps in shoulders with benign-appearing intra-articular portions viewed arthroscopically is significant, and long head of the biceps disease should also be considered in patients with painful rotator cuff disease and arthritic shoulder conditions.

Primary bicipital tendinitis seems to be rare, but it has been reported in volleyball players, swimmers, water polo players, tennis players, baseball players, and golfers.[189,192,194,199,203]

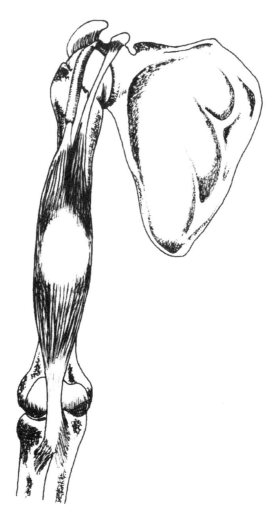

FIGURE 3.17 Biceps brachii muscle.

B. CLINICAL PICTURE AND DIAGNOSTICS

The most consistent complaint in primary bicipital tendinitis is severe pain in the area of the intertubercular groove. The pain increases gradually, usually without any trauma, and is associated with activity; it appears with frequent repetitions of the offending movement and disappears when resting. Typical clinical findings include pain caused by palpating the biceps tendon in its groove, as well as positive Speed's test and Yergason's sign.[194,199,203] In Speed's test, the examiner provides resistance to anteflexion of the arm during concomitant extension in the elbow and full supination of the forearm. In Yergason's test, resistance is provided against supination of the forearm during concomitant flexion of 90° in the elbow. A positive result is indicated when pain appears or intensifies in the intertubercular groove.

Bicipital tendinitis secondary to other pathological conditions in the shoulder appears to represent the more common form of this disorder.[191,207,210] Some authors state that it appears in more than 90% of the cases associated with impingement syndrome and anterior instability of the shoulder. When the condition occurs in association with other pathological conditions, it is termed secondary bicipital tendinitis.[192,203] For this reason, all diagnoses of bicipital tendinitis must be accompanied by a thorough and detailed clinical examination, including examinations for the stability of the shoulder and for impingement syndrome. According to Larson et al.[195] subacromial space injection, acromioclavicular joint injection, intra-articular injection, and injection of the biceps tendon are helpful in identifying such disorders as subacromial bursitis, acromioclavicular arthritis, injury to the glenohumeral joint, and bicipital tendinitis.

In addition to standard radiographic examinations of the shoulder, diagnosis of bicipital tendinitis requires special projections, e.g., the Fisk view, which enable the examiner to determine the size of the intertubercular groove.[185,200,203] This is important because short and narrow margins of the intertubercular groove are a well-known predisposition for developing recurrent dislocation of the tendon and consequent bicipital tendinitis.[180,203]

Arthrography of the shoulder is generally used for analysis of the tendon in the intertubercular groove. Recently, arthroscopy of the shoulder,[184,190,203] for the same purpose, has also been frequently performed. An enlarged tendon with characteristic changes (vacuoles) on the tendon sheath indicates bicipital tendinitis. Ultrasonography of the affected shoulder has also been recently used as an aid in recognizing changes in the biceps tendon (Figure 3.18). This has the added advantage of enabling examination of the tendon during movement.[187,197] Middleton et al.[197] found that tendinitis is characterized by heterogeneously structured tendon, edema of the tendon, and an enlargement of the tendon sheath.

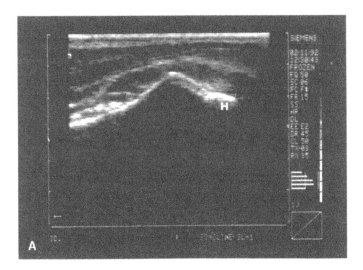

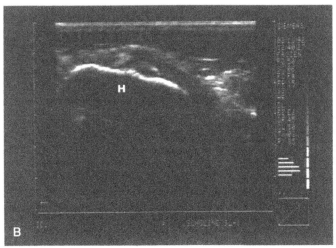

FIGURE 3.18 Longitudinal (A) and transversal (B) sonograms of the long head of the biceps muscle demonstrating tendonitis in a world champion kayak rider. H = humeral head.

C. Treatment

Non-operative treatment of primary bicipital tendinitis entails avoiding offending movements (modified rest), applying nonsteroidal anti-inflammatory medications,[182,183,209] and performing moderate stretching exercises. Deleterious effects of peribursal or intra-articular steroid infiltration appear minimal; but injections into the tendon or frequent, repetitive injections are contraindicated.[205] Good results are obtained when using a programmed therapy consisting of applying heat to the injured shoulder and performing stretching exercises for the shoulder (in abduction, adduction, and internal and external rotation). After the stretching exercises, the tender area is massaged with ice. In cases of secondary tendinitis, therapy for the primary disorder must also be carried out.[192,202,203]

Surgical treatment is indicated when the symptoms, despite completing nonsurgical therapy, persist for longer than 6 months. A number of surgical procedures are recommended in the medical literature.[208] The best results are obtained by performing tenodesis of the long head of the biceps.[181,186,188,204]

Post and Benca[203] describe 17 patients with primary bicipital tendinitis; 13 patients had tenodesis and 4 patients had transfer of the long head of the biceps to the origin of the conjoined tendon. Overall, excellent and good results were noted in 94% of both groups of patients when the long head of the biceps was tenodesed or transferred. Kumar and Satku[194] postulate on the basis of one case (treatment of a 40-year-old man with tenodesis of the long head of the biceps brachii in the bicipital groove, Hitchcock's operation) that resection of the stabilizing, intra-articular segment of the long head of the biceps in the Hitchcock's procedure allowed the short head to draw the humeral head proximally, resulting in the decrease in the acromiohumeral interval and recurrence of impingement. Becker and Cofield[181] followed 51 patients (54 shoulders) for an average of 13 years (2 to 23 years) after surgical tenodesis of the long head of the biceps brachii for the treatment of chronic tendinitis. At an average of 6 months postoperatively, some benefit was evident in all but three shoulders. However, after a longer follow-up, a satisfactory result was achieved in only 50% of patients; i.e., tenodesis of the long head of the biceps tendon was not an effective treatment for tendinitis over the long term.

Arthroscopic evaluation greatly improves the diagnosis and treatment of biceps tendon and related shoulder pathology. Routine tenodesis has been replaced by a more individualized approach, taking into consideration physiologic age, activity level, expectations, and exact shoulder pathology present.[202] New repair techniques are under development, and preservation of the biceps-labral complex is now preferred when possible. With advances in arthroscopy, the orthopedist can tailor treatment exactly to the pathology, minimizing morbidity and maximizing a successful outcome.

III. SLAP LESIONS

Superior glenoidal labrum lesion was first described and named SLAP (*Superior Labrum from Anterior to Posterior*) by Snyder et al.[150] The lesion originates behind the biceps muscle tendon anchor and extends anteriorly to half of the glenoid. The initial description of a lesion involving superior labrum was reported by Andrews et al.[2] in 1985 in high-level throwing athletes.

A. Etiopathogenesis

The most common mechanism of SLAP lesions is a fall or direct blow to the shoulder.[151] The second mechanism is due to traction with a sudden pull on the arm. Also, repetitive impacts or repetitive biceps tension from either throwing or overhead sports motion can produce a SLAP lesion.[2,33,88] The arthroscopic appearance of SLAP was described and classified by Snyder[150] into four groups and one complex (Figure 3.19):

Type I: The superior labrum demonstrates fraying and degeneration. The attachment of the labrum to the glenoid is intact. The biceps anchor is intact.

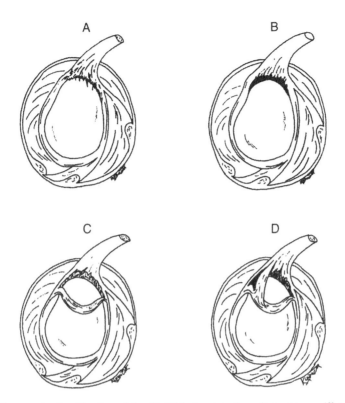

FIGURE 3.19 Arthroscopic classification of the SLAP lesion into four distinct types:[150] (A) type I; (B) type II; (C) type III; (D) type IV.

Type II: The superior labrum and biceps anchor are detached from the insertion on the superior glenoid, allowing the complex to arch away from the glenoid neck.

Type III: There is a bucket-handle tear of the meniscoid superior labrum. The remaining biceps tendon and labral rim attachment are intact. This is similar to a bucket-handle tear of the knee meniscus.

Type IV: There is a bucket-handle tear of the superior labrum with extension into the biceps anchor. The torn biceps tendon and the labral flap are displaced into the joint.

Complex: A combination of two or more SLAP types, most commonly a combination of types II and III or types II and IV.

B. Clinical Picture and Diagnostics

Patients complain of pain and mechanical symptoms such as catching, locking, popping, or grinding. There is no specific test to prove the SLAP lesion. MR imaging with gadolinium is recommended for imaging of delicate labrum pathology, but the most reliable diagnostic tool for SLAP lesions is arthroscopy.[30] Additionally, it is of utmost importance to thoroughly understand the arthroscopic anatomy and variations in the superior labral region.[33]

C. Treatment

Treatment of the SLAP lesion is based on correct identification and proper classification of the lesion. In type I the superior labrum is debrided back only to the stable rim. In type II the labrum and the anchor of the caput longum of the biceps muscle are fixated. In type III, with bucket-handle tear, the torn fragment is resected. In type IV lesions in younger patients, an attempt to reconstruct the biceps–labrum complex is recommended. In older patients, resection and tenodesis of the caput longum of the biceps muscle is performed. According to Imhoff et al.[77] long-term pain-free shoulder function in competitive athletes, throwers in particular, requires anatomical reconstruction of the originally unstable biceps, which is the cause of these lesions.

REFERENCES

Impingement Syndrome of the Shoulder and Slap Lesions

1. **Almekinders, L.C.** Impingement syndrome. *Clin. Sports Med.*, 2001; 20: 491–504.
2. **Andrews, J.R., Carson, W.G., and McLeod, W.D.** Glenoid labrum tears related to the long head of the biceps. *Am. J. Sports Med.*, 1985; 13: 337–341.
3. **Anzilotti, K.F., Jr., et al.** Rotator cuff strain: a post-traumatic mimicker of tendonitis on MRI. *Skel. Radiol.*, 1996; 25: 555–558.
4. **Arcand, M.A. et al.** Revision surgery after failed subacromial decompression. *Int. Orthop.*, 2000; 24: 61–64.
5. **Arroyo, J.S., Hershon, S.J., and Bigliani, L.U.** Special considerations in the athletic throwing shoulder. *Orthop. Clin. North Am.*, 1997; 28: 69–78.
6. **Bak, K.** Nontraumatic glenohumeral instability and coracoacromial impingement in swimmers. *Scand. J. Med. Sci. Sports*, 1996; 6: 132–144.
7. **Bak, K. and Faunl, P.** Clinical findings in competitive swimmers with shoulder pain. *Am. J. Sports Med.*, 1997; 25: 254–260.
8. **Bang, M.D. and Deyle, G.D.** Comparison of supervised exercise with and without manual physical therapy for patients with shoulder impingement syndrome. *J. Orthop. Sports Phys. Ther.*, 2000; 30: 126–137.
9. **Bateman, J.E.** Neurologic painful conditions affecting the shoulder. *Clin. Orthop.*, 1983; 173: 44–55.
10. **Baums, M.H. et al.** Synovial chondromatosis as an unusual cause for subacromial impingement in a tennis player. *Sportverletz. Sportschaden*, 2002; 16: 80–81.
11. **Belling Sorensen, A.K. and Jorgensen, U.** Secondary impingement in the shoulder: an improved terminology in impingement. *Scand. J. Med. Sci. Sports*, 2000; 10: 266–278.
12. **Bergman, A.G. and Fredericson, M.** Shoulder MRI after impingement test injection. *Skel. Radiol.*, 1998; 27: 365–368.
13. **Bigliani, L.U. et al.** The relationship of acromial architecture to rotator cuff disease. *Clin. Sports Med.*, 1991; 10: 823–838.
14. **Bigliani, L.U. et al.** Operative repair of massive rotator cuff tears: long-term results. *J. Shoulder Elbow Surg.*, 1992; 1: 120–130.
15. **Bigliani, L.U. et al.** Repair of rotator cuff tears in tennis players. *Am. J. Sports Med.*, 1992; 20: 112–117.
16. **Birtane, M., Calis, M., and Akgun, K.** The diagnostic value of magnetic resonance imaging in subacromial impingement syndrome. *Yonsei Med. J.*, 2001; 42: 418–424.
17. **Bjorkenheim, J.M. et al.** Subacromial impingement decompressed with anterior acromioplasty. *Clin. Orthop.*, 1990; 252: 150–155.
18. **Blevins, F.T.** Rotator cuff pathology in athletes. *Sports Med.*, 2001; 24: 205–220.
19. **Bollen, S.R.** Upper limb injuries in elite rock climbers. *J. R. Coll. Surg. Edinburgh*, 1990; 35(6 Suppl.): 18–20.
20. **Bolukbasi, S. et al.** Modified and classic acromioplasty for impingement of the shoulder. *Int. Orthop.*, 2002; 26: 10–12.
21. **Boult, M. et al.** Arthroscopic subacromial decompression with a holmium:YAG laser: review of the literature. *ANZ J. Surg.*, 2001; 71: 172–177.
22. **Brandt, T.D. et al.** Rotator cuff sonography: a reassessment. *Radiology*, 1989; 173: 323–327.
23. **Brooks, C.H., Rewell, W.J., and Heatley, F.W.** A quantitative histological study of the vascularity of the rotator cuff tendon. *J. Bone Joint Surg.*, 1992; 74B: 151–153.
24. **Brox, J.I. et al.** Arthroscopic surgery versus supervised exercises in patients with rotator cuff disease (stage II impingement syndrome): a prospective, randomized, controlled study in 125 patients with a 2^1/$_2$-year follow-up. *J. Shoulder Elbow Surg.*, 1999; 8: 102–111.

25. **Buchberger, D.J.** Introduction of a new physical examination procedure for the differentiation of acromioclavicular joint lesions and subacromial impingement. *J. Manipulative Physiol. Ther.,* 1999; 22: 316–321.

26. **Burke, W.S., Vangsness, C.T., and Powers, C.M.** Strengthening the supraspinatus: a clinical and biomechanical review. *Clin. Orthop.,* 2002; 402: 292–298.

27. **Butters, K.P. and Rockwood, C.A.** Office evaluation and management of the shoulder impingement syndrome. *Orthop. Clin. North Am.,* 1988; 194: 755–767.

28. **Calis, M. et al.** Diagnostic values of clinical diagnostic tests in subacromial impingement syndrome. *Ann. Rheum. Dis.,* 2000; 59: 44–47.

29. **Carson, W.G., Jr.** Rehabilitation of the throwing shoulder. *Clin. Sports Med.,* 1989; 8: 657–697.

30. **Chandani, V.P. et al.** Glenoid labral tears: prospective evaluation with MR imaging, MR arthrography and CT arthrography. *Am. J. Radiol.,* 1993; 161: 1229–1235.

31. **Chansky, H.A. and Iannotti, J.P.** The vascularity of the rotator cuff. *Clin. Sports Med.,* 1991; 10: 807–822.

32. **Checroun, A.J., Dennis, M.G., and Zuckerman, J.D.** Open versus arthroscopic decompression for subacromial impingement. A comprehensive review of the literature from the last 25 years. *Bull. Hosp. Joint Dis.,* 1998; 57: 145–151.

33. **Čičak, N., Klobucar, H., and Maric, D.** Overuse injury syndromes in the shoulder area. *Arh. Hig. Rada Toksikol.,* 2001; 52: 393–402.

34. **Clunie, G.P. et al.** Technetium-99m human immunoglobulin imaging in patients with subacromial impingement or adhesive capsulitis. *Clin. Rheumatol.,* 1998; 17: 419–421.

35. **Codeman, E.A.** Complete rupture of the supraspinatus tendon. Operative treatment with report of two successful cases. *Boston Med. Surg. J.,* 1911; 164: 708–710.

36. **Cofield, R.H.** Rotator cuff disease of the shoulder. *J. Bone Joint Surg.,* 1985; 67(A): 974–979.

37. **Cohen, R.B. and Williams, G.R., Jr.** Impingement syndrome and rotator cuff disease as repetitive motion disorders. *Clin. Orthop.,* 1998; 351: 95–101.

38. **Collins, R.A. et al.** Ultrasonography of the shoulder: static and dynamic imaging. *Orthop. Clin. North Am.,* 1987; 18: 351–361.

39. **Cone, R.O., III, Resnick, D., and Danzig, L.** Shoulder impingement syndrome. Radiographic evaluation. *Radiology,* 1984; 150: 29–33.

40. **Crues, J.V., III and Fareed, D.O.** Magnetic resonance imaging of shoulder impingement. *Top. Magn. Reson. Imaging,* 1991; 3: 39–49.

41. **Čičak, N., Matasovic, T., and Bajraktarevic, T.** Ultrasound guidance of needle placement for shoulder arthrography. *J. Ultrasound Med.,* 1992; 11: 135–137.

42. **Demirhan, M., Eralp, L., and Atalar, A.C.** Synovial chondromatosis of the subcoracoid bursa. *Int. Orthop.,* 1999; 23: 358–360.

43. **Edelson, G. and Teitz, C.** Internal impingement in the shoulder. *J. Shoulder Elbow Surg.,* 2000; 9: 308–315.

44. **Ellenbecker, T.S. and Derscheid, G.L.** Rehabilitation of overuse injuries of the shoulder. *Clin. Sports Med.,* 1989; 8: 583–604.

45. **Fritz, R.C.** Magnetic resonance imaging of sports-related injuries to the shoulder: impingement and rotator cuff. *Radiol. Clin. North Am.,* 2002; 40: 217–234.

46. **Frost, P. and Andersen, J.H.** Shoulder impingement syndrome in relation to shoulder intensive work. *Occup. Environ. Med.,* 1999; 56: 494–498.

47. **Fu, F.H., Harner, C.D., and Klein, A.H.** Shoulder impingement syndrome. A critical review. *Clin. Orthop.,* 1991; 269: 162–173.

48. **Fukuda, H.** Shoulder impingement and rotator cuff disease. *Curr. Orthop.,* 1990; 4: 225–232.

49. **Gerber, C.** Latissimus dorsi transfer for the treatment of irreparable tears of the rotator cuff. *Clin. Orthop.,* 1992; 275: 152–160.

50. **Gerber, C., Ternier, G., and Ganz, R.** The role of the coracoid process in the chronic impingement syndrome. *J. Bone Joint Surg.,* 1985; 67B: 703–708.

51. **Gerber, C. and Sebesta, A.** Impingement of the deep surface of the subscapularis tendon and the reflection pulley on the anterosuperior glenoid rim: a preliminary report. *J. Shoulder Elbow Surg.,* 2000; 9: 483–490.

52. **Giombini, A., Rossi, F., Pettrone, F.A., and Dragoni, S.** Posterosuperior glenoid rim impingement as a cause of shoulder pain in top level waterpolo players. *J. Sports Med. Phys. Fitness*, 1997; 37: 273–278.

53. **Glockner, S.M.** Shoulder pain: a diagnostic dilemma. *Am. Fam. Physician*, 1995; 15: 1677–1687.

54. **Glousman, R.E.** Instability versus impingement syndrome in the throwing athlete. *Orthop. Clin. North Am.*, 1993; 24: 89–99.

55. **Godefroy, D. et al.** Shoulder imaging: what is the best modality? *J. Radiol.*, 2001; 82: 317–332.

56. **Gotoh, M. et al.** Interleukin-1-induced subacromial synovitis and shoulder pain in rotator cuff diseases. *Rheumatology* (Oxford), 2001; 40: 995–1001.

57. **Graichen, H. et al.** Technique for determining the spatial relationship between the rotator cuff and the subacromial space in arm abduction using MRI and three-dimensional image processing. *Magn. Reson. Med.*, 1998; 40: 640–643.

58. **Graichen, H. et al.** Three-dimensional analysis of shoulder girdle and supraspinatus motion patterns in patients with impingement syndrome. *J. Orthop. Res.*, 2001; 19: 1192–1198.

59. **Gratz, S. et al.** Arthroscintigraphy in suspected rotator cuff rupture. *Nuklearmedezin,* 1998; 37: 272–278.

60. **Greenfield, B. et al.** Posture in patients with shoulder overuse injuries and healthy individuals. *J. Orthop. Sports Phys. Ther.*, 1995; 21: 287–295.

61. **Gumina, S. et al.** The morphometry of the coracoid process — its aetiologic role in subcoracoid impingement syndrome. *Int. Orthop.*, 1999; 23: 198–201.

62. **Habermeyer, P.** Sehnenrupturen in Schulterbereich. *Orthopade,* 1989; 18: 257–267.

63. **Halbrecht, J.L., Tirman, P., and Atkin, D.** Internal impingement of the shoulder: comparison of findings between the throwing and nonthrowing shoulders of college baseball players. *Arthroscopy,* 1999; 15: 253–258.

64. **Hancock, R.E. and Hawkins, R.J.** Applications of electromyography in the throwing shoulder. *Clin. Orthop.*, 1996; 330: 84–97.

65. **Hawkins, R.J. and Kennedy, J.C.** Impingement syndrome in athletes. *Am. J. Sports Med.,* 1980; 8: 151–157.

66. **Hawkins, R.J., Misamore, G.W., and Hobelka, P.E.** Surgery of full thickness rotator cuff tears. *J. Bone Joint Surg.,* 1985; 67A: 1349–1355.

67. **Hawkins, R.J. and Abrams, J.S.** Impingement syndrome in the absence of cuff tear (stages 1 and 2). *Orthop. Clin. North Am.,* 1987; 18: 373–383.

68. **Hawkins, R.J., Chris, T., Bokor, D. et al.** Failed anterior acromioplasty. A review of 51 cases. *Clin. Orthop.,* 1989; 243: 106–111.

69. **Hawkins, R.J. et al.** Arthroscopic subacromial decompression. *J. Shoulder Elbow Surg.,* 2001; 10: 225–230.

70. **Hayes, P.R. and Flatow, E.L.** Attrition sign in impingement syndrome. *Arthroscopy,* 2002; 18: E44

71. **Hebert, L.J. et al.** Scapular behavior in shoulder impingement syndrome. *Arch. Phys. Med. Rehabil.,* 2002; 83: 60–69.

72. **Hedtmann, A. and Fett, H.** Ultrasound diagnosis of the rotator cuff. *Orthopade,* 2002; 31: 236–246.

73. **Holder, J. et al.** Rotator cuff disease: assessment with MR arthrography versus standard MR imaging in 36 patients with arthroscopic confirmation. *Radiology,* 1992; 182: 431–436.

74. **Howell, S.M. et al.** Classification of the role of the supraspinatus muscle in shoulder function. *J. Bone Joint Surg.,* 1986; 68(A): 398–404.

75. **Hyvonen, P. et al.** Supraspinatus outlet view in the diagnosis of stages II and III impingement syndrome. *Acta Radiol.,* 2001; 42: 441–446.

76. **Imhoff, A. and Ledermann, T.** Arthroscopic subacromial decompression with and without the Holmium:YAG-laser. A prospective comparative study. *Arthroscopy,* 1995; 11: 549–556.

77. **Imhoff, A.B. et al.** Superior labrum pathology in the athlete. *Orthopade,* 2000; 29: 917–927.

78. **Ingvarsson, T., Hagglund, G., and Johnsson, R.** Anterior acromioplasty. A comparison of two techniques. *Int. Orthop.*, 1996; 20: 290–292.

79. **Itoi, E. and Tabata, S.** Conservative treatment of rotator cuff tears. *Clin. Orthop.,* 1992; 275: 165–173.

80. **Jerosch, J., Castro, W.H., and Sons, H.V.** Das sekundare Impingement-Syndrom beim Sportler. *Sportverletz Sportschaden,* 1990; 4: 180–185.

81. **Jerosch, J. and Asshewer, J.** Kernspintomographische Veranderungen der Supraspinatussehne beim Impingement-Syndrom des Sportlers. *Sportverletz Sportschaden,* 1991; 5: 12–16.
82. **Jobe, C.M.** Superior glenoid impingement. Current concepts. *Clin. Orthop.,* 1996; 330: 98–107.
83. **Jobe, C.M.** Superior glenoid impingement. *Orthop. Clin. North Am.,* 1997; 28: 137–143.
84. **Jobe, F.W. and Jobe, C.M.** Painful athletic injuries of the shoulder. *Clin. Orthop.,* 1983; 173: 117–124.
85. **Jobe, F.W. and Bradley, J.P.** Rotator cuff injuries in baseball. Prevention and rehabilitation. *Sports Med.,* 1988; 6: 378–387.
86. **Jobe, F.W.** Throwing injuries in the athlete, in *Orthopaedic Knowledge Update 3.* Philadelphia: American Academy of Orthopaedic Surgeons, 1990; 293–302.
87. **Jobe, W.J. et al.** The shoulder in sports, in *The Shoulder,* Rockwood, C.A. and Matsen, F.A., III, Eds. Philadelphia: W.B. Saunders, 1990; 961–990.
88. **Jobe, W.W. et al.** Anterior capsulolabral reconstruction of the shoulder in athletes in overhand sports. *Am. J. Sports Med.,* 1991; 19: 428–434.
89. **Jones, J.H.** Swimming overuse injuries. *Phys. Med. Rehabil. Clin. North Am.,* 1999; 10: 77–94.
90. **Kameyama, O. et al.** Medical check of competitive canoeists. *J. Orthop. Sci.,* 1999; 4: 243–249.
91. **Kitay, G.S. et al.** Roentgenographic assessment of acromial morphologic condition in rotator cuff impingement syndrome. *J. Shoulder Elbow Surg.,* 1995; 4: 441–448.
92. **Kruger-Franke, M. et al.** Stress-related clinical and ultrasound changes in shoulder joints of handball players. *Sportverletz. Sportschaden,* 8: 166–169.
93. **Kujat, R.** Impingement syndrome of the shoulder. *Unfallchirurg,* 1986; 89: 409–417.
94. **Lee, S.U. and Lang, P.** MR and MR arthrography to identify degenerative and posttraumatic diseases in the shoulder joint. *Eur. J. Radiol.,* 2000; 35: 126–135.
95. **Levy, H.J., Gardner, R.D., and Lemak, L.J.** Arthroscopic subacromial decompression in the treatment of full-thickness rotator cuff tears. *Arthroscopy,* 1991; 7: 8–13.
96. **Lindblom, K.** Arthrography and roentgenography in ruptures of the tendon of the shoulder joint. *Acta Radiol.,* 1939; 20: 548.
97. **Lindblom, K.** On pathogenesis of ruptures of the tendon aponeurosis of the shoulder joint. *Acta Radiol.,* 1939; 20: 563–577.
98. **Lindblom, K. and Palmer, I.** Ruptures of the tendon aponeurosis of the shoulder joint — the so-called supraspinatus ruptures. *Acta Chir. Scand.,* 1939; 82: 133–142.
99. **Lo, Y.P., Hsu, Y.C., and Chan, K.M.** Epidemiology of shoulder impingement in upper arm sports events. *Br. J. Sports Med.,* 1990; 24: 173–177.
100. **Lyons, A.R. and Tomlinson, J.E.** Clinical diagnosis of tears of the rotator cuff. *J. Bone Joint Surg.,* 1992; 74B: 414–415.
101. **MacDonald, P.B., Clark, P., and Sutherland, K.** An analysis of the diagnostic accuracy of the Hawkins and Neer subacromial impingement signs. *J. Shoulder Elbow Surg.,* 2000; 9: 299–301.
102. **MacGillivray, J.D. et al.** Multiplanar analysis of acromion morphology. *Am. J. Sports Med.,* 1998; 26: 836–840.
103. **Machner, A. et al.** Revisions after arthroscopic interventions in the subacromial space. *Z. Orthop. Ihre Grenzgeb.,* 2000; 138: 104–109.
104. **Martin-Hervas, C. et al.** Ultrasonographic and magnetic resonance images of rotator cuff lesions compared with arthroscopy or open surgery findings. *J. Shoulder Elbow Surg.,* 2001; 10: 410–415.
105. **McCann, P.D. and Bigliani, L.U.** Shoulder pain in tennis players. *Sports Med.,* 1994; 17: 53–64.
106. **McConville, O.R. and Iannotti, J.P.** Partial-thickness tears of the rotator cuff: evaluation and management. *J. Am. Acad. Orthop. Surg.,* 1999; 7: 32–43.
107. **McFarland, E.G. et al.** Internal impingement of the shoulder: a clinical and arthroscopic analysis. *J. Shoulder Elbow Surg.,* 1999; 8: 458–460.
108. **McMaster, W.C.** Swimming injuries. An overview. *Sports Med.,* 1996; 22: 332–336.
109. **Meister, K.** Internal impingement in the shoulder of the overhand athlete: pathophysiology, diagnosis, and treatment. *Am. J. Orthop.,* 2000; 29: 433–438.
110. **Middleton, W.D.** Status of rotator cuff sonography. *Radiology,* 1989; 173: 307–309.
111. **Morrison, D.S., Frogameni, A.D., and Woodworth, P.** Non-operative treatment of subacromial impingement. *J. Bone Joint Surg. Am. Vol.,* 1997; 79: 732–737.
112. **Nash, H.L.** Rotator cuff damage: reexamining the causes and treatments. *Phys. Sportsmed.,* 1988; 16: 128–135.

113. **Neer, C.S., II.** Anterior acromioplasty for the chronic impingement syndrome in the shoulder. *J. Bone Joint Surg.,* 1972; 54(A): 41.

114. **Neer, C.S.** Impingement lesions. *Clin. Orthop.,* 1983; 173: 70–77.

115. **Neer, C.S., Craig, E.V., and Fukuda, H.** Cuff tear arthropathy. *J. Bone Joint Surg.,* 1983; 65(A): 1232–1244.

116. **Neviaser, J.S.** Ruptures of the rotator cuff of shoulder. New concepts in the diagnosis and operative treatment of chronic ruptures. *Arch. Surg.,* 1971; 102: 483–485.

117. **Neviaser, R.J.** Tears of the rotator cuff. *Orthop. Clin. North Am.,* 1980; 11(2): 295–306.

118. **Neviaser, T.J.** Arthroscopy of the shoulder. *Orthop. Clin. North Am.,* 1987; 18: 361–373.

119. **Neviaser, T.J.** The role of the biceps tendon in the impingement syndrome. *Orthop. Clin. North Am.,* 1987; 18: 383–387.

120. **Nirshl, R.P.** Shoulder tendinitis, in *AAOS Symposium on Upper Extremity Injuries in Athletes,* Pettrone, F.A., Ed. St. Louis: C.V. Mosby, 1986; 322–337.

121. **Ogilvie-Harris, D.J. and D'Angelo, G.** Arthroscopic surgery of the shoulder. *Sports Med.,* 1990; 9: 120–128.

122. **Paley, K.J. et al.** Arthroscopic findings in the overhand throwing athlete: evidence for posterior internal impingement of the rotator cuff. *Arthroscopy,* 2000; 16: 35–40.

123. **Park, T.S. et al.** Roentgenographic assessment of acromial morphology using supraspinatus outlet radiographs. *Arthroscopy,* 2001; 17: 496–501.

124. **Patel, V.R. et al.** Arthroscopic subacromial decompression: results and factors affecting outcome. *J. Shoulder Elbow Surg.,* 1999; 8: 231–237.

125. **Paulson, M.M., Watnik, N.F., and Dines, D.M.** Coracoid impingement syndrome, rotator interval reconstruction, and biceps tenodesis in the overhead athlete. *Orthop. Clin. North Am.,* 2001; 32: 485–493.

126. **Petje, G. et al.** Radiographic evaluation of the acromion in impingement syndrome: comparison with arthroscopic findings in 147 shoulders. *Acta Orthop. Scand.,* 2000; 71: 609–612.

127. **Pieper, H.G., Quack, G., and Krahl, H.** Secondary impingement of the rotator cuff in overhead sports caused by instability of the shoulder joint. *Croat. Sports Med. J.,* 1992; 7: 24–28.

128. **Pieper, H.G., Quack, G., and Krahl, H.** Impingement of the rotator cuff in athletes caused by instability of the shoulder joint. *Knee Surg. Sports Traumatol. Arthrosc.,* 1993; 1: 97–99.

129. **Plafki, C. et al.** Local anesthetic injection with and without corticosteroids for subacromial impingement syndrome. *Int. Orthop.,* 2000; 24: 40–42.

130. **Plancher, K.D., Litchfield, R., and Hawkins, R.J.** Rehabilitation of the shoulder in tennis players. *Clin. Sports Med.,* 1995; 14: 111–137.

131. **Post, M., Silver, R., and Singh, M.** Rotator cuff tear: diagnosis and treatment. *Clin. Orthop.,* 1983; 173: 78–91.

132. **Post, M. and Cohen, J.** Impingement syndrome. Review of late stage 2 and early stage 3 lesions. *Clin. Orthop.,* 1986; 207: 126–132.

133. **Radke, S., Kenn, W., and Gohlke, F.** MRI of the shoulder. Degenerative changes and rotator cuff tears. *Orthopade,* 2001; 30: 484–491.

134. **Rafii, M. and Minkoff, J.** Advanced arthrography of the shoulder with CT and MR imaging. *Radiol. Clin. North. Am.,* 1998; 36: 609–633.

135. **Rahme, H. et al.** The subacromial impingement syndrome. A study of results of treatment with special emphasis on predictive factors and pain-generating mechanisms. *Scand. J. Rehabil. Med.,* 1998; 30: 253–262.

136. **Rathburn, J.B. and McNab, I.** The microvascular pattern of the rotator cuff. *J. Bone Joint Surg.,* 1970; 52: 540–553.

137. **Read, J.W. and Perko, M.** Shoulder ultrasound: diagnostic accuracy for impingement syndrome, rotator cuff tear, and biceps tendon pathology. *J. Shoulder Elbow Surg.,* 1998; 7: 264–271.

138. **Reddy, A.S. et al.** Electromyographic analysis of the deltoid and rotator cuff muscles in persons with subacromial impingement. *J. Shoulder Elbow Surg.,* 2000; 9: 519–552.

139. **Resnick, D.** Shoulder imaging. Perspective. *Magn. Reson. Imaging Clin. North Am.,* 1997; 5: 661–665.

140. **Ribarić, G., Pećina, M., and Bojanić, I.** Impingement sindrom ramena. *Basketball Med. Per.,* 1988; 3: 15–23.

141. **Rockwood, C.A. and Lyons, F.R.** Shoulder impingement syndrome: diagnosis, radiographic evaluation, and treatment with a modified Neer acromioplasty. *J. Bone Joint Surg. Am. Vol.*, 1994; 76: 473–474.

142. **Roye, R.P., Grana, W.A., and Yates, C.K.** Arthroscopic subacromial decompression: two- to seven-year follow-up. *Arthroscopy*, 1995; 11: 301–306.

143. **Saha, A.K.** Mechanism of shoulder movements and a plea of the recognition of "zero position" of glenohumeral joint. *Clin. Orthop.*, 1983; 173: 3–10.

144. **Sahlstrand, T.** Operations for impingement of the shoulder. Early results in 52 patients. *Acta Orthop. Scand.*, 1989; 60: 45–48.

145. **Scheib, J.S.** Diagnosis and rehabilitation of the shoulder impingement syndrome in the overhand and throwing athlete. *Rheum. Dis. Clin. North Am.*, 1990; 16: 971–988.

146. **Schiepers, P. et al.** The role of arthroscopy in subacromial pathology. Retrospective study of a series of arthroscopic acromioplasties. *Acta Orthop. Belg.*, 2000; 66: 438–448.

147. **Schroder, J. et al.** Open versus arthroscopic treatment of chronic rotator cuff impingement. *Arch. Orthop. Trauma Surg.*, 2001; 121: 241–244.

148. **Seil, R. et al.** Extracorporeal shockwave therapy in tendinosis calcarea of the rotator cuff: comparison of different treatment protocols. *Z. Orthop. Ihre Grenzgeb.*, 1999; 137: 310–315.

149. **Small, N.C.** Complications in arthroscopy: the knee and other joints. *Arthroscopy*, 1986; 2: 253–258.

150. **Snyder, S.J. et al.** SLAP lesions of the shoulder. *Arthroscopy*, 1990; 6: 274–279.

151. **Snyder, S.J., Banas, M.P., and Karzel, R.P.** An analysis of 140 injuries to the superior glenoid labrum. *J. Shoulder Elbow Surg.*, 1995; 4: 243–248.

152. **Sonnery-Cottet, B. et al.** Results of arthroscopic treatment of posterosuperior glenoid impingement in tennis players. *Am. J. Sports Med.*, 2002; 30: 227–232.

153. **Spangehl, M.J. et al.** Arthroscopic versus open acromioplasty: a prospective, randomized, blinded study. *J. Shoulder Elbow Surg.*, 2002; 11: 101–107.

154. **Speen, K.P., Lohnes, J., and Garrett, W.E., Jr.** Arthroscopic subacromial decompression: results in advanced impingement syndrome. *Arthroscopy*, 1991; 7: 291–296.

155. **Steinbeck, J. et al.** Outcome of endoscopic subacromial decompression operation in tendinitis and partial rupture of the rotator cuff. *Z. Orthop. Ihre Grenzgeb.*, 1998; 136: 8–12.

156. **Stelzle, F.D., Gaulrapp, H., and Pforringer, W.** Injuries and overuse syndromes due to rock climbing on artificial walls. *Sportveletz. Sportschaden*, 2000; 14: 128–133.

157. **Stephens, S.R. et al.** Arthroscopic acromioplasty: a 6- to 10-year follow-up. *Arthroscopy*, 1998; 14: 382–388.

158. **Struhl, S.** Anterior internal impingement: an arthroscopic observation. *Arthroscopy*, 2002; 18: 2–7.

159. **Suenaga, N. et al.** Coracoacromial arch decompression in rotator cuff surgery. *Int. Orthop.*, 2000; 212–216.

160. **Swen, W.A. et al.** Sonography and magnetic resonance imaging equivalent for the assessment of full-thickness rotator cuff tears. *Arthritis Rheum.*, 1999; 42: 2231–2238.

161. **Tasu, J.P. et al.** MR evaluation of factors predicting the development of rotator cuff tears. *J. Comput. Assist. Tomogr.*, 2001; 25: 159–163.

162. **Throling, J. et al.** Acromioplasty for impingement syndrome. *Acta Orthop. Scand.*, 1985; 56: 147–148.

163. **Tibone, J.E. et al.** Shoulder impingement syndrome in athletes treated by an anterior acromioplasty. *Clin. Orthop.*, 1985; 198: 134–140.

164. **Ticker, J.B., Fealy, S., and Fu, F.H.** Instability and impingement in the athlete's shoulder. *Sports Med.*, 1995; 19: 418–426.

165. **Traughber, P.D. and Goodwin, T.E.** Shoulder MRI: arthroscopic correlation with emphasis on partial tears. *J. Comput. Assist. Tomogr.*, 1992; 16: 129–133.

166. **Tyler, T.F., Nicholas, S.J., Roy, T., and Gleim, G.W.** Quantification of posterior capsule tightness and motion loss in patients with shoulder impingement. *Am. J. Sports Med.*, 2000; 28: 668–673.

167. **Uhthoff, H.K. and Sarkar, K.** Classification and definition of tendinopathies. *Clin. Sports Med.*, 1991; 10: 707–720.

168. **Vahlensieck, M. et al.** Shoulder MRI: the subacromial/subdeltoid bursa fat stripe in healthy and pathologic conditions. *Eur. J. Radiol.*, 1992; 14: 223–227.

169. **Van Holsbeeck, E. et al.** Shoulder impingement syndrome. *Acta Orthop. Belg.*, 1991; 57: 25–29.

170. **Valadie, A.L., III, et al.** Anatomy of provocative tests for impingement syndrome of the shoulder. *J. Shoulder Elbow Surg.*, 2000; 9: 36–46.

171. **Walch, G. et al.** Traitement chirurgical des epaules douloureuses par lesions de la coiffe et du long biceps en fonction des lesions. Reflexions sur le concept de Neer. *Rev. Rheum. Mal. Osteo-Articulaires*, 1991; 58: 247–257.

172. **Walch, G. et al.** Impingement of the deep surface of the supraspinatus tendon on the posterosuperior glenoid rim: an arthroscopic study. *J. Shoulder Elbow Surg.*, 1992; 1: 238–245.

173. **Wang, H.K. and Cochrane, T.A.** A descriptive epidemiological study of shoulder injury in top level English male volleyball players. *Int. J. Sports Med.*, 2001; 22: 159–163.

174. **Warner, J.J., Kann, S., and Maddox, L.M.** The "arthroscopic impingement test." *Arthroscopy*, 1994; 10: 224–230.

175. **Wasilewski, S.A. and Frankl, U.** Rotator cuff pathology. Arthroscopic assessment and treatment. *Clin. Orthop.*, 1991; 267: 65–70.

176. **Watson, M.** The refractory painful arc syndrome. *J. Bone Joint Surg.*, 1978; 60B: 544–546.

177. **Wilbourn, A.J.** Electrodiagnostic testing of neurologic injuries in athletes. *Clin. Sports Med.*, 1990; 9: 229–247.

178. **Yanai, T., Hay, J.G., and Miller, G.F.** Shoulder impingement in front-crawl swimming: I. A method to identify impingement. *Med. Sci. Sports Exerc.*, 2000; 32: 21–29.

179. **Ynagisawa, K. et al.** Vascular endothelial growth factor (VEGF) expression in the subacromial bursa is increased in patients with impingement syndrome. *J. Orthop. Res.*, 2001; 19: 448–455.

Bicipital Tendinitis

180. **Agins, H.J. et al.** Rupture of the distal insertion of the biceps brachii tendon. *Clin. Orthop.*, 1988; 234: 34–38.

181. **Becker, D.A. and Cofield, R.H.** Tenodesis of the long head of the biceps brachii for chronic bicipital tendinitis. *J. Bone Joint Surg.*, 1989; 71: 376–381.

182. **Bonafede, R.P. and Bennett, R.M.** Shoulder pain. Guidelines to diagnosis and management. *Postgrad. Med.*, 1987; 82: 185–189.

183. **Calabro, J.J., Londino, A.V., Jr., and Eyvazzadeh, C.** Sustained-release indomethacin in the management of the acute painful shoulder from bursitis and/or tendinitis. *Am. J. Med.*, 1985; 79: 32–38.

184. **Ciullo, J.V. and Stevens, G.G.** The prevention and treatment of injuries to the shoulder in swimming. *Sports Med.*, 1989; 7: 182–204.

185. **Cone, R.O. et al.** The bicipital groove: radiographic, anatomic and pathologic study. *Am. J. Roentgenol.*, 1983; 141: 781–788.

186. **Crenshaw, A.H. and Kilgore, W.E.** Surgical of bicipital tendosynovitis. *J. Bone Joint Surg.*, 1966; 48(A): 1496–1502.

187. **Čičak, N. and Buljan, M.** Diagnostic ultrasound of the shoulder, in *Diagnostic Ultrasound of the Locomotor System*, Matasovic, T., Ed. Zagreb: Skolska Knjiga, 1990; 155–179.

188. **Dines, D., Warren, R.F., and Inglis, A.E.** Surgical treatment of lesions of the long head of the biceps. *Clin. Orthop.*, 1982; 164: 165–169.

189. **Eakin, C.L. et al.** Biceps tendon disorders in athletes. *J. Am. Acad. Orthop. Surg.*, 1999; 7: 300–310.

190. **Gachter, A. and Seeling, W.** Schulterarthroskopie. *Arthroskopie*, 1988; 1: 162–170.

191. **Goldman, A.B.** Calcific tendinitis of the long head of the biceps brachii distal to the glenohumeral joint: plain film radiographic findings. *Am. J. Roentgenol.*, 1989; 153: 1011–1016.

192. **Jobe, F.W. and Brodley, J.P.** The diagnosis and nonoperative treatment of shoulder injuries in athletes. *Clin. Sports Med.*, 1989; 8: 419–438.

193. **Johnson, L.L.** The shoulder joint: an arthroscopist's perspective of anatomy and pathology. *Clin. Orthop.*, 1987; 223: 113–125.

194. **Kumar, V.P. and Satku, K.** The Hitchcock procedure. A cause for failure: a case report. *Clin. Orthop.*, 1992; 275: 161–164.

195. **Larson, H.M., O'Connor, F.G., and Nirschl, R.P.** Shoulder pain: the role of diagnostic injections. *Am. Fam. Physician*, 1996; 53: 1637–1647.

196. **Lupo, S.-C. and Di Biabo, T.M.** La tendinopatia del capo lungo del bicipite brachiale negli atleti participanti pallavolo. *Med. Sport*, 1987; 40: 131–140.

197. **Middleton, W.D., Reinus, W.R., and Totty, W.G.** Ultrasonographic evaluation of the rotator cuff and biceps tendon. *J. Bone Joint Surg.,* 1986; 68(A): 440–450.

198. **Murthi, A.M., Vosburg, C.L., and Neviaser, T.J.** The incidence of pathologic changes of the long head of the biceps tendon. *J. Shoulder Elbow Surg.,* 2000; 9: 382–385.

199. **Neviaser, R.J.** Lesions of the biceps and tendinitis of the shoulder. *Orthop. Clin. North Am.,* 1980; 11: 334–340.

200. **Neviaser, R.J.** Painful shoulder conditions. *Clin. Orthop.,* 1983; 173: 63–69.

201. **Patton, W.C. and McCluskey, G.M., III.** Biceps tendinitis and subluxation. *Clin. Sports Med.,* 2001; 20: 505–529.

202. **Pfahler, M., Branner, S., and Refior, H.J.** The role of bicipital groove in tendopathy of the long biceps tendon. *J. Shoulder Elbow Surg.,* 1999; 8: 419–424.

203. **Post, M. and Benca, P.** Primary tendinitis of the long head of the biceps. *Clin. Orthop.,* 1989; 246: 117–125.

204. **Slatis, P. and Aalto, K.** Medial dislocation of the tendon of the long head of the biceps brachii. *Acta Orthop. Scand.,* 1979; 50: 73–77.

205. **Smith, D.L. and Campbell, S.M.** Painful shoulder syndromes: diagnosis and management. *J. Gen. Intern. Med.,* 1992, 7: 328–339.

206. **Uhthoff, H.K. and Sarkar, K.** Classification and definition of tendinopathies. *Clin. Sports Med.,* 1991; 10: 707–720.

207. **Veldman, P.H. and Gortis, R.J.** Shoulder complaints in patients with reflex sympathetic dystrophy of the upper extremity. *Arch. Phys. Med. Rehabil.,* 1995; 76: 239–242.

208. **Walch, G., Boilean, P., Noel, E., Liotard, J.P., and Dejour, H.** Traitement chirurgical des epaules doulouremses par lesions de la coiffe et du long biceps en fonction des lesions. Reflexions sur le concept de Neer. *Rev. Rheum. Mal. Osteo-Articulaires,* 1991; 58: 247–257.

209. **Wober, W. et al.** Comparative efficacy and safety of the non-steroidal antiinflammatory drugs nime-sulide and diclofenac in patients with acute subdeltoid bursitis and bicipital tendinitis. *Int. J. Clin. Pract.,* 1998; 52: 169–175.

210. **Zuckerman, J.D. et al.** The painful shoulder: Part II. Intrinsic disorders and impingement syndrome. *Am. Fam. Physician,* 1991; 43: 497–512.

4 Elbow

I. HUMERAL EPICONDYLITIS (TENNIS ELBOW)

Humeral epicondylitis is an enthesitis that manifests at the origin of the forearm extensors on the lateral epicondyle (lateral or radial epicondylitis), or at the origin of the forearm flexors and pronator teres on the medial epicondyle (medial or ulnar epicondylitis).

A. HISTORY

The first description of symptoms related to epicondylitis was given in 1873 by the German physician Runge,[31] who associated this condition with extended use of the arm in writing. In 1882, Morris used the phrase *lawn tennis arm.* A year later, Mayor[31] introduced the term *tennis elbow* in a paper in the *British Medical Journal.* In 1896, a German study documented symptoms of lateral epicondylitis in workers in a variety of occupations, including bricklayers, carpenters, plumbers, bakers, shoemakers, and violinists.[11] Bernhard[31] first noted the correlation between tenderness and pain and the excessive use of the forearm extensors. In 1910, Franke introduced the term *humeral epicondylitis.*[27]

Lateral epicondylitis occurs seven to ten times more frequently than medial epicondylitis.[25,26,67,94,98,128,130,138] Humeral epicondylitis is equally common in both sexes, manifests usually between the ages of 30 and 50, and occurs four times more frequently in individuals in their 40s. The dominant arm is most often affected. Bilateral involvement is rare.

Lateral epicondylitis is commonly called *tennis elbow,* whereas medial epicondylitis has a variety of names: synonimes epitrochleitis, javelin thrower's elbow, and pitcher's elbow. Some authors[16,35] have called both lateral and medial epicondylitis tennis elbow. Nirschl recognizes lateral epicondylitis as *lateral tennis elbow,* medial epicondylitis as *medial tennis elbow,* and triceps tendinitis as *posterior tennis elbow.*[78–82]

Although humeral epicondylitis is referred to in medical nomenclature by a number of names associated with different sports, in 95% of the cases in clinical practice it is encountered as an occupational hazard in nonathletes, primarily computer users, bricklayers, shoemakers, cooks, truck drivers, surgeons, dentists, and in other workers who perform repeated contractions of the extensor and supinator muscles (in lateral epicondylitis) or flexor and pronator muscles (in medial epicondylitis). In fact, tennis elbow is usually caused by activities other than tennis.[83,90,112] Professions in which repeated contractions are performed against a resisting force are particularly prone to development of humeral epicondylitis. In athletes, who account for 5% of the cases in clinical practice, humeral epicondylitis is most often found in tennis players, javelin throwers, bowlers, fencers, golfers, rock climbers, hockey players, and handball players.[17,18,21,37,43,51,74,95,100,115,117,121]

Allander[2] reported an incidence of 1 to 5% of lateral epicondylitis in a population of 15,268 people between the ages of 31 and 74. In a group of women between the ages of 42 and 46 years, he reported an incidence of 10%, which is remarkably high when compared to the annual incidence of 1% or less. According to Verhaar[124] epidemiological studies show an incidence of tennis elbow between 1 and 2%. The prevalence of tennis elbow in women between 40 and 50 years of age is 10%. Half the patients with tennis elbow seek medical attention. Luopajaravi et al.[72] reported on a risk-prone population of factory workers and sales assistants with an average age of 39 years. The incidence was 3%. Kivi[61] studied a population of 7600 manual workers and diagnosed humeral epicondylitis in 88 workers (50 males and 38 females). Lateral epicondylitis was diagnosed in 74 workers (84%), and medial epicondylitis was diagnosed in 14 cases (16%). The mean age of the afflicted workers was 43 years.

A study performed by Gruchow and Palletier[45] analyzed 532 tennis players (278 males and 254 females), between the ages of 20 and 60 years. Their results indicated that age and the amount of daily playing time are correlated to the development of lateral epicondylitis and that the incidence and recurrence of symptoms rises proportionally with age. Lateral epicondylitis was diagnosed in 24.8% of the players under 40 years of age and in 57.4% of the players older than 40 years. Further analysis showed that players older than 40 years are twice as likely to develop tennis elbow when compared to players younger than 40 years and that players older than 40 years who play more than 2 h/day on average have a 3.5 times greater risk of developing lateral epicondylitis. Their study indicated no significant difference between the incidence and recurrence of symptoms with regard to the weight of the racket and the material from which it is made. However, some authors believe that the increased incidence of tennis elbow in players is directly attributable to the materials from which modern rackets are made. With wooden rackets, vibrations that occur when the ball is hit tend to be absorbed, whereas modern rackets, which are made from metal, graphite, and fiberglass, do not absorb vibrations as effectively.[135] The grip size of the racket can also be a cause for development or recurrence of tennis elbow. A grip larger than $4^{1}/_{2}$ in. can lead, especially in older players, to the development of lateral epicondylitis. The grip strength in patients with tennis elbow is influenced by elbow position.[29] Some authors emphasize that players with more playing experience have a higher incidence of tennis elbow, which they attribute to the greater amount of daily playing time of experienced players. In contrast, Nirschl's[81] study shows that inexperienced tennis players have a higher incidence of tennis elbow because of improper stroking technique. Priest et al.[97] analyzed the incidence of humeral epicondylitis in a population of tennis players and obtained results similar to those of Gruchow and Palletier[45] with one interesting exception. Their study showed that professional and semiprofessional tennis players had a higher incidence of medial epicondylitis, which they attributed to the strenuous movements those players performed while serving. O'Dwyer and Howie[84] reported on 95 cases of medial epicondylitis in 83 patients and found 90% were related to work and only 10% to sport or leisure activities. Surgery was needed in 12%, which compared with less than 4% of patients with lateral epicondylitis over the same period. The results of open release of the common flexor origin were good, with only one exception.

B. ETIOPATHOGENESIS

To understand the development of lateral epicondylitis, consider the backhand stroke in tennis. While performing this stroke, the forearm extensors are contracted to stabilize the wrist and to hold the racket. Repetitive concentric contractions, which occur if the stroke is improperly performed, shorten these muscles as they maintain tension to stabilize the wrist and produce a force that is transmitted via the muscles to their origin on the lateral epicondyle. These repetitive concentric contractions produce chronic overload of the bone–tendon junction, which in turn leads to decreased vascularization of the junction and overstimulation of free nerve endings. An aseptic inflammatory reaction results.

To understand the development of medial epicondylitis, consider the mechanics of baseball pitching. The specialized technique used in baseball pitching produces a large valgus stress across the elbow, which leads to overstretching of the medial collateral ligament and tension in the bone–tendon junction of the muscles that have their origin on the medial epicondyle. Baseball pitchers, while throwing the ball, extend the arm at the elbow; at the same time, they pronate the forearm and produce a palmar flexion of the wrist just prior to releasing the ball to obtain horizontal control of the pitch. Constant repetition of this movement in practice and competition can result in strain of the medial collateral ligament or overuse of the forearm flexors and pronator teres.

In all cases of lateral epicondylitis, the origin of the extensor carpi radialis brevis muscle is afflicted.[26,39,53,54,67,80,82] The origins of the extensor digitorum communis and extensor carpi radialis

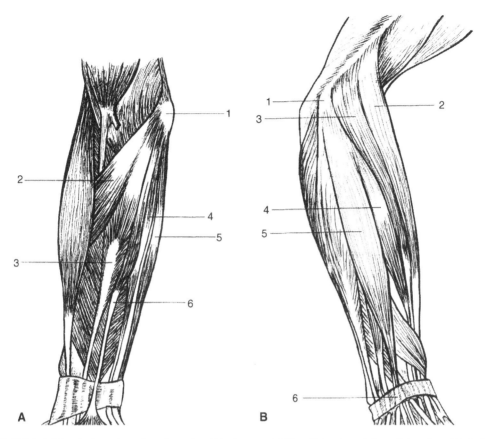

FIGURE 4.1 Muscle insertion sites from the (A) ulnar and (B) radial epicondylus of the ulna. (A) 1: Epicondylus ulnaris (medialis); 2: pronator teres muscle; 3: flexor carpi radialis muscle; 4: flexor digitorum superficialis muscle; 5: flexor carpi ulnaris muscle; 6: palmaris longus muscle. (B) 1: Epicondylus radialis (lateralis); 2: brachioradialis muscle; 3: extensor carpi radialis brevis muscle; 4: extensor carpi radialis longus muscle; 5: extensor digitorum communis muscle; 6: retinaculum extensorum.

muscles are affected in 35% of the cases. The extensor carpi ulnaris is rarely involved. In all cases of medial epicondylitis, the origins of the pronator teres and flexor carpi radialis muscles are affected, whereas the origin of the flexor carpi ulnaris muscle is affected in only 10% of the cases[63,80,82] (Figure 4.1).

Coonrad and Hooper[25] have theorized that macroscopic or microscopic tears in the muscle origin are the likely cause of symptoms in tennis elbow, and Kibler[59] considers tennis elbow a consequence of gradual degeneration on a cellular and tissue level. We do not agree. In our opinion, the sequence of events is that overuse leads to avascularization of the affected muscle origin, which leads to overstimulation of the free nerve ends and results in aseptic inflammation. Further repetition of offending movements causes angiofibroblastic hyperplasia of the origin. Then in the final stage, partial or complete rupture of the tendon occurs. Angiofibroblastic hyperplasia prevents healing, allowing the aseptic inflammation to continue with ultimate damage to the tendon origin. Nirschl states that the degree of angiofibroblastic hyperplasia is correlated to the duration and severity of symptoms.[79–81] The afflicted tendon origin is gray and resembles immature fibrous tissue; it is shiny, edematose, and easily crumbles. Histological analysis reveals the characteristic invasion of fibroblasts and vascular tissue, which is the typical picture of angiofibroblastic hyperplasia. Regan et al.[99] compared the histopathologic features from 11 patients who were treated surgically for lateral epicondylitis to similar tissue from 12 cadaveric specimens. The surgical specimens were interpreted as abnormal in all 11 specimens, and all 12 of the control specimens were reported as being without histologic abnormality. Vascular proliferation was present in 10 of the 11 surgical patients, and focal hyaline degeneration was recorded in all 11 of the surgical specimens. These data suggest that chronic refractory lateral epicondylits is a degenerative rather than an inflammatory process. This may account for the lack of response to rest and anti-inflammatory medication. Ljung et al.[71] consider that substance P and calcitonin gene-related peptide expression at the origin of the extensor carpi radialis brevis muscle have implications for the etiology of tennis elbow.

C. CLINICAL PICTURE AND DIAGNOSTICS

The main symptoms consist of pain and tenderness at the lateral epicondyle (in lateral epicondylitis) or at the medial epicondyle (in medial epicondylitis). In most cases, pain is characterized by a gradual onset that, after prolonged repetition of provoking movements, intensifies to the level of severe pain, restricting basically all activity. A sudden onset of pain is usually associated with one very strenuous movement, i.e., when throwing a heavy object. In lateral epicondylitis, tenderness is produced by palpation on the extensor muscles origin on the lateral epicondyle. In some cases, the pain can spread along the radial side of the forearm to the wrist and, in rare cases, even to the third and fourth fingers. The pain can be very intense, preventing the patient from turning a key in a lock or even picking up a pencil.

According to Warren,[130] there are four stages in the development of this injury with regard to the intensity of the symptoms.

1. Faint pain a couple of hours after the provoking activity.
2. Pain at the end of or immediately after the provoking activity.
3. Pain during the provoking activity, which intensifies after ceasing that activity.
4. Constant pain, which prohibits any activity.

During physical examination, pain is provoked by palpation on the extensor muscle origin on the lateral epicondyle. The pain will typically intensify if the patient extends the elbow while the examiner palpates the tender area.

The following tests are used to improve localization of the exact area of tenderness and to achieve a better assessment of the intensity of the pain on the lateral epicondyle:

1. Extending the wrist against resistance while the forearm is in full pronation and extended at the elbow; produces pain at the lateral epicondylar origin. This test was described by Mills[11] in 1928.
2. Extending the middle finger against resistance with the forearm in pronation and the elbow extended; produces pain in the same area. This test was described by Roles and Maudsley[103] (Figure 4.2).
3. The "chair test." This test employs a small chair weighing approximately 4 kg with an opening on the seat of the chair. The patient pushes his or her fingers through the opening and attempts to lift the chair with an extended elbow and pronated forearm. The pain will usually appear during the act of lifting. Failing that, the patient should further extend the wrist, and if the test is positive, the pain will either appear for the first time or intensify.
4. Gardner's "stress test."[40] The examiner tries to flex the patient's wrist against the force of the patient's contracted extensor muscles. The elbow is in extension and the forearm in full pronation. In lateral epicondylitis, flexion and extension are usually complete. However, in some chronic cases, hypertrophy of the extensor muscles is visible, and the patient will lack 5 to 15° of wrist extension.[11,19,81,82,138]

Other test strategies are also useful. An electromyographic analysis and an investigation of intervention strategies have been attempted in patients with lateral or medial epicondylitis of the

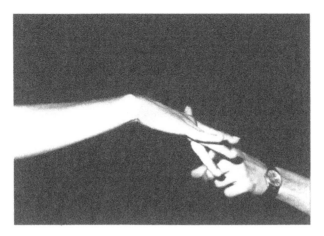

FIGURE 4.2 Extension test for the flexed middle finger in the metacarpophalangeal joint against resistance.

elbow.[41,57,101] Routine anteroposterior and lateral elbow radiographs are usually normal. Calcification of the soft tissues about the lateral epicondyle is occasionally present. Leach and Miller[67] reported an incidence of 22% and Pomerance[96] of 16% of cases with calcification in a studied population suffering from lateral epicondylitis. MR imaging evaluation is very useful in diagnosis and especially in differential diagnosis in patients with lateral or medial epicondylitis of the elbow.[14,23,34,37,49,50,88,91,116,119] Sonographic examination[24] and laser Doppler imaging[32] are recommended for investigating epicondylitis. Thermography of the afflicted elbow can be a very useful aid in diagnosing lateral epicondylitis.[9,63,108,122] Binder et al.[9] reported that thermography of the afflicted elbow in 53 out of 56 patients (95%) with diagnosed lateral epicondylitis demonstrated a localized area of greater heat ("hot spot") near the lateral epicondyle with a center that is 1 to 3°C higher than the normal isotherm.

In medial epicondylitis, the area of greatest tenderness is located at the origin of the flexor muscles on the medial humeral epicondyle. In some cases, the pain radiates along the ulnar side of the forearm to the wrist and occasionally even into the fingers. Grip strength is diminished and provokes pain. During physical examination, resisted flexion of the wrist with the elbow extended and the forearm in supination will produce pain in the medial epicondyle area.[11,67,138] In chronic medial epicondylitis, muscle function and pain measures show a lesser impaired function of the arm than in chronic lateral epicondylitis.[92,93]

Medial epicondylitis in a throwing athlete is differentiated from a chronic medial ligamentous strain by placing the wrist in flexion and the forearm in pronation and then gently applying a valgus stress to the slightly (10 to 20°) flexed elbow. If done gently, this should not be painful if the problem is medial epicondylitis alone. With medial collateral ligament strain or partial rupture, the test will be painful and may demonstrate, in cases of rupture, medial instability of the elbow.

A biomechanically based evaluation framework can be used to document all the clinical symptoms.[60]

D. DIFFERENTIAL DIAGNOSIS

In cases of lateral epicondylitis resistant to non-operative treatment, differential diagnosis must take into account radial tunnel syndrome, which some authors call *resistant tennis elbow*.[48,103] The radial tunnel, with a length less than 5.0 cm, begins proximally at the level of the capitellum of the humerus, which is its posterior wall, and continues to the distal end of the supinator muscle. There are five possible causes of compression in this tunnel: (1) abnormal fibrous band in front of the radial head, (2) a "fan" of radial recurrent vessels, (3) the sharp tendinous origin of the extensor carpi radialis brevis, (4) the arcade of Frohse, and (5) a fibrous band at the distal edge of the supinator muscle. The most common cause of compression is a fibrous arcade of Frohse. Ritts et al.[102] reported that the arcade of Frohse was the cause of 69.4% of the cases of radial tunnel syndrome. Spinnerr's research[89] shows that the arcade of Frohse is absent in fetuses and that only 30% of the mature population have it. Some authors differentiate compression at the arcade of Frohse as a separate syndrome, which they call the *supinator muscle syndrome*.[10,22,89]

In radial tunnel syndrome, there may be a spectrum of complaints, including pain, paresthesias, and weakness. Motor deficit is not nearly as common as in posterior interosseous nerve syndrome. The most common symptom is a dull pain in the posterolateral area of the forearm, which sometimes spreads to the dorsal side of the wrist. The pain increases during repeated movements of pronation and extension of the forearm if the wrist is palmarly flexed.

Physical examination must include carefully localizing the point of tenderness. Maneuvers that aggravate or reproduce the patient's symptoms should be carried out, and the most useful test is resisted forearm supination (with the elbow in flexion of 90° and the forearm in full pronation). This maneuver will worsen or reproduce the symptoms. Extension of the middle finger against resistance with the elbow in complete extension may result in similar symptoms, but not with the same frequency as the resisted forearm supination test.

Although the clinical features of radial tunnel syndrome are quite characteristic, it is often confused with lateral epicondylitis. Werner[132] reported that the radial tunnel syndrome is found with lateral epicondylitis in 5% of the cases; in contrast, Beenisch and Wilhelm[10] reported that preoperative tests found supinator muscle syndromes together with lateral epicondylitis in 53% of their patients.

Differential diagnostics of medial epicondylitis should also take into account compressive neuropathy of the median and ulnar nerves in the area of the elbow.[52]

The median nerve is vulnerable to compression as it passes under the lacertus fibrosis or bicipital aponeurosis, through the opening between the heads of the pronator teres muscle, through one of the heads of the pronator teres muscle (pronator teres syndrome), and below the fibrous arch of the flexor digitorum superficialis muscle in which case the anterior interosseous nerve is affected (anterior interosseous syndrome or Kiloh-Nevin syndrome).[55,89] Compressive neuropathy of the median nerve in the elbow area is usually characterized by a dull, diffuse pain in the proximal part of the forearm, which increases during activity and typically decreases when resting.[55] The area of greatest tenderness is usually located above the point of compression.

The ulnar nerve is vulnerable to compression in the elbow area as it passes through the ulnar groove or between the two heads of the flexor carpi ulnaris muscle (cubital tunnel syndrome).[38,43,89] The early stages of ulnar nerve entrapment of the elbow are characterized by paresthesias on the ulnar aspect of the forearm and in the ring and small finger. Sensory changes definitely precede motor changes; however, a careful evaluation of the intrinsic musculature of the hand is essential to detect any weakness. Because of the functional ceasing of the adductor pollicis muscle, Froment's symptom appears. This symptom is characterized by flexion in the interphalangeal joint of the thumb when the patient tries to grip a piece of paper between thumb and forefinger. The same symptoms can be caused by dislocation of the ulnar nerve (luxatio nervi ulnaris) from its groove during elbow flexion. The dislocation can be caused by the shallowness of the groove due to the ripping of the epicondylo-olecranon ligament, the valgus position of the elbow, or congenital abnormalities of the humeral epicondyles. During flexion and extension of the elbow, the nerve slips from its groove and slides toward the volar. In most cases, it is squeezed against the medial epicondyle, leading to compression and stretching of the nerve.

Nirschl[80–82] has reported on associated medial epicondylitis with compressive neuropathy of the ulnar nerve (in 60% of his cases), that differential diagnosis should always take into account the possibility of ulnar nerve compression whenever a patient localizes the area of greater pain in the vicinity of the ulnar groove. This is especially important in cases with unstable medial collateral ligaments. According to Grana[43] medial epicondylitis and ulnar nerve problems are common in the throwing athlete, resulting from the tremendous valgus stress that occurs during the acceleration phase of pitching.

E. TREATMENT

The wide variety of treatments, especially such non-operative treatments as local injection treatment,[4,5,47,73,109,110,113,126] laser therapy,[8,120] acupuncture,[33,75] shock waves, [62,64,104,105,129] bandage,[107,111,136] glycosaminoglycan polysulfate injection,[1] treatment with fluoroquinolone antibiotics,[68] or with botulinum toxin,[76] or with topical diclofenac,[15] stretching exercises,[92,111] coupled with the published results, indicates that as yet, no definite type of treatment is universally endorsed including the wide variety of surgical treatments. Endoscopic (arthroscopic) therapy[6,44,87] or percutaneous release of the common extensor origin for tennis elbow[46,137] are becoming more common in clinical practice.

1. Non-Operative Treatment

Our approach to non-operative treatment is based on the following principles: relieving pain, controlling inflammation, and monitoring further activity. Following these principles, we have compiled a program for non-operative treatment of lateral epicondylitis, which we have divided into three phases. The therapy should start as soon as possible, ideally, as soon as the first symptoms appear. One of the most common mistakes is to ignore the early symptoms and continue on as before, repeating offending activities with the same intensity. We agree with Solveborn,[112] "The earlier the treatment, the better."

a. The First Phase

Eliminating painful activities and resting from work or athletic activities are the most important aspects of this phase. While avoiding painful activities, the patient should continue to perform normal, active movements with other parts of the symptomatic extremity to avoid stiffness and other complications. Of oral nonsteroidal anti-inflammatory agents, we generally recommend agents from the oxicamic family (piroxicam) administered in the highest daily doses.

Icing or other types of cryotherapy should be applied three times per day for 15 min. This lessens the pain by reducing the conductibility of the sensory nerves. Ice also reduces the inflammatory response by decreasing the level of chemical activity and by vasoconstriction, which reduces the swelling. Elevation of the extremity is indicated if an edema of the wrist or fingers is present. In this phase, we also recommend wearing a plastic splint for the wrist ("wrist splint"). A volar splint with the wrist in 20° of extension will usually permit functional use of the hand while preventing overuse of wrist extensors.

b. The Second Phase

The main feature of this phase is stretching exercises. The underlying principle of this phase is that, by lengthening the tendon during relaxation, we can reduce its stretching during offending movements. Stretching exercises for the extensor muscles of the wrist and fingers should be performed in the following manner: Fully extend the elbow and palmarly flex the wrist. While applying pressure with the other hand, increase the palmar flexion as much as possible but stop at the first painful sensation (Figure 4.3). Remain in the point of maximum nonpainful extension for a period of 15 to 25 s. This exercise is repeated four to five times a day with two series of ten exercises in each session; the patient should always stop at the first sign of pain. In this phase of therapy, the patient should also perform isotonic exercises, once a day, according to the following plan:

1. Stretching exercises — Hold for 15 to 25 s; repeat 10 times.
2. Isotonic exercises — Perform three series of 15 repetitions.
3. Stretching exercises — Hold for 15 to 25 s; repeat 10 times.
4. Icing — Massage the tender area with ice or crushed ice for 10 to 15 min.

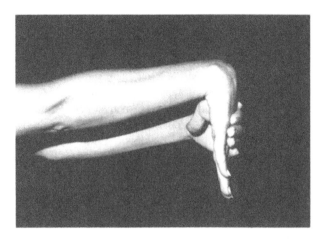

FIGURE 4.3 Passive stretching of the extensor muscles of the lower arm.

Isotonic exercises are performed in the following manner: Place the forearm on a table in a position of full pronation with the wrist hanging over the edge; in this position, perform extension and flexion movements of the wrist. In the beginning phase, the patient should perform the exercise slowly, counting to six after each flexion (the eccentric phase of contraction) and to three after each extension of the wrist (the concentric phase of contraction). When these movements become painless, the patient should gradually increase the speed and resistance. Increasing the speed of the exercises has the effect of increasing the loading on the tendon, while the gradual increase of outside resistance leads to progressive strain of the tendon, resulting in an increase of its stretching strength. The outside resistance is accomplished by lifting small weights — at first 0.5 kg, and then slowly progressing to 5 kg. The maximum weight should not exceed 10% of the patient's body weight.

As already noted, besides stretching and isotonic exercises, the patient should also perform isometric exercises. A good example is the following: Place a rubber band around the gathered fingers and thumb; then perform extension of the fingers against force. The exercise is repeated three times a day with 50 repetitions in each series while gradually increasing the tightness of the rubber band. A second useful exercise is to extend the arm at the elbow and abduct the forearm to a horizontal position. An elastic tube or tennis ball is placed in the hand and the patient proceeds to squeeze the object alternately with greater and lesser strength. This exercise is begun in the third week of treatment and is performed three times a day with 50 repetitions.

In the first 2 weeks of therapy, stimulation by high-voltage galvanic stimulator is also administered. This produces a piezoelectric effect that promotes tissue healing and enhances localized blood flow. In some patients, it also creates an analgesic effect.

Once all offending movements become painless, the patient can return to his or her normal daily activities. However, heavy physical work and athletic activities should be avoided. In all activities, the patient should wear a non-elastic elbow brace ("counterforce brace") (Figure 4.4). This brace plays the role of a secondary muscle attachment site and relieves tension on the attachment at the lateral epicondyle. The brace is applied firmly around the forearm (below the head of the radius) and is tightened enough so that, when the patient contracts the wrist extensors, he or she does not fully contract the muscles. Schauss et al.[107] on the basis of an experimental study concluded that to be effective these bandages must, from a technical standpoint, be of a strap construction to build up adequate pressures. This phase lasts for 6 to 8 weeks. If the pain recurs or worsens, the intensity of the exercise program is reduced. If the pain persists, the patient is returned to the first phase of treatment. Lewis et al.[70] investigated effects of manual work on recovery from lateral epicondylitis.

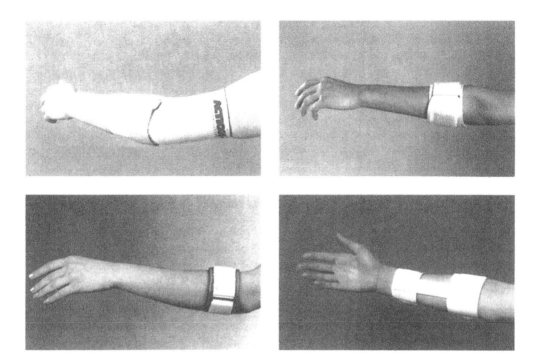

FIGURE 4.4 Various types of counterforce braces.

c. The Third Phase

The patient gradually returns to all activities, but continues to perform stretching exercises and to strengthen the affected muscle groups. A non-elastic elbow brace should be worn during all strenuous activities.

Recurrence of the symptoms is frequent if exercises are not repeated daily to increase the resistance gradually. The patient should be made aware that before any athletic or strenuous activity is undertaken, a long warm-up period of the affected muscle group, including stretching exercises, is necessary. Once the activity is finished, stretching exercises and cryotherapy must be performed.

To avoid recurrence in cases with work-related etiologies, patients should lighten the weight of their work tools or reduce the frequency of the offending movements. Failing that, rest periods should be increased and the time lengthened to allow relaxation of the muscles; this is to reduce the risk of recurrence. With tennis players, prevention of lateral epicondylitis is accompanied by correcting improper stroking techniques and methods of holding the racket, choosing the optimal shape, material, and weight of the racket, enlarging the grip, and reducing racket string tension.

We believe that local corticosteroid injections should be avoided as long as possible and used only in resistant cases that do not respond to more conservative measures. In these cases, as many as three injections deep into the subcutaneous fat tissue can be administered. The injections should not be repeated more than three times because the progressive response to each injection is reduced and the risk of possible complications (subcutaneous atrophy, weakening of the surrounding tissues) increases. Care must be taken not to administer the injection into the tendon because of the increase in pressure in the bradiotroph tissue and because of the possibility of a tendon rupture, which is an unwanted side effect.

Lateral epicondylitis is generally treated with physiotherapy or corticosteroid injections. Dutch clinical guidelines recommend a wait-and-see policy. Smidt et al.[109] compared the efficacy of these approaches. They randomly assigned 185 patients and at 6 weeks, corticosteroid injections were significantly better than all other therapy options for all outcome measures. Success rates were 92% compared with 47% for physiotherapy and 32% for wait-and-see policy. However, the recurrence rate in the injection group was high. Long-term differences between injections and physiotherapy were significantly in favor of physiotherapy. Physiotherapy had better results than wait-and-see policy, but differences were not significant. Solveborn et al.[113] in a prospective, randomized, double-blind study of tennis elbow treated 109 patients with a single injection of steroid with either lidocaine or bupivacaine. The steroid injection treatment, regardless of which local anesthetic was given, presented a typical pattern, with symptoms relieved quickly in weeks and then deterioration for many patients at 3 months, indicating a tendency to recurrence. Patients who had not been treated earlier in any way had a more favorable prognosis, as did those with a history of epicondylalgia of up to 3 months. Verhaar et al.[126] performed a prospective, randomized trial on 106 patients to compare the effects of local corticosteroid injections vs. physiotherapy as advocated by Cyriax in the treatment of tennis elbow. They conclude that at 6 weeks, treatment with corticosteroid injections was more effective than Cyriax physiotherapy, and they recommend it because of its rapid action, reduction of pain, and absence of side effects. In a recent published review article Smidt et al.[110] conclude that for short-term outcomes (6 weeks), statistically significant and clinically relevant differences were found on pain, global improvement, and grip strength for corticosteroid injection compared to placebo, local anesthetic, and conservative treatments. For intermediate (6 weeks to 6 months) and long-term outcomes (more than 6 months), no statistically significant or clinically relevant results in favor of corticosteroid injections were found. So, it is not possible to draw a firm conclusion. Much better-designed, conducted, and reported randomized controlled trials with intermediate and long-term follow-up are needed. An attempted meta-analysis for the treatment of lateral epicondylitis showed that there were too many methodological differences to allow a quantitative meta-analysis.[66] According to Chumbley et al.[20] basic treatment principles are described by the acronym PRICEMM: protection, rest, ice, compression, elevation, medication, and modalities (physical therapy).

2. Surgical Treatment

The symptoms of humeral epicondylitis will prove to be resistant in 5 to 10% of patients. In those cases, surgical treatment is indicated.[7,12,25,28,30,36,42,56,58,65,67,69,77–82,85,86,98,106,114,118,123,125,127,131,133,134,137] Surgical treatment is indicated when symptoms persist for longer than 6 months and significantly disable the patient from performing normal working or athletic activities despite an adequately carried out non-operative treatment. It is also indicated in cases with frequent recidives and incomplete remissions. A relative indication may be present in athletes for whom the amount of time spent out of competition can be crucially important. Different surgical techniques and their modification have been proposed for treating humeral epicondylitis. A review of the literature shows that the most commonly used techniques are modifications of the Hohmann and Bosworth methods.

When dealing with lateral epicondylitis, we use the following modification of the Hohmann method. A curvilinear incision is made over the area of the lateral epicondyle. The deep antebrachial fascia is incised, revealing the lateral epicondyle. The tendinous origin of the extensor carpi radialis brevis muscle is part sharply and part bluntly freed from the lateral epicondyle. Using a surgical chisel, the epicondyle is decorticated while the surrounding, less vital structures are excised. Hemostasis is performed after which the wound is closed by layers. Postoperative immobilization is carried out with six layers of sheet cotton and a light circumferential long arm cast with the elbow at 90° and the wrist in functional position. Nirschl[79] reported a 75% success rate using this technique, and Stotz et al.[118] reported a 65% success-to-failure ratio.

Recent knowledge into the etiopathogenesis of humeral epicondylitis has instigated Coonrad and Hooper[25] to develop a new operative method that has been slightly modified by Nirschl and Pettrone.[79] The procedure begins with a lateral 5-cm-long incision over the lateral epicondyle. The deep fascia is incised and gently separated, revealing the tendinous origin of the common extensor. Because the origin of the extensor carpi radialis brevis muscle is usually the affected site, the extensor carpi radialis longus muscle is gently lifted to reveal the affected origin. Excision of the affected tendon origin of the extensor carpi radialis brevis muscle is performed, and in some cases, part of the tendon origin of the extensor carpi radialis longus is excised as well. Excision of part of the extensor digitorum communis muscle is very rarely indicated. When necessary, a small opening is made through the synovium for inspection of the radiohumeral joint. Part of the periosteum is removed using an osteotome, or four to five holes are drilled with a small drill down to the spongeous bone. The tendons are then reattached at this site after previously being longitudinally joined. The wound is closed by layers. Postoperative immobilization is carried out with a light circumferential long arm cast with the elbow at 90° and the forearm in a neutral position. Total elevation of the extremity above shoulder level is necessary for 3 days. Mobilization is initiated after 5 to 7 days after which intense rehabilitation is begun. Nirschl and Pettrone[79] reported excellent results using this method without any residual pain contraction or loss of muscle strength in 97.7% of their cases, and Coonrad[26] reported excellent results obtained using this method in all of his patients.

In the last 15 years, percutaneous tenotomy of the extensor muscles in lateral epicondylitis or the flexor muscles in medial epicondylitis has been frequently performed.[7,42,46,123,137] The procedure is done in the following manner. The forearm is placed on the operating table in supination while the elbow is in 90° flexion. The posterior edge of the lateral epicondyle is palpated, and an impression is made 1 cm from the edge toward the middle of the epicondyle on the skin with the thumb. The skin and deeper tissue overlying the epicondyle are infiltrated with a local anesthetic. Using a No. 11 blade (tenotome), a puncture incision is made through the skin to the bone, and the tendinous origin of the common extensors is freed from the bone. The release is carried down from the proximal to the distal portion of the epicondyle and parallel with the axis of the humerus. The skin is closed with one stitch, and dry sterile dressing is placed on the wound.

A similar procedure is performed on the medial side of the elbow for medial epicondylitis. When releasing the muscles, extreme caution must be taken to prevent damage to the ulnar nerve. To avoid this complication, the index finger of the surgeon's hand is kept in the ulnar groove during the release. Baumgard and Schwartz[7] reported excellent results in 91.4% of the patients on whom a percutaneous tenotomy of the extensor muscles was performed and in 84% of the patients on whom a percutaneous tenotomy of the flexor muscles was performed. Yeger and Turner[137] performed percutaneous tenotomy of the extensor muscles in 109 patients. In 102 of these (93.5%), the results were excellent. The advantages of this operative method, as noted by different authors,[7,42,46,137] lie in the simplicity of the procedure. The procedure does not require hospitalization, entails very rare postoperative complications, and allows a quick return to normal working activity (on average, 9 days). In athletes and manual workers, however, this procedure is not indicated, in our opinion, because postoperative complications may reduce grip strength.

Anatomical and clinical research has shown that the entire lateral epicondylar region is innervated only by radial nerve branches. Based on these investigations Wilhelm[133,134] has developed a surgical procedure for complete denervation, which is indicated only in resistant cases of tennis elbow. The results of this procedure also depend on simultaneous indirect decompression of the posterior interosseous nerve. Excellent or good results were obtained in 90% on average. Stangl and Freilinger[114] use the same Wilhelm denervation operation in epicondylitis humeri radialis. Epicondylar resection with anconeus muscle transfer for chronic lateral epicondylitis is also recommended.[3]

Organ et al.[86] undertook a retrospective analysis of 34 patients (35 elbows) who had undergone prior failed surgical intervention for lateral tennis elbow. At revision surgery, findings included residual tendinosis of the extensor carpi radialis brevis tendon in 34 of 35 elbows. Salvage surgery included excision of pathologic tissue of the extensor carpi radialis brevis tendon origin combined with excision of the excessive scar tissue and repair of the extensor aponeurosis when necessary; 83% of the elbows had good or excellent results at follow-up from 17 months to 17 years.

Today, arthroscopic (endoscopic) treatment of lateral epicondylitis is recommended.[6,44,87] Arthroscopic release offers several potential advantages over open techniques. It preserves the common extensor origin by addressing the lesion directly. It allows for an intra-articular examination for possible chondral lesions, loose bodies, and other disorders such as an inflamed lateral synovial fringe. It also permits a shorter postoperative rehabilitation period and an earlier return to work.[6]

II. POSTERIOR IMPINGEMENT SYNDROME OF THE ELBOW

Repetitive, sudden, forceful extension of the elbow present in many athletic activities — baseball, handball, tennis, and throwing sports — can lead to development of the posterior impingement syndrome of the elbow.[140,141,145,148,150] These movements are characterized by the violent collision of the olecranon against the olecranon fossa. In addition to the posterior impingement syndrome of the elbow, these movements can also lead to the development of triceps tendinitis, apophysitis of the olecranon (which can be likened to Osgood-Schlatter disease), and stress fracture of the olecranon (Figure 4.5). Awaya et al.[139] describe MR imaging findings in patients with elbow synovial fold syndrome. A synovial fold extending from the posterior fat pad in the elbow is a frequent finding on MR imaging. The patients present clinically with symptoms mimicking an intra-articular body. The characteristic symptom of posterior impingement syndrome of the elbow is a sharp pain that manifests when the elbow snaps into full extension during activity.[140] The tenderness is localized to the posterior or posterior medial side of the elbow. The patient also complains of reduced mobility, i.e., inability to extend the elbow fully. Crepitations are frequent during movements of the elbow; in some cases, "stiffness" and a diffuse pain accompanied by a swelling of the elbow are also

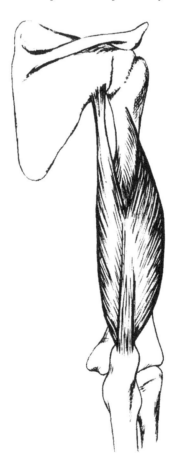

FIGURE 4.5 Triceps brachii muscle.

present. During physical examination, pain is discovered over the posterior or posteromedial area of the olecranon. Pain can also be induced with a strong passive extension of the elbow. The valgus stress test of the elbow will also produce characteristic pain during the last 5 to 10° of elbow extension. In cases of triceps tendinitis, pain will appear during extension against resistance.

Radiographic examination can show what movements provoke collision of the bony parts in the elbow and existence or absence of loose bodies in the elbow. Radiographic examination will also show bony osteophytes on the posteromedial aspect of the olecranon. Cortical thickening of the olecranon fossa, which can be found in both symptomatic and asymptomatic patients, is explained as a physiological adaptation of bone to repetitive stress. Ferrara et al.[142-144] found that plain film and ultrasound were sufficient for the detection of chronic lesions of the elbow. MRI did not add significant findings.

Initial treatment consists of reducing stress to the elbow joint (relative rest) and alleviating the pain, swelling, and inflammation. This is accomplished by temporarily ceasing athletic activities, using nonsteroidal anti-inflammatory drugs, and icing the affected area. Taping, with the aim of preventing full extension and valgus of the elbow (adhesive tape applied to the anterior side of the elbow), can enable the patient to resume athletic activities without pain.

During rehabilitation, exercises that strengthen the elbow flexors (biceps, brachialis, and brachioradialis) should be performed to prevent the maximal extension of the elbow. Stretching exercises of the extensor muscles (triceps) should also be performed. According to Wilson et al.,[151] good results from surgical treatment are short term, and clinical symptoms often recur. Surgical treatment consists of removing the bony osteophytes, performing an osteotomy of the tip of the olecranon, or performing a debridement of the olecranon and olecranon fossa. The last can be performed arthroscopically.[141,142,144-147,149,151]

III. MEDIAL TENSION/LATERAL COMPRESSION SYNDROME

Medial tension/lateral compression syndrome is a term used to describe a complex of overuse injuries of the elbow characterized by tenderness, reduced mobility, and the inability to throw a ball without pain. Medial tension/lateral compression syndrome is caused by repetitive valgus stress at the elbow.[153,155,156,159-161] The act of throwing a ball causes a strong valgus stress, which leads to stretching of the structures on the medial side of the elbow and at the same time to compression of the lateral side of the joint. Because of this etiology and because of its high frequency in baseball players, medial tension/lateral compression syndrome is also known in the medical literature as *pitcher's elbow* in mature athletes and *Little League elbow* in younger athletes (Figure 4.6).

The syndrome is characterized by extra-articular changes on the medial side of the elbow. In most cases, these changes consist of enthesitis of the wrist flexors and pronator teres on the medial epicondyle of the humerus (medial epicondylitis). Less common are ruptures of these muscles or avulsion fracture of the medial epicondyle. Strain or rupture of the ulnar collateral ligament of the elbow is another frequent symptom. In older athletes, a bony spike on the tip of the ulna (ulnar traction spur) is sometimes found. Blohm et al.[155] present a case of an acute traction apophysitis, "Little League elbow," in an adolescent badminton player. Some authors believe that compression of the ulnar nerve in this area can also result from the same repetitive stretching movements.

On the lateral side of the elbow, compression causes intra-articular damage. Degenerative changes of the elbow and loose bodies are characteristically found in older athletes, whereas osteochondritis dissecans of the humeral capitulum is typical in younger athletes. Osteochondritis results from repeated valgus stresses incurred while throwing a ball, but also from improper throwing technique. Podesta et al.[166] present a case of a 7-year-old Little League pitcher with the diagnosis of distal humeral epiphyseal separation.

Radiographic examination is routinely used to diagnose osteochondritis (Figure 4.7). In the beginning stages, a tomogram can also be indicated. Osteochondritis is seen as an area of greater

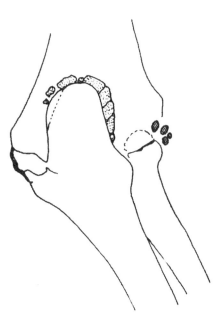

FIGURE 4.6 Medial tension/lateral compression syndrome of the elbow.

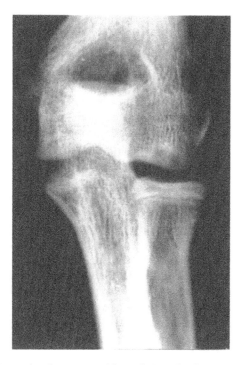

FIGURE 4.7 Radiograph of a top-level gymnast with medial tension/lateral compression syndrome.

radiolucency, fragmentation, and deformation of the capitellum.[160] MR imaging allows clear depiction of the muscles, tendons, ligaments, bones, cartilage, nerves, and vessels that compose the elbow. MR arthrography can be a valuable supplementary technique for optimizing evaluation of intra-articular structures, including the undersurfaces of the collateral ligaments.[158,159] Arthroscopic surgical treatment[153,156] is the method generally preferred today when dealing with early stages of osteochondritis; the aim is to prevent degenerative changes in the elbow, loose bodies, angular deformation of the radial head, and reduced mobility. McManama et al.[165] review 14 patients who underwent elbow arthrotomy for osteochondritis of the capitellum. They conclude that after a failure of conservative therapy surgical treatment, including removal of the intra-articular loose bodies, excision of capitellar lesions, and curettage to bleeding bone, can be expected to produce pain relief and improvement in joint motion. Kiyoshige et al.[163] treated seven young male baseball players with osteochondritis dissecans of the capitellum using closed-wedge osteotomy. This procedure was established by Yosh in 1986 for treatment of Little League elbow.[163] The follow-up study of 7 to 12 years revealed minimal osteoarthritic change and suggests that the treatment is useful for such injuries.

On the posterior side of the elbow, the repetitive collisions of the olecranon against the olecranon fossa produce degenerative changes on the olecranon — in most cases, a bony spur or loose joint bodies. Lowery et al.[164] report three cases of painful persistence of the olecranon epiphyseal plate in adolescent pitchers. Tenderness of the tip on the medial side of the olecranon is diagnosed during physical examination and must be considered in differential diagnosis. A typical symptom of this syndrome, also known as posterior impingement syndrome, is a sharp pain felt during sudden, passive extension in the elbow. Surgical treatment is indicated in most cases.

REFERENCES

Humeral Epicondylitis

1. **Akermark, C. et al.** Glycosaminoglycan polysulfate injections in lateral humeral epicondylalgia: a placebo-controlled double-blind trial. *Int. J. Sports Med.*, 1995; 16: 196–200.
2. **Allander, E.** Prevalence, incidence and remission rates of some common rheumatic diseases or syndromes. *Scand. J. Rheumatol.*, 1974; 3: 145–153.
3. **Almquist, E.E., Necking, L., and Bach, A.W.** Epicondylar resection with anconeus muscle transfer for chronic lateral epicondylitis. *J. Hand Surg. (Am.)*, 1998; 23: 723–731.
4. **Altay, T., Gunal, I., and Ozturk, H.** Local injection treatment for lateral epicondylitis. *Clin. Orthop.*, 2002; 398: 127–130.
5. **Assendelft, W.J. et al.** Corticosteroid injections for lateral epicondylitis a systematic overview. *Br. J. Gen. Pract.*, 1996; 46: 209–216.
6. **Baker, C.L., Jr., et al.** Arthroscopic classification and treatment of lateral epicondylitis: two-year clinical results. *J. Shoulder Elbow Surg.*, 2000; 9: 475–482.
7. **Baumgard, S.H. and Schwartz, D.R.** Percutaneous release of the epicondylar muscles for humeral epicondylitis. *Am. J. Sports Med.*, 1982; 10: 233–236.
8. **Basford, J.R., Sheffield, C.G., and Cieslak, K.R.** Laser therapy: a randomized, controlled trial of the effects of low intensity Nd:YAG laser irradiation on lateral epicondylitis. *Arch. Phys. Med. Rehabil.*, 2000; 81: 1504–1510.
9. **Binder, A., Parr, G., Page Thomas, P., and Hazleman, B.** A clinical and thermographic study of lateral epicondylitis. *Br. J. Rheumatol.*, 1983; 22: 77–81.
10. **Beenisch, J. and Wilhelm, K.** Die epicondylitis humeri lateralis. *Fortschr. Med.*, 1985; 103: 417–419.
11. **Bojanić, I. et al.** Epicondylitis humeri. *Basketball Med. Per.*, 1988; 3: 69–81.
12. **Boyd, H.B. and McLeod, A.C.** Tennis elbow. *J. Bone Joint Surg.*, 1973; 55(A): 1183–1187.
13. **Boyer, M.I. and Hastings H., II.** Lateral tennis elbow: "Is there any science out there?" *J. Shoulder Elbow Surg.*, 1999; 8: 481–491.
14. **Bredella, M.A. et al.** MR imaging findings of lateral ulnar collateral ligament abnormalities in patients with lateral epicondylitis. *Am. J. Roentgenol.*, 1999; 173: 1379–1382.
15. **Burnham, R. et al.** The effectiveness of topical diclofenac for lateral epicondylitis. *Clin. J. Sport Med.*, 1998; 8: 78–81.
16. **Cabot, A.** Tennis elbow. *Orthop. Rev.*, 1987; 16: 69–73.
17. **Caldwell, G.L., Jr., and Safran, M.R.** Elbow problems in the athlete. *Orthop. Clin. North Am.*, 1995; 26: 465–485.
18. **Chen, F.S., Rokito, A.S., and Jobe, F.W.** Medial elbow problems in the overhead-throwing athlete. *J. Am. Acad. Orthop. Surg.*, 2001; 9: 99–113.

19. **Chop, W.M., Jr.** Tennis elbow. *Postgrad. Med.*, 1989; 86: 301–308.
20. **Chumbley, E.M., O'Connor, F.G., and Nirschl, R.P.** Evaluation of overuse elbow injuries. *Am. Fam. Physician*, 2000; 61: 691–700.
21. **Ciccotti, M.G. and Charlton, W.P.** Epicondylitis in the athlete. *Clin. Sports Med.*, 2001; 20: 77–93.
22. **Coenen, W.** Über ein diagnostisches Zeichen bei der sogenannten Epicondylitis humeri radialis. *Z. Orthop.*, 1986; 124: 323–326.
23. **Coel, M., Yamada, C.Y., and Ko, J.** MR imaging of patients with lateral epicondylitis of the elbow (tennis elbow): importance of increased signal of the anconeus muscle. *Am. J. Roentgenol.*, 1993; 161: 1019–1021.
24. **Connell, D. et al.** Sonographic examination of lateral epicondylitis. *Am. J. Roentgenol.*, 2001; 176: 777–782.
25. **Coonrad, R.W. and Hooper, R.W.** Tennis elbow: its course, natural history, conservative and surgical management. *J. Bone Joint Surg.*, 1973; 55(A): 1177–1182.
26. **Coonrad, R.W.** Tennis elbow. *Instr. Course Lect.*, 1986; 35: 94–101.
27. **Cyriax, J.H.** The pathology and treatment of tennis elbow. *J. Bone Joint Surg.*, 1936; 18: 921–940.
28. **Čurković, B. and Domljan, Z.** Radijalni epikondilitis. *Lijec. Vjesn.*, 1982; 104: 362–364.
29. **De Smet, L. and Fabry, G.** Grip strength in patients with tennis elbow. Influence of elbow position. *Acta Orthop. Belg.*, 1996; 62: 26–29.
30. **Dobyns, J.H.** Musculotendinous problems at the elbow, in *Surgery of the Musculoskeletal System*, McCollister, E.C., Ed. New York: Churchill Livingstone, 1983; 211–232.
31. **Emery, S.E. and Gifford, J.F.** 100 years of tennis elbow. *Contemp. Orthop.*, 1986; 12: 53–58.
32. **Ferrel, W.R., Balint, P.V., and Sturrock, R.D.** Novel use of laser Doppler imaging for investigating epicondylitis. *Rheumatology* (Oxford), 2000; 39: 1214–1217.
33. **Fink, M. et al.** Acupuncture in chronic epicondylitis: a randomized control trial. *Rheumatology* (Oxford), 2002; 41: 205–209.
34. **Fritz, R.C.** MR imaging of sports injuries of the elbow. *Magn. Reson. Imaging Clin. North Am.*, 1999; 7: 51–72.
35. **Froimson, A.I.** Tenosynovitis and tennis elbow, in *Operative Hand Surgery*, Green, D.P., Ed. New York: Churchill Livingstone, 1982; 1507–1521.
36. **Friedlander, H.L., Reid, R.L., and Cape, R.F.** Tennis elbow. *Clin. Orthop.*, 1967; 51: 109–116.
37. **Gaary, E.A., Potter, H.G., and Altchek, D.W.** Medial elbow pain in the throwing athlete: MR imaging evaluation. *Am. J. Roentgenol.*, 1997; 168: 795–800.
38. **Gabel, G.T. and Morrey, B.F.** Operative treatment of medial epicondylitis. Influence of concomitant ulnar neuropathy at the elbow. *J. Bone Joint Surg. (Am.)*, 1995; 77: 1065–1069.
39. **Garden, R.S.** Tennis elbow. *J. Bone Joint Surg.*, 1961; 43(B): 100–106.
40. **Gardner, R.C.** Tennis elbow: diagnosis, pathology and treatment. *Clin. Orthop.*, 1970; 72: 248–253.
41. **Glazebrook, M.A. et al.** Medial epicondylitis. An electromyographic analysis and an investigation of intervention strategies. *Am. J. Sports Med.*, 1994; 22: 674–679.
42. **Goldberg, G.D., Alroham, E., and Siegel, I.** The surgical treatment of chronic lateral humeral epicondylitis by common extensor release. *Clin. Orthop.*, 1988; 223: 208–212.
43. **Grana, W.** Medial epicondylitis and cubital tunnel syndrome in the throwing athlete. *Clin. Sports Med.*, 2001; 20: 541–548.
44. **Grifka, J., Boenke, S., and Kramer, J.** Endoscopic therapy in epicondylitis radialis humeri. *Arthroscopy*, 1995; 11: 743–748.
45. **Gruchow, H.W. and Palletier, B.S.** An epidemiologic study of tennis elbow. *Am. J. Sports Med.*, 1979; 7: 234–238.
46. **Grundberg, A.B. and Dobson, J.F.** Percutaneous release of the common extensor origin for tennis elbow. *Clin. Orthop.*, 2000; 376: 137–140.
47. **Hay, E.M. et al.** Pragmatic randomised controlled trial of local corticosteroid injection and naproxen for treatment of lateral epicondylitis elbow in primary care. *Br. Med. J.*, 1999; 319: 964–968.
48. **Heyse-Moore, G.H.** Resistant tennis elbow. *J. Hand Surg.*, 1984; 9: 64–66.
49. **Ho, C.P.** Sports and occupational injuries of the elbow: MR imaging findings. *Am. J. Roentgenol.*, 1995; 164: 1465–1471.
50. **Ho, C.P.** MR imaging of tendon injuries in the elbow. *Magn. Reson. Imaging Clin. North Am.*, 1997; 5: 529–543.

51. **Holtzhausen, L.M. and Noakes, T.D.** Elbow, forearm, wrist and hand injuries among sport rock climbers. *Clin. J. Sport Med.,* 1996; 6:196–203.

52. **Howard, F.M.** Controversies in nerve entrapment syndromes in the forearm and wrist. *Orthop. Clin. North Am.,* 1986; 17: 375–381.

53. **Janda, J. and Koudela, K.** Skelletmuskelbeteiligung bei der Enthesopatie des Epicondylus lateralis humeri. *Z. Orthop.,* 1988; 126: 105–107.

54. **Jobe, F.W. and Ciccotti, M.G.** Lateral and medial epicondylitis of the elbow. *J. Am. Acad. Orthop. Surg.,* 1994; 2: 1–8.

55. **Johnson, R., Spinner, M., and Shrewsbury, M.M.** Median nerve entrapment syndrome in the proximal forearm. *J. Hand Surg.,* 1979; 4: 48–51.

56. **Kaplan, E.B.** Treatment of tennis elbow (epicondylitis) by denervation. *J. Bone Joint Surg.,* 1959; 41(A): 147–151.

57. **Kelley, J.D. et al.** Electromyographic and cinematographic analysis of elbow function in tennis players with lateral epicondylitis. *Am. J. Sports Med.,* 1994; 22: 359–363.

58. **Khashaba, A.** Nirschl tennis elbow release with or without drilling. *Br. J. Sports Med.,* 2001; 35: 200–201.

59. **Kibler, W.B.** Pathophysiology of overload injuries around the elbow. *Clin. Sports Med.,* 1995; 14: 447–457.

60. **Kibler, W.B.** Clinical biomechanics of the elbow in tennis: implications for evaluation and diagnosis. *Med. Sci. Sports Exerc.,* 1994; 26: 1203–1206.

61. **Kivi, P.** The etiology and conservative treatment of humeral epicondylitis. *Scand. J. Rehabil. Med.,* 1982; 15: 37–41.

62. **Ko, J.Y, Chen, H.S., and Chen, L.M.** Treatment of lateral epicondylitis of the elbow with shock waves. *Clin. Orthop.,* 2001; 387: 60–67.

63. **Koudela, K. and Novak, B.** Entezopatia epicondyli humeri lateralis: termographic a termometrie loketniho kloubu. *Acta Chir. Orthop. Traumatol. Cech.,* 1985; 52: 415–416.

64. **Krischek, O. et al.** Extracorporeal shockwave therapy in epicondylitis humeri ulnaris or radialis — a prospective, controlled, comparative study. *Z. Orthop. Ihre Grenzgeb.,* 1998; 136: 3–7.

65. **Kurvers, H. and Verhaar, J.** The results of operative treatment of medial epicondylitis. *J. Bone Joint Surg. (Am.),* 1995; 77: 1374–1379.

66. **Labelle, H. et al.** Lack of scientific evidence for the treatment of lateral epicondylitis of the elbow. An attempted meta-analysis. *J. Bone Joint Surg. (Br.),* 1992; 74: 646–651.

67. **Leach, R.E. and Miller, J.K.** Lateral and medial epicondylitis of the elbow. *Clin. Sports Med.,* 1987; 6: 259–272.

68. **Le Huec, J.C. et al.** Epicondylitis after treatment with fluoroquinolone antibiotics. *J. Bone Joint Surg. Br. Vol.,* 1995; 77: 293–295.

69. **Leppilahti, J. et al.** Surgical treatment of resistant tennis elbow. A prospective randomised study comparing decompression of the posterior interosseous nerve and lengthening of the tendon of the extensor carpi radialis brevis muscle. *Arch. Orthop. Trauma Surg.,* 2001; 121: 329–332.

70. **Lewis, M. et al.** Effects of manual work on recovery from lateral epicondylitis. *Scand. J. Work Environ. Health,* 2002; 28: 109–116.

71. **Ljung, B.O., Forsgren, S., and Friden, J.** Substance P and calcitonin gene-related peptide expression: the extensor carpi radialis brevis muscle origin: implication for the etiology of tennis elbow. *J. Orthop. Res.,* 1999; 17: 554–559.

72. **Luopajaravi, T. et al.** Prevalence of tenosynovitis and other injuries of the upper extremities in repetitive work. *Scand. J. Work Environ. Health,* 1979; 5: 48–55.

73. **Madan, S. and Jowett, R.L.** Lateral epicondylalgia: treatment by manipulation under anesthetic and steroid injection and operative release. *Acta Orthop. Belg.,* 2000; 66: 449–454.

74. **Maloney, M.D., Mohr, K.J., and El Attrache, N.S.** Elbow injuries in the throwing athlete. Difficult diagnoses and surgical complications. *Clin. Sports Med.,* 1999; 18: 795–809.

75. **Molsberger, A. and Hille, E.** The analgesic effect of acupuncture in chronic tennis elbow pain. *Br. J. Rheumatol.,* 1994; 33: 1162–1165.

76. **Morre, H.H., Keizer, S.B., and van Os, J.J.** Treatment of chronic tennis elbow with botulinum toxin. *Lancet,* 1997; 349: 1746.

77. **Neviaser, T.J. et al.** Lateral epicondylitis: results outpatient surgery and immediate motion. *Contemp. Orthop.,* 1985; 11: 43–46.

78. **Nirschl, R.O.** Tennis elbow. *Orthop. Clin. North Am.,* 1973; 4: 787–800.

79. **Nirschl, R.O. and Pettrone, F.A.** Tennis elbow. *J. Bone Joint Surg.,* 1979; 61(A): 832–839.

80. **Nirschl, R.P.** Sports and overuse injuries to the elbow, in *The Elbow and Its Disorders,* Morrey, B.F., Ed. Philadelphia: W.B. Saunders, 1985; 309–341.

81. **Nirschl, R.P.** Tennis elbow (epicondylitis): surgery and rehabilitation of the professional athlete, in *AAOS Symposium on Upper Extremity Injuries in Athletes,* Pettrone, F.A., Ed. St. Louis: C.V. Mosby, 1986; 244–265.

82. **Nirschl, R.P.** Prevention and treatment of elbow and shoulder injuries in the tennis player. *Clin. Sports Med.,* 1988; 7: 289–308.

83. **Noteboom, T. et al.** Tennis elbow: a review. *J. Orthop. Sports Phys. Ther.,* 1994; 19: 357–366.

84. **O'Dwyer, K.J. and Howie, C.R.** Medial epicondylitis of the elbow. *Int. Orthop.,* 1995; 19: 69–71.

85. **Ollivierre, C.O., Nirschl, R.P., and Pettrone, F.A.** Resection and repair for medial tennis elbow. A prospective analysis. *Am. J. Sports Med.,* 1995; 23: 214–221.

86. **Organ, S.W. et al.** Salvage surgery for lateral tennis elbow. *Am. J. Sports Med.,* 1997; 25: 746–750.

87. **Owens, B.D., Murphy, K.P., and Kulko, T.R.** Arthroscopic release for lateral epicondylitis. *Arthroscopy,* 2001; 17: 582–587.

88. **Patten, R.M.** Overuse syndromes and injuries involving the elbow: MR imaging findings. *Am. J. Roentgenol.,* 1995; 164: 1205–1211.

89. **Pećina, M., Krmpotić-Nemanić, J., and Markiewitz, A.D.** *Tunnel Syndromes. Peripheral Nerve Compression Syndromes,* 3rd ed. Boca Raton, FL: CRC Press, 2001.

90. **Pedersen, L.K. and Jensen, L.K.** Relationship between occupation and elbow pain, epicondylitis. *Ugeskr. Laeg.,* 1999; 161: 4751–4755.

91. **Pfahler, M. et al.** Magnetic resonance imaging in lateral epicondylitis of the elbow. *Arch. Orthop. Trauma Surg.,* 1998; 118: 121–125.

92. **Pienimaki, T. et al.** Long-term follow-up of conservatively treated chronic tennis elbow patients. A prospective and retrospective analysis. *Scand. J. Rehabil. Med.,* 1998; 30: 159–166.

93. **Pienimaki, T. et al.** Associations between pain, grip strength, and manual tests in the treatment evaluation of chronic tennis elbow. *Clin. J. Pain,* 2002; 18: 164–170.

94. **Penners, W. et al.** Epicondylitis humeri — Tennis-Ellenbogen. *Forschr. Med.,* 1977; 95: 1587–1592.

95. **Plancher, K.D., Halbrecht, J., and Lourie, G.M.** Medial and lateral epicondylitis in athlete. *Clin. Sports Med.,* 1996; 15: 283–305.

96. **Pomerance, J.** Radiographic analysis of lateral epicondylitis. *Shoulder Elbow Surg.,* 2002; 11: 156–157.

97. **Priest, J.D., Braden, V., and Gerberich, J.G.** The elbow and tennis. *Phys. Sportsmed.,* 1980; 8: 80–88.

98. **Regan, W.D.** Lateral elbow pain in the athlete: a clinical review. *Clin. J. Sports Med.,* 1991; 1: 53–58.

99. **Regan, W. et al.** Microscopic histopathology of chronic refractory lateral epicondylitis. *Am. J. Sports Med.,* 1992; 20: 746–749.

100. **Rettig, A.C.** Elbow, forearm and wrist injuries in the athlete. *Sports Med.,* 1998; 25: 115–130.

101. **Riek, S., Carson, R.G., and Wright, A.** A new technique for the selective recording of extensor carpi radialis longus and brevis EMG. *J. Electromyogr. Kinesiol.,* 2000; 10: 249–253.

102. **Ritts, G.D., Wood, M.B., and Lindscheid, R.L.** Radial tunnel syndrome. *Clin. Orthop.,* 1987; 219: 201–205.

103. **Roles, N.C. and Maudsley, R.H.** Radial tunnel syndrome: resistant tennis elbow as a nerve entrapment. *J. Bone Joint Surg.,* 1972; 54(B): 499–508.

104. **Rompe, J.D. et al.** Analgesic effect of extracorporeal shock-wave therapy on chronic tennis elbow. *J. Bone Joint Surg. (Br.),* 1996; 78: 233–237.

105. **Rompe, J.D. et al.** Low-energy extracorporeal shock wave therapy for persistent tennis elbow. *Int. Orthop.,* 1996; 20: 23–27.

106. **Routson, G.W. and Gingras, M.** Surgical treatment of tennis elbow. *Orthopaedics,* 1981; 4: 769–772.

107. **Schauss, S. et al.** Effectiveness of epicondylitis bandages from the biomechanical viewpoint — an experimental study. *Z. Orthop. Ihre Grenzgeb.,* 2000; 138: 492–495.

108. **Shilo, R., Engel, J., Farin, I., and Horochowski, H.** Thermography as a diagnostic aid in tennis elbow. *Handchirurgie,* 1976; 8: 101–103.

109. **Smidt, N. et al.** Corticosteroid injections, physiotherapy, or a wait-and-see policy for lateral epicondylitis: a randomised controlled trial. *Lancet,* 2002; 359: 657–662.

110. **Smidt, N. et al.** Corticosteroid injections for lateral epicondylitis: a systematic review. *Pain,* 2002; 96: 23–40.

111. **Solveborn, S.A.** Radial epicondylalgia ("tennis elbow"): treatment with stretching or forearm band. A prospective study with long-term follow-up including range-of-motion measurements. *Scand. J. Med. Sci. Sports,* 1997; 7: 229–237.

112. **Solveborn, S.A.** "Tennis elbow" is usually caused by other than tennis. The earlier the treatment the better; spontaneous remission occur often within 8–13 months. *Lakartidningen,* 1999; 96: 483–485.

113. **Solveborn, S.A. et al.** Cortisone injection with anesthetic additives for radial epicondylalgia (tennis elbow). *Clin. Orthop.,* 1995; 316: 99–105.

114. **Stangl, P.C. and Freilinger, G.** Long-term results of the Wilhelm denervation operation in epicondylitis humeri radialis (tennis elbow). *Handchir. Mikrochir. Plast. Chirurg.,* 1993; 25: 121–123.

115. **Stelzle, F.D., Gaulrapp, H., and Pforringer, W.** Injuries and overuse syndromes due to rock climbing on artificial walls. *Sportverletz. Sportschaden,* 2000; 14: 128–133.

116. **Steinborn, M. et al.** Magnetic resonance imaging of lateral epicondylitis of the elbow with a 0.2-T dedicated system. *Eur. Radiol.,* 1999; 9(7): 1376–1380.

117. **Stockard, A.R.** Elbow injuries in golf. *J. Am. Osteopath. Assoc.,* 2001; 101: 509–516.

118. **Stotz, R., Firkowiez, M., and Muller, J.** Beitrag zur operativen Therapie der Epicondylitis humeri radialis. *Helv. Chir. Acta,* 1984; 51: 189–193.

119. **Sugimoto, H. and Ohsawa, T.** Ulnar collateral ligament in the growing elbow: MR imaging of normal development and throwing injuries. *Radiology,* 1994; 192: 417–422.

120. **Tam, G.** Low power laser therapy and analgesic action. *J. Clin. Laser Med. Surg.,* 1999; 17: 29–33.

121. **Theriault, G. and Lachance, P.** Golf injuries. An overview. *Sports Med.,* 1998; 26: 43–57.

122. **Thomas, D. et al.** Computerized infrared thermography and isotopic bone scanning in tennis elbow. *Ann. Rheum. Dis.,* 1992; 51: 103–107.

123. **Vangsness, C.T. and Jobe, F.W.** Surgical treatment of medial epicondylitis. *J. Bone Joint Surg.,* 1991; 73(B): 409–411.

124. **Verhaar, J.A.** Tennis elbow. Anatomical, epidemiological and therapeutic aspects. *Int. Orthop.,* 1994; 18: 263–267.

125. **Verhaar, J. et al.** Lateral extensor release for tennis elbow. A prospective long-term follow-up study. *J. Bone Joint Surg. (Am.),* 1993; 75: 1034–1043.

126. **Verhaar, J.A. et al.** Local corticosteroid injection versus Cyriax-type physiotherapy for tennis elbow. *J. Bone Joint Surg. Br. Vol.,* 1996; 78: 128–132.

127. **Vogt, J.C.** Long term result of surgical treatment of epicondylitis. A propos of 26 cases. *J. Chirurg.,* 1994; 131: 358–362.

128. **Wadswort, T.G.** Tennis elbow: conservative, surgical and manipulative treatment. *Br. Med. J.,* 1987; 294: 621–624.

129. **Wang, C.J. and Chen, H.S.** Shock wave therapy for patients with lateral epicondylitis of the elbow: a one- to two-year follow-up study. *Am. J. Sports Med.,* 2002; 30: 422–425.

130. **Warren, R.F.** Tennis elbow (epicondylitis): epidemiology and conservative treatment, in *AAOS Symposium on Upper Extremity Injuries in Athletes,* Pettrone, F.A., Ed. St. Louis: C.V. Mosby, 1986; 233–243.

131. **Wanivenhaus, A., Kickinger, W., and Zweymuller, K.** Die Epicondylitis humeri radialis unter besonderer Berücksichtigung der Operation nach Wilhelm. *Wien. Klin. Wochenschr.,* 1986; 98: 338–341.

132. **Werner, C.O.** Lateral elbow pain and posterior interosseous nerve entrapment. *Acta Orthop. Scand.,* 1979; 174(Suppl.): 1–110.

133. **Wilhelm, A.** Tennis elbow: treatment of resistant cases by denervation. *J. Hand Surg. (Br.),* 1996; 21: 523–533.

134. **Wilhelm, A.** Treatment of therapy refractory epicondylitis lateralis humeri by denervation. On the pathogenesis. *Handchir. Mikrochir. Plast. Chir.,* 1999; 31: 291–302.

135. **Wilson, J.F. and Davis, J.S.** Tennis racket shock mitigation experiments. *J. Biomech. Eng.*, 1995; 117: 479–484.

136. **Wuori, J.L. et al.** Strength and pain measures associated with lateral epicondylitis bracing. *Arch. Phys. Med. Rehabil.*, 1998; 79: 832–837.

137. **Yerger, B. and Turner, T.** Percutaneous extensor tenotomy for chronic tennis elbow. *Orthopaedics*, 1985; 8: 1261–1263.

138. **Yocum, L.A.** The diagnosis and nonoperative treatment of elbow problems in the athlete. *Clin. Sports Med.*, 1989; 8: 439–451.

Posterior Impingement Syndrome of the Elbow

139. **Awaya, H. et al.** Elbow synovial fold syndrome: MR imaging findings. *Am. J. Roentgenol.*, 2001; 177: 1377–1381.

140. **Baker, C.L., Jr. and Jones, G.L.** Arthroscopy of the elbow. *Am. J. Sports Med.*, 1999; 27: 251–264.

141. **Billi, A. et al.** Joint impingement syndrome: clinical features. *Eur. J. Radiol.*, 1998; 27(Suppl. 1): 39–41.

142. **Eriksson, E. and Denti, M.** Diagnostic and operative arthroscopy of the shoulder and elbow joint. *Ital. J. Sports Trauma*, 1985; 7: 165–188.

143. **Ferrara, M.A. and Marcelis, S.** Ultrasound of the elbow. *J. Belg. Radiol.*, 1997; 80: 122–123.

144. **Ferrara, M.A. et al.** Modifications of the elbow induced by the practice of handball on radiography, US and MRI. *J. Belg. Radiol.*, 1999; 82: 222–227.

145. **Garrick, G.J. and Requa, R.K.** Epidemiology of women's gymnastics injuries. *Am. J. Sports Med.*, 1980; 8: 261–264.

146. **Garrick, G.J. and Webb, R.D.**, *Sports Injuries: Diagnosis and Management*, Philadelphia: W.B. Saunders, 1990.

147. **Micheli, L.J. et al.** Elbow arthroscopy in the pediatric and adolescent population. *Arthroscopy*, 2001; 17: 694–699.

148. **Moskal, M.J., Savoie, F.H., III, and Field, L.D.** Elbow arthroscopy in trauma and reconstruction. *Orthop. Clin. North Am.*, 1999; 30: 163–177.

149. **Nirschl, R.P.** Prevention and treatment of elbow and shoulder injuries in the tennis player. *Clin. Sports Med.*, 1988; 7: 289–308.

150. **Ogilvie-Harris, D.J., Gordon, R., and MacKay, M.** Arthroscopic treatment for posterior impingement in degenerative arthritis of the elbow. *Arthroscopy*, 1995; 11: 437–443.

151. **Wilson, F.D. et al.** Valgus extension overload in the pitching elbow. *Am. J. Sports Med.*, 1983; 11: 83–88.

152. **Woods, G.W.** Elbow arthroscopy. *Clin. Sports Med.*, 1987; 6: 557–564.

Medial Tension/Lateral Compression Syndrome

153. **Andrews, J.R. and Carson, W.G.** Arthroscopy of the elbow. *Arthroscopy*, 1985; 1: 97–107.

154. **Barnes, D.A. and Tullos, H.S.** An analysis of 100 symptomatic baseball players. *Am. J. Sports Med.*, 1978; 6: 62–67.

155. **Blohm, D., Kaalund, S., and Jakobsen, B.W.** "Little League elbow" — acute traction apophysitis in an adolescent badminton player. *Scand. J. Med. Sci. Sports*, 1999; 9: 245–247.

156. **Caldwell, G.L. and Safran, M.R.** Elbow problems in the athlete. *Orthop. Clin. North Am.*, 1995; 26: 465–485.

157. **Clain, M.R. and Hershman, E.B.** Overuse injuries in children and adolescents. *Phys. Sportsmed.*, 1989; 17: 111–123.

158. **Cotten, A., Boutin, R.D., and Resnick, D.** Normal anatomy of the elbow on conventional MR imaging and MR arthrography. *Semin. Musculoskel. Radiol.*, 1998; 2: 133–140.

159. **Desharnais, L., Kaplan, P.A., and Dussault, R.G.** MR imaging of ligamentous abnormalities of the elbow. *Magn. Reson. Imaging Clin. North Am.*, 1997; 5: 515–528.

160. **Garrick, G.J. and Webb, R.D.**, *Sports Injuries: Diagnosis and Management*. Philadelphia: W.B. Saunders, 1990.

161. **Ireland, M.L. and Andrews, J.R.** Shoulder and elbow injuries in the young athletes. *Clin. Sports Med.,* 1988; 7: 473–494.

162. **Kocher, M.S., Waters, P.M., and Micheli, L.J.** Upper extremity injuries in the paediatric athlete. *Sports Med.,* 2000; 30: 117–135.

163. **Kiyoshige, Y.** Closed-wedge osteotomy for osteochondritis dissecans of the capitellum. A 7- to 12-year follow-up. *Am. J. Sports Med.,* 2000; 28: 534–537.

164. **Lowery, W.D., Jr., et al.** Persistence of the olecranon physis: a cause of "Little League elbow." *J. Shoulder Elbow Surg.,* 1995; 4: 143–147.

165. **McManama, G.B., Jr., et al.** The surgical treatment of osteochondritis of the capitellum. *Am. J. Sports Med.,* 1985; 13: 11–21.

166. **Podesta, L., Sherman, M.F., and Bonamo, J.R.** Distal humeral epiphyseal separation in a young athlete: a case report. *Arch. Phys. Med. Rehabil.,* 1993; 74: 1216–1218.

5 Forearm and Hand

The wrist and hand comprise a large number of tendons and play an important role in work and sports; thus, overuse injuries are quite common in these regions. The injuries are often characterized by tendinitis or tenosynovitis.[6,21,26,58,90] Principal symptoms are pain and tenderness in the affected tendon or tendons. Pain increases with passive extension of the tendon or with contraction of the appropriate muscle against resistance.[40] The most common overuse injury of the wrist joint is known as *de Quervain disease* and is characterized by inflammation of the tendons passing through the fibro-osseous tunnel of the first dorsal compartment of the wrist at the level of the radial styloid, i.e., m. abductor pollicis longus and m. extensor pollicis brevis. Flexor carpi ulnaris tendinitis is a relatively common overuse wrist injury in athletes, whereas flexor carpi radialis tendinitis occurs much more rarely. Rowers and weight lifters, to a greater degree than other athletes, often suffer from intersection syndrome, also known as *oarsman's wrist*. Dorsal radiocarpal impingement syndrome is common in gymnasts, which, in sports medicine, is often referred to as *gymnast's wrist*. Trigger finger may also be included in overuse wrist syndromes. Long-term sports or working activity may cause the development of nerve entrapment syndromes — carpal tunnel and Guyon's tunnel in particular.

Actually, overuse injuries of the forearm and hand are large problems for people who work with computer keyboards ("crippled by computer"). The problem, more commonly known as *repetitive stress injury* (RSI), now strikes an estimated 185,000 U.S. office and factory workers a year. The cases account for more than half of U.S. occupational illnesses, compared with about 20% a decade ago.

I. DE QUERVAIN DISEASE

De Quervain disease implies inflammation of the tendons of the abductor pollicis longus muscle and the extensor pollicis brevis muscle as they pass through the first dorsal compartment of the wrist, about 3 cm proximal to the radial styloid (Figure 5.1). Thickening of tendinous membranes leads to stricture of the lumen of the first carpal canal. Also, thickening of the tendons distally from the narrowed compartment may often be noticed. After passing through the first carpal compartment, the tendons bend at a certain angle, which is somewhat larger in females; this angulation is accentuated by wrist ulnar deviation.[4] As a result, frequent repetitive ulnar abduction of the wrist causes irritation of tendons and their membranes. Naturally, irritation may be caused by altered osseous surface of the radial styloid as well.[15] In athletes, manual workers,[62,86] physical laborers, and especially drummers,[23] in whom the activity of the thumb is particularly emphasized, tenosynovitis of the first carpal compartment usually takes place. De Quervain disease develops more often when engaging in racket sports (tennis, squash),[72,90] but is also seen in athletic throwing disciplines, volleyball,[10] and rock climbing,[34,65] as well as in pianists.[20,61] The condition is more common in females (seven to nine times) than in males because of the greater tendinous angulation and greater range of ulnar wrist abduction in females. In 1895, de Quervain reported on five women with stenosing tendovaginitis.[19,84] However, in the 13th edition of *Gray's Anatomy* (1893), there is a description of identical changes in the first carpal compartment called *washerwoman's sprain*.[46]

According to Clarke et al.,[17] the term *stenosing tenovaginitis,* or *tenosynovitis,* is a misnomer; they argue that on the basis of histopathological investigations de Quervain disease is a result of intrinsic degenerative mechanisms rather than extrinsic, inflammatory mechanisms.

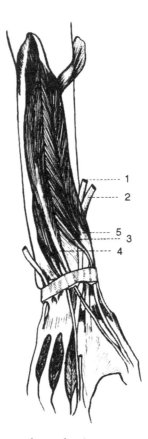

FIGURE 5.1 Muscles of the first three carpal tunnels. (1) extensor carpi radialis brevis muscle; (2) extensor carpi radialis longus muscle; (3) extensor pollicis brevis muscle; (4) extensor pollicis longus muscle; (5) abductor pollicis longus muscle.

Clinically, pain is dominant with this condition, especially in the area of the radial styloid.[54] Patients also complain of pain on ulnar deviation and closing of the hand. Pain may radiate to the proximal forearm or distally into the thumb. The pain becomes progressively worse so that patients eventually are unable to use their hand. On physical examination, there is localized tenderness and often soft-tissue swelling at the radial styloid. There may be palpable thickening, ganglion cyst formation, and crepitus over the first dorsal compartment. Diagnosis is confirmed on the basis of a positive Finkelstein's test (Figure 5.2). In this maneuver, the patient's wrist is passively ulnar-deviated while the thumb is held adducted in the palm. A positive test is indicated by pain in the region of the radial styloid. The test may also be positive in patients with basal thumb-joint (carpometacarpal, scaphoidotrapeziotrapezoidal, or radioscaphoid joints) arthrosis or intersection syndrome. To minimize false-positive tests, the ulnar deviation stress should be applied to the metacarpal of the index finger. Only rarely can radiographic examination reveal irregularity of osseous surface or thickening of the periosteum in the region of the first carpal compartment.

Even if de Quervain disease is also known as stenosing tendovaginitis, clinical finding of a trigger thumb is extremely rare in this condition.[1,81] Trigger thumb usually develops as the extensor pollicis brevis tendon passes in a separate fibrous compartment through the first carpal canal. Research has shown evidence of partial or complete septation of the dorsal compartment of the wrist in about 40% of people[36,41] and in Asians in 77.5% of wrists.[50] This fact is important, especially in view of operative treatment of de Quervain disease. In diagnosis of de Quervain disease it is possible to use different diagnostic imaging techniques, i.e., ultrasonography,[27,51,57,76] magnetic resonance imaging,[28] and scintigraphy,[70] but ultrasound examination appears to be the most appropriate and

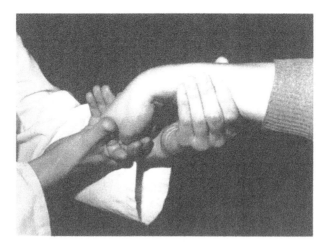

FIGURE 5.2 Finkelstein's test.

advantageous method as it reveals involvement of the sheaths and tendons in the simplest, most complete, and least expensive manner. In differential diagnosis of de Quervain disease it is particularly important to identify an associated Wartenberg's radial nerve entrapment syndrome.[44]

Initial treatment is always non-operative and entails avoidance of aggravating activity, reduction of overall activity, and administration of nonsteroid anti-inflammatory medication.[9] Immobilization of the forearm, wrist, and thumb (to the distal interphalangeal skin fold) in a splint (the so-called thumb spica splint) causes symptoms to disappear in more than 70% of patients.[89] Local administration of corticosteroids and anesthetics into the first carpal compartment is also part of non-operative treatment.[5,43,63,67,82,93] This brings dramatic relief, although unfortunately only temporarily, as it cannot prevent the disease from recurring. Generally, steroid injections should be limited to two or three injections over a 6-month period; usually, the second and third injections are less effective than the initial one. In an advanced stage of de Quervain disease, characterized by marked stenosis and thickening of tendinous membranes, surgical treatment is the only recourse available.[2,3,33,52,74,83,88,92] Surgery consists of decompression and release of the first dorsal compartment and also obligatory removal of the altered segments of tendinous membranes. Either a transverse or longitudinal incision may be used. Care should be taken to avoid any undue traction on the radial sensory nerve. The compartment should be released on its dorsal aspect to prevent subluxation of the tendons volarly with the thumb motion. Failure of surgical treatment is usually ascribed to inability to identify such possible anatomic abnormalities as the presence of a separate fibro-osseous canal for each tendon or the presence of multiple tendons of the abductor pollicis longus muscle.[48] Quite often during surgery only the abductor pollicis longus tendon is decompressed while the extensor pollicis brevis tendon remains intact in its separate compartment; this is the most common cause of repetitive complaints. Wetterkamp et al.[83] within a period of 6 years operated on 109 patients with de Quervain disease. Of the patients, 82% recovered completely and 18% had slight residual complaints, e.g., stress-dependent discomfort and irritations of the superficial radial nerve. For treatment of recurrent de Quervain tendonitis Wilson et al.[88] used the distally based radial forearm fascia-fat flap to create a fascial tube. In a study of Ta et al.[74] the cure rate of surgery, defined as the percentage of patients without postoperative complication, was 91%, with 88% of patients indicating full satisfaction.

II. TENOSYNOVITIS OF OTHER DORSAL COMPARTMENTS

In addition to the first dorsal compartment, tenosynovitis may develop in all other dorsal compartments of the wrist (Figure 5.3). Most often this occurs in the sixth compartment through which

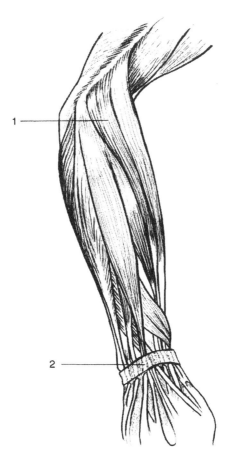

FIGURE 5.3 Radial and dorsal muscles of the forearm. (1) Lateral epicondyle; (2) extensor retinaculum.

the extensor carpi ulnaris tendon passes,[18,71] and second most often in the second compartment through which the extensor carpi radialis longus and brevis tendons pass. Tenosynovitis in the second carpal compartment should not be mistaken for oarsman's wrist (intersection syndrome). Tenosynovitis of the fourth and fifth carpal compartment is extremely rare. Individuals presenting with extensor tenosynovitis and lacking a history of direct trauma or overuse should be evaluated for systemic inflammatory disease, such as rheumatoid arthritis. Signs of fourth-compartment tenosynovitis included dorsal wrist pain with normal wrist motion, localized swelling, and tenderness over the fourth dorsal compartment. Conservative treatment may fail owing to intrusion of an anomalous muscle belly into the fourth dorsal compartment. The musculotendinous junction of the extensor indicis proprius protrudes into, or entirely through, the fourth dorsal compartment in 75% of individuals.[23] Ritter and Inglis[64] first reported hypertrophy of this muscle and secondary tenosynovitis in two athletes. Swelling distal to the extensor retinaculum may be a manifestation of hypertrophy of an extensor digitorum brevis manus muscle. This rare muscle originates from the wrist capsule or the base of the metacarpals and inserts into the extensor hood of the index and middle fingers. Tenosynovitis of the third carpal compartment, through which the extensor pollicis longus tendon passes, usually develops as a consequence of changes in the radius following malunion after fractures so that rupture of the extensor pollicis longus tendon often occurs. Tenosynovitis of the extensor pollicis longus and subsequent rupture of the tendon were first reported in Prussian drummers,[23] hence the name "drummer boy's palsy." The extensor pollicis longus is at risk of developing tenosynovitis as it passes around Lister's tubercule and any activity, either occupational or sports related, that requires repetitive thumb and wrist motion can induce tenosynovitis. Fulcher et al.[24] have occasionally seen this rare entity in squash players. Stenosing tenosynovitis of the fifth dorsal compartment has been reported after wrist trauma and rarely after overuse. An anomalous muscle belly may be found protruding into the fifth dorsal compartment and multiple slips of the extensor digiti quinti can be expected in 93% of individuals.

As a rule, treatment is non-operative. Only in the tenosynovitis of the sixth carpal compartment (extensor carpi ulnaris muscle) is surgery required due to thickening of the membranes or formation of calcifications. Steffens and Koob[71] have collected 28 cases of stenosing tenosynovitis over the dorsum of the wrist in the sixth compartment. All 28 patients had local infiltration with cortisone, but only 8 patients obtained complete relief; 18 of 20 patients obtained complete relief of their symptoms after surgical release of the sixth compartment. In 7 of the 15 patients described by Crimmins and Jones[18] initial treatment consisting of splinting and steroid injection failed and surgical release of the sixth compartment was required. All but one patient had a good or excellent result. Sports injuries often cause lesions in the sixth carpal compartment, specifically in terms of the sixth compartment ulnar wall rupture; this usually leads to recurrent subluxation of the extensor carpi ulnaris tendon.[12,47,66] The rupture may occur upon sudden supination, ulnar deviation, and volar flexion. It has been reported in tennis players, golfers, and weight lifters. The patient usually complains of a clicking sensation with forearm rotation, and subluxation of the extensor carpi ulnaris can be visibly palpated and observed. On supination with wrist ulnar deviation, the tendon often displaces with an audible snap when moved in the ulnar and palmar directions. On pronation, it relocates into its normal sulcus. The condition must be differentiated from recurrent subluxation of the distal radioulnar joint. Recurrent subluxation of the extensor carpi ulnaris tendon is treated surgically because reconstruction of the sixth carpal compartment is necessary on the dorsal wrist aspect; it is usually performed by using the extensor retinaculum. The extensor carpi ulnaris can be stabilized by creating a sling of extensor retinaculum or with a free retinacular graft.

III. INTERSECTION SYNDROME (OARSMAN'S WRIST)

Intersection syndrome is an overuse syndrome known by various other terms: peritendinitis crepitans, abductor pollicis longus bursitis, squeaker's wrist, oarsman's wrist, and crossover tendinitis. The condition usually develops at the site where the tendons of the extensor pollicis brevis and abductor pollicis longus (muscles of the first dorsal compartment of the wrist) pass across the extensor carpi radialis longus muscle and the extensor carpi radialis brevis muscle (the muscles of the second dorsal compartment of the wrist) (Figure 5.1 and Figure 5.3). The typical repetitive wrist motions (extension and radial deviation) cause inflammation of the bursa (according to some authors) normally found there; according to others, this develops as a result of a long-term friction and degenerative changes in abductor pollicis muscle and extensor pollicis brevis muscle bellies or hypertrophy of the same muscles bellies, with these muscles causing pressure on the underlying radial wrist extensors. In one 4-year prospective study the prevalence of intersection syndrome was found to be 0.37% of all patients with arm or hand pain.[60] Athletes who suffer from this disorder more often than others are rowers, canoeists, weight lifters, tennis players, indoor racket sportsmen,[68] hockey players, and athletic throwers. Painful crepitation with wrist movement as well as weak pinch and diminished grasp are the major symptoms. On physical examination, palpatory tenderness and soft-tissue swelling over the radiodorsal aspect of the distal forearm about 6 to 8 cm proximal to the Lister's tubercle are found.[30] The crepitus, which in some instances may be more like a "squeak," is palpable and audible; this usually occurs during wrist motion and upon palpation of the painful site. Non-operative treatment consists of avoidance of aggravating activity, immobilization in a splint, and nonsteroidal anti-inflammatory medication.[86] Direct steroid injection may be indicated and is usually curative. Intersection syndrome responds favorably to conservative treatment;[32,60,91] operative exploration and excision of the bursa are rarely required. If performed, surgery should be followed by prolonged protection from the aggravating stresses. Wulle[91] performs synoviectomy and incision of the thick fascia of the abductor pollicis longus muscle.

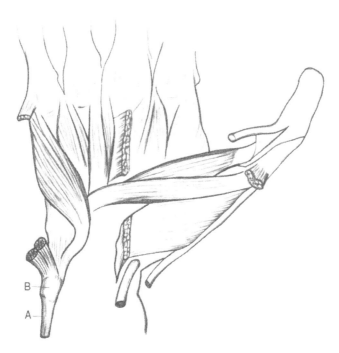

FIGURE 5.4 The relationship of the ulnar carpal flexor tendon muscle (A) to the pisiform bone (B).

IV. FLEXOR CARPI ULNARIS TENDINITIS

In view of the importance of muscle in wrist motions, flexor carpi ulnaris tendinitis is a relatively frequent condition that affects athletes, especially those involved in golf and racket sports, and others who engage in activities involving repetitive wrist motions. Tenderness and a painful tendon in the wrist joint increase with wrist flexion and ulnar deviation against resistance. The flexor carpi ulnaris tendon ends at the pisiform bone, while the pisohamate and pisometacarpal ligament attach the pisiform bone to the hamate and fifth metacarpal bone. It actually means that the flexor carpi ulnaris tendon ends at the hamate and metacarpal bone, while the pisiform bone, similar to the sesamoid bone, is an integral part of the tendon itself (Figure 5.4). A synovial sac (bursa) may be found between the tendon and pisiform bone; the pisiform bone also joins with the triquetrum bone. The pisiform bone may become the source of pain, also described as *enthesitis ossis pisiform* by those who consider the flexor carpi ulnaris muscle to be attached to the pisiform bone.[53] However, pain and tenderness in the pisiform bone region may be caused by irritation of the above-mentioned bursa in such a way that it envelops the pisiform bone so that bursitis may be the issue. Also, degenerative changes may take place between the pisiform bone and the triquetrum bone (osteoarthritis). During wrist flexion, when the examiner moves the pisiform bone radially and ulnarly, pain and occasionally crepitus will occur ("pisotriquetral grind test"). Paley et al.[59] examined 216 case reports published in the world medical literature and concluded that in 44.6% of cases, the patients suffered from enthesitis m. flexor carpi ulnaris or enthesitis of the pisiform bone, while in the remaining cases the patients had primary or secondary osteoarthritis in the pisotriquetral joint.

Treatment of flexor carpi ulnaris tendinitis consists of avoidance of aggravating motions, i.e., rest, immobilization of the wrist in a splint, and administration of nonsteroidal anti-inflammatory drugs and physical therapy. In the case of pisiform bone enthesitis, bursitis, or arthrosis in the pisotriquestral joint that do not respond to non-operative treatment procedures, surgery may be contemplated in the form of pisiform bone excision.[14] The pisiform bone is removed subperiosteally, preserving the continuity of the flexor carpi ulnaris tendon; during this procedure, lysis of peritendinous adhesions is also performed if they are present. Some authors[24] recommend the addition of a 5-mm Z-plasty lengthening of the flexor carpi ulnaris tendon. At times, calcium deposits may be found either adhering to or within the tendon, and these should also be removed.

V. FLEXOR CARPI RADIALIS TENDINITIS

Flexor carpi radialis tendinitis occurs much more rarely than tendinitis of the ulnar aspect of the wrist joint, primarily because the motion of the wrist joint in its radial aspect is much more limited when compared with the ulnar side. In the case of flexor carpi radialis tendinitis, wrist flexion against resistance and passive extension causes pain in the affected tendon. The flexor carpi radialis muscle (Figure 5.5) at about the midportion of the forearm continues into the tendon that passes over the carpal root in a separate compartment formed laterally and dorsally by the scaphoid and trapezoid bones, palmarly by the flexor retinaculum, and medially (ulnarly) by the carpi radiatum ligament; this is also a borderline case of carpal tunnel.[8] The tendon inserts into the palmar surface of the base of the second metacarpal bone. When passing through its own osseofibrous canal, the tendon is surrounded by the synovial sheath (vagina synovialis). Accordingly, clinical symptoms of stenosing tenosynovitis of the flexor carpi radialis may occasionally develop. Synovitis may be visible and palpable just proximal to the wrist crease overlying the flexor carpi radialis tendon. Untreated synovitis can cause restrictive adhesions that may produce pain on passive wrist extension. Rupture of the tendon may be the end result of invasive synovitis. The tendon stump and the surrounding inflammatory tissue may present as a tender mass at the wrist flexion creases and may

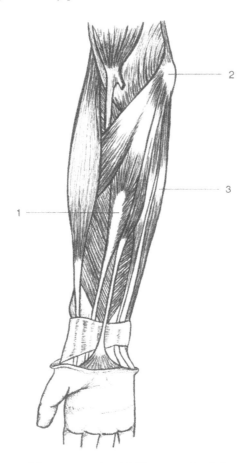

FIGURE 5.5 The palmar group of forearm muscles. (1) Flexor carpi radialis muscle, (2) epicondylus ulnaris (medialis), (3) flexor carpi ulnaris muscle.

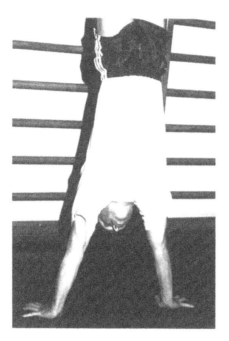

FIGURE 5.6 A cause of gymnast's wrist.

be confused with a palmar carpal ganglion. These symptoms may require surgical treatment in terms of canal decompression. Surgical release should be carried far enough distally to assure that the tunnel has been completely decompressed.[25] In the majority of cases, tendinitis and tenosynovitis of the flexor carpi radialis are treated non-operatively (wrist immobilization, anti-inflammatory agents, and corticosteroid injections).

VI. DORSAL RADIOCARPAL IMPINGEMENT SYNDROME (GYMNAST'S WRIST)

Repetitive wrist dorsiflexion, especially when performed with an extra load or force as in gymnastics during beam exercises, floor exercises (Figure 5.6), or jumping, may cause the formation of impingement syndrome in the dorsal aspect of the radiocarpal joint; this is often the reason for pain in the wrist joint in gymnasts.[26,29,35,39] Dorsal radiocarpal impingement syndrome is of twofold significance: (1) it causes discomfort and inability to perform exercises, and (2) in its differential diagnosis, it is of utmost importance not to overlook other possible causes of pain in the wrist joint, especially the possibility of fractures of the carpal bones, tears of the triangular fibrocartilage cartilage complex, ulnar impaction syndrome, dorsal wrist capsulitis, distal radius physeal injury, dorsal wrist ganglion, and stress fracture. Studies have indicated that 73% of gymnasts experience wrist pain, and it can also occur in participants in racket sports, golf,[56] weight lifting, martial arts, biking, and softball.[40] Pain in the dorsal aspect of the wrist root is the most characteristic sign of the disorder, and its onset is associated with an athletic or work activity. In cases when symptoms persist for a longer period of time, reduced and painful dorsal flexion of the wrist in regular everyday activities commonly results. In gymnasts dorsal wrist pain described as an intense pain across the dorsum of the wrist exacerbated by hyperextension is most likely a capsulitis. The onset of dorsal wrist pain is usually insidious and tends to increase with activity. Pain may occur with vaulting, floor exercise, or pommel horse maneuvers during which the wrist is forced into hyperdorsiflexion with compression or torsion. During the pommel horse exercise, the gymnast uses the wrist as a rigid structure to support his body weight. The wrist is subjected to high-intensity impact and stress from repetition. During the front scissors maneuver, the wrist may bear loads averaging 1 to 1.5 times body weight. The duration of the exercise and the force generated during a dismount maneuver increase the risk of injury.[29]

Clinical examination reveals pain and tenderness along the dorsal aspect of the radiocarpal joint, and pain may be elicited by a sudden dorsiflexion of the joint. Painful and limited dorsal flexion of the hand joint is a common finding. Radiology is helpful in differential diagnosis of the impingement syndrome, especially because of the possibility of carpal bone fractures, aseptic necrosis of carpal bones and their stress fractures, injuries of distal radial epiphysis, and subluxation of the lunate bone. Only in exceptional cases will radiograms of the wrist joint in lateral and neutral positions and also at full dorsal flexion show that osseous contact really exists between the radius and carpal bones, causing dorsiflexion block in the wrist joint. Bone scans help to differentiate stress fracture and are recommended as an obligatory diagnostic procedure if the symptoms persist after 2 weeks of treatment for dorsal radiocarpal impingement syndrome. Rest, application of ice, and nonsteroidal anti-inflammatory medication are essential for treatment. Relative rest means a limited wrist dorsiflexion that can be achieved by specially designed dorsal immobilization of the wrist using the so-called gym cuff or a special adhesive bandage for the joint.

Rehabilitation is aimed at strengthening the wrist flexor muscles to achieve dynamic limitation of the joint dorsiflexion. The extension exercises aimed at achieving a greater range of motion need not always yield the expected results. In the majority of cases, appropriate resting, symptomatic therapy, and physical therapy lead to cessation of the symptoms.

VII. TRIGGER FINGER

When active flexion or extension of the finger is either difficult or impossible, the condition is known as *trigger finger*. If flexion or extension of the finger is actively performed with difficulty or if, when performed passively, a clicking sound is heard, the finger is behaving as if it were pulling a trigger, as shown in Figure 5.7. Stenosing tendovaginitis of flexor tendons (most often of the middle finger, then the thumb, and the ring finger) is the pathoanatomic background. Thickening or widening of the flexor tendon has been found at its passing through the tendinous sheath compartment on the palmar aspect of the finger in the region of the metacarpophalangeal joint (Figure 5.7). However, sometimes the width of the tendon is normal but the compartment is narrow

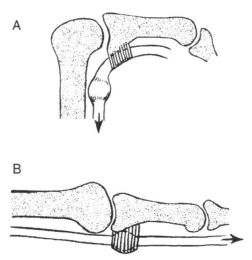

FIGURE 5.7 Trigger finger. (A) During finger flexion, the thickening of the tendon is situated proximally to the annular ligament. (B) During extension, the entrance is difficult due to the thickening; at a certain point (snapping), it enters under the annular ligament.

because the sheath is thickened. Katzman et al.[38] found that 31% of patients had radiographic abnormalities that were currently clinically significant. No radiographic finding changed management. Patients with stenosing flexor tenosynovitis without a history of injury or inflammatory arthritis do not need routine radiographs. Color Doppler ultrasound examinations may offer the opportunity to study the dynamic characteristic of tendons.[13]

The lesion occurs more often in women and is common in the right hand. Some authors ascribe this condition to chronic trauma, thus justifying its classification as an overuse syndrome, [75,80,90] and others think that trigger finger is not always work related.[37,77] About 19% of climbers have evidence of a digital pulley injury, and this type of the injury is known as "climber's finger."

Non-operative treatment consisting of rest splinting,[45] or corticosteroid injections into the tendon sheath, may be successful[11,22,42,55] Treatment of trigger fingers with a local injection of steroids is a simple and safe procedure, but the risk of recurrence in the first year is considerable.[79] The study of Benson and Ptaszek[7] suggests that surgical management may be the next best option in patients with trigger finger who continue to be symptomatic after a single injection. When the surgery is required[49] it is performed by a longitudinal discission of the tendon sheath in the region of the metacarpophalangeal joint. Surgical division of the A1 pulley can be performed percutaneously[16,31,73] or by open release.[78,87] Although steroid injections should remain the initial remedy for most trigger fingers, surgical intervention is highly successful when conservative treatment fails and should be considered for patients desiring quick and definitive relief from this disability.[78]

REFERENCES

1. **Alberton, G.M. et al.** Extensor triggering in de Quervain's stenosing tenosynovitis. *J. Hand Surg. Am.*, 1999; 24: 1311–1314.
2. **Alexander, R.D. et al.** The extensor pollicis brevis entrapment test in the treatment of de Quervain's disease. *J. Hand Surg. Am.*, 2002; 27: 813–816.
3. **Apimonbutr, P. and Budhraja, N.** Intra-operative "passive gliding" technique for de Quervain disease: a prospective study. *J. Med. Assoc. Thailand*, 2001; 84: 1455–1459.
4. **Arons, M.S.** De Quervain's release in working women: a report of failures, complications, and associated diagnosis. *J. Hand Surg.*, 1987; 12A: 540–544.
5. **Backstrom, K.M.** Mobilization with movement as an adjunct intervention in a patient with complicated de Quervain's tenosynovitis: a case report. *J. Orthop. Sports Phys. Ther.*, 2002; 32: 86–94.
6. **Batt, M.E.** A survey of golf injuries in amateur golfers. *Br. J. Sports Med.*, 1992; 26: 63–65.
7. **Benson, L.S. and Ptaszek, A.J.** Injection versus surgery in the treatment of trigger finger. *J. Hand Surg. Am.*, 1997; 22: 138–144.
8. **Bishop, A.T., Gabel, G.T., and Carmichael, S.W.** Flexor carpi radialis tendinitis. Part I: Operative anatomy. *J. Bone Joint Surg. Am.*, 1994; 76: 1009–1014.
9. **Bilić, R., Kolundćić, R., and Jelić, M.** Overuse injuries syndromes of the hand, forearm and elbow. *Arh. Hig. Rada Toksikol.*, 2001; 52: 403–414.
10. **Briner, W.W., Jr. and Kacmar, L.** Common injuries in volleyball. Mechanisms of injury, prevention and rehabilitation. *Sports Med.*, 1997; 24: 65–71.
11. **Buch-Jaeger, N. et al.** The results of conservative management of trigger finger. A series of 169 patients. *Ann. Chir. Main Memb. Super.*, 1992; 11: 189–193.
12. **Burkhart, S.S., Wood, M.B., and Linschied, R.L.** Posttraumatic recurrent subluxation of the extensor carpi ulnaris tendon. *J. Hand Surg.*, 1982; 7: 1–3.
13. **Buyruk, H.M. et al.** Doppler ultrasound examination of hand tendon pathologies. A preliminary report. *J. Hand Surg. Br.*, 1996; 21: 469–473.
14. **Carrol, R.E. and Coyle, M.P.,** Dysfunction of the pisotriquetral joint: treatment by excision of the pisiform. *J. Hand Surg.*, 1985; 10A: 703–707.
15. **Chien, A.J. et al.** Focal radial styloid abnormality as a manifestation of de Quervain's tenosynovitis. *Am. J. Roentgenol.*, 2001; 177: 1383–1386.
16. **Cihantimur, B., Akin, S., and Ozcan, M.** Percutaneous treatment of trigger finger. 34 fingers followed 0.5–2 years. *Acta Orthop. Scand.*, 1998; 69: 167–168.

17. **Clarke, M.T. et al.** The histopathology of de Quervain's disease. *J. Hand Surg. Br.*, 1998; 23: 732–734.
18. **Crimmins, C.A. and Jones, N.F.** Stenosing tenosynovitis of the extensor carpi ulnaris. *Ann. Plast. Surg.*, 1995; 35: 105–107.
19. **de Quervain, F.** On a form of chronic tendovaginitis by Dr. Fritz de Quervain in la Chaux-de-Fonds, 1895. *Am. J. Orthop.*, 1997; 26: 641–644.
20. **De Smelt, L., Ghyselen, H., and Lysens, R.** Incidence of overuse syndromes of the upper limb in young pianists and its correlation with hand size, hypermobility and playing habits. *Chir. Main*, 1998; 17: 309–313.
21. **Dobyns, J.H.** Short-shrift problems: a grab bag of athletic injuries, in *AAOS Symposium on Upper Extremity Injuries in Athletes,* Pettrone, F.A., Ed. St. Louis: C.V. Mosby, 1986; 170–173.
22. **Finsen, V. and Sandbu, H.** Injection therapy of trigger finger. *Tidsskr. Nor. Laegeforen,* 2001; 121: 3406–3407.
23. **Fry, N.J.H.** Overuse syndrome in musicians: prevention and management. *Lancet,* 1986; 1: 728–731.
24. **Fulcher, M.S., Kiefhaber, T.R., and Stern, P.J.** Upper-extremity tendinitis and overuse syndromes in the athlete. *Clin. Sports Med.*, 1998; 17: 433–448.
25. **Gabel, G.T., Bishop, A.T., and Wood, M.B.** Flexor carpi radialis tendinitis: II. Results of operative treatment. *J. Bone Joint Surg. Am. Vol.,* 1994; 76: 1015–1018.
26. **Garrick, J.G. and Webb, D.R.** *Sports Injuries: Diagnosis and Management.* Philadelphia: W.B. Saunders, 1990.
27. **Giovagnorio, F., Andreaoli, C., and De Cicco, M.L.** Ultrasonographic evaluation of de Quervain disease. *J. Ultrasound Med.*, 1997; 16: 685–689.
28. **Glajchen, N. and Schweitzer, M.** MRI features in de Quervain's tenosynovitis of the wrist. *Skel. Radiol.*, 1996; 25: 63–65.
29. **Greis, P.E., Weiss, R.J., and Burks, T.R.** Gymnastics, in *Sports Injuries*, 2nd ed., Fu, H.F. and Stone, D.A., Eds. Philadelphia: Lippincott/Williams & Wilkins, 2001; 472–473.
30. **Grundberg, A.B. and Reagan, D.S.** Pathologic anatomy of the forearm: intersection syndrome, *J. Hand Surg.,* 1985; 10A: 299–302.
31. **Ha, K.I., Park, M.J., and Ha, C.W.** Percutaneous release of trigger digits. *J. Bone Joint Surg. (Br.),* 2001; 83: 75–77.
32. **Hanlon, D.P. and Luellen, J.R.** Intersection syndrome: a case report and review of the literature. *J. Emerg. Med.*, 1999; 17: 969–971.
33. **Harvey, F.J., Harvey, P.M., and Horsley, M.W.** De Quervain's disease: surgical or nonsurgical treatment. *J. Hand Surg.,* 1990; 15A: 83–87.
34. **Holtzhausen, L.M. and Noakes, T.D.** Elbow, forearm, wrist and hand injuries among sport rock climbers. *Clin. J. Sport Med.*, 1996; 6: 196–203.
35. **Howse, C.** Wrist injuries in sport. *Sports Med.*, 1994; 17: 163–175.
36. **Jackson, W.T. et al.** Anatomical variations in the first extensor compartment of the wrist. *J. Bone Joint Surg.,* 1986; 68A: 923–926.
37. **Kasdan, M.L. et al.** Trigger finger: not always work related. *J. Ky. Med. Assoc.*, 1996; 94: 498–499.
38. **Katzman, B.M. et al.** Utility of obtaining radiographs in patients with trigger finger. *Am. J. Orthop.*, 1999; 28: 703–705.
39. **Kulund, D.N.**, *The Injured Athlete,* 2nd ed. Philadelphia: J.B. Lippincott, 1988.
40. **Koh, T.J., Grabiner, M.D., and Weiker, G.G.** Technique and ground reaction forces in the back handspring. *Am. J. Sports Med.*, 1992; 20: 61–66.
41. **Lacey, T., Goldstein, L.A., and Tobin, C.E.** Anatomical and clinical study of the variations in the insertions of the abductor pollicis longus tendon, associated with stenosing tendovaginitis. *J. Bone Joint Surg.,* 1951; 33A: 347–350.
42. **Lambert, M.A., Morton, R.J., and Sloan, J.P.** Controlled study of the use of local steroid injection in the treatment of trigger finger and thumb. *J. Hand Surg. (Br.)*, 1992; 17: 69–70.
43. **Lane, L.B., Boretz, R.S., and Stuchin, S.A.** Treatment of de Quervain's disease: role of conservative management. *J. Hand Surg. (Br.)*, 2001; 26: 258–260.
44. **Lanzetta, M. and Foucher, G.** Association of Wartenberg's syndrome and de Quervain's disease: a series of 26 cases. *Plast. Reconstr. Surg.*, 1995; 96: 408–412.
45. **Lindner-Tons, S. and Ingell, K.** An alternative splint design for trigger finger. *J. Hand Ther.*, 1998; 11: 206–208.

46. **Loomis, L.K.** Variations of stenosing tenosynovitis at the radial styloid process. *J. Bone Joint Surg.*, 1951; 33A: 340–346.

47. **Loty, B., Memier, B., and Mazas, F.** Luxation traumatique isolée du tendon cubital posterieur. *Rev. Chir. Orthop.*, 1986; 72: 219–222.

48. **Louis, D.S.** Incomplete release of the first dorsal compartment — a diagnostic test. *J. Hand Surg.*, 1987; 12A: 87–88.

49. **Lyu, S.R.** Closed division of the flexor tendon sheath for trigger finger. *J. Bone Joint Surg.*, 1992; 74B: 418–420.

50. **Mahakkanukrauh, P. and Mahakkanukrauh, C.** Incidence of a septum in the first dorsal compartment and its effects on therapy of de Quervain's disease. *Clin. Anat.*, 2000; 13: 195–198.

51. **Marini, M. et al.** De Quervain's disease: diagnostic imaging. *Chir. Organi Mov.*, 1994; 79: 219–223.

52. **Mellor, S.J. and Ferris, B.D.** Complications of a simple procedure: de Quervain's disease revisited. *Int. J. Clin. Pract.*, 2000; 54: 76–77.

53. **Mikić, Z., Somer, T., Tubić, M., and Ercegan, G.** Entezitis piriformne kosti. *Med. Pregl.*, 1985; 523–525.

54. **Moore, J.S.** De Quervain's tenosynovitis. Stenosing tenosynovitis of the first dorsal compartment. *J. Occup. Environ. Med.*, 1997; 39: 990–1002.

55. **Murphy, D., Failla, J.M., and Koniuch, M.P.** Steroid versus placebo injection for trigger finger. *J. Hand Surg. (Am.)*, 1995; 20: 628–631.

56. **Murray, P.M. and Cooney, W.P.** Golf-induced injuries of the wrist. *Clin. Sports Med.*, 1996; 15: 85–109.

57. **Nagaoka, M., Matsuzaki, H., and Suzuki, T.** Ultrasonographic examination of de Quervain's disease. *J. Orthop. Sci.*, 2000; 5: 96–99.

58. **Osterman, L.A., Moskow, L., and Low, D.W.** Soft-tissue injuries of the hand and wrist in racquet sports. *Clin. Sports Med.*, 1988; 7: 329–348.

59. **Paley, D., McMurtry, R.Y., and Cruickshank, B.** Pathologic condition of the pisiform and pisotriquetral joint. *J. Hand Surg.*, 1987; 12A: 110–119.

60. **Pantukosit, S., Petchkrua, W., and Stiens, S.A.** Intersection syndrome in Buriram Hospital: a 4-year prospective study. *Am. J. Phys. Med. Rehabil.*, 2001; 80: 656–661.

61. **Parlitz, D., Perschel, T., and Altenmuller, E.** Assessment of dynamic finger forces in pianists: effects of training and expertise. *J. Biomech.*, 1998; 31: 1063–1067.

62. **Piligian, G. et al.** Evaluation and management of chronic work-related musculoskeletal disorders of the distal upper extremity. *Am. J. Indust. Med.*, 2000; 37: 75–93.

63. **Rankin, M.F. and Rankin, E.A.** Injection therapy for management of stenosing tenosynovitis (de Quervain's disease) of the wrist. *J. Natl. Med. Assoc.*, 1998; 90: 474–476.

64. **Ritter, M.A. and Inglis, A.E.** The extensor indicis proprius syndrome. *J. Bone Joint Surg.*, 1969; 51(8): 1645–1648.

65. **Rohrbough, J.T., Mudge, M.K., and Schilling, R.C.** Overuse injuries in the elite rock climber. *Med. Sci. Sports Exerc.*, 2000; 32: 1369–1372.

66. **Rowland, S.A.** Acute traumatic subluxation of the extensor carpi ulnaris tendon at the wrist. *J. Hand Surg.*, 1986; 11A: 809–811.

67. **Sakai, N.** Selective corticosteroid injection into the extensor pollicis brevis tenosynovium for de Quervain's disease. *Orthopaedics*, 2002; 25: 68–70.

68. **Silko, G.J. and Cullen, P.T.** Indoor racquet sports injuries. *Am. Fam. Physician*, 1994; 50: 374–380.

69. **Silver, J.K. and Rozmaryn, L.M.** Overuse tendinitis of the intrinsic muscles. *Orthopedics*, 1998; 21: 891–894.

70. **Sopov, W. et al.** Scintigraphy of de Quervain's tenosynovitis. *Nucl. Med. Commun.*, 1999; 20: 175–177.

71. **Steffens, K. and Koob, E.** Diagnosis and therapy of tendovaginitis of the extensor carpi ulnaris (stenosis of the 6th extensor compartment). *Z. Orthop. Ihre Grenzgeb.*, 1994; 135: 437–440.

72. **Stroede, C.L., Noble, L., and Walker, H.S.** The effect of tennis racket string vibration dampers on racket handle vibrations and discomfort following impacts. *J. Sports Sci.*, 1999; 17: 379–385.

73. **Stothard, J. and Kumar, A.A.** Safe percutaneous procedure for trigger finger release. *J. R. Coll. Surg. Edinb.*, 1994; 39: 116–117.

74. **Ta, K.T., Eidelman, D., and Thomson, J.G.** Patient satisfaction and outcomes of surgery for de Quervain' s tenosynovitis. *J. Hand Surg. (Am.),* 1999; 24: 1071–1077.

75. **Tanaka, S., Petersen, M., and Cameron, L.** Prevalence and risk factors of tendinitis and related disorders of the distal upper extremity among U.S. workers: comparison to carpal tunnel syndrome. *Am. J. Indust. Med.,* 2001; 39: 328–335.

76. **Trentanni, C. et al.** Ultrasonic diagnosis of de Quervain's tenosynovitis. *Radiol. Med.* (Torino), 1997; 93: 194–198.

77. **Trezies, A.J. et al.** Is occupation an aetiological factor in the development of trigger finger? *J. Hand Surg. Br.,* 1998; 23: 539–540.

78. **Turowski, G.A., Zdankiewicz, P.D., and Thomson, J.G.** The results of surgical treatment of trigger finger. *J. Hand Surg. Am.,* 22: 145–149.

79. **van Ijsseldijk, A.L. et al.** Topical corticosteroid injection for trigger finger: good short-term results, but fairly high risk of recurrence. *Ned. Tijdschr. Geneeskd,* 1998; 142: 457–459.

80. **Verdon, M.E.** Overuse syndromes of the hand and wrist. *Prim. Care,* 1996; 23: 305–319.

81. **Viegas, S.F.** Trigger thumb of de Quervain's disease. *J. Hand Surg.,* 1986; 11A: 235–237.

82. **Weis, A.P., Akelman, E. and Tabatabai, M.** Treatment of de Quervain's disease. *J. Hand Surg. (Am.),* 1994; 19: 595–598.

83. **Wetterkamp, D., Rieger, H., and Brug, E.** Surgical treatment and results of healing of de Quervain stenosing tenovaginitis. *Chirurg,* 1996; 67: 740–743.

84. **Wetterkamp, D., Rieger, H., and Brug, E.** 100 years tendovaginitis stenosans de Quervain — review of the literature and personal results. *Handchir. Mikrochir. Plast. Chir.,* 1997; 29: 214–217.

85. **Williams, J.G.** Surgical management of traumatic non-infective tenosynovitis of the wrist extensors. *J. Bone Joint Surg.,* 1977; 59B: 408–410.

86. **Williams, R. and Westmorland, M.** Occupational cumulative trauma disorders of the upper extremity. *Am. J. Occup. Ther.,* 1994; 48: 411–420.

87. **Wilhelmi, B.J. et al.** Trigger finger release with hand surface landmark ratios: an anatomic and clinical study. *Plast. Reconstr. Surg.,* 2001; 108: 908–915.

88. **Wilson, I.F., Schubert, W., and Benjamin, C.I.** The distally based radial forearm fascia-flap for treatment of recurrent de Quervain's tendonitis. *J. Hand Surg. (Am.),* 2001; 26: 506–509.

89. **Witt, J., Pess, G., and Gelberman, R.H.** Treatment of de Quervain tenosynovitis. A prospective study of the results of injection of steroids and immobilization in a splint. *J. Bone Joint Surg.,* 1991; 73A: 219–222.

90. **Wood, M.B. and Dobyns, J.H.** Sports-related extraarticular wrist syndromes. *Clin. Orthop.,* 1986; 202: 93–102.

91. **Wulle, C.** Intersection syndrome. *Handchir. Mikrochir. Plast. Chir.,* 1993; 25: 48–50.

92. **Yuasa, K. and Kiyoshige, Y.** Limited surgical treatment of de Quervain's disease: decompression of only the extensor pollicis brevis subcompartment. *J. Hand Surg. (Am.),* 1998; 23: 840–843.

93. **Zingas, C., Failla, J.M., and van Holsbeeck, M.** Injection accuracy and clinical relief of de Quervain's tendinitis. *J. Hand Surg. (Am.),* 23: 89–96.

Part III

Spine

6 Low Back Pain

I. LOW BACK PAIN IN ATHLETES

In the context of this book, among the numerous factors that cause low back pain, emphasis should be placed on chronic overuse of the lumbosacral area, which manifests itself in some occupations and in professional and nonprofessional athletes. For this reason, we are including cases of low back pain resulting from excessive chronic overuse of the lumbosacral area whose clinical picture corresponds to that of overuse syndromes. This includes some forms of spondylolysis and spondylolisthesis, low back pain in gymnasts, low back pain in some cases of scoliosis and kyphosis, and myofibrositis. Low back pain is the ailment of the century in modern, technological, highly advanced societies. Viewed from a statistical point of view, all adults suffer from low back pain at least three times in their life. This, of course, also implies that out of three adults, one will suffer nine times in his or her lifetime. According to some statistics, between 50 and 80% of the population in developed industrial countries suffers, or has suffered, from low back pain.[41] The diagram of strain placed upon the lumbar vertebrae in various positions of the body clearly indicates that the frequency of low back pain in modern societies results in part from the way of life and work habits practiced in these societies[59,82] (Figure 6.1). Loss resulting from absence from work and cost of treatment for low back pain is enormous. To illustrate this, we will cite two examples. The first comes from the U.S. where in one calendar year, loss resulting from low back pain treatment and absence from work was approximated at $14 billion. This is the reason why innovative approaches to prevent and treat low back pain in workers are mandatory. The sports medicine approach for aggressive rehabilitation offers a possible solution.[40] The other example comes from the U.K. where in 1 year the number of working days lost because of low back pain exceeded £13 million. This clearly indicates that low back pain is also a socioeconomic problem.[35,60]

Low back pain is a term used to describe subjective feelings of pain and tenderness felt in the lumbar or, generally speaking, lower spine. As the term implies, the essence of this syndrome lies in the subjective feeling of pain, which can be of different intensity suffered by patients in a very individual manner. A variety of terms are used to describe this painful condition. *Lumbago* is an old expression used to describe acute pain in the lumbar spine area. Today the term *painful lumbar syndrome* is preferred and generally used to describe the same condition. The painful lumbar syndrome can be of vertebral origin, meaning the pain manifests itself exclusively in the area in which it originates — in other words, in the lumbar spine area. If painful symptoms manifest themselves in regions far from the spine, e.g., in the lower extremities, the term *vertebrogenic painful lumbar syndrome* is applied (e.g., lumboischialgia).

When dealing with this condition, one should always bear in mind that low back pain is just a syndrome, i.e., a number of different symptoms, and not a disease in the specific meaning of the word. The pain that is subjectively felt by patients is simply a manifestation of some pathological substrate.[67,68] Very few painful conditions have such a wide variety of possible causative factors as low back pain. The sophisticated methods of modern diagnostics coupled with an increasing amount of knowledge regarding the biomechanics of the spine have enabled researchers to delineate a large, and steadily increasing number of possible causative factors for low back pain.[16] We present a table (Table 6.1) of possible causative factors of low back pain based on our own experience and that of other researchers as reported in the medical literature. Even a cursory examination of Table 6.1 will reveal that the cause of low back pain is extremely difficult to detect, which explains why

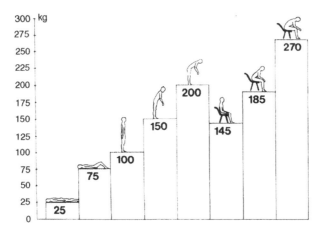

FIGURE 6.1 Diagram of the strain placed on the lumbar spine in various positions.

some patients change physicians a number of times before the correct diagnosis is ultimately reached. In everyday clinical practice, the most commonly encountered syndrome is the painful vertebral lumbar syndrome caused by degenerative changes in the area of the lumbar disk and small joints. From a clinical point of view, back pain can manifest in either the acute or chronic stage with the particulars of the clinical picture depending principally on the pathological substrate that led to the development of the syndrome.[14] Treatment in most cases (95 to 98%) is non-operative. It inevitably begins with non-operative treatment except in cases where an evident pathological substrate that demands surgical intervention is the cause. Examples of the latter include tumors, unstable fractures of the spine, and other similar causes. Although the majority of intervertebral disk injuries can be treated conservatively, the decision to follow an aggressive conservative vs. surgical course in any given individual must be made on an individual case basis.[100] Spinal fusion rarely is indicated for the athlete with internal disk disruption and no evidence of instability.[10] When treating athletes with episodes of acute low back pain, pain modulation and return to daily function are the primary treatment goals. When treating athletes with episodes of chronic low back pain, return to sport and prevention of recurrence are the primary treatment goals.[22] As part of the non-operative treatment of painful lumbar syndrome and as an important factor in preventing its development, special emphasis is placed on lifestyle and working habits. For this reason, special "schools" for people suffering from low back pain have been opened to teach people how to live and cope with their disease. Although physical therapy, chiefly hydrogymnastics and kinesitherapy, plays an important role in non-operative treatment of low back pain, the physician should always keep in mind that some exercises, especially dynamic exercises, increase the strain on the lumbal vertebrae[82] (Figure 6.2). Electrophysiological, kinesiological, and biomechanical research has increased our knowledge of kinesitherapy of painful lumbar syndrome. In kinesitherapy, programs with a conspicuous role are reserved for isometric exercises and stretching exercises such as for the hamstrings. Stretching exercises are performed with the purpose of affecting lumbar lordosis.[53] Kinesitherapy programs should be individualized with special consideration given to age, sex, bone, ligament, and muscle status of the lumbar spine.[93] The exercises should gradually increase and at all times be adapted to the stage of the disease and to the muscle strength and fitness of the patient.

Low back pain in both professional and nonprofessional athletes corresponds to the general clinical picture of this syndrome and has the same possible causative factors.[13] However, low back pain is unique in professional and nonprofessional athletes in that a clear distinction must be drawn between cases in which a normal and healthy spine is subjected to excessive strain caused by athletic activities resulting in low back pain and cases in which endogenous factors such as sacralization or lumbalization of the lower spine cause low back pain in athletes who take part in

**TABLE 6.1
Low Back Pain**

Congenital and developmental anomalies
   Facet tropismus
   Transitional vertebra
      Sacralization of the lumbar vertebra
      Lumbalization of the sacral vertebra
   Spina bifida
   Congenital scoliosis and kyphosis
   Scheuermann disease
   Spondylolysis and spondylolisthesis
Inflammations
   Rheumatic (arthritis rheumatoides, spondylitis ankylosans — Bechterew disease)
   Infections
      Acute (osteomyelitis — spondylitis pyogenes)
      Chronic (osteomyelitis chronica, spondylitis tuberculosa, spondylitis mykosa)
Trauma
   Overstrains in lumbar spine
      Acute (injuries)
      Chronic (damage)
   Subluxation of small joints (facet syndrome)
   Infractions and fractures (vertebral body and processes)
   Subluxations of sacroiliac joints
   Spondylosis and spondylolisthesis
   Post-traumatic kyphosis
Degenerative changes
   Osteochondrosis and spondylosis
   Spondylarthrosis
   Discopathia
   Nerve root entrapment syndrome
   Interspinous arthrosis
   Sacroiliac arthrosis
Tumors
Metabolic disorders
   Osteoporosis
   Osteomalacia
   Paget disease
   Kummel disease
Mechanical
   Postural low back pain
   Decrease or increase of lumbar lordosis
   Instability of the spine
   Scoliosis (more than 30°)
   Retroposition of lumbar vertebra
   Muscular changes (myofibrositis, myogelosis, hypertonus)
   Static disorders of the feet
   Abnormal biomechanics of the hip joints (subluxation, luxation, contracture)
   Inequality of the legs
   Abnormal biomechanics of the sacroiliac joints
   Venter pnedulus
Vascular diseases
Irradiation of the pain from visceral organs

TABLE 6.1 (Continued)
Low Back Pain

Gynecological diseases (inflammations, dismenorrhea, descensus, prolapse or
    retroflexion of the uterus)
Diseases of the gastroenterological system
Diseases of the urogenital system
Abscessus subphrenicus
Diseases of the splenium
Psychogenic

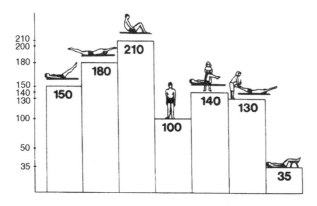

FIGURE 6.2 Diagram of the strain placed on the lumbar spine during some dynamic exercises.

normal, nonexcessive athletic activities. The worst possible combination is when an athlete suffering from abnormal low back architecture (abnormal endogenous factors) takes part in excessive and high-risk athletic activities (abnormal exogenous factors). Table 6.2 shows the possible combinations between the condition of the spine and the strain placed on the spine during various athletic activities. Different views are proposed in the current medical literature regarding the risk potential of various sports for developing low back pain and the specific high-risk movements that place excessive strain on the spine.[24,31,39,54,77,86,90] Kujala et al.[49] suggest that lengthy training duration predisposes young athletes to low back pain. The problem of low back pain in young, adolescent, or college athletes has been investigated by many authors.[3,7,27,28,46,49–52,56,58,61,63,75] In one of their studies, Kujala et al.[52] investigated the prognosis of low back pain and the association of clinical symptoms and anatomic findings among young athletes.

The causes of prolonged back pain among young athletes are usually established by imaging studies. Knowledge of anatomic abnormalities may help in tailoring training programs and avoiding the progression of changes during growth. Simple restriction of painful activities usually leads to good recovery. According to Micheli and Wood[58] there are significant differences in the major

TABLE 6.2
Low Back Pain in Athletes

Spine	Strain
Normal	Abnormal (excessive)
Abnormal	Normal
Abnormal	Abnormal (excessive)

TABLE 6.3
High-Risk Sports for Developing Low Back Pain

Vertical	Flexion/Extension	Rotation
Horseback riding	Football	Tennis and racket sports
Gymnastics	Soccer	Golf
Skydiving	Gymnastics	Aerobics
Waterskiing	Diving	
Jogging on hard surfaces	Hockey	
	Field hockey	

causes of low back pain in young athletes compared with causes of low back pain in the general adult population, for example, 47% of the 100 adolescents were ultimately shown to have a spondylolysis stress fracture of the pars interarticularis and only 5% of adult subjects were found to have a spondylolysis associated with low back pain. A stress fracture of the ala of the sacrum was identified on bone scan and computerized tomography (CT) scan in two teenage female athletes with low back pain that limited athletic activity. The lesions healed with rest.[27] A review of the literature yielded 29 cases of sacral stress fractures in athletes, mainly runners, but Shah and Stewart[80] described a case of a sacral stress fracture causing low back pain in a volleyball player. Garces et al.[20] recommend scintigraphy in early diagnosis of stress fracture of the lumbar spine in athletes. Scintigraphy showed increased uptake in 17 of 33 athletes complaining of back pain of more than 1 month duration and with normal radiography of the lower spine. Interestingly, no difference in prevalence or severity of back pain was seen between different phases of the menstrual cycle or between users and nonusers of oral contraceptives; that is, the data of the Brynhildsen et al.[7] study do not support the hypothesis that low back pain is influenced by hormonal fluctuations during the menstrual cycle or by use of oral contraceptives. The most frequently mentioned high-risk sports for developing low back pain are shown in Table 6.3.

To successfully treat athletes suffering from low back discomfort, the sports medicine specialist must be aware of the psychological impact of low back pain on athletes. Commonly, the injured patient (athlete) wishes to return to activity immediately, with very little respect for or knowledge of the biology of healing. In the face of low back pain, the realities of human fragility become obvious, perhaps for the first time. This particular type of injured athlete requires constant counseling from the sports medicine consultant. The patient must also be made aware that, in some cases, the healing process can be quite long, and in other cases complete healing is unobtainable. Patients should be counseled to try to adapt their lifestyle and athletic activities to the limitations imposed by the condition of their spine. Green et al.[25] concluded that a warm-up followed by bench rest does lead to an increase in stiffness of the lumbar spine, suggesting this practice is not in the best interest of reducing the risk of back injury or optimal performance. According to Harvey and Tanner,[28] lumbar spine pain accounts for 5 to 8% of athletic injuries.

Although back pain is not the most common injury, it is one of the most challenging for the sports physician to diagnose and treat. A thorough history and physical examination are usually more productive in determining a diagnosis and guiding treatment than are imaging techniques. Flory et al.[19] recommend isokinetic back testing in the athletes as a way of preventing the development of severe problems among the athletes developing low back pain. A different and more in-depth approach is needed when treating an athlete suffering from low back pain than when treating a sedentary subject with the same pathology. In fact, pain symptoms may frequently arise only when there is functional overloading, whereas pain is absent or not disabling in normal daily activity.[34] Treatment is also different for the athlete because complete functional recovery must take place in as short a period of time as possible, and it will often have to be finalized in relation to sports-related commitments.

Of the many possible causes of low back pain, we will mention only those that are thought to result from chronic injuries, i.e., from overuse. We will begin with congenital or developmental anomalies, which at first glance, may appear to be contradictory to the above. However, we would like to reiterate at this point that congenitally abnormal spines (an abnormal endogenous factor) can be damaged by repeated microtraumas and thus result in the classical clinical picture of overuse syndrome.

II. SPONDYLOLYSIS AND SPONDYLOLISTHESIS

Spondylolysis is a condition that is present in approximately 6% of individuals, but it has been reported in up to 50% of athletes with back pain.[87] This condition is essentially a break in bone continuity resulting from a defect in the junction between the superior and inferior processus articularis; it is most often encountered in the fifth and fourth lumbar vertebra. This junction is known as the *pars interarticularis* or *isthmus* (Figure 6.3). The defect in the bone is usually fibrocartilaginous in nature. Most authors agree that spondylolysis can be caused by other than congenital factors. Spondylolysis can be caused by trauma and can also result as a consequence of overuse syndrome — from stress fractures. This is especially frequent in female gymnasts. Spondylolisthesis is a condition in which the defect in the vertebral arch causes the slipping of the vertebra in the forward projection. Spondylolysis is, in most cases, asymptomatic and can be detected only by roentgenographic examination. Special slanted oblique projections of the spine are taken, which in positive cases show the figure of the "Scottish terrier" with an abnormally extended neck, indicating a defect in the isthmus of the vertebral arch (Figure 6.4). Advanced imaging with single photon emission computed tomographic (SPECT) bone scintigraphy, CT, and magnetic resonance (MR) imaging may be needed to ascertain the acuity of the lesion, assist in identifying a particular pars lesion as potentially symptomatic, and to exclude other spinal pathology that may be present.[83,85,96] Rossi and Dragoni[76] report the results of the retrospective study of 473 cases of spondylolysis observed on 3505 plain films of the lumbar spine performed on athletes with low back pain. The analysis of the results showed the following:

1. The incidence of spondylolysis was higher in athletes (13.49%) than in the general population (4 to 7%).
2. The incidence of spondylolysis was higher in the distal portion of the lumbar spine (in 81.40% of cases L5 was involved).
3. In 52% of cases, spondylolysis was associated with spondylolisthesis — the latter of Grade 1 according to Meyerding's classification in 74.39% of cases.
4. Bilateral and single-segment forms prevailed.
5. The incidence of spondylolysis differed in the various sports according to the specific mechanical stimulation involved.

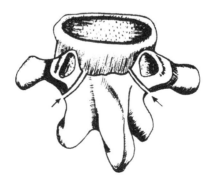

FIGURE 6.3 Localization of the spondylolytic defect in the vertebral arch (arrows).

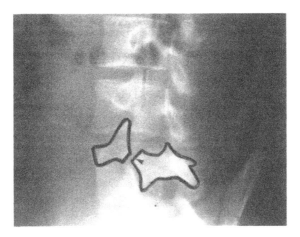

FIGURE 6.4 Figure of a "Scottish terrier."

Although spondylolysis or listhesis is a frequent injury in athletes, mainly in weight lifters, wrestlers, gymnasts, divers, and ballet dancers, it is infrequently reported in swimmers.[62] In many sports that are dominated by females (gymnastics, dancing, figure skating), the athletes carry a high risk of having spondylolysis or a stress fracture. Idiopathic scoliosis and spondylolysis can be common back problems in female athletes.[65] Half of all pediatric athletic patients with back pain is related to disturbances of the posterior elements of the spine including spondylolysis, which presents as low back pain aggravated by activity, frequently with minimal physical findings.[74] Congeni et al.[9] examined the natural course of athletically active young people with back pain and a diagnosis of spondylolysis (stress fracture of the pars interarticularis of the facet joint of the lumbar spine). The study group included 40 patients with low back pain and diagnosis of spondylolysis by nuclear medicine study. CT scans were performed to help determine long-term treatment and prognosis. Of the patients, 45% demonstrated chronic nonhealing fractures, 40% demonstrated acute fractures in various stages of healing, and 15% demonstrated no obvious fractures. Some authors believe that spondylolysis can, by itself and without the presence of spondylolisthesis, cause low back pain. Treatment is most often non-operative. Surgical fixation and bone transplantation of the vertebral arch is very rarely indicated.[6]

Abraham et al.[1] describe the scintigraphic appearance of both a symptomatic and asymptomatic *retroisthmic cleft* in two athletes with low back pain. This lesion, which involves lamina, is the least common of the neural arch defects of which spondylolysis is the most common.

Spondylolisthesis is a term used to define the slippage of the body of the vertebra above a caudally located vertebra (Figure 6.5). The slippage, in most cases, is directed in the forward direction, but it can also be directed in the backward projection. The three principal causes of spondylolisthesis are (1) congenital lack of the processus articularis (which is very rare), (2) spondylolysis, and (3) degenerative changes (arthrosis) on the facet joints. Spondylolisthesis caused by degenerative changes on the facet joints (Figure 6.6) is also called *pseudospondylolisthesis* (false spondylolisthesis) because the slippage of the vertebral body is relatively very slight.[15,36,79] The slippage can appear between any two vertebra, although, in most cases, it is limited to the area between the fourth and fifth lumbar vertebra. Slippage in the backward direction (retrolisthesis) is frequent and is called *retropositio*.[36] Neurological side effects are rare in pseudospondylolisthesis. Spondylolisthesis caused by spondylolysis is characterized by the fact that the vertebral body, together with the pedicles (the origins of the vertebral arch from the vertebral body), slips forward together with the processus articularis superiores, which has the effect of displacing the entire spine above that vertebra in the forward direction (Figure 6.5). The lamine and the processus articularis inferiores remain behind in their normal anatomical position. Four grades of spondylolisthesis are recognized by Meyerding, depending on the amount (length) of the forward slipping of the vertebral body. Grade 1 is defined by a 0

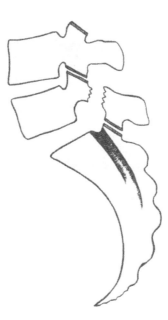

FIGURE 6.5 Spondylolisthesis of the fifth lumbar vertebra due to spondylolysis in the arch of the same vertebra.

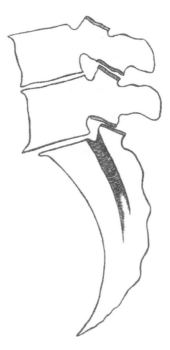

FIGURE 6.6 Pseudospondylolisthesis due to arthrosis of the small vertebral joint.

to 25% of the posteroanterior vertebral body length of the caudally located vertebra slipping in the forward direction. Grade 2 is defined by 25 to 50%, Grade 3 by 50 to 75%, and Grade 4 by 75% and more vertebral body length forward slippage. In cases when the fifth lumbar vertebra slips over the edge of the sacrum into the pelvis, the term *spondyloptosis* is applied.

The clinical picture of spondylolisthesis caused by an inherited lack of the processus articularis in children and adolescents is characterized by neurological side effects. In pseudospondylolisthesis, the symptoms usually manifest in mature and older patients and are characterized by a painful lower back of vertebral origin. Spondylolisthesis caused by spondylolysis can be both symptomatic and asymptomatic. The symptomatology in this case depends on the amount of vertebral body slippage. The most frequently encountered symptom is low back pain, but in some cases the root of the nerve can also be affected, causing lumboischialgia. In clinical diagnostics, the "sign of the step" is characteristic. This sign is best seen by tracing the spinous processus with the tip of the finger in the cranial to caudal direction. At one point (the point of the forward slipping of the affected vertebral body), the finger encounters a displacement in the form of a step (Figure 6.5). Depending on the degree of forward slipping, other clinical symptoms can also be seen: the trunk of the patient becomes shorter while the rib arches tend to move closer to the cristae illiacae; in a standing position, the hands reach more distally toward the knees; lumbar lordosis is more pronounced; and the hips are in a flexed position. If painful symptoms are present, they usually appear and/or intensify in a standing or sitting position.

Treatment depends on the gravity of the symptoms, the age of the patient, and the progression of the spondylolisthesis (if the slippage of the vertebral body continues). In most cases, treatment is conservative and consists of physical therapy, wearing of braces, and adapting the patient's lifestyle and working habits to the limitations imposed by the condition of his or her spine. Conservative treatment should always be attempted before surgery, which is indicated when neurological side effects are apparent or when the patient suffers intense pain. If pain persists in combination with an intact intervertebral disk of the slipped segment, Hasler and Dick[29] recommend a direct repair of the pars interarticularis instead of an intersegmental fusion. Patients with low-grade spondylolisthesis (Meyerding 1, 2) require repeated radiological follow-up during growth because of the inherent risk of slip progression. If a slip of more than 50% is detected before the end of growth, operative treatment is indicated. High-grade spondylolisthesis (Meyerding 3, 4) leads to anterior shift of the whole trunk, kyphosis of the slipped vertebra with subsequent compensatory lumbar hyperlordosis, and flattening of the thoracic spine. Pelvic flexion is clinically evident. Reduction of the slipped and kyphotic vertebra with correction of the spinal, sacral, and pelvic profile is recommended and preferable to simple fusion *in situ*. Surgical treatment consists of fusion (spondylodesis) of the affected spinal segments with concomitant bone transplantation.

III. MYOFIBROSITIS

Among the mechanical causes of low back pain (caused primarily by continuous exposure to mechanical strain), an important place is reserved for changes in the paravertebral musculature in the form of hypertonus and the appearance of small knots. These changes are known under the general term *fibrositis,*[35] although some authors refer to them as *miogeloses* (as if the muscle has changed from a gel state into a solid, i.e., raw egg vs. hard-boiled egg). Histological analysis, however, has failed to prove the presence of fibrositis knots in the muscle. The clinical picture is characterized by the presence of pain in the paravertebral lumbar muscles. This pain is often correlated with the weather, especially changes in weather (a climatic factor). Other, less precisely localized "rheumatic" pains can also be present in other parts of the body.

Physical examination reveals localized tenderness of the affected muscle to palpation. All other clinical or radiological indicators are absent. Movements of the spine are unhindered and a true spasm of the muscles is lacking. Treatment is empirical and consists of physiotherapy accompanied by massage and exercises, especially stretching exercises.

IV. LOW BACK PAIN IN GYMNASTS

Low back pain, especially in female gymnasts, is a specific sports injury. Most authors today agree that the aggressive factors in gymnastics are the excessive movements in which increased retroflexion is most important.[21,23] The excessive flexibility of the spine results from the generalized excessive mobility of the complete locomotor system, which is a prerequisite for serious gymnastic training and also the result of the training. The excessive mobility of, primarily, the lumbar spine is a consequence of the "stretching" of the stabilizing system of the spine. The static and dynamic strain placed on the excessively mobile spine, particularly the lumbar area, leads to excessive lumbar curvature, hyperlordosis.[94] At first, this hyperlordosis is limited to relatively infrequent episodes, principally during gymnastic routines, but as time goes on hyperlordosis becomes habitual (Figure 6.7). Hyperlordosis represents a biomechanical imbalance in which the center of strain is shifted toward the posterior structures of the vertebrae.[42] The harm of this newly developed situation is best understood when one recognizes that the defensive mechanism of the lumbar spine to this excessive strain is flexion, shifting the center of the strain to the anterior, more massive structures of the vertebrae. Excessive strain also activates the adaptive mechanism of bone tissue — hypertrophy. The first phase of bone hypertrophy is an increase in osteoclastic activity, which prepares the affected area for new hypertrophic bone. During the osteoclastic phase, the bone is exceptionally vulnerable so that intensive training and hyperlordosis are among the prime biomechanical factors in the development of this ailment. The intensity of training, length and duration of training, and the class of competition are also directly correlated with the development of this syndrome. The study of Ohlen et al.[64] showed that 1° of the total sagittal lumbar mobility was lost for every 1° of increased lordosis. Low back pain was reported by 20% of the female gymnasts, and these girls had a significantly larger lordosis than girls with no history of low back pain. The female gymnasts who typically seek counsel from physicians are, in most cases, athletes who have been training for a number of years, who train more than 18 h/week, and who belong to the highest class of competition. The most commonly reported symptom is paravertebral pain, usually unilaterally, in the area of the thoracolumbar junction and the lumbar spine. The dominant symptom is pain. Quite frequently, this is the only symptom present, in spite of extensive diagnostic procedures, and the only sign the physician has that some disorder is present. The principal characteristic of the pain is that it is induced by sporting activities and is progressive. In the beginning phase of the ailment, the pain appears when gymnasts begin their routine, and eases as soon as they stop training. In later stages, the pain persists for a short time after training is finished, whereas the terminal phase is characterized by pain that persists the whole day.

Pain is the only unique and lasting symptom of this disorder. Other symptoms and signs vary, depending on the pathohistological base of the disorder: spondylolysis, protrusion or prolapse of the intervertebral disk, fracture of the vertebra, or spondylogenic pain.[21] Spondylolysis is the most frequent disorder that causes low back pain in female gymnasts.[21,23] The pathological changes are pain in female gymnasts,[21,23] which are usually located on the fourth and fifth lumbar vertebrae. Spondylolysis caused by excessive athletic activity is almost always stable, and very rarely (almost never) progresses into spondylolisthesis of the first degree. This possible development should, however, always be kept in mind during physical examination and diagnostic procedures, especially when the consulted sports medicine specialist encounters a varied and rich symptomatology. The reason is that spondylolysis has, with the exception of pain, practically no other symptoms. Neurological disorders appear only in the terminal phases of spondylolisthesis. In most cases, low back pain induced by gymnastic activity, especially in those activities in which retroflexion is dominant (exercises on the floor, exercises on the beam, landings after jumping over the vault), is the only symptom of spondylolysis.

Back muscles, in principle, show no signs of muscle spasm. The mobility of the spine is in order, and the gymnast will typically touch the floor with both her palms while in a standing position with no difficulty. Because of the generally decreased mobility of people with spine disorders, this exercise will seem to show that everything is in order. However, the physician should be careful, and try to determine whether this is a case of "relative loss" of mobility. The physician should anamnestically try to determine if there is a subjective feeling of loss of mobility, and then ask the patient to perform a flexion test from the hip from a horizontal position. The gymnast will typically

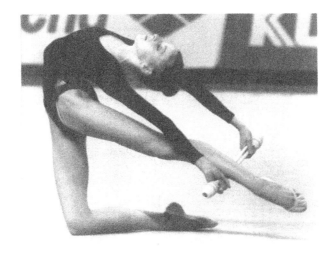

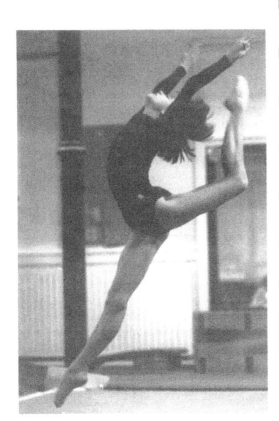

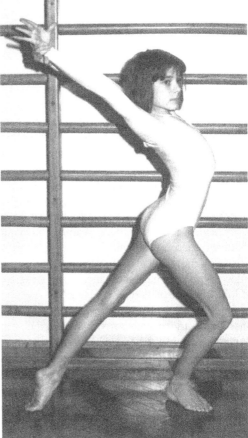

FIGURE 6.7 Characteristic attitudes and hyperlordosis in gymnasts.

flex her extended foot in the hip for 90°, which is a normal finding in untrained and "not-loosened-up" patients. Normal flexion for a highly trained, hypermobile female gymnast consists of a 120 to 130° flexion, which represents a relative loss of mobility of 30 to 40° (Figure 6.8). This relative loss of mobility is caused by the excessive tightness of the knee tendons (hamstrings). The hyperextension test can be used to provoke pain. The test is carried out by having the patient stand

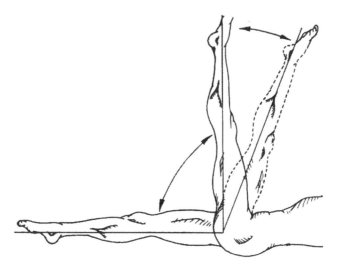

FIGURE 6.8 Test of hip flexion performed from a lying position. The hip flexion may reach 120° to 130° in the trained female gymnast. Untrained individuals and gymnasts with decreased mobility achieve hip flexion of only 90°.

on one foot and perform hyperextension (maximal possible retroflexion). The appearance of pain on the ipsilateral side is a strong indicator of spondylolysis. In addition to this indicator, retroflexion is almost always painful, a fact that is used to provoke pain during extension against pressure from a flexed position. The appearance of pain is a strong indicator of spondylolysis. In a roentgeno-graphic analysis of the lumbar spine of 100 young female gymnasts engaged in high-level compe-tition, the incidence of pars interarticular defects was 11% and 6% had spondylolisthesis.[33] This is four times higher than in their non-athletic female peers.

A complete radiological examination is especially important and should in fact be a routine examination in gymnasts with low back pain. Persistent back pain beyond 2 weeks warrants a complete evaluation, careful history and physical examination, four-view radiographic assessment of the spine, and, if necessary, bone scans or other more advanced techniques to make a specific diagnosis of the cause of the pain.[57] A complete radiological examination consists of one antero-posterior, one lateral, and two oblique images of the spine. The anteroposterior image registers the "upside-down Napoleon hat" phenomenon, a radiographic indicator of well-developed spondylolis-thesis of the fifth lumbar vertebra. The effect is caused by the projection of the slipped body of the fifth lumbar vertebra. The lateral radiogram is used to evaluate the stability of the spondylolysis — in other words, to determine if slippage of the vertebral body has occurred.[11]

Radiographic images taken from an oblique projection are crucially important as this is the only projection in which the pars interarticularis is clearly visible. The pars interarticularis, as we have already mentioned, is the area in which spondylolysis typically develops (Figure 6.9). A negative radiological result with persisting low back pain indicates the need for scintigraphic examination (Figure 6.10). An increased amount of the radioactive isotope coupled with positive anamnestic and clinical findings is a strong indication for a possible diagnosis of spondylolysis. Research has shown that a suspect scintigraphic finding, in a couple of months, turns into radio-graphically visible spondylolysis. A positive scintigraphic finding, without concomitant anamnestic or clinical confirmation, is not a sufficient criterion for positive diagnosis of spondylolysis or for prescribing therapy. On the other hand, however, negative radiological and scintigraphic findings do not rule out the possibility of spondylolysis, as some cases have shown a marked increase in the severity of existing symptoms and the appearance of new, previously not-present symptoms. For this reason, pain, as the most persistent and most unique symptom, must be regarded as the fundamental criterion and best orientation for prescribing and evaluating the success of therapy.

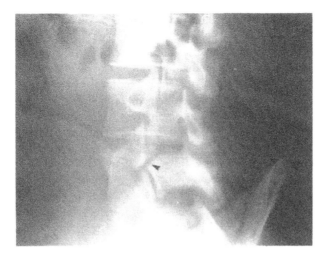

FIGURE 6.9 Roentgenogram of spondylolysis in a top-level gymnast.

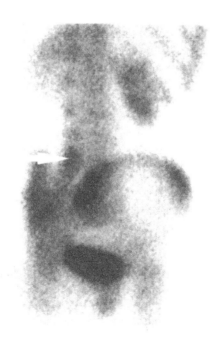

FIGURE 6.10 Bone scan demonstrating spondylolysis (arrow).

On the other hand, in the study of Falter and Hellerere[18] despite the radiologically pathological findings, the gymnasts were mainly asymptomatic. This could be due to the hypertrophied dorsispinal and abdominal musculature, which compensates for the pathological osseous structure. Inconsistency between radiographs and clinical observation can be noted according Guillodo et al.[26] and spontaneous consolidation of spondylolysis and pecicular fracture can occur despite the practice of the gymnastics 15 h/week.

Therapy for this overuse syndrome, as for other overuse syndromes, consists of rest for the overstrained tissue. The way this is to be accomplished when low back pain is caused by spondylolysis is at present controversial. One group of authors believes that spondylolysis, from the very beginning, should be treated as a fracture, and hence immobilized. To this effect, plastic braces are prescribed with a position of 0° lumbar lordosis. This treatment is prescribed with the aim of lessening the strain on the posterior structures of the vertebra. The brace is worn 23 h/day while the remaining hour is, apart from satisfying the physiological needs of the patient, used for physical therapy: strengthening exercises for the abdominal and pelvic muscles, stretching exercises for the lower extremities, and exercises for correcting lumbar hyperlordosis. The brace is worn for a period of 6 months, or until the initially positive scintigraphic finding turns negative. Mention must be made that an initial negative, "cold" scintigraphic finding, which indicates a decreased reparatory potential of the bone tissue, should not be taken as an absolute counterindication for prescribing the plastic brace. In a number of cases, such a cold scintigraphic finding resulted, after application of the plastic brace, in a well-healed case of spondylolysis. At 3 to 4 weeks after the initial application of the brace, most patients become asymptomatic. In this period during the hours when the patient is not wearing the brace (these can be increased to 2 to 3 h/day) light gymnastic activity is allowed with the exception of exercises performed on the beam and landing practice. The appearance of any symptoms is an absolute counterindication for any activity.

Under the influence of therapy, about one third of the positive scintigraphic findings become negative; this indicates complete bone healing. In such cases, complete sports activities, under full strain, are allowed. Such a result has a favorable long-term prognosis. However, in about 90% of the cases in which complete bone healing is not accomplished within 6 months, pain and any other present symptoms also disappear. This is also considered an adequate indicator for complete return to full sports activities. The reasoning behind this is that the stability of spondylolysis, despite induced strain, very rarely turns into spondylolisthesis. Cases in which complete bone healing is not obtained have a less favorable prognosis and a higher risk of recurrence of the symptoms. In this case, the same therapy should be repeated. Quite understandably, some athletes will lack the necessary patience and willpower to undergo therapy again. In all probability, they will continue with their gymnastic activities despite the discomfort; as a consequence, the ailment will progress. It will cease to be associated with only athletic activities and will become a permanent fixture in everyday life. In such situations, on rare occasions, spondylolisthesis can develop. As conservative therapy in this case is usually not adequate, surgical treatment is indicated. After such treatment, a return to the sports scene is usually possible after 1 year.

Contrary to the above-mentioned group of authors who believe that a brace should be applied immediately, there exists a second group of authors with a different opinion based on the knowledge of the stability of spondylolisthesis. This group believes that there is no need for the application of a brace before physical therapy and rest are utilized. A brace, according to this group of authors, should be applied only if this form of therapy produces no results.

Compression syndrome, or protrusion or prolapse of the intervertebral disk (Figure 6.11), is a less frequent cause of low back pain in gymnasts. In younger athletes, protrusion or prolapse of the intervertebral disk is not preceded by degenerative changes.[47] The main cause is excessive athletic activity. The clinical picture differs with regard to that seen in older patients. In most cases, pain is not the dominant symptom. In fact, it is minimal. In the majority of cases, the gymnast, or the trainer, notice a loss of flexibility in the knee tendons (hamstrings), or the beginning of an antalgic

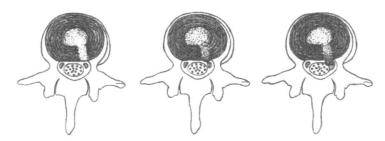

FIGURE 6.11 The stage of prolapse of the annulus fibrosus and protrusion of the nucleus pulposus in the area of spinal nerve root.

position of the spine. Clinical examination reveals a positive Lasegue, irradiation in the area of the sciatic nerve, and decreased mobility of the spine in flexion and when straightening up from a flexed to an upright stance. These maneuvers, as well as flexion in the hip with an extended knee, will typically provoke pain. Neurological side effects as well as clearly seen muscle weakness are extremely rare but possible symptoms.[37] Clinical examination includes a complete radiological examination, CT, electromyoneurography, myelography, and MR imaging. Tertti et al.[89] performed MR imaging on 35 young competitive gymnasts and 10 control subjects to detect the number of degenerated disks and other lumbar disorders. The results indicate that despite the excessive range of motion and strong axial loading of the lumbar spine that are associated with gymnastic maneuvers, incurable primary damage to the intervertebral disks is uncommon in young gymnasts during growth.

A proven compression syndrome demands treatment according to established principles. The therapy is based on relieving the affected area by lying in a neutral position. Analgesics, usually aspirin, can also be prescribed as well as cryotherapy and transcutaneous electrostimulation. In younger individuals, a positive response to this treatment is usually seen after about 2 weeks, but this does not by any means indicate that a return to full athletic activities is allowed. Moreover, a general recommendation is that active exercise should cease for a period of 6 to 12 months after a confirmed diagnosis of compression syndrome. During this interval, the patient is advised to wear a somewhat more flexible brace, constructed with 15° lumbar lordosis; this allows the patient to remain mobile, active, and able to attend school. If after 3 weeks of applied conservative therapy there is no improvement or if, before that time limit, progressive neurological side effects have manifested (such as urinary or anal incontinence), decompression is strongly indicated. The decompression can be carried out either surgically or by injecting chymopapain into the intervertebral disk. Posterolateral fusion of the affected interarticular joints is also recommended in the following cases: if there are radiological indications of the degeneration of the intervertebral disk; if there are radiological or scintigraphic indications of spondylolysis; or if there is anamnestic information of chronic pain in the lumbar spine before the rupture of the disk.

Successful therapy, and by this we imply a full return to sports activities under full strain, is achieved somewhat less frequently than in cases of spondylolysis or fracture. Restitution allowing a complete return to athletic activities is attained in about 50% of the cases.

Spondylogenic pain is the probable diagnosis reached by exclusion after a detailed physical examination has ruled out the possibility of spondylolysis, fracture of the vertebra, and prolapse and protrusion of the disk as other possible causative factors. Symptoms include pain, a hyperlordotic stance, tightness of the hamstrings, lumbodorsal fasciae, and flexors of the hip; in most cases, a relative weakness of the abdominal musculature can also be a symptom. Physical therapy as described in the therapy of spondylosis represents the basic therapeutic treatment in patients with spondylogenic pain. Often, this therapy completely eliminates pain and reduces the curvature of the lumbar lordosis to normal limits. In cases that do not respond to this treatment, the same exercise program is adhered to with the concomitant use of a brace constructed with 0° lumbar lordosis with an open front. The brace is worn for a period of 2 to 3 months. If after this period of time there is no evident improvement, a complete physical reexamination is indicated, and the physician should also consult with the trainer and parents of the gymnast. It is possible that, for some reason, the child is "running" into the disease and that the present symptomatology is the result of a conversive neurosis (psychogenic etiology of low back pain).

In addition to these causes of low back pain, which are connected with athletic activities, the physician should consider causes that are not initiated by sports activities. More rare, but differentially diagnostic causes include osteogenic sarcomas, sacroileitus, and discitis.

A special problem is *low back pain in elite rhythmic gymnasts*. Rhythmic gymnastics is a sport that blends the athleticism of a gymnast with the grace of a ballerina. The sport demands both the coordination of handling various apparatus and the flexibility to attain positions not seen in any other sport.[32] To attain perfection and reproducibility of their routines, the athletes must practice and repeat the basic elements of their routine thousands of times. In so doing, the athlete places herself at risk for a myriad of overuse injuries, the most common of which is low back pain. In the prospective study of Hutchinson[32] 86% of the gymnasts complained of back pain. Konermann and Sell[43] examined 24 former female artistic gymnasts of the German national team for spinal deformities after the end of their athletic career. During their athletic career 15 gymnasts complained of low back pain, which persisted in 7 after finishing their athletic activities. In the study of Wismach and Krause[97] 64% of the artistic gymnasts complained of back pain during competitive sports, and even after having given it up, 61% still complained. According to Tanchev et al.[88] a tenfold higher incidence of scoliosis was found in rhythmic gymnastic trainees (12%) than in their normal coevals (1.1%). Delay in menarche and generalized joint laxity are common in rhythmic trainees. The results strongly suggest the important etiologic role of a "dangerous triad": generalized joint laxity, delayed maturity, and asymmetric spinal loading. It would appear that rhythmic gymnasts are at relatively increased risk of suffering low back complaints secondary to their sport.

The presence of low back pain in gymnasts should be treated as a serious problem.[23] Low back pain syndrome is characterized by its progressive nature. It begins as a slight, barely perceptible pain and continually progresses until the pain and discomfort in the terminal stages of the disease can terminate the sports career of the patient and permanently endanger her health. Therefore, it is mandatory to perform a detailed clinical examination of all gymnasts who experience low back pain for a period of longer than 2 weeks. After treatment and rehabilitation, it is equally important to resume athletic activities gradually and to control the level of strain to which the patient is exposed.

V. SCOLIOSIS AND SPORTS

The question often arises: Can people with structural scoliosis of the spine take part in athletic activities? To answer the question it is essential to recognize some important facts. First, one must have a clear concept of what athletic activities mean. In other words, the physician should differentiate physical education in school and recreational sports from highly competitive professional sports. With regard to scoliosis, the physician should take into account the natural history,[12] degree of deformation, etiology of the scoliosis, and age of the patient.[81] The aforementioned facts indicate that there is no general answer to the question. If such an answer were demanded, it would in all probability have to be affirmative. In other words, patients with structural scoliosis of the spine are allowed to take part in athletic activities. Furthermore, taking an active part in athletic activities is recommended and can in some cases represent a form of therapy in treating scoliosis.[8,17,30,38,70] To highlight our opinion on this matter, we would like to cite the opinion of Stagnara,[84] who believes that active participation in athletic activities should be incorporated in the therapy recommended for patients with scoliosis. Athletic activities should be incorporated in a kinesitherapy program. Without them, therapy would be tedious and boring for the patient.[44] Athletic activities generally improve or stabilize the general state of the organism and have a beneficial effect on a number of vital functions, especially on the cardiorespiratory system.[2] According to the same author, the criteria that allow a recommendation for taking part in athletic activities depend upon the severity of the scoliosis and the age and sex of the patient.[84]

Generally speaking, the following is preferable:

- Recommend a sport that is performed outdoors (or at least partially connected to spending some time out of the house or office) and that places some sort of effort on the cardio-respiratory system (e.g., basketball, volleyball, jogging.).
- Prohibit dangerous sports (skydiving, rugby, judo).
- Exclude athletic activities that demand a high level of specialized technical skills and are connected with physical attributes and considerable strength. These may be beyond the capabilities of the scoliotic patient and may thus discourage the patient from taking part.
- Choose sports in which the patients can participate for long periods of time, preferably all their lives, such as walking, hiking, bicycling, tennis.

Stagnara[84] particularly emphasizes the importance of swimming, which has the advantage of placing the spine in a medium free from strain caused by gravitational forces. It also enables the maintenance of correct posture combined with significant physical activity and respiration and, depending on the style of swimming recommended, can force the spine into a position that corrects the deviation. However, we feel it is important to mention that placing the spine in a horizontal position in water does not generate muscle activity in the functional positions of greatest importance to the patient, i.e., when sitting and standing. Furthermore, it is by no means certain that the muscle quality best adapted to the therapeutic idea of extended postural correction is achieved.[84] A special question is the advisability of "asymmetric" sporting activities. Stagnara points out that it is impossible to correct a toracal scoliotic deviation by swimming continually with a sidestroke. On the other hand, some athletic activities, due to the constant repetition of asymmetrical movements, can overdevelop one extremity or one side of the body; this cannot be a cause of scoliosis and cannot in all probability worsen existing scoliosis.[84] Tennis players, even professional tennis players, do not develop structural scoliosis, but simply develop a stronger right or left arm. The beneficial effects of a sporting activity such as tennis outweigh by far the physician's possible doubts about the harmful side effects.[72] With regard to physical education in school, we believe that, as a general rule, children with structural scoliosis less than 30° should be encouraged to participate actively in all athletic activities, as this is without doubt more beneficial to the child than physical inactivity. The imposed limit of 30° is not arbitrarily determined. Studies have shown that in patients who suffer from scoliosis greater than 30°, the afflicted biomechanics can, without regard to the etiology of the scoliosis, lead to an increase of the curvature of the spine. When dealing with school-age patients whose scoliosis is greater than 30°, the physician should consider excusing the child from physical education. In collaboration with professor Kristofic, who has a special interest in kinesitherapy of scoliosis, we present a schematic representation and diagram of the differential participation of children in physical education[48,72] with regard to the amount of scoliotic curvature present in the spine of the child (Table 6.4). Examination of Table 6.4 shows that we have taken, as the limit for unrestricted participation in physical education, the amount of structural scoliosis not

---

TABLE 6.4
Physical Education Program Recommendations Regarding Scoliosis

Scoliosis (°)	Physical Education
≤10	Physical education program without limitation
11–20	Physical education program without limitation Supervision/regular medical control
21–30	Partial exemption from the so-called "lineal program" Exemption of jumps over athletic or gymnastic device; some flexibility exercises on the floor — whirling, handstand position, etc.; athletic disk throwing, shot putting, etc.; lifting and carrying Capable of participating in a special exercise program, if organized Activity of choice: swimming, volleyball, basketball, running, tennis, table tennis, etc. Kinesitherapy within a medical center (facultative)
31–50	Total exemption from physical education until the end of treatment Capable of participating in a special exercise program, provided the program is conducted by instructors trained in kinesitherapy Activity of choice: swimming, volleyball, basketball Kinesitherapy within a medical center
≥51	Permanent exemption from physical education; special exercise programs are not anticipated, although if technically and professionally available, they would be desirable Optional activity of choice: swimming, walking Kinesitherapy within a medical center

exceeding 20°. The reason we have chosen the limit of 20°, and not 30°, is that we believe not only should the current amount of scoliosis be taken into account, but the physician should also keep in mind the evolutionary character of the disease, i.e., the prognosis. This can be evaluated only by a specially educated orthopedic specialist (who is a specialist in scoliosis), while the practical implementation of the prescribed program is left to the physical education instructor.[45] Precisely because of the discrepancy in the level of expertise between the orthopedic specialist and the physical education instructor, we have taken a lower degree of spinal curvature as the limit for unrestrained physical activity. In view of this, we offer some alternative suggestions, such as partial exception from physical education or exercising under special programs if the setup of these programs is feasible.[48,72] Athletic activities outside of school programs are also recommended with the stipulation that children with scoliosis exceeding 20° should be encouraged to participate in "useful" sports to correct the spine. This is particularly important when one takes into account that today active participation and competition in athletic activities begins at a very early age.

Some authors recommend that patients with scoliosis avoid the following sports: throwing (in athletics), fencing, and rowing. This opinion is compatible with the known statistics relative to pathological changes in the vertebrae and professional sports. Pathological changes in vertebrae are encountered in professional athletes with the following distribution: gymnasts (50%), divers (40%), and rowers (50%). There are no precise statistical data on the frequency of pathological changes in wrestlers and weight lifters, but empirical evidence shows that athletes who take part in these sports are also prone to develop scoliotic changes in the spine. The objective of Watson's study[92] was to investigate possible relationships between the incidence of sports injury and the existence of body mechanical defects in soccer players. The results suggest that intervention to improve body mechanics would be likely to reduce the incidence of sports injuries in football. In the study of Boldori et al.[4] on 3765 students of the fourth- and sixth-grade classes of primary schools the prevalence of kyphosis, hyperlordosis, and back asymmetry in children playing and not playing sports were compared. The incidence of hyperlordosis was significantly lower in boys playing soccer, whereas the incidence of back asymmetry was higher in girls playing basketball. Swimming was the best sport for females whereas males who swan registered a higher incidence of hyperkyphosis compared to the control group.

The discussion of scoliosis and sports involves, in our opinion, four points: (1) sports activities and idiopathic scoliosis; (2) sports in the treatment of idiopathic scoliosis; (3) physical education of school children with idiopathic scoliosis; and (4) sports activities in surgically treated patients with idiopathic scoliosis.

To deal with the first of these points, we decided to see whether professional athletes with scoliosis of the spine feel any difficulties and constraints in sports activities or in everyday life. We examined all the students at the School of Physical Education of the University of Zagreb; the total was 541: 353 males and 188 females (aged 19 to 25 years). All were anthropometrically measured and clinically examined by forward bending tests; moreover, all clinically positive cases for scoliosis of the spine were checked radiologically. All the examinees were also asked to fill out a special questionnaire concerning the presence of any spine complaints during their course of studies or engagement in a selected professional sports activity. On clinical examination, scoliosis of the spine was detected in 18.3% of the subjects. After radiography, 12.05% of the subjects could be said to have scoliosis proper, while only 2.3% of the subjects had scoliosis with a Cobb angle exceeding 10°. The presence of pain or any complaints during sports activities are reviewed in Table 6.5 for scoliotic subjects and the control group, i.e., subjects presenting with no scoliosis of the spine.

Regarding the incidence of scoliosis in our subjects, the results match the incidence established in the general population.[55] It should, however, be noted that our subjects had engaged in sports since their early youth, a fact that also later had a bearing on their choice of course of study. In terms of the occurrence of pain or difficulties in everyday life or in athletic activities, there were no differences between scoliotic and nonscoliotic subjects. All our scoliotic subjects followed their

TABLE 6.5
Presence of Pain or Complaints in the Spine

Pain/Complaints	Scoliosis (%)		
	Yes	No	Total
Male			
Yes	21.8	22.1	78
No	78.2	77.9	275
Total	100.0	100.0	353
Female			
Yes	37.2	37.2	70
No	62.8	62.8	118
Total	100.0	100.0	188

course of study normally and engaged in professional sports. No one consulted a doctor or discontinued his or her engagement in sports activity, even for a short period of time, because of scoliosis of the spine. This clearly demonstrates that scoliosis was not felt and was not considered by any means as an obstacle to engaging in intensive sports activities. Our study can also provide an indirect answer to the third point raised earlier, i.e., physical education in scoliotic children. It is our view that scoliotic children with an angle of up to 30° feel no constraints as far as physical education in school is concerned. Regarding sports activities in surgically treated patients with idiopathic scoliosis, it is our view that sports activities can be permitted, even up to the highest level, 1 year after surgery. We base this opinion on the fact that we have had examples of surgically treated patients engaging in professional competitive sports such as table tennis (Figure 6.12), handball, volleyball, etc. Of course, it should be noted that each patient should be considered individually.[99] According to Rubery and Bradford[78] the majority of surgically treated patients were returned to gym class between 6 months and 1 year after surgery. Contact sports were generally withheld until 1 year after surgery. Hopf et al.[30] recommend that operated patients begin sport activities 1 year postoperatively. For patients with a fused spine the number of the remaining lumbar moving segments and the deformity are essential for the exercise load. If there are fewer than three

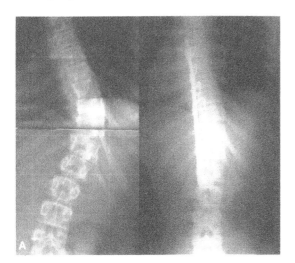
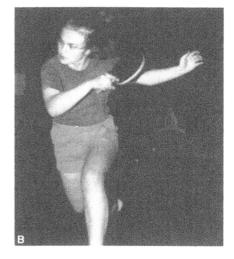

FIGURE 6.12 (A) Scoliosis in top-level table tennis player. Preoperative and postoperative roentgenogram. (B) One year after the surgery.

free lumbar segments all kinds of sport with axial and rotationary burdens are not recommended.[91] The study of Parsch et al.[66] revealed that over the long term, patients with idiopathic scoliosis suffer impairment of their sports activities compared with age-matched controls. The main reasons for this are functional impairment and the frequency of back pain. Sports activity is more restricted after extended spinal fusion than after non-operative treatment. Therefore, our general answer to whether individuals with scoliosis of the spine may engage in sports is affirmative, although we are aware that this matter will require additional extensive research if we are to be strictly accurate and more selective than we are today in answering the question raised by scoliosis and sports.

In summary, we feel that it is important to stress once again that any physical activity is preferable to physical inactivity for the patient with scoliosis.

VI. JUVENILE (ADOLESCENT) KYPHOSIS — SCHEUERMANN DISEASE AND SPORTS

Juvenile (adolescent) kyphosis represents a special clinical entity characterized by an increased, somewhat inferiorly positioned thoracal kyphosis, which in most cases is accompanied by radiologically visible wedge-shaped vertebrae (Figure 6.13). Currently, the criteria for diagnosing Scheuermann kyphosis are (1) incorrect superior and inferior epiphyseal rings of the vertebral body, (2) decrease of the intervertebral disk space, (3) the presence of one or more vertebra wedged for 5° or more, and (4) an increase of thoracal kyphosis to more than 40°. The etiology of the disease is, as yet, not completely known. The most commonly mentioned cause is thought to be avascular necrosis of the cartilaginous apophyseal rings of the body of the vertebra. This is why this disease is often categorized in the juvenile osteochondrosis group of diseases (epiphysitis and apophysitis). It is quite obvious that the causative factor of this disease is the discrepancy between the strain placed on and the weight-bearing capabilities of the epiphyseal rings of the body of the vertebra. In this context, the question of continued athletic activities presents with regard to the manifestation and possible worsening of the adolescent kyphosis of the spine. An increased frequency of radiologic abnormalities in the thoracolumbar spine has been reported among young athletes in various sports. To evaluate the incidence of these abnormalities in young elite skiers, Rachbauer et al.[73] compared 120 skiers younger than 17 years old with a random sample of 39 control subjects. The elite alpine

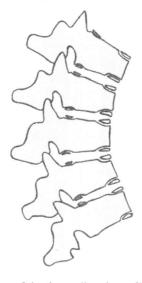

FIGURE 6.13 Schematic roentgenogram of the thoracalis spinae affected by Scheuermann disease.

skiers and ski jumpers demonstrated a significantly higher rate of anterior endplate lesions than did the control subjects. Strenuous physical activity is known to cause structural abnormalities in the immature vertebral body. Concern that exposure to years of intense athletic training may increase the risk of developing adolescent hyperkyphosis in certain sports, as well as the known association between hyperkyphosis and adult-onset back pain, led Wojtys et al.[98] to examine the association between cumulative hours of athletic training and the magnitude of the sagittal curvature of the immature spine. A sample of 2270 children between 8 and 18 years of age were studied. The results in these young athletes showed that a larger angle of thoracic kyphosis and lumbar lordosis were associated with greater cumulative training time. Biedert et al.[5] describe a 14-year-old female gymnast whose complaint was that of chronic low back pain. Radiographs and CT showed both lumbar manifestations of Scheuermann disease and an osseous destruction of the S1 vertebral body. The authors suggest that this is a sacral component of Scheuermann disease.

When evaluating the ability of patients suffering from Scheuermann disease to participate in athletic activities, two completely different and controversial viewpoints exist. One holds that the patient should be allowed to continue any and all athletic activities without any constraint, whereas the other holds that the patient should be forbidden all sports activities.[71] The reason for this difference in opinion is not only in the unclear genesis of this disease, but also in the inability to diagnose precisely the development of the disease. The obvious questions concerning this dilemma are (1) to what degree do athletic activities have a beneficiary effect on the disease? (2) can latent Scheuermann disease manifest in patients who participate in sports? and (3) will the disease show an inclination to worsen in patients who participate in athletic activities (athletic activities as an unfavorable factor)? First, we review all the possible positive effects that participating in sports activities can have on juvenile kyphosis. The positive effects include: "immobilizing" the spine in a functionally correct position caused by a correct stance, strengthening the muscles of the body, decreasing myostatic decompensation, increasing psychological functions such as will and energy, and increasing stamina and general condition, resulting from correct breathing technique and strengthening of the heart and vascular system; this will increase the patient's ability to participate in sports activities. Statistical analysis from the University Hospital in Heidelberg has shown that out of a total sample of 5504 athletes, 437 (7.8%) seek treatment because of pathological changes in the spine. Abstaining from athletic activities was recommended to only one patient. Orthopedic evaluation in professional athletes has shown that out of a total sample of 580 cases from 34 different sports, Scheuermann disease was found in 18.9% of the cases while an oval back was indicated in 16.8% of the sample. These changes, which frequently appear together, were therefore present in 35.7% of the sample. A recommendation for abstaining from athletic activities was issued in only eight cases. Numerous athletes have often continued training without any discomfort for a number of years despite having certain characteristics of Scheuermann disease. On the other hand, it is necessary to cite the opinion of Sward.[87] Because of the increased interest in physical fitness and because athletes start their training at younger ages, the risk for injuries to the growing individual has increased. The spine, as with the rest of the skeleton, is at greater risk of injury during growth, especially during the adolescent growth spurt. Back pain is more common among athletes participating in sports with high demands on the back than among other athletes and non-athletes. Disk degeneration, defined as disk height reduction on conventional radiographs and reduced disk signal intensity on MR imaging, has been found in a higher frequency among wrestlers and gymnasts than non-athletes. Abnormalities of the vertebral bodies including abnormal configuration, Schmorl's nodes, and apophyseal changes are common among athletes. These abnormalities are similar to those found in Scheuermann disease. Athletes with these types of abnormalities have more back pain than those without.

Therefore, we feel it is imperative to develop a uniform system of classification for patients suffering from juvenile kyphosis, and a uniform set of criteria concerning the advisability of athletic activity in patients with this syndrome. We believe that kyphotic changes in the spine should be classified into three basic stages:

1. Functional stage — at the end of the first decade of life, characterized by a kyphotic posture, but no radiologically visible changes characteristic of Scheuermann disease
2. Florid stage — between the ages of 12 and 14 years, characterized by a fully developed clinical picture and characteristic radiological findings
3. Late stage (or the stage following recovery from Scheuermann disease) — in patients over 18 years of age; generally referred to as discomforts and pains felt as a consequence of degenerative changes in the spine

Because of the complexity of the problem, other factors such as the precise localization of the disease, the expected level of strain, and the athletic activity in which the patient is participating bear considerable weight when reaching the final evaluation.[44] Taking this into account, it is quite logical that a relatively more developed juvenile kyphosis located more distally will have a worse prognosis. In the following, we are mainly concerned with the intensity of the strain and the effect of various athletic activities on different stages of the disease.

In the first stage of the disease, unrestricted individual (partly adapted) athletic activities are allowed. However, physical examinations (at least twice a year) are mandatory. In the event of any pain or discomfort, a consultation with the examining physician is necessary. This is followed by a reduction in the level of strain placed on the spine and in some cases a complete cessation of athletic activities (Table 6.6).

With patients in the second stage of the disease, athletic activities are forbidden to those who complain of pain or discomfort, in which case special, targeting medical gymnastics is prescribed. For the remaining patients (those who do not feel any pain or discomfort and who usually make up around 80% of the cases), athletic activities (with certain restrictions) are allowed (Table 6.7). Table 6.8 illustrates which athletic activities have a positive effect and which have a negative effect on the course of the disease.[71]

Of the sports with a general positive effect on the course of the disease, special attention should be given to the problem of horseback riding as an integral part of, or as an addition to, physical therapy of Scheuermann disease. Data provided by Harms[71] indicate that horseback riding can be an ideal addition to physical therapy of juvenile kyphosis. When the correct riding technique is employed and the patient is correctly sitting on the horse, the ischial tuberosities of the rider are in direct contact with the saddle while the hips are in a gently flexed position. At the same time, the patient's pelvis is continually and rhythmically turned over, which is the basic aim of medical

---

TABLE 6.6
Functional Stage of Kyphosis (Kyphotic Posture)

The level of strain placed upon the spine is unrestricted if the following is adhered to:
• Regular physical examination (at least twice a year)
• In the event of pain, a reduction in the level of strain

TABLE 6.7
Florid Stage of the Disease

In cases where pain or discomfort is felt (20% of the cases)
• All athletic activities are forbidden
• Specific (targeting) medical gymnastics is carried out
In cases with no pain (80% of the cases)
• Reduced activity with regard to bending compression and hyperextension of the spine

TABLE 6.8
Effect of Athletic Activities on the Course of the Disease

Athletic Activity	Positive Effect on the Development of the Disease	Negative Effect on the Development of the Disease
Swimming	Backstyle	Butterfly style
	Breaststroke with proper breathing technique	High jumps into water
Bicycling	At the recreational level (with high steering and back support)	At the competitive level
Gymnastics	Exercises that do not bend the spine	Exercises that include bending the spine
Athletics		All jumps (because of bending of the spine); weight lifting
Rowing		Because of bending and general strain on the spine
Games that use a ball: volleyball, basketball, soccer, tennis	Exercises all, for developing the body	

gymnastics. As a consequence of this, the rider is forced to adapt automatically (by process of compensation), the thoracal curvature is straightened, and shoulder girdle is placed into a correct position. During the rhythmic movements produced by the walking, trotting, and galloping of the horse, the pelvis is forced to perform alternating movements of bending and straightening, which is an ideal way to strengthen the back muscles, to loosen up, and to relax, i.e., unblock, the spine. Thus, we believe that horseback riding is an ideal activity, and from the patient's point of view an almost unconscious method of performing medical gymnastics. However, the physician should be careful when placing strain (particularly when the strain placed upon the spine is vertical as in horseback riding) on the spine of patients with extreme defects of the spine. These cases are relatively rare, but nonetheless the practicing physician should bear in mind that excessive vertical strain can negatively affect the already damaged disks. In such cases, horseback riding should be allowed only after an orthopedic brace is correctly put in place. Follow-up of patients who have used horseback riding as part of their therapy for juvenile kyphosis, in varying degrees, has shown that no pain or discomfort has appeared as a result of worsening of the disease, and also that there has been no increase in the curvature of the spine.

The third stage of the disease, characterized by the state of the patient once he or she has recovered from the disease, demands a differential evaluation (Table 6.9). An important fact to keep in mind is that patients belonging to the second group should, by all means, correctly perform their prescribed exercises for strengthening the muscles of the trunk (these exercises are performed solely as a means of increasing the patient's stamina). With patients who belong to the third group, the physician should differentiate between those who suffer daily pain and those who suffer only when exposed to excessive levels of strain. The physician should, likewise, differentiate between patients whose discomforts are caused by muscle insufficiency and those in whom pain is the result of degenerative changes. If the pain is present on a daily basis or if it appears after 30 min or longer periods of standing or walking, the prescribed treatment is shown in Table 6.9. In cases where the pain is caused by degenerative changes in the spine, the patient is encouraged to participate in athletic activities primarily to strengthen the muscles of the trunk to have a corrective effect on the mobile part of the spine.[21] Such patients are also encouraged to participate in sports that mobilize the spine without exposing it to excessive strain (i.e., sports that involve the handling of a ball).

TABLE 6.9
Late Stage of the Disease or State after Recovery

Evaluation of the General State	Admissible Level of Strain
A. Immobilization in a correct position, strong muscles of the trunk, absence of pain	Unlimited
B. Immobilization in an incorrect position, strong muscles of the trunk, absence of pain	Limited level of strain (i.e., special training sessions)
C. Immobilization in an incorrect position, weak muscles of the trunk, pain is present	Same level of strain as under B
	Medical gymnastics is performed
Daily pain	Athletic activity with a positive effect on the disease is chosen
Caused by muscle insufficiency	
Caused by secondary degenerative changes	Reduced strain
	Medical gymnastics
Pain felt when under strain	Same level of strain as under B

After reviewing the current state of knowledge, as reported in the medical literature, we feel obliged to report that, in the vast majority of cases, patients who suffer from Scheuermann disease can participate in athletic activities under medical supervision.[71] Inherent in this supposition is that the physician is aware of the particular demands that each sport places on the patient. Excessive kyphosing and lordosing (spondylolysis and spondylolisthesis) of the spine should be avoided. Swimming, for instance, is a sport that is often recommended because of its therapeutic and beneficial effects on the patient. However, the physician should be aware that swimming, if performed in the butterfly style, or without the proper breathing technique, can have a negative effect on the further development of the disease. Three patients with backache aggravated by swimming the butterfly stroke were subsequently diagnosed as having Scheuermann kyphosis.[95] These patients were treated with conventional methods. However, they were allowed additional time out of the brace to participate in swimming and were encouraged to do so, but they withheld from the butterfly. An average of 27% correction of curvature was seen with an average follow-up of 1.6 years. Symptoms subsided in all cases. We should also keep in mind that in some athletic activities, particularly at the professional level, pathological changes of the vertebrae are relatively frequent: in gymnastic exercises (50%), high jumps into water (40%), and rowing (50%). Therefore, we advocate orthopedic examinations for adolescents before they take up a particular sport.

In conclusion, we report that patients suffering from Scheuermann disease can participate in athletic activities. The only prerequisite is close collaboration among the athlete, trainer, and sports physician. Other important facts that should be kept in mind are the timely choice of an adequate sport, individual adaptation of the level of strain placed on the patient, and an interdisciplinary collaboration between all consulted specialists.[71]

REFERENCES

1. **Abraham, T., Holder, L., and Silberstein, C.** The retroisthmic cleft. Scintigraphic appearance and clinical relevance in patients with low back pain. *Clin. Nucl. Med.*, 1997; 22: 161–165.
2. **Basmaijan, J. V.** *Therapeutic Exercise.* Baltimore: Williams & Wilkins, 1978.
3. **Bellah, R.D., Summerville, D.A., Treves, S.T., and Micheli, L.J.** Low-back pain in adolescent athletes: detection of stress injury to the pars interarticularis with SPECT. *Radiology*, 1991: 180: 509–512.
4. **Boldori, L., Da Solda, M., and Marelli, A.** Anomalies of the trunk. An analysis of their prevalence in young athletes. *Minerva Pediatr.*, 1999; 51: 259–264.

5. **Biedert, R.M, Friederich, N.F., and Gruhl, C.** Sacral osseous destruction in a female gymnast: unusual manifestation of Scheuermann's disease? *Knee Surg. Sports Traumatol Arthrosc.*, 1993; 1: 110–112.
6. **Blanda, J., Bethem, D., Moats, W., and Lew, M.** Defects of pars interarticularis in athletes: a protocol for nonoperative treatment. *J. Spinal Disord.*, 1993; 6: 406–411.
7. **Brynhildsen, J.O., Hammar, J., and Hammar, M.L.** Does the menstrual cycle and use of oral contraceptives influence the risk of low back pain? A prospective study among female soccer players. *Scand. J. Med. Sci. Sports*, 1997; 7: 348–353.
8. **Cecker, T.J.** Scoliosis in swimmers. *Clin. Sports Med.* 1986; 5: 149–157.
9. **Congeni, J., McCulloch, J., and Swanson, K.** Lumbar spondylolysis. A study of natural progression in athletes. *Am. J. Sports Med.*, 1997; 25: 248–253.
10. **Cooke, P.M. and Lutz, G.E.** Internal disc disruption and axial back pain in the athlete. *Phys. Med. Rehabil. Clin. North Am.*, 2000; 11: 837–865.
11. **Bradford, D.S., Lonstein, J.E., Moe, J., Ogilvie, J.W., and Winter, R.B.** *Moe's Textbook of Scoliosis and Other Spinal Deformities*, 2nd ed. Philadelphia: W.B. Saunders, 1987.
12. **Bunnel, W.P.** The natural history of idiopathic scoliosis. *Clin. Orthop.*, 1988; 229: 20–25.
13. **Densiger, R.H.** Biomechanical considerations for clinical application in athletes with low back pain. *Clin. Sports Med.*, 1989; 8: 703–715.
14. **Domljan, Z. and Curkovic, B.** Iliolumbalni sindrom. *Lije. Vjesn.*, 1983; 105: 105–107.
15. **Durrigl, P. and Durrigl, T.** Degenerativne afekcije vertebralnog dinamikog segmenta. *Reumatizam*, 1967; 5: 165.
16. **Durrigl, T.** Lumbalgije u okviru suvremene medicine rada. *Lije. Vjesn.*, 1961; 83: 1079–1082.
17. **Dubravić, S., Pećina, M., Bojanić, I., and Šimunjak, B.** Common orthopaedic problems in female athletes. *Croat. Sports Med. J.*, 1991; 6: 38–46.
18. **Falter, E. and Hellerere, O.** High performance gymnasts during the period of growth. *Morphol. Med.*, 1982; 2: 39–44.
19. **Flory, P.D., Rivenburgh, D.W., and Stinson, J.T.** Isokinetic back testing in the athlete. *Clin. Sports Med.*, 1993; 12: 529–546.
20. **Garces, G.L., Gonzalez-Montoro, I., Rasines, J.L., and Santonja, F.** Early diagnosis of stress fracture of the lumbar spine in athletes. *Int. Orthop.*, 1999; 23: 213–215.
21. **Gaspert, T. and Pećina, M.** Bolni sindromi kraljeznice kod gimnasticarki. *Koćarkaćki Med. Vjesn.*, 1988; 3: 63–68.
22. **George, S.Z. and Delitto, A.** Management of the athlete with low back pain. *Clin. Sports Med.*, 2002; 21: 105–120.
23. **Goldberg, M.J.** Gymnastic injuries. *Orthop. Clin. North Am.*, 1980; 11: 717–726.
24. **Granhed, H. and Morelli, B.** Low back pain among retired wrestlers and heavyweight lifters. *Am. J. Sports Med.*, 1988; 16: 530–533.
25. **Green, J.P., Grenier, S.G., and McGill, S.M.** Low-back stiffness is altered with warm-up and bench rest: implications for athletes. *Med. Sci Sports Exerc.*, 2002; 34: 1076–1078.
26. **Guillodo, Y., Botton, E., Saraux, A., and Le Goff, P.** Contralateral spondylolysis and fracture of the lumbar pedicle in an elite female gymnast: a case report. *Spine*, 2000; 25: 2541–2543.
27. **Haasbeek, J.F. and Green, N.E.** Adolescent stress fractures of the sacrum: two case reports. *J. Pediatr. Orthop.*, 1994; 14: 336–338.
28. **Harvey, J. and Tanner, S.** Low back pain in young athletes. A practical approach. *Sports Med.*, 1991; 12: 394–406.
29. **Hasler, C. and Dick, W.** Spondylolysis and spondylolysthesis during growth. *Orthopade*, 2002; 31: 78–87.
30. **Hopf, C., Felske-Adler, C., and Heine, J.** Empfehlungen zur sportlichen Betätigung von Patienten mit idiopathischen Skoliosen. *Z. Orthop.*, 1991; 129: 204–207.
31. **Horne, J., Cockshott, W.P., and Shannon, H.S.** Spinal column damage from water ski jumping. *Skel. Radiol.*, 1987; 16: 612–616.
32. **Hutchinson, M.R.** Low back pain in elite rhythmic gymnasts. *Med. Sci. Sports Exerc.*, 1999; 31: 1686–1688.
33. **Jackson, D.W., Wiltse, L.L., and Cirincoine, R.J.** Spondylolysis in the female gymnast. *Clin. Orthop.*, 1976; 117: 68–73.

34. **Jacchia, G.E., Butler, U.P., Innocenti, M., and Capone, A.** Low back pain in athletes: pathogenetic mechanisms and therapy. *Chir. Organi Mov.*, 1994; 79: 47–53.
35. **Jajic, I. et al.** *Lumbalni Bolni Sindrom.* Zagreb: Skolska Knjiga, 1984.
36. **Junghanns, H.** *Wirbelsaule und Beruf.* Stuttgart: Hipokrates Verlag, 1980.
37. **Jusic, A.** Klinicka electromioneurografija i neuromuskularne bolesti. Zagreb: JUMENA, 1981.
38. **Jarrouse, Y.** Quel sport pour quel rachis? in *Muscles, Tendons et Sport,* Benezis, C., Simeray, J., and Simon, L., Eds. Paris: Masson, 1990; 73–77.
39. **Keene, J.S. and Drummond, D.S.** Mechanical back pain in the athlete. *Compr. Ther.*, 1985; 11: 7–14.
40. **Keane, G.P. and Saal, J.A.** The sports medicine approach to occupational low back pain. *W. J. Med.*, 1991; 154: 525–527.
41. **Kelsey, J.H. and White, A.A.** Epidemiology and impact of low back pain. *Spine*, 1980; 5: 133.
42. **Keros, P. et al.** *Functional Anatomy of Locomotor System.* Zagreb: Medicinska Naklada, 1968.
43. **Konermann, W. and Sell, S.** The spine: a problem area in high performance artistic gymnastics. A retrospective analysis of 24 former artistic gymnasts of the German A team. *Sportverletz. Sportschaden*, 1992; 6: 156–160.
44. **Korbelar, P., Kuera, M., and Sazima, V.** Abweichungen der Wirbelsaule in der sportmedizinischen Praxis. *Sportverletz. Sportschaden,* 1988; 2: 69–71.
45. **Kovacic, S., Ed.** *Scoliosis and Kyphosis.* Zagreb: Medicinska Naklada, 1977.
46. **Kraft, D.E.** Low back pain in the adolescent athlete. *Pediatr. Clin. North Am.* 2002; 49: 643–653.
47. **Kramer, J.** Intervertebral disk diseases: causes, diagnosis, treatment and prophylaxis. Stuttgart: G. Thieme, 1982.
48. **Kristofic, I. and Pećina, M.** Ciljana primjena programa preventivnih vjezbi u djece sa skoliozom kraljeznice. *Acta Med.,* 1982; 8: 33–36.
49. **Kujala, U.M., Salminen, J.J., Taimela, S. et al.** Subject characteristics and low back pain in young athletes and nonathletes. *Med. Sci. Sports Exerc.,* 1992; 24: 627–632.
50. **Kujala, U.M., Taimela, S., Erkintalo, M. et al.** Low-back pain in adolescent athletes. *Med. Sci. Sports Exerc.*, 1996; 28: 165–170.
51. **Kujala, U.M., Taimela, S., Oksanen, A., and Salminen, J.J.** Lumbar mobility and low back pain during adolescence. A longitudinal three-year follow-up study in athletes and controls. *Am. J. Sports Med.*, 1997; 25: 363–368.
52. **Kujala, U.M., Kinnunen, J., Helenius, P. et al.** Prolonged low-back pain in young athletes: a prospective cases series study of findings and prognosis. *Eur. Spine J.*, 1999; 8: 480–484.
53. **Lee, C.K.** Office management of low back pain. *Orthop. Clin. North Am.,* 1988; 19: 797–804.
54. **Locke, S. and Allen, G.D.** Etiology of low back pain in elite boardsailors. *Med. Sci. Sports Exerc.,* 1992; 24: 964–966.
55. **Loncar-Dusek, M., Pećina, M., and Prebeg, Z.** A longitudinal study of growth velocity and development of secondary gender characteristics versus onset of idiopathic scoliosis. *Clin. Orthop.,* 1991; 270: 278–282.
56. **Mahlamaki, S., Soimakallio, S., and Mischelsson, J.E.** Radiological findings in the lumbar spine of 39 young cross-country skiers with low back pain. *Int. J. Sports Med.*, 1988; 9: 196–197.
57. **Micheli, L.J.** Back injuries in gymnastics. *Clin. Sports Med.*, 1985; 4: 85–93.
58. **Micheli, L.J. and Wood, R.** Back pain in young athletes. Significant differences from adults in causes and patterns. *Arch. Pediatr. Adolesc. Med.*, 1995; 149: 15–18.
59. **Nachemson, A.** Lumbar intradiscal pressure. *Acta Orthop. Scand. Suppl.,* 1960; 43: 1.
60. **Nachemson, A.** Work for all, for those with low back pain as well. *Clin. Orthop.,* 1983; 179: 77.
61. **Nadler, S.F., Wu, K.D., Galski, T., and Feinberg, J.H.** Low back pain in college athletes. A prospective study correlating lower extremity overuse or acquired ligamentous laxity with low back pain. *Spine*, 1998; 23: 828–833.
62. **Nyska, M., Constantini, N., Cale-Benzoor, M. et al.** Spondylolysis as a cause of low back pain in swimmers. *Int. J. Sports Med.*, 2000; 21: 375–379.
63. **Ogon, M., Riedl-Huter, C., Sterzinger, W. et al.** Radiologic abnormalities and low back pain in elite skiers. *Clin. Orthop.*, 2001; 390: 151–162.
64. **Ohlen, G., Wredmark, T., and Spamgfort, E.** Spinal sagittal configuration and mobility related to low back pain in the female gymnast. *Spine*, 1989; 14: 847–850.

65. **Omey, M.L., Micheli, L.J., and Gerbino, P.G., II.** Idiopathic scoliosis and spondylolysis in the female athlete. Tips for treatment. *Clin. Orthop.*, 2000; 372: 74–84.

66. **Parsch, D., Gartner, V., Brocai, D.R. et al.** Sports activity of patients with idiopathic scoliosis at long-term follow-up. *Clin. J. Sport Med.*, 2002; 12: 95–98.

67. **Pećina, M.** Piriformis sindrom u diferencijalnoj dijagnostici bolnih kriza. *Acta Orthop. Iugosl.*, 1975; 6: 196–200.

68. **Pećina, M.** Contribution of the etiological explanation of the piriformis syndrome. *Acta Anat.* (Basel), 1979; 105: 181–187.

69. **Pećina, M., Ed.** *Scoliosis and Kyphosis*. Zagreb: University Press Liber, 1983.

70. **Pećina, M., Dubravčić-Šimunjak, S., Bojanić, I., and Janković, S.** Scoliosis and sports. *Acta Med. Croat.*, 1993; 47: 189–191.

71. **Pećina, M. and Kovac, V.** Morbus Scheuermann and sports. *Sportsko-Med. Objave*, 1983; 20: 123–129.

72. **Pećina, M. and Kristofic, I.** Tjelesni odgoj u prevenciji i lijecenju skolioticnih drzanja i skolioza. *Fiz. Kult.*, 1983; 3: 93–105.

73. **Rachbauer, F., Sterzinger, W., and Eibl, G.** Radiographic abnormalities in the thoracolumbar spine of young elite skiers. *Am. J. Sports Med.*, 2001; 29: 446–449.

74. **Ralston, S. and Weir, M.** Suspecting lumbar spondylolysis in adolescent low back pain. *Clin. Pediatr.* Philadelphia, 1998; 37: 287–293.

75. **Reid, D.A. and McNair, P.J.** Factors contributing to low back pain in rowers. *Br. J. Sports Med.*, 2000; 34: 321–322.

76. **Rossi, F. and Dragoni, S.** Lumbar spondylolysis and sports. The radiological findings and statistical considerations. *Radiol. Med.* (Torino), 1994; 87: 397–400.

77. **Roy, S.H., De Luca, C.J., Snyder-Mackler, L. et al.** Fatigue, recovery, and low back pain in varsity rowers. *Med. Sci. Sports Exerc.*, 1990; 22: 463–469.

78. **Rubery, P.T. and Bradford, D.S.** Athletic activity after spine surgery in children and adolescents: results of a survey. *Spine*, 2002; 27: 423–427.

79. **Schmorl, G. and Junghans, H.** *Die Gesunde und die kranke Wirbelsaule in Rontgenbild und Klinik.* Stuttgart: G. Thieme, 1968.

80. **Shah, M.K. and Stewart, G.W.** Sacral stress fractures: an unusual cause of low back pain in an athlete. *Spine*, 2002; 27: E104–108.

81. **Sires, A.** Rachis de l'enfant et sport: de la prevention a la pratique, in *Muscles, Tendons et Sport,* Benezis, C., Simeray, J., and Simon, L., Eds. Paris: Masson, 1990; 289–295.

82. **Spengler, D.M.** Low back pain: assessment and management. New York: Grune & Stratton, 1982.

83. **Stablker, A., Paulus, R., Steinborn, M. et al.** Spondylolysis in the developmental stage: diagnostic contribution of MRI. *Fortschr. Gebiete Rontg. Bildg. Verf.*, 2000; 172: 33–37.

84. **Stagnara, P.** *Les Deformations du Rachis.* Paris: Masson, 1985.

85. **Standaert, C.J., Herring, S.A., Halpern, B., and King, O.** Spondylolysis. *Phys. Med. Rehabil. Clin. North Am.*, 2000; 11: 785–803.

86. **Stanish, W.** Low back pain in athletes: an overuse syndrome. *Clin. Sports Med.*, 1987; 6: 321–344.

87. **Sward, L.** The thoracolumbar spine in young elite athletes. Current concepts on the effects of physical training. *Sports Med.*, 1992; 13: 357–364.

88. **Tanchev, P.I., Dzherov, A.D., Parushev, A.D. et al.** Scoliosis in rhythmic gymnasts. *Spine*, 2000; 25: 1367–1372.

89. **Tertti, M., Paajanen, H., Kujala, U.M. et al.** Disc degeneration in young gymnasts. A magnetic resonance imaging study. *Am. J. Sports Med.*, 1990; 18: 296–298.

90. **Verni, E., Prosperi, L., Lucaccini, C. et al.** Lumbar pain and fin swimming. *J. Sports Med. Phys. Fitness.*, 1999; 39: 61–65.

91. **von Strempel, A., Scholz, M., and Daentzer, M.** Sports capacity of patients with scoliosis. *Sportverletz. Sportschaden*, 1993; 7: 58–62.

92. **Watson, A.W.** Sports injuries in footballers related to defects of posture and body mechanics. *J. Sports Med. Phys. Fitness*, 1995; 35: 289–294.

93. **Weiker, G.G.** Evaluation and treatment of common spine and trunk problems. *Clin. Sports Med.*, 1989; 8: 399–417.

94. **White, A.A. and Panjabi, M.M.** *Clinical Biomechanics of the Spine.* Philadelphia: J.B. Lippincott, 1978.
95. **Wilson, F.D. and Linseth, R.E.** The adolescent "swimmer's back." *Am. J. Sports Med.*, 1982; 10: 174–176.
96. **Wirtz, D.C., Wildberger, J.E., Rohrig, H., and Zilkens, K.W.** Early diagnosis of isthmic spondylolysis with MRI. *Z.. Orthop. Grenzgeb.*, 1999; 137: 508–511.
97. **Wismach, J. and Krause, D.** Spinal changes in artistic gymnasts. *Sportverletz. Sportschaden*, 1988; 2: 95–99.
98. **Wojtys, E.M., Ashton-Miller, J.A., Huston, L.J., and Moga, P.J.** The association between athletic training time and the sagittal curvature of the immature spine. *Am. J. Sports Med.*, 2000; 28: 490–498.
99. **Wood, K.B.** Spinal deformity in the adolescent athlete. *Clin. Sports Med.*, 2002; 21: 77–92.
100. **Young, J.L., Press, J.M., and Herring, S.A.** The disc at risk in athletes: perspective on operative an nonoperative care. *Med. Sci. Sports Exerc.*, 1997; 29: S222–S232.

Part IV

Lower Extremities

7 Hip and Thigh

I. GROIN PAIN

A. GROIN STRAIN

Painful groin syndrome is generally considered the most frequent overuse syndrome in some athletic activities, e.g., soccer.[78,79] The term *groin pain,* itself, clearly indicates the site and the principal symptom of the syndrome. However, neither the site nor the pain is precisely defined. When considering the location and anatomic structures affected by overuse, together with the locations and characteristics of pain, the location might be precise, but it could also be a case of diffuse vague pain in the groin region, small pelvis, and upper leg regions. The term *syndrome* is fully justified; indeed, the symptoms are numerous and so are the causes of pain in the groin region. Hence, it is not surprising that the modern medical literature abounds with terms defining pain in the groin region: necrotic osteitis pubis, anterior pelvic joint syndrome, traumatic pubic osteitis, Pierson syndrome, gracilis muscle syndrome, pubic stress symphysitis, pubic symphysis osteoarthropathy, symphysitis, pubic chondritis, and post-traumatic necrosis of the pubic bone.[71,78] These terms and expressions have commonly been used to describe adductor tendinitis, rectus abdominis tendinitis, avulsion injuries of the adductor tendons, postoperative changes without infection in the symphysis region, and a number of arthrotic changes. According to Morelli and Smith[61] groin injuries comprise 2 to 5% of all sports injuries, and adductor strains and osteitis pubis are the most common musculoskeletal causes of groin pain in athletes.

To understand the painful groin syndrome, one should bear in mind all the muscles that insert in the symphysis region. These muscles attach to the upper and lower branches of the pubic bones, to the inguinal ligament, to the branch of the ischium, to the small trochanter, and to the iliac crest (Table 7.1). Also, it should not be forgotten that the groin region is the crossroad of two muscle systems: (1) the trunk muscles, primarily the abdominal muscles, and (2) the muscles of the lower extremity (Figure 7.1), primarily the upper leg muscles, especially the adductor muscles (Figure 7.2). The pelvic region and the hips carry large static and dynamic weight so that both the static and dynamic positions of the pelvis in space ensure equilibrium (balance) of those muscles that are either inserted into or originate from the pelvic bones, especially in the groin region. In general considerations of overuse syndrome development, it is stated that the balance of antagonist muscles and coordination of agonists are essential to prevent the syndrome. When we think that the activity and equilibrium of muscles originating from or being inserted into the groin region may also be disturbed because of changes in the lumbar spine or the hip joint, the knee joint, the sacroiliac joints, and the symphysis, it is no wonder that multiple possibilities exist for the development of overuse syndrome affecting certain anatomic structures in the groin region. In addition, it is important to recognize that the groin region is the site of the inguinal canal located above the inguinal ligament, of the lacuna nervorum and vasorum beneath the inguinal ligament, and of the femoral and obturator canals. Of course, these are the openings through which the anatomic structures for the lower extremity pass. Therefore, the groin region is justly referred to as the Gibraltar of the lower extremity. All of the above-mentioned information clearly shows that the painful groin syndrome cannot be attributed solely to one particular anatomic structure in the region but, rather, that the approach to the syndrome, in prevention, diagnosis, or treatment, should be based on the idea of multiple causative factors contributing to development of the syndrome.[78,79] It is precisely the approach we have assumed although we distinguish between painful groin

TABLE 7.1
Insertion and Origin of Muscles in the Groin Region

Lig. inguinale	M. obliquus abdominis externus
	M. obliquus abdominis internus
Ramus superior	M. rectus abdominis
Ossis pubis	M. obliquus abdominis externus
	M. obliquus abdominis internus
	M. transversus abdominis
	M. pyramidalis
	M. pectineus
	M. adductor longus
	M. adductor brevis
Ramus inferior	M. adductor brevis
Ossis pubis	M. gracilis
	M. cremaster
Ramus ossis ischii	M. adductor magnus
Tuber ossis ischii	M. adductor magnus
	M. semitendinosus
	M. semimembranosus
	M. biceps femoris (caput longum)
Trochanter minor	M. iliopsoas
Spina iliaca anterior superior	M. sartorius
Spina iliaca anterior inferior	M. rectus femoris

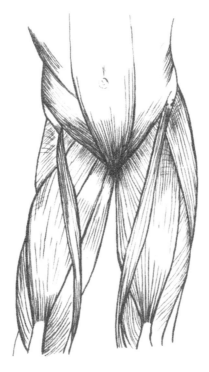

FIGURE 7.1 The groin area is the crossroads of the trunk and lower extremity muscles.

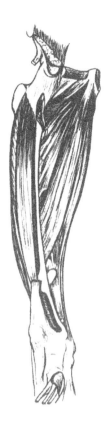

FIGURE 7.2 Adductors of the thigh.

syndrome in a narrow sense and painful groin syndrome in a wider sense, for which "pain in the groin" seems to be a more appropriate term because the pain may arise from different pathological conditions in and around the groin region.

Painful groin syndrome in a narrow sense primarily implies tendinitis of the adductor muscles — the long adductor muscle and the gracilis muscle in the first instance, as well as the abdominal muscles, especially the rectus abdominis and pyramidalis muscles. Long-lasting tendinitis of these muscles may evolve into a general and vague picture of diffuse pain in the pubic bones and the symphysis region.

1. Etiopathogenesis

Bones, muscles, and tendons are the structures within which changes characteristic of a painful overuse syndrome commonly develop.[31,49,59,62,72,77–79] According to Martens et al.,[59] the load-bearing capacity of a tendon and tendinous attachment differs from individual to individual. The limits of this capacity may be influenced by external and internal factors. The internal factors include insufficiency of the paravertebral and abdominal muscles, hip joint disorders, inequality of leg length, disorders in the sacroiliac joint, and foot deformities. The external factors include injuries in the adductor region, injuries in the hip joint, and inadequate athletic training.[59] Several authors have reported[10,30,41,42,64,94] that the cause of groin pain lies in the disproportion between the strength of the abdominal wall muscles and the strength of the lower extremity muscles, as well as in an uneven load on all attachments in the symphysis and groin region (Figure 7.3).

Durey and Boeda[20] report that the painful groin syndrome is an injury or, more precisely, a lesion characteristically occurring in soccer players, because the symphysis region is the point of attachment and the point of origin for groups of muscles with different functions, which are

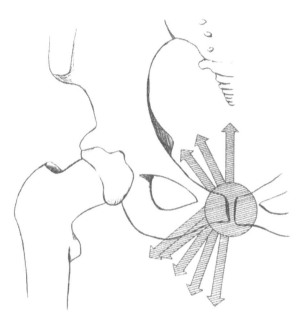

FIGURE 7.3 Graphic representation of the imbalance of strength between the abdominal muscles and muscles of the lower extremity.

especially active during soccer playing. Adductors are under strain when side blows are performed in soccer and also when striking a ball with the interior side of the foot. In addition, these groups of muscles are especially under strain when "sliding starts" are performed (Figure 7.4). In the course of attempting a start, lower extremities are placed wide apart. The parting point is the symphysis region where the abdominal muscles contract simultaneously to prevent falling backward. Janković[43] also states that during sliding starts the adductor muscles are involved to their maximum, resulting in strain, microtraumas, and eventually inflammation of the region surrounding the tendinous attachment.[49] In 78.2% of patients, clinical examination reveals weakness of oblique abdominal muscles, so that during the sliding starts the upper leg muscles, especially the adductors, become extremely strained.[43] Sudden acceleration or change in direction of movement and rough ground have been reported as other causes of adductor muscle overuse.[20,43]

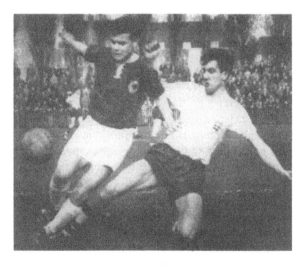

FIGURE 7.4 Maximal use of the adductor muscle, especially the gracilis muscle, is present in sliding tackles.

Anderson et al.[3,4] describe "thigh splints," also known as the adductor insertion avulsion syndrome, a painful condition affecting the proximal to mid femur at the insertion of the adductor muscles of the thigh. Symptoms of vague hip, groin, or thigh pain may be associated with stress-related changes in the proximal to mid femoral shaft (thigh splints). When interpreting magnetic resonance (MR) imaging studies of the pelvis in patients with theses symptoms, careful attention should be directed to this portion of the femur.

Ashby[5] considers chronic obscure groin pain as enthesopathy or "tennis elbow" of the groin. Among 49 patients with chronic obscure groin pain, enthesopathy at the pubic insertion of the inguinal ligament was the cause of pain in 30 patients (32 groins). Enthesopathy also occurred in five rectus and one adductor longus tendons.

Chronic pain on the ventral surface of the scrotum and the proximal ventromedial surface of the thigh especially in athletes has been diagnosed in various ways; recently, in Europe the concept of "sports hernia" has been advocated.[2] According to Fon and Spence[26] sports hernia is a debilitating condition that presents as chronic groin pain. A tear occurs at the external oblique abdominal muscle, which may result in an occult hernia. The diagnosis of sports hernia is difficult. The condition must be distinguished from the more common osteitis pubis and musculotendinous injuries, but according to Hackney[35] the sports hernia should be high on the list of differential diagnoses in chronic groin pain. Sports hernias can cause prolonged groin pain, and provide a difficult diagnostic dilemma. In athletes with prolonged groin pain, with increased pain during Valsalva maneuvers, and tenderness along the posterior inguinal wall and external canal, an insidious sports hernia should be considered. In cases of true sports hernia, treatment is by surgical reinforcement of the inguinal wall.[55] Lovell[54] reviewed 189 athletes with chronic groin pain to determine the prevalence of the underlying conditions. The most common pathology found was an incipient hernia (50% of cases). Fredberg et al.[27] present a review based on the results of 308 operations for unexplained, chronic groin pain suspected to be caused by an imminent, but not demonstrable, inguinal hernia, i.e., sports hernia. However, in 49% of cases hernia was also demonstrated on the opposite, asymptomatic groin side. In conclusion, the final diagnosis (and treatment) often reflects the specialty of the physician and the present literature does not supply proper evidence to support the theory that sports hernia constitutes a credible explanation for chronic groin pain.[3,27]

In a study published by Malycha and Lovell,[58] 50 athletes with chronic undiagnosed groin pain underwent surgical exploration and inguinal hernia repair. Operative findings revealed a significant bulge in the posterior inguinal wall in 40 athletes. Of the 50 athletes, 41 (93%) returned to normal activities. It is concluded that athletes with chronic groin pain who are unable to compete in active sport should be considered for routine inguinal hernia repair if no other pathology is evident after clinical examination and investigation.[26,58] Taylor et al.[87] also consider abdominal musculature abnormalities including inguinal hernias as a cause of groin pain in athletes.

Pilardeau et al.[75] term painful groin syndrome *the Lucy syndrome,* named after the fossil hominid remains of Australopithecus. The authors explain that the relatively more erect posture of modern humans, when compared to Australopithecus, has caused a change in the position of the pelvis, leading to lowering of the ischial bone tuberosity and to lifting of the symphysis and anterior pelvic aspect. This, in turn, has led to strain in the adductor muscles and in the rectus femoris muscle.

2. Epidemiology

Painful groin syndrome is most commonly found in soccer players.[16,20,42,43,74,79,83] Cabot[20] reported that 0.5% of 42,000 examined soccer players complained of pain in the groin. Ekstrand and Gillquist[23] conducted a 1-year follow-up study of 12 soccer teams. Their results show that 13% of injuries are located in the groin region and 2.73% of cases are injuries of the adductor muscle. Nielsen and Yde[65] studied 123 soccer players; according to their report, 2.75% of cases are attributed to groin tendinitis. In a study sample of 1475 soccer players examined by Janković,[43] 6.24% had painful groin syndrome. According to Gilmore[32] groin pain in the soccer athlete is a common problem accounting for 5% of soccer injuries. Kidron[46] considers that approximately 2.5% of all sports-related injuries are in the pelvic area.

In addition to soccer players, these injuries have also been reported in ice hockey, water polo, and handball players, fencers, high jumpers, bowlers, skaters, hurdlers, swimmers, and triathletes.[18,24,50,69,71,72,79,88]

3. Clinical Picture and Diagnostics

Painful groin syndrome is characterized by pain in the inguinal and lower abdominal regions. Often the pain develops gradually, and the athlete is unaware of its connection with any injury. As time goes by, the pain becomes more severe and irradiates into the upper leg adductor zone, the pubic region, and the perineum, spreading toward the hips and the anterior abdominal wall. Overuse only increases the pain. The pain restricts certain motions during training and the game, especially reducing the speed of the player. In adductor overuse, the pain occurs during sprinting, ball kicking, sliding starts, and pivoting.[20,43,59,94] Furthermore, the motion performed when entering or exiting a car may cause pain. In abdominal muscle overuse, the pain occurs in the lower abdominal region, especially during sprinting and sudden motion, e.g., a rapid change of direction when running.[59] Pain may appear bilaterally as well. In persistent cases, pain occurs simultaneously in the lower abdominal area and the adductor region.

Similar to other overuse syndromes, painful groin syndrome is also characterized by specific developmental stages. Initially, the pain is unilateral and appears shortly after the strain. It disappears until the time of the next training session so that it does not prevent the athlete from actively participating in training and matches. With time, the pain persists and is not relieved by the time of the next athletic event. During that period, even a minor strain may cause severe pain. Then the pain becomes bilateral, i.e., it occurs in the other groin. This causes greater difficulties for the athlete even in everyday life, especially when climbing up and down stairs or hills, rising from a sitting position, or attempting to get up from bed. Coughing, sneezing, defecation, urination, and sexual activity also cause pain in the groin.

The pain is not strictly limited to the origin or insertion of a given muscle but diffusely extends over a wider area, thus justifying the term pubalgia. This may be understood as a developmental stage of the adductor or rectus abdominis muscles tendinitis, but also of the gracilis and pyramidalis muscles tendinitis. These events confirm the complexity of a pathological condition, i.e., best described by the term painful groin syndrome. Mental difficulties of these patients should by all means be added to the clinical picture, for they are too often suspected of malingering.

Clinical examination reveals pain during palpation of the pubic bone occurring above the gracilis and adductor longus muscle attachments.[30,43,59] The patient feels pain during passive elevation of the foot at external rotation and in maximum abduction of the upper leg. When testing adductors, the patient lies on his or her back with slightly abducted lower extremities so that a fist may be inserted between the knees (Figure 7.5). The patient is then asked to hold the fist tightly by contracting the adductor muscles of the upper leg. This motion causes pain in the typical site of the upper leg adductor muscle attachment on the pubic bone.[43,74,79]

In tendinitis of the rectus abdominis muscles, pain following palpation appears in the region of the attachment to the ramus superior pubis (superior pubic branch). In a great number of patients, inspection of the abdominal wall reveals weakness of the oblique abdominal muscles. The so-called sausage and spindle-like prominences above the iliac crest and the inguinal ligament (in the literature commonly referred to as Malgaigne's sign) appearing during contraction of the abdominal muscles are also signs of abdominal wall weakness.[43]

For the testing of rectus abdominal muscles, the patient lies on his or her back and lifts the lower extremities at an angle of 45° from the surface (Figure 7.6). During these motions, pain occurs in the lower abdominal region and at the point of the muscle attachment to the pubic bone. The pain also appears when the patient is asked to sit up (Figure 7.7).

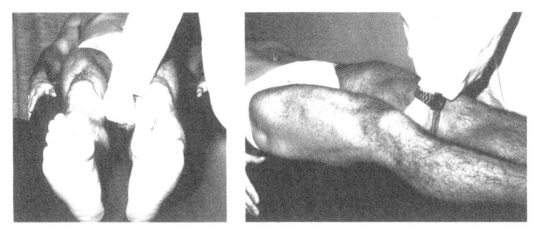

FIGURE 7.5 Two views of test for determining tenderness of the adductor muscles.

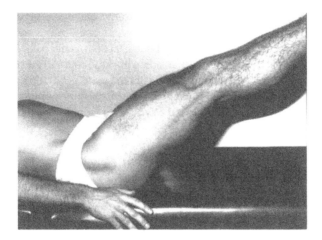

FIGURE 7.6 Test for the straight abdominal muscles: lift legs from the surface to form a 45° angle.

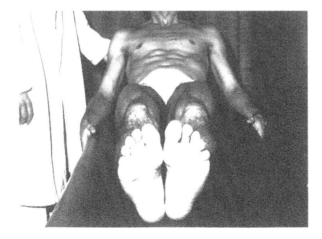

FIGURE 7.7 Test for the straight abdominal muscles: lift trunk from the surface.

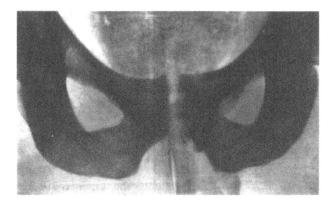

FIGURE 7.8 The first stage of radiologically visible changes in the pubic symphysis. Translucency is visible on the affected (painful) side of the groin.

When painful groin syndrome is identified, radiographic images of the pelvis, showing pubic bones, symphysis, and both hips, are necessary.[70] These enable the physician to rule out arthrotic changes in the hip, stress fractures and reactions of the pubis ramus and pubic symphysitis, pelvic avulsion injuries, and femoral stress fractures as causes of pain; it also enables rough analysis of sacroiliac joints and the caudal segment of the lumbosacral spine (discogenic pain, spondylolysis). Centered scans of the symphysis with the patient in a standing position first on one leg (the affected side) and then on the other leg are recommended. The scans may show pathological mobility of the symphysis, which is important because, during athletic activity (e.g., running, jumping, kicking), the symphysis moves cranially, caudally, anteriorly, posteriorly, and to a lesser degree, rotatively. These motions of the symphysis are especially observable in soccer players and long-distance walkers.[53]

According to Janković,[43] radiologically identified changes in the symphysis and pubic bones may be classified into four stages that correspond to the developmental stages of the painful groin syndrome clinical picture. During the first stage, the os pubis is characterized by larger, semioval or semicircular transparencies directed toward the symphyses (Figure 7.8). The transparencies are not limited strictly to the gracilis muscle attachment; they also appear at the attachments of the adductor longus and brevis muscles. In the gracilis muscle attachment to the counter pubic bone, rare osteolithic changes may be seen. Significant asymmetry of the symphyseal regions is absent at this stage. In the second stage, the symphyseal region is clearly asymmetrical (Figure 7.9). The pathological changes in the pubic bone show unclear borders. Scan of the distal symphyseal half

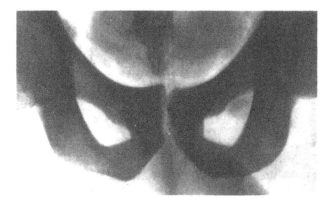

FIGURE 7.9 The second radiologically visible stage is characterized by asymmetry of the pubic symphysis and sawlike bone on the pathologically changed side.

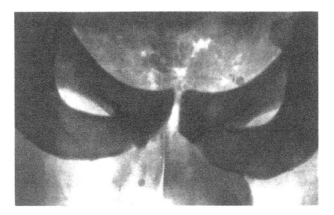

FIGURE 7.10 Shape of the pubis bones is irregular and undulating with clearly visible bone condensation (characteristic for the third radiological stage).

shows an oblique borderline of the bones with the disappearing symphyseal angle (bone) so that now it is an oblique line extending medially and proximally in the distal and lateral directions. The third stage is characterized by an irregularly undulated symphyseal region of both pubic bones, a partially protruded edge borderline, and a clear condensation of osseous structure (Figure 7.10). At the site of Cooper's pubic ligaments, a borderline swelling or borderline indentation of the osseous apposition may be seen bilaterally. The symphyseal fissure may be vertical or extremely oblique. The scan resembles that of a secondary osteoarthritis. In addition to the changes occurring in the symphyseal region during the third stage, the fourth stage is characterized by osseous areas assuming the form of lines or drops in the foramen obturatum area or symphyseal part of the pubic bone branch. According to the radiologic morphological criteria, these correspond to the finding of myositis ossificans.[94] The sclerosing bone regions are primarily found on the side showing an old post-traumatic pubic osteonecrosis (Figure 7.11).

Scintigraphy has proved highly valuable in the diagnosis. It helps to identify stress fracture and avulsions in the pubic branch region.[21,51] Le Jeune et al.[51] state that in the case of radiologically invisible changes in the symphysis and a negative scintigraphic finding, the diagnosis is long adductor muscle tendinitis.

Ultrasound diagnostics are very useful in differential diagnosis of acute trauma from overuse injuries (Figure 7.12).[8,45,68] Orchard et al.[68] found that dynamic ultrasound examination is able to

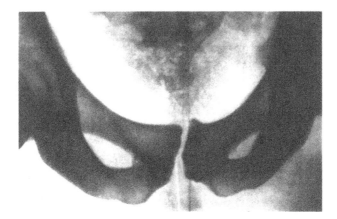

FIGURE 7.11 The fourth radiologically visible stage, in addition to the changes described in the third stage, is characterized by clearly visible radiological signs characteristic for post-traumatic osteonecrosis.

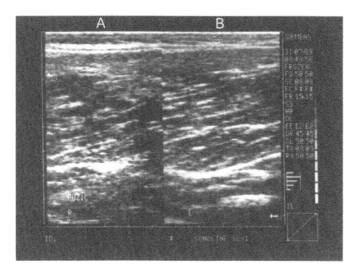

FIGURE 7.12 Sonogram shows partial rupture of adductor muscles. (A) Rupture; (B) normal muscles.

detect inguinal canal posterior wall deficiency in young males with no clinical signs of hernia. This condition is very prevalent in professional Australian Rules football players, including some who are asymptomatic. Ultrasonography is also a valuable method in the diagnosis of chronic tendon injuries in the groin.[45] Sonography can be used to depict changes in the tensor fascia lata, confirming the diagnosis and assessing the severity of the tendinopathy.[8]

If inguinal hernia is suspected as a cause of pain, herniography should be performed.[56,82,83,95]

The role of MR imaging (MRI) in diagnosis of groin pain in athletes is stressed by many authors.[7,19,22,47] MRI is a valuable method for evaluating discrete and ambiguous pelvic pain in athletes, particularly for identifying concomitant changes in the superior ramus, which may give rise to long-standing pain localized laterally in the groin.[22]

4. Treatment

Treatment of painful groin syndrome is as complex as the causes of its development. Similar to many other situations in medicine, the best possible treatment is based on elimination of causes and prevention of development of the syndrome. Because painful groin syndrome is not of unique etiology, it is very difficult to establish unique principles of treatment. However, in our opinion, treatment should always commence with non-operative procedures; only when these fail, strictly selective surgery should be contemplated, i.e., depending on the cause of the syndrome. The following are some common principles of non-operative treatment of painful groin syndrome regardless of its cause: (1) alleviate pain and control inflammation in the myotendinous apparatus; (2) hasten healing of the myotendinous apparatus; and (3) control further activities.

We emphasize that it is of utmost importance to commence treatment as early as possible, i.e., when the first symptoms occur.[71,78] Not paying due attention to initial symptoms and continuation with athletic activity at the same intensity are the most common mistakes. When an athlete contacts a physician during the initial stage of overuse syndrome development, training intensity should be decreased and all motions causing pain avoided (i.e., sudden acceleration or change of direction; an easy-going straight-line run is allowed). When the syndrome is at a later stage of development, the athlete should discontinue training altogether.

Local cryotherapy of the painful site is aimed at alleviating inflammation. Ice should be applied four to five times a day for 15 to 20 min (never directly on the skin). Before the activity, heparin or similar ointments together with techniques promoting local hyperemia, i.e., heating, are locally applied.[59,72,78,79] Anti-inflammatory nonsteroidal medications are given orally, also with the aim of relieving inflammation. Some authors[36,59,79] recommend local corticosteroid infiltrations. Stretching exercises should be commenced at the same time, starting with static stretching exercises for the adductor muscles. These exercises are performed such that the muscle is stretched to the point of pain and kept in the position for 15 to 20 s. The athlete should repeat the stretching exercises several times a day, at minimum three times. It is especially important that the stretching exercises do not cause additional pain. Along with the exercises, cryotherapy is recommended (local application of ice). Holmich et al.[38] recommend active physical training as treatment for long-standing adductor-related groin pain in athletes. An active training program with a program aimed at improving strength and coordination of the muscles acting on the pelvis, in particular the adductor muscles, is very effective in the treatment of athletes with long-standing adductor related groin pain. A distinct syndrome of lower-abdominal/adductor pain in male athletes appears correctable by a procedure designed to strengthen the anterior pelvic floor.[60]

Athletes with weak abdominal muscles should work on strengthening the muscles. Equal strengthening is required for both the rectus and oblique abdominal wall muscles.[72,74] The exercises should be performed several times a day. At the beginning, the exercises are repeated only a few times and without any load. Gradually, the number of repetitions and the load are increased. Athletes who have discontinued their specific training may engage in supplemental activities, purposely maintaining general physical fitness (bicycling, backstroke or freestyle swimming).

The purpose of rehabilitation is to preserve strength, elasticity, and contractual abilities of the tissues along with the improvement of mechanical and structural characteristics of the tissues. At the start of rehabilitation, isometric or static strengthening exercises for the adductor muscles are introduced.[36] When performing isometric exercises, the contraction force should not cause any pain. The training begins with only a few contractions daily; later, training gradually increases the number of contractions and the total load.

At the stage when isometric training may be performed without pain, dynamic strength training may be introduced. At the beginning of the adductor muscle dynamic training, the weight of the leg itself is used as a load. Gradually, the load may be increased by adding supplemental weight, although this should not be done too fast. Isokinetic training is actually best, although it requires special equipment (Cybex). Isokinetic training includes working at a constant speed and maximum resistance along the whole range of movement.

At the end of rehabilitation, athletes may return to their specific training. The common error is that many tend to resume full athletic engagement too soon, which may necessitate repeating the treatment. In such cases, instead of approximately 3 months, the treatment may be prolonged for 12 or more months. According to Lynch and Renstrom[55] patience is the key to obtain complete healing, because a return to sports too early can lead to chronic pain, which becomes increasingly difficult to treat. Fricker[29] states: "Patients should be reminded that there are no short cuts and precipitate return to sport is not worth the risk in most cases."

Operative treatment of painful groin syndrome, to a certain extent, depends on the attitude in approaching this complex problem.[10,30,41,43,81,94] Authors who consider tendinitis the most important feature of the painful groin syndrome recommend operative treatment in terms of disinsertion, i.e., cutting (tenotomy) of the adductor, gracilis, rectus abdominis, piramidalis, and other muscles. Authors who believe that painful groin syndrome is primarily caused by disproportion in strength between the abdominal wall muscles and the upper leg muscles, especially emphasizing weak abdominal muscles (oblique and transverse abdominal muscles in particular), recommend surgical strengthening of the anterior abdominal wall by the method applied for inguinal hernia, i.e., by the Bassini method.[64]

Gilmore's groin repair is very successful according to Brannigan et al.[14] They present results of 100 consecutive groin repairs in 85 young athletes, and 96% of their patients returned to competitive sport within 15 weeks. Laparoscopic preperitoneal hernia repair should be considered as a treatment modality in athletes presenting with chronic groin pain.[85] Azurin et al.[6] also state that endoscopic preperitoneal herniorrhaphy is an effective treatment for obscure groin pain when the pain is associated with an inguinal hernia; the procedure allows a short recovery time before return to full athletic activity. The "hockey groin syndrome," marked by tearing of the external oblique aponeurosis and entrapment of the ilioinguinal nerve, is successfully treated by ilioinguinal nerve ablation and reinforcement of the external oblique aponeurosis.[40]

We agree with the opinion of Quilles,[94] who in praising Bassini's modified operative methods, states: "It is more fair to enrich the poor than to impoverish the rich," meaning that it is better to strengthen or support the abdominal muscles than to weaken the adductor muscles by tenotomy. Nevertheless, on the basis of our experience, we have realized that sometimes the disequilibrium and difference are so great that muscular balance may be achieved only by a combination of "enriching the poor and impoverishing the rich." The fact is that in certain cases, besides strengthening the anterior abdominal wall, tenotomy of the adductor needs to be done, especially when tendinitis is clinically obvious, e.g., upper leg long adductor tendinitis. Tenotomy of the adductor longus tendon in the treatment of chronic groin pain in 16 male athletes was described by Akermark and Johansson.[1] All but 1 of the athletes returned to the same sport within a mean of 14 weeks after surgery. Similar to all other surgeries, postoperative rehabilitation procedure is essential here as well. On the second or third day following surgery, the patient gets up and starts with a moderate dose of static exercises for abdominal muscles accompanied by general physical therapy measures, such as breathing exercises, exercises for proper circulation in the lower extremities, etc. After the stitches are removed and the wound appears satisfactory, swimming, easy walking, and gradual increase in the intensity of exercises for strengthening of the abdominal wall muscles are recommended. A month after the operation (sometimes even 3 weeks after), the patient is allowed to run easily and to perform the exercises for abdominal wall muscles regularly, gradually increasing the load, but only to the pain limit. After 6 weeks (sometimes 5), a soccer player is allowed to begin ball training. After 8 weeks (sometimes 6), the player is allowed to participate in a training match, and after 10 to 12 weeks (sometimes 8) full participation in athletic activity is allowed. Eventually, it should be pointed out that when discussing treatment of painful groin syndrome, whether operative or non-operative, the approach should always be individualized. In this regard, it should be emphasized that procedures may and should be combined and that there is no unique scheme for painful groin treatment.

Prevention is of utmost importance, especially in young patients, and should be aimed at strengthening the abdominal muscles, particularly the obliques. Exercises for strengthening abdominal muscles are often done so that only the rectus abdominal muscles are strengthened. If exercises are exaggerated, tendinitis may result, i.e., painful groin syndrome may develop. We add here that stretching exercises should be intensified for the upper leg muscles and for the whole lower extremity muscle, especially before and after the athletic activity. The greatest mistake is made when the athlete, the coach, and the physician lose patience, and the athlete returns to full strain too soon, thus repeatedly causing the recurrence of painful groin syndrome. Such a course of events may continue for several years only to result in definite cessation of any engagement in athletic activities.

From the etiological, diagnostic, and therapeutic points of view, painful groin syndrome is further complicated by the many origins and insertions of muscles and tendons in the pelvis, hip joint, and proximal segment of the upper leg regions as well as the bursal sacs (synovial sacs), all of which may be the site of pathological changes in terms of overuse syndrome. The possibility of stress fracture of bones in these regions should be taken into account, and in younger persons, the possibility of epiphysiolysis and apophysitis should not be ruled out. Nerve entrapment syndromes are also of importance in differential diagnosis.[13,73,96]

B.   OSTEITIS PUBIS

The term osteitis pubis indicates that inflammatory changes are taking place, although in the majority of cases, no causative agent has been isolated (identified). A number of different terms have been used in the past with the purpose of avoiding the connotation of inflammation (e.g., osteitis necroticans pubis, syndroma rectus-adductor, traumatic inguino-leg syndrome, anterior pelvic joint syndrome, groin pain in athletes, osteoarthropathy of the pubic symphysis, traumatic pubic osteitis, Pierson syndrome, pubic chondritis, and post-traumatic osteonecrosis of the pubic bone.[80,92] However, these expressions were also used to denote pelvis stress fractures, adductor tendinitis, avulsion injuries of the adductor tendons, postoperative changes occurring without infection, stress changes in the symphyseal region, and various arthrotic changes. Major and Helms[57] have studied a group of athletes in whom stress injuries to the pubic symphysis are associated with changes in the sacroiliac joint as demonstrated by degenerative changes or in the sacrum as manifested as a sacral stress fracture. In a large number of cases, a link between osteitis pubis and urological problems has been described as well as postpartal complications.[71]

The condition was first reported in an athlete (fencer) in 1932 by Spinelli.[84] Only in the early 1960s, did significant study of the condition in athletes begin. Osteitis pubis has been reported in soccer players, U.S. football players, basketball players, long-distance runners (marathon), and long-distance walkers.[9,71,72,92,150] As Lloyd-Smith et al.[53] report on the basis of their research, the condition is more common in men. Osteitis pubis is seen particularly in those sports requiring sprinting and sudden changes of direction. Among the total number of osseous lesions in the pelvic bones, osteitis pubis ranks third in frequency (14% in males, 6.3% in females). These authors further report that in 43% of patients, varus alignment has been observed, and in 29% of cases different leg length has been found. So far, etiology is unknown. Steinbach et al.[86] report that venous obstructions caused by trauma might be the cause, whereas Goldstein and Rubin[33] report that osteitis pubis is caused by chronic infection, and Wheeler[90] ascribes pubic osteitis to aseptic necrosis.

The patient complains of pain in the lower abdomen and in the groin, but cannot link it to any known injury. At a later stage, the pain spreads in a fanlike manner into the adductor region. The principal characteristics of the pain are that its onset is linked to the athletic activity, then diminishes, and gradually disappears upon resting. The pain may also occur or become more intense when coughing, sneezing, or laughing.[93] Palpation during clinical examination causes pain along the pubic bone and the symphysis itself.

Radiography of the pelvis shows no changes in the initial phase of the disorder, but later on, the alterations are visible in the symphyseal region (fraying and sclerosis).[71]

Scintigraphic scan shows increased bilateral accumulation of radionuclides around the pubic bone even in the initial stage of the disease (Figure 7.13).[15,17] Scintigraphy helps in differential diagnosis, because in the case of avulsion or stress fracture in the pubic branch region, the accumulation of radionuclides is unilateral.[80] Le Jeune[51] reported that, in the case of a negative scintigraphic scan and positive clinical signs, adductor longus and rectus muscle tendinitis is usually in question.

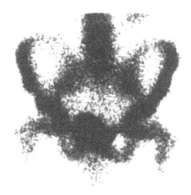

FIGURE 7.13 Bone scan demonstrating osteitis pubis.

MRI has proved to be a valuable diagnostic technique in detecting osteitic change as an area of low signal intensity on T1-weighted images and of high and homogeneous signal intensity on T2-weighted scans without fat suppression.[7] Only MRI can permit an accurate and early diagnosis of the different sports-related pubic conditions.[52] MRI is also a valuable tool in monitoring the alterations with reference to their response to treatment, which may also help return the athletes to their activities. Verrall et al.[89] concluded that athletes with groin pain and tenderness of the pubic symphysis and/or superior pubic ramus have clinical features consistent with the diagnosis of osteitis pubis. The increased signal intensity seen on MRI is due to pubic bone marrow edema, such that an association exists between the clinical features of osteitis pubis and the MRI finding of pubic bone marrow edema.

The treatment recommended is reduced athletic activity or complete rest if the pain is too severe. As supplementary activity, swimming may be recommended (free and backstroke only). Pearson[71] recommends administration of nonsteroidal anti-inflammatory medication in combination with corticosteroids (10 mg of prednisone daily for 10 days). Symphyseal corticosteroid injection is a useful technique for treatment of osteitis pubis in athletes.[39,66] We use a corticosteroid injection with 5 ml 2% lidocaine. The procedure is well tolerated and may facilitate early resumption of competitive activities. Prospects for recovery are very good. When athletic activities are avoided, the disease subsides spontaneously. However, the duration of the recovery process may be variable.

Mulhall et al.[63] reported of outcome with symphyseal curettage in cases refractory to conservative management of osteitis pubis in professional soccer players. Williams et al.[93] treated operatively seven rugby players with osteitis pubis and vertical instability at the pubic symphysis after non-operative treatment had failed to improve their symptoms. The vertical instability was diagnosed based on flamingo view radiographs showing greater than 2 mm of vertical displacement. Operative treatment consisted of arthrodesis of the pubic symphysis by bone grafting supplemented by a compression plate. At a mean follow-up of 52.4 months, all patients were free of symptoms and flamingo views confirmed successful arthrodesis with no residual instability of the pubic symphysis.

II. ILIOPSOAS TENDINITIS AND BURSITIS (PSOAS SYNDROME)

Iliopsoas muscle tendinitis is caused by frequent repetitive flexions in the hip joint (Figure 7.14). It is a relatively uncommon and unrecognized cause of anterior hip pain and anterior snapping hip, but it is common in weight lifters, skiers, oarsmen, football players, long and high jumpers, and hurdlers.[11,44,54,64,69] Bursitis of the iliopsoas is more common in gymnasts, wrestlers, and uphill runners. The principal clinical sign is pain in the groin region on the anterior aspect of the hip joint, in the small pelvis, and sometimes in the back as well; this is accounted for by the fact that tendinitis and bursitis of the iliopsoas develop as a result of hypertonic muscle and prolonged strain. Overuse or excessive strain may be the consequence of disturbed biomechanical relations in the lumbar spine and in the hip joint.

Initially, the pain is mild in intensity, but the repetitive strain makes the pain increasingly intense to the degree that the athletic activity becomes impossible. Often the patient cannot find the link between the pain and injury. Palpation of the tendinous attachment to the small trochanter causes pain. If when sitting a patient places the affected leg over the healthy one, i.e., with its heel touching the knee of the unaffected leg, a painful and tense iliopsoas muscle may be palpated. During flexion of the upper leg in the hip joint against resistance, pain occurs at the point of the muscle attachment. The motion should be attempted in a sitting position (Figure 7.15) because then the iliopsoas muscle is the chief and only flexor of the upper leg in the hip joint. Between the iliopsoas tendon and the anterior aspect of the hip joint articular capsule, there is a nut-sized synovial sac; when irritated, it produces a clinical picture of a typical bursitis, reaching its peak on the fourth or fifth day from the onset of pain during and after the athletic activity. Eventually, the activity has to be discontinued entirely.

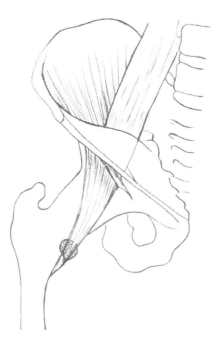

FIGURE 7.14 Insertion of the iliopsoas tendon to the lesser trochanter. Broken lines indicate bursa between the tendon and joint capsule.

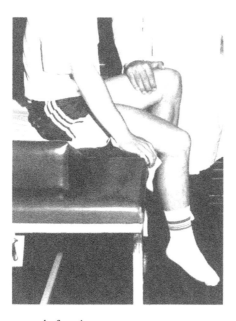

FIGURE 7.15 Test for iliopsoas muscle function.

In differential diagnosis, the following should also be considered: tendinitis of the adductor longus muscle and rectus femoris muscle; rupture and avulsion of the iliopsoas muscle, rectus femoris muscle, and adductor longus muscle;[12] and labrum lesions in the hip joint.[37] MR-arthrography is recommended in patients with clinical suspicion for labral lesions of the hip joint.[37] Rupture of the iliopsoas muscle is extremely rare. In most cases, the attachment of the muscle to the small trochanter is the rupture site. The injury most commonly occurs when the upper leg in flexion is forcibly extended. At the moment of injury, the athlete complains of severe pain in the groin region. After the injury, the upper leg is usually kept in flexion, adduction, and external rotation as this is the position of least pain.[74] Each attempt at extension and internal rotation causes severe pain as does active contraction of the muscles. At the site of the injury, pain occurs on palpation. In addition to ultrasound, radiographs should be taken and attention paid to the probability of the avulsion of the small trochanter.[25,91] These studies are especially important for the younger age groups as in these patients the epiphysis of the small trochanter is not yet united with the bone shaft. In the case of complete avulsion, surgery is the only recourse available.[34,67,72] Tendinitis of the iliopsoas muscle is treated non-operatively.

When the patient contacts a physician during the initial stage of the disorder, training should not be completely discontinued but only reduced in intensity. However, if the athlete contacts a physician at a later stage, a rest period of 3 to 4 weeks is necessary. During this time, the athlete may engage in substitute activities, such as swimming or riding a bicycle. The site of injury is treated with ice for at least 15 min, three to four times a day (the ice should not come into direct contact with the skin), and anti-inflammatory nonsteroidal drugs are administered orally. Renstrom et al.[79] recommend an additional local infiltration of corticosteroids followed by a 2-week rest. At the very beginning of treatment, stretching and static strengthening exercises without load or weight bearing should be commenced.[36] At a later stage, dynamic exercises for strengthening may be introduced, although care should be taken that the patient feels no pain. When pain is absent, even during maximum load, the athlete is ready to resume training at full intensity as required for participation in competition.

III. TENDINITIS OF THE RECTUS FEMORIS MUSCLE

Tendinitis of the rectus femoris muscle usually occurs as a result of prolonged, repetitive, and sudden increase in strengthening exercise training or intensive goal-shooting training, e.g., in soccer. The athlete feels pain in the region above the hip joint at the point where the rectus femoris muscle attaches anteriorly and inferiorly to the iliac spine. The patient is unable to associate the onset of pain with an injury. Pain appears on palpation of rectus femoris muscle tendon attachment. The pain may also be provoked by resisting upper leg flexion and lower leg extension.

In differential diagnosis, the following should be taken into consideration: rupture or avulsion of the rectus femoris muscle or iliopsoas muscle, tendinitis of the iliopsoas muscle or adductor longus muscle, stress fracture of the femoral neck, changes in the hip joint (e.g., arthrosis, rheumatoid arthritis, osteochondritis dissecans, loose body in a joint, synovitis), and bursitis.[74,79] Calcific tendinitis at the site of origin of the rectus femoris muscle is a rare lesion.[76] Presumed to be formed by deposition of hydroxyapatite crystals, this entity may be confused with other lesions such as os acetabuli or post-traumatic abnormalities. The characteristic location and appearance of the calcifications in a symptomatic patient with no history of trauma should allow diagnosis and subsequent symptomatic therapy.[76] Calcification of the reflected tendon of the rectus femoris muscle often closely resembles osteoarthritis of the hip.[169] Pain in the groin region may develop as a consequence of the rupture at the attachment point or in the proximal third of the rectus femoris muscle. At the moment of injury, the pain is so severe that the athlete is compelled to discontinue activity. If complete rupture takes place, the muscle cannot be contracted. During palpation of the injured site, pain appears, and often a defect may be palpated on the belly of the muscle. Upper leg flexion against resistance causes pain at the site of the injury. Pain in the muscle during extension of the lower leg against resistance is an additional sign of the trauma.

Ultrasound will confirm the diagnosis and enable evaluation of the severity of injury (Figure 7.16). Radiographs should also be taken to rule out bone avulsion.

Complete rupture, especially if in combination with avulsion fracture, is treated operatively.[67] Partial rupture is usually treated non-operatively; during the initial stage, rest, cryotherapy, compression, elevation, and nonsteroidal anti-inflammatory medication are prescribed. Rehabilitation

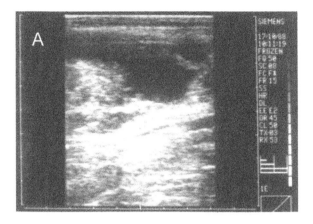

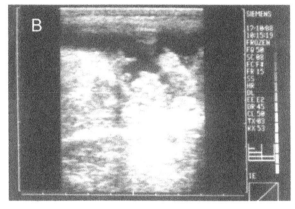

FIGURE 7.16 Sonogram showing rupture with hematoma of rectus femoris muscle. (A) Relaxation; (B) contraction.

in terms of strengthening the muscles may begin when pain and swelling disappear.[48] Treatment of rectus femoris muscle tendinitis is very similar to the treatment of overuse syndromes, e.g., tendinitis of the iliopsoas muscle.

IV. HIP EXTERNAL ROTATOR SYNDROME

Although rare, external hip rotator syndrome presents a complicated problem, with regard to both diagnosis and treatment.[99] It is most frequently found in hurdlers and ballet dancers where the symptoms consist of a vague pain in the buttocks and the greater trochanter area. The inflexibility of the hip external rotators (Figure 7.17), primarily the piriformis, gemellus superior, and gemellus inferior muscles, together with the internal rotation contracture of the hip, is thought to lead to chronic overuse of these muscles.

To locate the exact area of pain, the upper leg is maximally and externally rotated during physical examination; pressure is applied to the greater trochanter area, producing intense pain. Differential diagnosis must take into account the possibility of piriformis muscle syndrome[73,104] and trochanteric bursitis, which can be confirmed by ultrasound. Piriformis muscle syndrome is described in Chapter 13, Nerve Entrapment Syndromes.

Non-operative treatment of short external hip rotator syndrome is based on stretching exercises for the afflicted muscle groups and neighboring muscles, with the aim of increasing their flexibility and concurrently the flexibility of the whole hip. Other non-operative measures include rest, ice, and nonsteroidal anti-inflammatory drugs. Steroid injections can also be administered.

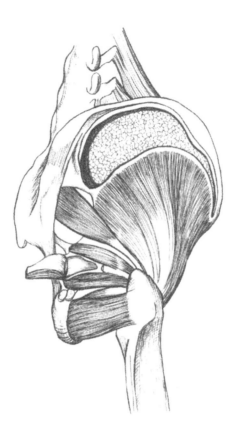

FIGURE 7.17 External rotator muscles of the hip.

V. GLUTEUS MEDIUS SYNDROME

Gluteus medius syndrome is characterized by pain involving the buttock, lateral hip, groin, or the sacroiliac joint. The patient may also report dysestesia and numbness in the buttock or posterior aspect of the thigh. Prolonged sitting may exacerbate pain. The pain can be caused by overuse and inflammation of gluteus medius muscle or of the sciatic nerve, which is immediate adjacent. Kellgren[102] in 1938 was the first to report on referred pain from the gluteus medius. Activities with high hip abductor demand have been associated with gluteus medius syndrome, especially in martial arts, cycling, aerobics, and dance. Usually, symptoms are elicited only during sports participation, but gradually these symptoms can become present during the patient's routine daily activities. Green et al.[98] report on a 24-year-old male amateur cyclist who had numbness and tingling localized to a small region on the superior portion of the right buttock. The area involved demonstrated paresthesia to light touch sensory evaluation. Manual-resisted muscle testing created soreness in the lumbosacral area and buttock. Trigger points were identified in the right gluteus medius. During physical examination, hip abductor strength should be compared with the contralateral extremity. A full neurological exam is essential to rule out neurological causes. Palpation in the buttock region and over the gluteus medius muscle can discover trigger points or tenderness to palpation on or around the muscle. Regarding trigger points, Njoo and Van der Does[103] consider that the clinical usefulness of trigger points is increased when localized tenderness and the presence of either jump sign or patient recognition of the pain complaint are used as criteria to establish the presence of trigger points in the gluteus medius muscle. Other physical findings in gluteus medius syndrome may include limited stretch range of muscle, presence of a taut, palpable band in muscle, and referred pain produced by direct palpation of trigger points. Kingzett-Taylor et al.[100] performed 250

MRI examinations of the hip for the evaluation of buttock, lateral hip, or groin pain. Examination revealed that 8 patients had complete retracted tears of the gluteus medius, 14 patients had partial tears, and MR findings were consistent with tendinosis in 13 patients. The gluteus minimus muscle was also involved in 10 patients. MRI is the imaging technique of choice in differentiating the cause of hip pain in athletes.[105]

Differential diagnosis of the gluteus medius syndrome includes sciatica, radiculopathy, greater trochanteric bursitis, iliotibial band syndrome, quadratus femoris tendinitis,[101] sacroiliac joint dysfunction, and especially piriformis syndrome, but also the pelvic compartment syndrome.[97]

Stretching exercises of the gluteus medius, gluteus maximus, gluteus minimus, and the piriformis is recommended in conservative treatment of patients with gluteus medius syndrome. Cold packs, ultrasound, and other modalities can be incorporated into the physical therapy program. The physician should try to modify the aggravating movements and elements in the athlete's sport, for example, seat size or positioning of cyclist. Injection with anesthetics and corticosteroids has been diagnostic as well therapeutic. In rare cases, surgical debridement of a chronic tendinosis is an available option.[102]

VI. SNAPPING HIP SYNDROME

Snapping hip syndrome is a symptom complex characterized by an audible snapping sensation, which is usually, but not necessarily, associated with hip pain during certain movements of the hip joint. A number of different etiologies, both intra-articular and extra-articular, have been described.[117,125,127,130] Intra-articular causes for the snapping hip include loose bodies, osteocartilaginous exostosis, osteochondromatosis, and subluxation of the hip.[121,128] The most frequent extra-articular cause of the snapping hip is the snapping of the iliotibial band over the greater trochanter. For a long time, this was considered to be the only extra-articular cause of snapping hip syndrome, but further research has uncovered other extra-articular etiologies. These include the snapping of the iliopsoas tendon over the iliopectineal eminence of the pelvis, the iliofemoral ligaments over the femoral head, and the tendinous origin of the long head of the biceps femoris muscle over the ischial tuberosity. Taking into account the localization of the causes for snapping hip, we recognize three different snapping hip syndromes: medial (internal), lateral (external), and posterior snapping hip syndrome (Table 7.2).

Medial (internal) snapping hip syndrome is caused either by the snapping of the iliopsoas tendon over the iliopectineal eminence of the pelvis, as described by Nunziata and Blumenfeld[120] in 1951, or by the snapping of the iliofemoral ligaments over the femoral head, as reported by Howse[113] in 1972. This type of snapping hip syndrome is frequently found in ballet dancers.[125] When leaving the pelvis, the iliopsoas tendon lies in a groove between the anterior-inferior iliac

TABLE 7.2
Extra-Articular Causes of Snapping Hip

Localization	Etiology
Medial (internal)	Iliofemoral ligament over femoral head
	Iliopsoas tendon over the anterior-inferior iliac spine
	Iliopsoas tendon over the iliopectineal eminence
	Iliopsoas tendon over the bony ridge on the lesser trochanter
Lateral (external)	Iliotibial band over the greater trochanter
	Gluteus maximus tendon over the greater trochanter
Posterior	Tendinous origin of the long head of the biceps femoris muscle over the ischial tuberosity

spine laterally and the iliopectineal eminence medially. From there, the tendon inserts on the lesser trochanter passing over an anteromedially placed bony ridge. The snapping of the iliopsoas tendon occurs when the hip is extended from a flexed, abducted, and externally rotated position. The snapping can take place over the anterior-inferior iliac spine, the iliopectioneal eminence, or at the point where the iliopsoas tendon passes over the bony ridge on the lesser trochanter. In addition to an audible snapping sound, this movement is also, in some cases, accompanied by a painful sensation in the frontal hip area.

Wunderbaldinger et al.[129] evaluated the diagnostic value and significance of various imaging techniques for demonstrating the underlying causative pathology of clinically suspected internal snapping hip syndrome. The underlying causative pathology could be established in 37% of patients by the use of conventional radiographs alone and in 46% of patients by ultrasonography alone, and in combination in 83% of the patients. When MRI was used, a causative pathology was found in all patients (100%).

Differential diagnosis includes consideration of psoas bursitis. Frequent movements of the iliopsoas tendon can lead to irritation of the iliopsoas bursa situated between the iliopsoas tendon and the anterior hip capsule; communication exists between them in about 15% of adult hips.[127] This irritation is accompanied by pain in the frontal hip area, which increases typically with resisted hip flexion. Psoas muscle syndrome, which consists of psoas bursitis, enthesitis, and tenosynovitis of the iliopsoas muscle, is therefore a clinical entity that should be differentiated from snapping hip syndrome.

Treatment of medial (internal) snapping hip syndrome depends on whether the syndrome is asymptomatic, accompanied only by audible snapping sounds, or whether it is associated with hip pain. Non-operative treatment consists of reduction of (or temporary cessation of) painful activities and movements, nonsteroidal anti-inflammatory medication, and stretching exercises.[127] Good results are sometimes obtained by steroid injections. Surgical treatment is indicated in those patients whose painful symptoms persist after prolonged non-operative therapy. The operative procedure consists of resection of the lesser trochanter bony prominence, transection of the tendinous slip at the level of the groove between the iliopectineal eminence and anterior-inferior iliac spine, and/or partial or total release of the iliopsoas tendon.[118,121,127]

Jacobson and Allen[115] referred 18 patients with 20 symptomatic hips and all patients underwent lengthening of the iliopsoas tendon. Lengthening of the iliopsoas tendon was accomplished by step cutting of the tendinous portion of the iliopsoas. All patients, except one, had a marked reduction in the frequency of snapping after tendon lengthening, and 14 of 20 hips had no snapping postoperatively. Gruen et al.[112] present 11 patients (12 hips) surgically treated by lengthening of the iliopsoas tendon through a true ilioinguinal approach. All 11 patients had complete postoperative mitigation of their snapping hip, and 9 reported excellent pain relief. Although non-operative measures are usually successful in the treatment of internal snapping hip, surgical tendon lengthening is a viable approach in cases refractory to non-operative therapy.

Lateral (external) snapping hip syndrome is the most frequent and, consequently, the best-known snapping hip syndrome. It is caused by the slipping of the iliotibial band over the posterior part of the greater trochanter (Figure 7.18), and is frequent in runners, dancers, and basketball players.[114,121,125–127] It can be asymptomatic or accompanied by pain, which is especially intense in those cases that develop trochanteric bursitis. In addition to the audible snapping phenomenon, the symptomatic form is characterized by pain in the region of the greater trochanter, which sometimes radiates to the buttocks and/or lateral thigh. The snapping can best be observed by placing the palm of one's hand on the greater trochanter area of the patient during walking. Another maneuver that will consistently reproduce the patient's symptoms is to have the patient stand on the healthy leg and imitate running motions on the affected side. In some cases, the snapping can only be demonstrated by having the patient lie on the unaffected side with a large pad under the pelvis so that the affected hip is in adduction. Keeping the knee in extension, which tightens the fascia lata, the affected hip is then actively flexed and extended. The iliotibial band can then be felt to flip anteriorly

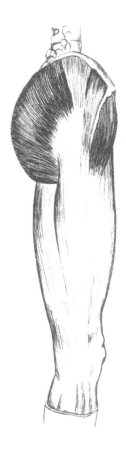

FIGURE 7.18 Iliotibial band.

over the greater trochanter as the hip is flexed. The most common cause of the slipping of the iliotibial band over the greater trochanter is its excessive tightness (shortening), which can result from leg length discrepancies, pelvic tilt, or certain activities such as habitual running on the sides of roads. In the last case, the disorder occurs on the "downside leg," because the drainage pitch of the road causes increased tension in the iliotibial band in this extremity. Tightness of the iliotibial band is diagnosed using Ober's test. Excessive tightness of the iliotibial band causes greater friction between the band, the greater trochanter, and the bursa that is normally located there; this in turn leads to chronic trochanteric bursitis. Characteristic symptoms of this bursitis include intense pain in the greater trochanter area and limping.

Conventional sonographic studies can identify signs of tendinitis, bursitis, or synovitis. Dynamic sonographic studies reveal the cause of snapping hip in most patients.[109,123] Snapping hip is characterized on sonography by a sudden abnormal displacement of the snapping structure. Choi et al.[109] found that dynamic sonography was helpful in the diagnosis of external snapping hip syndrome; it showed real-time images of sudden abnormal displacement of the iliotibial band or the gluteus maximus muscle overlying the greater trochanter as a painful snap during hip motion.

Non-operative treatment of lateral (external) snapping hip syndrome consists of rest, avoidance of painful movements, iliotibial band stretching exercises, strengthening of the hip flexors, buttocks, hamstrings, hip rotation muscles, and quadriceps, nonsteroidal anti-inflammatory medication, and correction of the disturbed biomechanical relationships of the lower extremities (arch supports, adequate shoes, etc.). Injections of local anesthetics and soluble steroids are also sometimes effective.[119]

In refractory cases that do not respond to non-operative therapy, surgical treatment is indicated. Numerous operative procedures have been described. Operative procedures include resection of a

TABLE 7.3
Operations for Painful Snapping Hip

Author (Year)	Operation	Ref.
Dickinson (1928)	Simple release of the band	48
Orlandi et al. (1981)	Incision of the band and suturing of the cut ends to the greater trochanter	48
Bruckl et al. (1984)	Diagonal notching of the band and fixation of band to the greater trochanter	49
Fery and Sommelet (1988)	Cruciate incision of the band over the greater trochanter and the four flaps produced are sutured back on themselves or to adjacent structures	51
Asai and Tonnis (1979)	V-Y-plasty	47
Dederich (1983)	Z-plasty	50
Brignall and Stainsby (1991)	Z-plasty	48
Larsen and Johansen (1986)	Resection of the posterior half of the band	54
Zoltan et al. (1986)	Excision of an ellipsoid-shaped portion of the band overlying the greater trochanter	62

large portion of the greater trochanter or various surgical alterations of the iliotibial band. The latter include the simple release of the iliotibial band, the release and fixation of the cut ends of the band to the greater trochanter, lengthening of the band, and excision of a portion of the band in the greater trochanter area (Table 7.3).[106–108,110,111,123–127] We have successfully used the operative procedure described by Zoltan et al.[130] on our patients (Figure 7.19). The procedure consists of excising an ellipsoid-shaped portion of the band overlying the greater trochanter; we have termed this procedure as *fenestration* of the iliotibial band.[122] Kim et al.[116] have treated three patients with Z-plasty of the iliotibial band, but only one of three patients was able to return to full activities.

Posterior snapping hip syndrome is caused by the snapping of the tendinous origin of the long head of the biceps femoris muscle over the proximal part of the ischial tuberosity. Rask[124] has described cases in which the subluxation of this tendon was accompanied by an audible snapping sound, a condition that he termed *snapping bottom*. Differential diagnosis must include consideration of developed bursitis in this area and enthesitis of the tendon, which we classify as part of the hamstring syndrome. Treatment is usually non-operative.

VII. HAMSTRING SYNDROME

Hamstring syndrome is a condition that affects muscles of the posterior thigh, primarily the semitendinosus, semimembranosus, and biceps femoris muscles (Figure 7.20). It is frequent in sprinters, hurdlers, and both long and high jumpers, but can also be found in other athletes, especially those who engage in rapid acceleration and short intense sprinting, such as baseball players, football players, tennis players, water-skiers, dancers, and others.[131,142,157,158,165,168] Hamstring syndrome is caused either by the overuse of the muscles at their insertion on the ischial tuberosity or by the partial or total rupture of an individual muscle. It is a very common sports injury and numerous studies have been devoted to determining the causative factors and possible preventive measures of this typical self-induced injury. One of the reasons for this attention is the well-documented propensity of this syndrome to recur (as epitomized by the old saying "once a strain, always a strain"). Although hamstring injuries are common in athletes, the distribution and location of such injuries have not been well defined. De Smet and Best[136] used MRI to determine the frequency of injury by muscle, involvement of one or more muscles, and location of injuries within the musculotendinous unit. The biceps femoris is the most commonly injured hamstring muscle and the

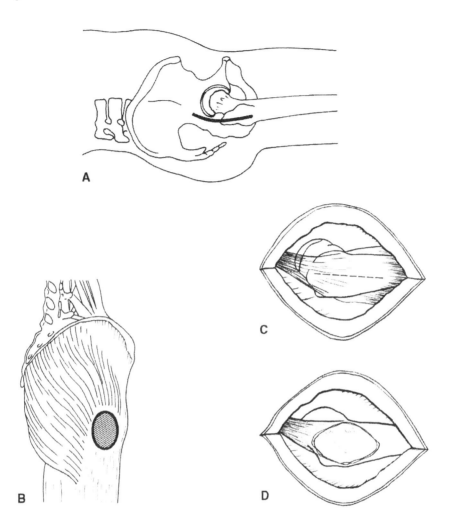

FIGURE 7.19 Schematic representation of the operative procedure described by Zoltan et al.[130] — fenestration of the iliotibial band. (A) Area of the greater trochanter projection; (B) skin incision; (C and D) ellipsoid-shaped excision of the iliotibial band overlying the greater trochanter.

semitendinosus is the second most commonly injured. Although hamstring injuries often involve one muscle injured proximally, multiple muscles were involved in 33% of athletes and the injuries were distal in 40% of athletes. All intramuscular injuries occurred at the musculotendinous junction, either at the ends of the muscle or within the muscle belly.[136]

A. ETIOPATHOGENESIS

Numerous authors have tried to determine the predisposing factors that might cause the hamstring muscle group to become strained.[172] O'Neil[172] summarizes some of these factors, such as fatigue, poor posture, improper warm-up, overuse, abnormal muscle contraction, improper conditioning, magnesium imbalance, sepsis, and anatomical variations, as primary causes leading to hamstring strain. The results of the study of Hennessey and Watson[144] indicate that, while differences in hamstring flexibility are not evident between injured and noninjured groups, poorer low back posture was found in the injured group. Regular monitoring of posture in athletes is therefore recommended. Most authors today agree that the basic causative reason for development of hamstring syndrome is muscle strength imbalance between the hamstring muscle group and the quadriceps femoris

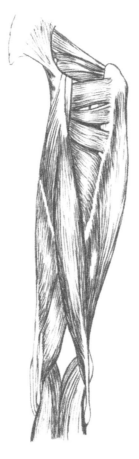

FIGURE 7.20 Posterior thigh muscles — hamstring muscles.

muscle. The normal biomechanics of the lower extremity depends on smoothly coordinated recip-
rocal action between the quadriceps and the hamstring muscle group. Unusual stress is placed on
the quadriceps and hamstrings mechanism at certain points within the range of motion, which
suddenly precipitates injury. Hamstring syndrome will develop, in various forms, when there is a
relative weakness of the hamstring muscle group in relationship to the quadriceps femoris muscle.
The relationship between the hamstring muscle group and the quadriceps femoris muscle has
changed during evolution. Pilardeau et al.[162,163] speculate that the hamstring syndrome is caused by
the still inadequate adaptation of modern humans to an upright position. For this reason, they
classify hamstring syndrome as belonging to *Lucy syndrome*, as described above. The osseous
remains of Lucy, an Australopithecus who lived approximately 3 million years ago, indicate that
she walked in a semi-crouch with habitually flexed knees. The upright position modern humans
has caused a permanent elongation of the posterior thigh muscles and at the same time has shortened
the quadriceps muscle in relation to the Australopithecus.

Studies have indicated that the hamstring muscles should have at least 60% of the strength of
the quadriceps[170] in athletes; this is often not the case with the hamstrings, which have 40%, and
sometimes even less, of the strength of the quadriceps. Unlike the quadriceps, however, hypotrophy
of the hamstring muscles is not readily visible, and unlike the unstable knee syndrome, weakened
hamstring muscles do not cause severe clinical symptoms. This is one of the basic reasons strengthening of the hamstring muscle group does not receive enough attention. Hamstring-to-quadriceps
muscle strength ratios change during movements in the hip and knee joint. This is further complicated by the fact that the hamstring muscles are primarily biarticular structures that act on both of

these joints. During a 60° flexion of the knee, the quadriceps-to-hamstring strength ratio corresponds to 2:1. A ratio of 3:1 is considered a predisposition to hamstring strain. At a 30° knee flexion, the quadriceps-to-hamstring strength ratio becomes 1:1. During the last 20° of this flexion, the mechanical efficiency of the quadriceps muscle in extending the knee begins to decline. However, extension of the knee is enhanced at this point by the synergistic action of the gastrocnemius and hamstring muscles, creating a paradoxical extension moment at the knee in a closed kinetic chain. This example best illustrates the complex relationship existing between the quadriceps and the hamstring muscle group. Hamstring syndrome can also develop as a result of strength deficit between the right and left hamstring muscle groups. A 10% or greater muscle strength deficit between the two sides is also thought to be a predisposition for hamstring strain. According to Yamamoto[177] imbalance of the bilateral legs, hamstring strength, and the ratio of the flexor to extensor were shown to be parameters related to the occurrence of hamstring strains. Sprinters with a history of hamstring injury differed from uninjured runners, in that they were weaker in eccentric contractions and in concentric contractions at low velocities.[146]

In addition to relative or absolute weakness of the hamstring muscles, another and fairly frequent cause of hamstring syndrome is decreased flexibility of these muscles. The flexibility of the hamstring muscles is determined by a number of individual characteristics, including sex, age, type and duration of athletic activity, and the specific types of training programs (during the season and offseason). Flexibility of the hamstring muscles is commonly measured by the Well's "sit-and-reach" test (Figure 7.21). The sit-and-reach test calls for the athlete to bend forward while sitting, in an effort to reach to or beyond the toes with the ankles supported in a neutral position. Performance is measured on a ruler placed in front of the athlete's toes. The basic problem with this test is that, while it does present a general picture of trunk flexion capability, the results are dependent on the mobility of multiple joints and the extensibility of various soft-tissue structures. The test also does not allow for the relative length of body segments (i.e., in the case of basketball players) or for unilateral conditions. A more appropriate test for the flexibility of the hamstring muscle group has been described by Wallace (Figure 7.22). The athlete is positioned supine with both hips and knees extended. The athlete flexes the tested hip and knee to 90°, stabilizing the thigh in that position with the hands. From this position, the athlete attempts to straighten the knee into full extension. Decreased flexibility is demonstrated by the number of degrees the athlete lacks from completing full extension of the knee. There are several modifications of the classic sit-and-reach test.[145]

The speed at which various muscle fibers contract is also a factor that can contribute to the development of hamstring syndrome. Histochemical studies[138] indicate that the hamstring muscles have a relatively high proportion of type 2 fibers, which are involved with exercises of higher intensity and force production. Strength at high velocities of movement or power can be measured by the high-speed stress test. Aided by various types of testing equipment, of which the Cybex II is most commonly used, the strength of the hamstring muscles and the hamstring-to-quadriceps muscle strength ratio are isokinetically determined. This test also allows evaluation of the muscle strength torque curve, which typically decreases in size. Isokinetic studies have shown that the

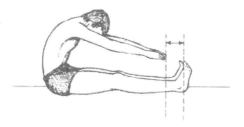

FIGURE 7.21 Well's test (sit-and-reach test).

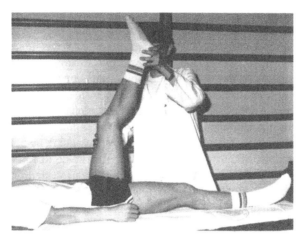

FIGURE 7.22 Wallace's test.

quicker loss of strength in the hamstring muscles, when compared to the quadriceps, is a factor that can predispose an athlete to hamstring strain. However, Bennell et al.[133] using a Kin-Com isokinetic dynamometer at angular velocities of 60 and 180 deg/s concluded that isokinetic muscle strength testing was not able to directly discriminate Australian Rules football players at risk for a hamstring injury.

In summary, the causes of hamstring strains have been attributed to various factors, the most important of which are muscle strength. This includes both the quadriceps-to-hamstring muscle strength ratio and the strength deficit between the right and left hamstring muscle groups. It also includes the flexibility of both the hamstring muscles and the lower extremities. Generally, when observing levels of flexibility and strength within an athletic population, attention should be directed toward individual variation with respect to such factors as age, level of maturity, sex, specific event or position, and demands that a particular activity place on the individual. An athlete who is below the standards of a specific group of players in flexibility and muscle strength should not be allowed to compete with that group of players as this predisposes the individual to hamstring injury. Studies have shown[142,158] that a combination of testing on the Cybex II and moderate training and/or rehabilitation (also with the aid of Cybex II) can help prevent development of the hamstring syndrome in athletes or its recurrence in already injured athletes.

B. CLINICAL PICTURE AND DIAGNOSTICS

Clinical features of hamstring syndrome that have resulted from overuse of the hamstring muscles at the point of their insertion at the ischial tuberosity include constant pain in the lower gluteal area, which radiates down the posterior thigh to the popliteal area. The pain typically increases during the performance of forcible or sudden movements, which stretch the hamstring muscles (i.e., in sprinting or hurdling). Another characteristic complaint is pain felt while sitting, e.g., while driving a car or sitting during lectures. The pain is often relentless, causing the patient to change position or stand up for relief.

During physical examination, the pain can be reproduced by applying pressure to the ischial tuberosity area. In some cases, it is possible to palpate the tautness of the hamstring muscles. Various clinical tests that cause the stretching of the hamstring muscles also induce pain in the ischial tuberosity area.[147] One of the most common tests has the patient stand by a table and lift the outstretched affected leg on the table. Bending the body forward produces intense pain at the site of the ischial tuberosity. Well's and Wallace's tests also produce pain in the same area. Pećina[161] uses the more exact "shoe wiping" test (Figure 7.23), which consists of having the patient imitate movements typically used when wiping shoes on a doormat. The hip and knee are in a position of

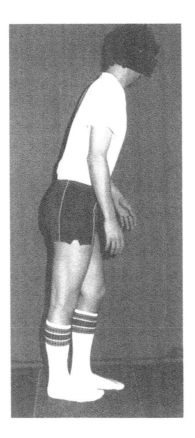

FIGURE 7.23 Doormat sign.

maximal extension while the hamstring muscles are in retroflexion in the hip. While performing these movements, the hamstring muscles are stretched and, at the same time, in motion, which gives an additional value to this test; this enables the patient to score positive even when scoring negative on other tests. A positive score is indicated by pain in the ischial tuberosity area or along one of the hamstring muscles. Another frequently used test has the patient lie in a prone position with legs extended in the knees and attempt to flex the knee of the afflicted leg. The examiner holds the leg by the ankle and applies a gradually increasing amount of resisting pressure to the flexion, which, at a given degree of flexion and resisting pressure to that flexion, produces pain in the ischial tuberosity area. Research done at our department indicates that this is a less reliable test than tests incorporating passive stretching of the hamstring muscles. The best test, in our opinion, is the shoe-wiping test according to Pećina; this test combines testing the hamstring muscles in a stretched position and in motion. Any diagnosis of hamstring syndrome should include a neurological examination because differential diagnosis includes ruling out the possibility of spinal sciatica. Radiological, electrodiagnostic (EMG), computerized tomographic (CT), and MRI examinations can be used to achieve this. Piriformis syndrome presents a special problem in differential diagnosis.[74,75] Gluteal pain is the most frequent symptom of this syndrome, although in this case, the tenderness is located more proximally at the buttock, over the belly of the piriformis muscle. Pain caused by resisted abduction in conjunction with external rotation of the thigh (Pace's sign) and the test for piriformis syndrome, according to Pećina et al.,[160] are commonly used tests for this syndrome. The latter test is performed by having the patient stand in an upright position with the afflicted leg maximally rotated internally and then bending forward. This typically causes pain as the ischiadicus is stretched over the passively extended piriformis. The test can also be performed in a lying position with the patient supine with the leg maximally and internally rotated and extended

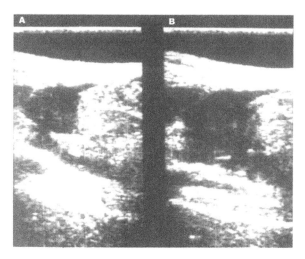

FIGURE 7.24 Sonogram of the posterior thigh demonstrating hematoma in the biceps femoris muscle. (A) Relaxation; (B) contraction.

in the knee. Pain is produced by trying to lift the afflicted leg from the surface. Ischiogluteal bursitis also causes buttock pain similar to that of hamstring syndrome. It differs from it in that the pain is also felt at rest, and patients have difficulties in finding a comfortable position at night. Chronic compartment syndrome also causes pain in the posterior thigh, especially during exercise, but there is no gluteal pain while sitting.

Hamstring syndrome, as we have already mentioned, can also be caused by a partial rupture of one of the hamstring muscles. Most authors agree that the most commonly ruptured muscle is the biceps femoris. Patients usually remember the exact moment they heard the sound, or felt the "tearing," or simply felt a sharp pain in the posterior thigh. Depending on the degree of rupture, which some authors divide into slight, moderate, and severe, the patient can, in some cases, resume athletic activities. However, the pain will intensify during the following 3 to 6 h in moderate and slight ruptures and during the following 30 min in severe ruptures. Careful physical examination of the patient can reveal the exact location of the injury, which corresponds to the area of greatest pain. All movements causing greater stretching of the injured muscle typically produce pain along the whole muscle. In severe cases, visible bleeding on the skin will appear with characteristic changes in color from blue to brown descending all the way down to the knee. Street and Burks[171] reported an unusual case of chronic complete hamstring avulsion causing foot drop.

Ultrasound examination has greatly facilitated diagnosis.[137,143,153,155] Detailed ultrasound examination of the injured muscle, in both the longitudinal and transverse projections, and in a relaxed and contracted state, can reveal a hematoma in the muscle visible in the shape of a diffusely limited area of irregular shape (Figure 7.24). Ultrasound examination can also reveal fibrous scar tissue caused by previous hamstring muscle tear or tears. In younger patients, roentgenographic diagnosis is also indicated because avulsions of the ischial tuberosity are possible, which manifests with similar symptoms. MRI is very helpful in detecting injury site, extent, and characteristics and can also predict the time period an athlete will be disabled and help define the best treatment planning.[134–136,164,176]

C. Treatment

Treatment of injured hamstring muscles can best be summarized with the old saying "the best treatment is prevention." This applies both to injuries resulting from overuse at the insertion of the muscles on the ischial tuberosity and from rupture of the muscle. Hartig and Henderson[141] have reported that increasing hamstring flexibility decreases lower extremity overuse injuries in military basic trainees. However, once an injury does take place, the initial therapy is based on the principles of RICE (*r*est, *i*ce, *c*ompression, and *e*levation).[179] After 24 to 36 h, ice is removed and heat is applied to the injured area. This quickens the circulation to help the healing process. The results of the study of Taylor et al.[173] suggest that adequate hamstring stretching can occur without the use of a superficial thermal modality. After a couple of days during which the pain gradually recedes, the patient begins stretching exercises. The proper execution of these exercises is of the greatest importance. The patient must remain in the position of greatest nonpainful extension for 15 s. To date, limited information exists describing a relatively new stretching technique, dynamic range of motion (DROM). The results of the study performed by Bandy et al.[132] suggest that, although both static stretch and DROM will increase hamstring flexibility, a 30-s static stretch was more effective than the newer technique, DROM, for enhancing flexibility. Given that a 30-s static stretch increased range of motion more than two times that of DROM, the use of DROM to increase flexibility of muscle must be questioned.[132] On the other hand, according to Halbertsma et al.[140] the increased range of motion, i.e., the extensibility of the hamstrings, results from an increase in stretch tolerance. At this stage of treatment, nonsteroidal anti-inflammatory drugs can also be used. Strengthening of the hamstring muscles is also part of the rehabilitation process. Garrick and Webb[139] note that the greatest mistake is to concentrate solely on stretching exercises. The hamstring muscles, just as all other muscles, regain their normal functional flexibility only, and at the same time, when they regain their normal muscle strength. There is no better example for the saying "a weak muscle is a tightened muscle" than an injured hamstring muscle that has been inadequately rehabilitated. Another important factor in the rehabilitation process is advising both the athlete and the trainer that an unnecessarily quick return to full training accompanied by inadequate warm-ups while ignoring stretching exercises before and after training can, and often does, lead to the recurrence of a hamstring injury.[178] The return to normal training depends on the severity of the injury, and the final decision can be made only after a careful assessment of the whole rehabilitation program based on day-to-day examinations.

Treatment of hamstring syndrome that has developed as a result of overuse at its origin on the ischial tuberosity is usually non-operative. It consists of a rehabilitation program of stretching exercises and strengthening of the hamstring muscles.[154,174] Physical procedures commonly applied to all chronic overuse syndromes are also applicable, as are nonsteroidal anti-inflammatory drugs. The study of Reynolds et al.[167] does not support the use of nonsteroidal anti-inflammatory drugs in the treatment of acute hamstring muscle injuries. On rare occasions, corticosteroids are locally applied. The impression of Levine et al.[152] is that intramuscular corticosteroid injection hastens players' return to full play and lessens the game and practice time they miss. According to Upton et al.[175] thermal pants may play a role in preventing recurrent hamstring injuries but other factors such as inadequate preseason training and incomplete rehabilitation after injury are likely to be more significant risk factors for injury.

Surgical treatment as recommended by Puranen and Orava[165] consists of cutting and dividing the tendinous tissue near the site of origin of the hamstring muscles without loosening the muscles from the ischial tuberosity. After division, the tendon ends should be completely separated from each other. The sciatic nerve must also be freed from any tendinous parts of the hamstring muscle. Puranen and Orava[166] reported that 52 of the 59 operated patients were completely relieved following this operation. According to Kujala et al.[149] after first aid with rest, compression, cold, and elevation, the treatment of hamstring muscle injury must be tailored to the grade of injury. Experimental studies have shown that a short period of immobilization is needed to accelerate formation of the granulation tissue matrix following injury. The length of immobilization is, however, dependent on the grade of injury and should be optimized so that the scar can bear the pulling forces operating on it without re-rupture. Mobilization, on the other hand, is required to regain the original strength of the muscle and to achieve good final results in resorption of the connective tissue scar and recapillarization of the damaged area. Another important aim of immobilization — especially in sports medical practice — is to avoid muscle atrophy and loss of strength and extensibility, which rapidly result from prolonged immobilization. Complete ruptures with loss of function should be operated on, as should cases resistant to conservative therapy in which, in the late phase of repair, the scar and adhesions prevent the normal function of the hamstring muscle. Urgent surgical treatment is recommended in cases with total or nearly total soft-tissue hamstring muscle insertion rupture.[148,156] Kurosawa et al.[151] reported two cases with complete avulsion of the hamstring tendons from the ischial tuberosity and in one of these two cases the less satisfactory results of non-operative treatment were clearly shown in both isokinetic muscle force evaluation and sports activities.

REFERENCES

Groin Pain

1. **Akermark, C. and Johansson, C.** Tenotomy of the adductor longus tendon in the treatment of chronic groin pain in athletes. *Am. J. Sports Med.*, 1992; 20: 640–643.
2. **Akita, K. et al.** Anatomic basis of chronic groin pain with special reference to sports hernia. *Surg. Radiol. Anat.*, 1999; 21: 1–5.
3. **Anderson, K., Strickland, S.M., and Warren, R.** Hip and groin injuries in athletes. *Am. J. Sports Med.*, 2001; 29: 521–533.
4. **Anderson, M.W., Kaplan, P.A., and Dussault, R.G.** Adductor insertion avulsion syndrome (thigh splints): spectrum of MR imaging features. *Am. J. Roentgenol.*, 2001; 177: 673–675.
5. **Ashby, E.C.** Chronic obscure groin pain is commonly caused by enthesopathy: "tennis elbow" of the groin. *Br. J. Surg.*, 1994; 81: 1632–1634.
6. **Azurin, D.J. et al.** Endoscopic preperitoneal herniorrhaphy in professional athletes with groin pain. *J. Laparoendosc. Adv. Surg. Tech. A*, 1997; 7: 7–12.
7. **Barile, A.** Groin pain in athletes: role of magnetic resonance. *Radiol. Med.*, 2000; 100: 216–222.
8. **Bass, C.J. and Connell, D.A.** Sonographic findings of tensor fascia lata tendinopathy: another cause of anterior groin pain. *Skel. Radiol.*, 2002; 31: 143–148.
9. **Batt, M.E., McShane, J.M., and Dillingham, M.F.** Osteitis pubis in collegiate football players. *Med. Sci. Sports Exerc.*, 1995; 27: 629–633.
10. **Benezis, C.** Syndrome de surmenage inguino-pubiens, in *Microtraumatologie du Sport,* Rodineau, J. and Simon, L., Eds. Paris: Masson, 1990.
11. **Biundo, J.J., Jr., Irwin, R.W., and Umpierre, E.** Sports and other soft tissue injuries, tendinitis, bursitis, and occupation-related syndromes. *Curr. Opin. Rheumatol.*, 2001; 13: 146–149.
12. **Booher, J.M. and Thibdeau, G.A.** *Athletic Injury Assessment.* St. Louis: Mosby College Publishing, 1986.
13. **Bradshaw, C., McCrory, P., Bell, S., and Brukner, P.** Obturator nerve entrapment. A cause of groin pain in athletes. *Am. J. Sports Med.*, 1997; 25: 402–408.
14. **Brannigan, A.E., Kerin, M.J., and McEntee, G.P.** Gilmore's groin repair in athletes. *J. Orthop. Sports Phys. Ther.*, 2000; 30: 329–332.
15. **Briggs, R.C., Kolbjornsen, P.H., and Southal, R.C.** Osteitis pubis, Tc-99m MDP, and professional hockey players. *Clin. Nucl. Med.*, 1992; 17: 861–863.
16. **Brunet, B., Imbert, J.C., and Brunet-Guedj, E.** Les pubalgies: etiopathogenie, diagnostic et traitement medical, in *Muscles, Tendons et Sport,* Benezis, C., Simeray, J., and Simon, L., Eds. Paris: Masson, 1990.
17. **Burke, G., Joe, C., Levine, M., and Sabio, H.** Tc-99-m bone scan in unilateral osteitis pubis. *Clin. Nucl. Med.*, 1994; 19: 535.
18. **Collins, K. et al.** Overuse injuries in triathletes. A study of the 1986 Seafair Triathlon. *Am. J. Sports Med.*, 1989; 17: 675–680.
19. **De Paulis, F. et al.** Sports injuries in the pelvis and hip: diagnostic imaging. *Eur. J. Radiol.*, 1998; 27: 49–59.
20. **Durey, A. and Breda, A.** *Medicine du Football.* Paris: Masson, 1978.
21. **Ekberg, O. et al.** Long standing groin pain in athletes. A multidisciplinary approach. *Sports Med.*, 1988; 6: 56–61.

22. **Ekberg, O., Sjoberg, S., and Westlin, N.** Sports-related groin pain: evaluation with MR imaging. *Eur. Radiol.*, 1996., 6: 52–55.

23. **Ekstrand, J. and Gillquist, J.** Soccer injuries and their mechanisms: a prospective study. *Med. Sci. Sports Exerc.*, 1983; 15: 267–270.

24. **Estwanik, J.J., Sloane, B., and Rosenberg, M.A.** Groin strain and other possible causes of groin pain. *Phys. Sportsmed.*, 1990; 18: 54–65.

25. **Fernbach, S.K. and Wilkinson, R.H.** Avulsion injuries of the pelvis and proximal femur. *AJR*, 1981; 158: 581–584.

26. **Fon, L.J. and Spence, R.A.** Sportsman's hernia. *Br. J. Sports Med.*, 2000; 87: 545–552.

27. **Fon, L.J. and Spencer, R.A.** Sportsman's hernia. *Br. J. Surg.*, 2000; 87: 545–552.

28. **Fredberg, U. and Kissmeyer-Nielsen, P.** The sportsman's hernia — fact or fiction? *Scand. J. Med. Sci. Sports*, 1996; 6: 201–204.

29. **Fricker, P.A.** Management of groin pain in athletes. *Br. J. Sports Med.*, 1997; 31: 97–101.

30. **Fricker, A.P., Taunton, J.E., and Ammann, W.** Osteitis pubis in athletes. Infection, inflammation or injury? *Sports Med.*, 1991; 12: 266–279.

31. **Gibbon, W.W.** Groin pain in athletes. *Lancet*, 1999; 353: 1444–1445.

32. **Gilmore, J.** Groin pain in the soccer athlete: fact, fiction, and treatment. *Clin. Sports Med.*, 1998; 17: 787–793.

33. **Goldstein, A.E. and Rubin, S.W.** Osteitis pubis following suprapubic prostatectomy: results with deep roentgen therapy. *Am. J. Surg.*, 1947; 74: 480–487.

34. **Grisogono, V.** *Sports Injuries.* London: John Murray, 1984.

35. **Hackney, R.G.** The sports hernia: a cause of chronic groin pain. *Br. J. Sports Med.*, 1993; 27: 58–62.

36. **Hess, G.P. et al.** Prevention and treatment of overuse tendon injuries. *Sports Med.*, 1989; 8: 371–384.

37. **Hofmann, S. et al.** Clinical and diagnostic imaging of labrum lesions in the hip joint. *Orthopaede*, 1998; 27: 681–689.

38. **Holmich, P. et al.** Effectiveness of active physical training as treatment for long-standing adductor-related groin pain in athletes: randomised trial. *Lancet*, 1999; 353: 439–443.

39. **Holt, M.A. et al.** Treatment of osteitis pubis in athletes. Results of corticosteroid injections. *Am. J. Sports Med.*, 1995; 23: 601–606.

40. **Irshad, K. et al.** Operative management of "hockey groin syndrome": 12 years of experience in National Hockey League players. *Surgery*, 2001; 130: 759–764.

41. **Jaeger, J.H.** La pubalgie, hypothese pathogenique, techniques operatoires, casuistique, resultats et indications. *Sport Med.*, 1982; 21: 28–32.

42. **Jaeger, J.H.** La pubalgie, in *Lesions Traumatiques des Tendons chez le Sportif*, Catonne, Y. and Saillant, G., Eds. Paris: Masson, 1992.

43. **Janković, G.** Mehanika i etiopatogeneza nastanka oste´cenja u podru´c ju simfize kod nogometa, in. *Magisterij.* Zagreb: Medicinski fakultet Sveućilićta u Zagrebu, 1976.

44. **Johnston, C.A. et al.** Iliopsoas bursitis and tendinitis. A review. *Sports Med.*, 1998; 25: 271–283.

45. **Kalebo, P. et al.** Ultrasonography of chronic tendon injuries in the groin. *Am. J. Sports Med.*, 1992; 20: 634–639.

46. **Kidron, A.** Groin pain in sport. *Harefuah*, 2001; 140: 1095–1099.

47. **Kneeland, J.B.** MR imaging of sports injuries of the hip. *Magn. Reson. Imaging Clin. North Am.*, 1999; 7: 105–115.

48. **Kulund, D.N.** *The Injured Athlete*, 2nd ed. Philadelphia: J.B. Lippincott, 1988; 423–425.

49. **La Cava, G.** L'enthesite ou maladie des insertions. *Press Med.*, 1959; 67: 9.

50. **Lacroix, V.J. et al.** Lower abdominal pain syndrome in National Hockey League players: a report of 11 cases. *Clin. J. Sports Med.*, 1998; 8: 5–9.

51. **Le Jeune, J.J. et al.** Pubic pain syndrome in sportsmen: comparison of radiographic and scintigraphic findings. *Eur. J. Nucl. Med.*, 1984; 9: 250–253.

52. **Liebert, P.L., Lombardo, J.A., and Belhobek, G.H.** Acute posttraumatic pubic symphysis instability in an athlete. *Phys. Sportsmed.*, 1988; 16: 87–90.

53. **Lloyd-Smith, R. et al.** A survey of overuse and traumatic hip and pelvic injuries in athletes. *Phys. Sportsmed.*, 1985; 13:131–141.

54. **Lovell, G.** The diagnosis of chronic groin pain in athletes: a review of 189 cases. *Aust. J. Sci. Med. Sport*, 1995; 27: 76–79.

55. **Lynch, S.A. and Renstrom, P.A.** Groin injuries in sport: treatment strategies. *Sports Med.*, 1999; 28: 137–144.
56. **Macarthur, D.C. et al.** Herniography for groin pain of uncertain origin. *Br. J. Surg.*, 1997; 84: 684–685.
57. **Major, N.M. and Helms, C.A.** Pelvic stress injuries: the relationship between osteitis pubis (symphysis pubis stress injury) and sacroiliac abnormalities in athletes. *Skel. Radiol.*, 1997; 26: 711–717.
58. **Malycha, P. and Lovell, G.** Inguinal surgery in athletes with chronic groin pain: the "sportsman's" hernia. *Aust. N.Z. J. Surg.*, 1992; 62: 123–125.
59. **Martens, M.A., Hansen, L., and Mulier, J.C.** Adductor tendinitis and muscles rectus abdominis tendopathy. *Am. J. Sports Med.*, 1987; 15: 353–356.
60. **Meyers, W.C. et al.** Management of severe lower abdominal or inguinal pain in high-performance athletes. *Am. J. Sports Med.*, 2000; 28: 2–8.
61. **Morelli, V. and Smith, V.** Groin injuries in athletes. *Am. Fam. Physician*, 2001; 64: 1405–1414.
62. **Muckle, D.S.** Associated factors in recurrent groin and hamstring injuries. *Br. J. Sports Med.*, 1982; 16: 37–39.
63. **Mulhall, K.J. et al.** Osteitis pubis in professional soccer players: a report of outcome with symphyseal curettage in cases refractory to conservative management. *Clin. J. Sport Med.*, 2002; 12: 179–181.
64. **Nešović, B.** Bolni sindrom simfize kod sportista i mogućnosti njegovog lijećenja, in *Povrede u Sportu i Njihovo Lijećenja,* Beograd: SFKJ 1988; 104–113.
65. **Nielsen, A.B. and Yde, J.** Epidemiology and traumatology of injuries in soccer. *Am. J. Sports Med.*, 1989; 17: 803–807.
66. **O'Connell, M.J. et al.** Symphyseal cleft injection in the diagnosis and treatment of osteitis pubis in athletes. *Am. J. Roentgenol.*, 2002; 179: 955–959.
67. **O'Donoghue, D.H.** *Treatment of Injuries to Athletes,* 4th ed. Philadelphia: W.B. Saunders, 1984.
68. **Orchard, J.W. et al.** Groin pain associated with ultrasound finding of inguinal canal posterior wall deficiency in Australian Rules footballers. *Br. J. Sports Med.*, 1998; 32: 134–39.
69. **O'Toole, M.L. et al.** Overuse injuries in ultraendurance triathletes. *Am. J. Sports Med.*, 1989; 17: 514–518.
70. **Pavlov, H.** Roentgen examination of groin and hip pain in the athlete. *Clin. Sports Med.*, 1987; 6: 829–843.
71. **Pearson, R.L.** Osteitis pubis in a basketball player. *Phys. Sportsmed.*, 1988; 16: 69–72.
72. **Pećina, M. and Bojanić, I.** Overuse injuries in track and field athletes. *Croat. Sports Med. J.*, 1991; 6: 24–37.
73. **Pećina, M., Krmpotić-Nemanić, J., and Markiewitz, A.D.** *Tunnel Syndromes. Peripheral Nerve Compression Syndromes,* 3rd ed. Boca Raton, FL: CRC Press, 2001.
74. **Peterson, L. and Renstrom, P.** *Sports Injuries: Their Prevention and Treatment.* London: Martin Dunitz, 1988.
75. **Pilardeau, P. et al.** Le syndrome de Lucy. *J. Traumatol. Sport,* 1990; 7: 171–175.
76. **Pope, T.L., Jr. and Keats, T.E.** Case report 733. Calcific tendinitis of the origin of the medial and lateral heads of the rectus femoris muscle and the anterior iliac spin (AIIS). *Skel. Radiol.*, 1992; 21: 271–272.
77. **Renstrom, P.A.** Tendon and muscle injuries in the groin area. *Clin. Sports Med.*, 1992; 11: 815–831.
78. **Renstrom, P. and Johanson, R.** Overuse injuries in sports: a review. *Sports Med.*, 1985; 2: 316–333.
79. **Renstrom, P. and Peterson, L.** Groin injuries in athletes. *Br. J. Sports Med.*, 1980; 14: 30–36.
80. **Rold, J.F. and Rold, B.A.** Pubic stress symphysitis in a female distance runner. *Phys. Sportsmed.*, 1986; 14: 61–65.
81. **Schneider, P.G.** Leistenschmerz: operative Therapiemöglichkeiten. *Orthopade,* 1980; 9: 190–192.
82. **Smedberg, S.G. et al.** Herniography in the diagnosis of obscure groin pain. *Acta Chir. Scand.,* 1985; 151: 663–667.
83. **Smedberg, S.G. et al.** Herniography in athletes with groin pain. *Am. J. Surg.,* 1985; 149: 378–382.
84. **Spinelli, A.** Una nuova malattia sportiva: la pubalgia degli schermitori. *Ortop. Traumatol. Appar. Mot.,* 1932; 4: 111–127.
85. **Srinivasan, A. and Schuricht, A.** Long-term follow-up of laparoscopic preperitoneal hernia repair in professional athletes. *J. Laparoendosc. Adv. Surg. Tech. A.,* 2002; 12: 101–106.

86. **Steinbach, H.L., Petrakis, N.L., Gilfillan, R.S., and Smith, D.R.** Pathogenesis of osteitis pubis. *J. Urol.,* 1955; 74: 840–846.

87. **Taylor, D.C. et al.** Abdominal musculature abnormalities as a cause of groin pain in athletes. Inguinal hernias and pubalgia. *Am. J. Sports Med.,* 1991; 19: 239–242.

88. **Tonsoline, P.A.** Chronic adductor tendinitis in a female swimmer. *J. Orthop. Sports Phys. Ther.,* 1993; 18: 629–633.

89. **Verrall, G.M., Slavotinek, J.P., and Fon, G.T.** Incidence of pubic bone marrow oedema in Australian rules football players: relation to groin pain. *Br. J. Sports Med.,* 2001; 35: 28–33.

90. **Wheeler, W.K.** Periostitis pubis following suprapubic cystotomy. *J. Urol.,* 1941; 45: 467–475.

91. **Wiese, H. et al.** An unusual swelling in the groin. *Eur. J. Radiol.,* 1990; 10: 156–158.

92. **Wiley, J.J.** Traumatic osteitis pubis: the gracillis syndrome. *Am. J. Sports Med.,* 1983; 11: 360–363.

93. **Williams, P.R., Thomas, D.P., and Downes, E.M.** Osteitis pubis and instability of the pubic symphysis. When nonoperative measures fail. *Am. J. Sports Med.,* 2000; 28: 350–355.

94. **Witvoet, J.** *Lesions Osteotendineuses des Sportifs.* Conf. d'Enseignement, No. 19. Paris: Expansion Scientifique Française, 1979.

95. **Yilmazlar, T. et al.** The value of herniography in football players with obscure groin pain. *Acta Chir. Belg.,* 1996; 96: 115–118.

96. **Ziprin, P., Williams, P., and Foster, M.E.** External oblique aponeurosis nerve entrapment as a cause of groin pain in the athlete. *Br. J. Surg.,* 1999; 86: 566–568.

Hip External Rotator Syndrome and Gluteus Medius Syndrome

97. **Bosch, U. and Tscherne, H.** The pelvic compartment syndrome. *Arch. Orthop. Trauma Surg.,* 1992; 111: 314–317.

98. **Green, B.N., Johnson, C.D., and Maloney, A.** Effects of altering cycling technique on gluteus medius syndrome. *J. Manipulative Physiol. Ther.,* 1999; 22: 108–113.

99. **Hunter, S.C. and Poole, R.M.** The chronically inflamed tendon. *Clin. Sports Med.,* 1987; 6: 371–387.

100. **Kingzett-Taylor, A. et al.** Tendinosis and tears of gluteus medius and minimus muscles as a cause of hip pain: MR imaging findings. *Am. J. Roentgenol.,* 1999; 173: 1123–1126.

101. **Klinkert, P., Jr. et al.** Quadratus femoris tendinitis as a cause of groin pain. *Br. J. Sports Med.,* 1997; 31: 348–349.

102. **Melamed, H. and Hutchinson, M.R.** Soft tissue problems of the hip in athletes. *Sports Med. Arthrosc. Rev.,* 2002; 10: 168–175.

103. **Njoo, K.H. and Van der Does, E.** The occurrence and inter-rater reliability of myofascial trigger points in the quadratus lumborum and gluteus medius: a prospective study in non-specific low back pain patients and controls in general practice. *Pain,* 1994; 58: 317–323.

104. **Pećina, M.** Piriformis syndrome in differential diagnosis of low back pain. *Acta Orthop. Iugosl.,* 1975; 6: 196–200.

105. **Shin, A.Y. et al.** The superiority of magnetic resonance imaging in differentiating the cause of hip pain in endurance athletes. *Am. J. Sports Med.,* 1996; 24: 168–176.

Snapping Hip Syndrome

106. **Asai, H. and Tonnis, D.** Die Verlängerung des Tractus iliotibialis zur Behandlung der schnappenden Hufte. *Orthop. Praxis,* 1979; 15: 128–130.

107. **Brignall, C.G. and Stansby, G.D.** The snapping hip. Treatment by Z-plasty. *J. Bone Joint Surg.,* 1991; 73B: 253–254.

108. **Bruckl, R. et al.** Zur operativen Behandlung der schnappenden Hufte. *Z. Orthop.,* 1984; 122: 308–313.

109. **Choi, Y.S. et al.** Dynamic sonography of external snapping hip syndrome. *J. Ultrasound Med.,* 2002; 21: 753–758.

110. **Dederich, R.** Die schnappende Hufte Erweiterung des Tractus Iliotibialis durch Z-plastik. *Z. Orthop.,* 1983; 121: 168–170.

111. **Fery, A. and Sommelet, J.** La hanche a ressaut: resultats tardifs de vingt-trois cas operes. *Int. Orthop. (SICOT),* 1988; 12: 277–282.

112. **Gruen, G.S., Scioscia, T.N., and Lowenstein, J.E.** The surgical treatment of internal snapping hip. *Am. J. Sports Med.*, 2002; 30: 607–613.
113. **Howse, A.J.G.** Orthopaedists aid ballet. *Clin. Orthop.*, 1972; 89: 52–63.
114. **Jacobs, M. and Young, R.** Snapping hip phenomenon among dancers. *Am. Correct. Ther. J.*, 1978; 32: 92–98.
115. **Jacobson, T. and Allen, W.C.** Surgical correction of the snapping iliopsoas tendon. *Am. J. Sports Med.*, 1990; 18: 470–474.
116. **Kim, D.H. et al.** Coxa saltans externa treated with Z-plasty of the iliotibial tract in a military population. *Mil. Med.*, 2002; 167: 172–173.
117. **Larsen, E. and Johansen, J.** Snapping hip. *Acta Orthop. Scand.*, 1986; 57: 168–170.
118. **Lyons, J.C. and Peterson, L.F.A.** The snapping iliopsoas tendon. *Mayo Clin. Proc.*, 1984; 59: 327–329.
119. **Melamed, H. and Hutchinson, M.R.** Soft tissue problems of the hip in athletes. *Sports Med. Arthrosc. Rev.*, 2002; 10: 168–175.
120. **Nunziata, A. and Blumenfeld, I.** Cadeva a restorte. A proposito de una variedad. *Prensa Med. Argent.*, 1951; 38: 1997–2001.
121. **O'Neill, D.B. and Micheli, L.J.** Overuse injuries in the young athlete. *Clin. Sports Med.*, 1988; 7: 591–610.
122. **Pećina, M., Bojanić, I., and Hašpl, M.** The snapping hip. *Hip Int.*, 1994; 4: 133–136.
123. **Pelsser, V. et al.** Extraarticular snapping hip: sonographic findings. *Am. J. Roentgenol.*, 2001; 176: 67–73.
124. **Rask, M.R.** Snapping bottom: subluxation of the tendon of the long head of the biceps femoris muscle. *Muscle Nerve*, 1980; 3: 250–251.
125. **Reid, D.C.** Prevention of hip and knee injuries in ballet dancers. *Sports Med.*, 1988; 6: 295–307.
126. **Sammarco, J.G.** Diagnosis and treatment in dancers. *Clin. Orthop.*, 1984; 187: 176–187.
127. **Schaberg, J.E., Harper, M.C., and Allen, W.C.** The snapping hip syndrome. *Am. J. Sports Med.*, 1984; 12: 361–365.
128. **Weyer, R. and Tonnis, D.** Eine Untersuchungsmethode zum Machweis der schnappenden Hufte. *Z. Orthop.*, 1980; 118: 895–896.
129. **Wunderbaldinger, P. et al.** Efficient radiological assessment of the internal snapping hip syndrome. *Eur. Radiol.*, 2001; 11: 1743–1747.
130. **Zoltan, D.J., Clancy, W.G., Jr., and Keene, J.S.** A new operative approach to snapping hip and refractory trochanteric bursitis in athletes. *Am. J. Sports Med.*, 1986; 14: 201–204.

Hamstring Syndrome

131. **Askling, C. et al.** Sports related hamstring strains — two cases with different etiologies and injuries sites. *Scand. J. Med. Sci. Sports*, 2000; 10: 304–307.
132. **Bandy, W.D., Irion, J.M., and Briggler, M.** The effect of static stretch and dynamic range of motion training on the flexibility of hamstring muscles. *J. Orthop. Sports Phys. Ther.*, 1998; 27: 295–300.
133. **Bennell, K. et al.** Isokinetic strength testing does not predict hamstring injury in Australian Rules footballers. *Br. J. Sports Med.*, 1998; 32: 309–314.
134. **Brandser, E.A. et al.** Hamstring injuries: radiographic, conventional tomographic, CT, and MR imaging characteristics. *Radiology*, 1995; 197: 257–262.
135. **Clanton, T.O. and Coupe, K.J.** Hamstring strains in athletes: diagnosis and treatment. *J. Am. Acad. Orthop. Surg.*, 1998; 6: 237–248.
136. **De Smet, A.A. and Best, T.M.** MR imaging of the distribution and location of acute hamstring injuries in athletes. *Am. J. Roentgenol.*, 2000; 174: 393–399.
137. **Fornage, B.D. and Rifkin, M.D.** Ultrasound examination of tendons. *Radiol. Clin. North Am.*, 1988; 26: 87–107.
138. **Garret, W.E., Califf, J.C., and Bassett, F.H., III.** Histochemical correlates of hamstring injuries. *Am. J. Sports Med.*, 1984; 12: 98–103.
139. **Garrick, J.G. and Webb, D.R.** *Sports Injuries: Diagnosis and Management.* Philadelphia: W.B. Saunders, 1990.

140. **Halbertsma, J.P., van Bolhuis, A.I., and Goeken, L.N.** Sport stretching: effect on passive muscle stiffness of short hamstrings. *Arch. Phys. Med. Rehabil.*, 1996; 77: 688–692.

141. **Hartig, D.E. and Henderson, J.M.** Increasing hamstring flexibility decreases lower extremity overuse injuries in military basic trainees. *Am. J. Sports Med.*, 1999; 27: 173–176.

142. **Heiser, T.M. et al.** Prophylaxis and management of hamstring muscle injuries in intercollegiate football players. *Am. J. Sports Med.*, 1984; 12: 368–370.

143. **Hannesschlager, G. and Rudelberger, W.** Real-Time-Sonographie bei sportspezifischen Sehnenverletzungen. *Sportverletz. Sportschaden*, 1988; 2: 133–146.

144. **Hennessey L. and Watson, A.W.** Flexibility and posture assessment in relation to hamstring injury. *Br. J. Sports Med.*, 1993; 27: 243–246.

145. **Hui, S.S. and Yuen, P.Y.** Validity of the modified back-saver sit–and–reach test: a comparison with other protocols. *Med. Sci. Sports Exerc.*, 2000; 32: 1655–1659.

146. **Jonhagen, S., Nemeth, G., and Eriksson, E.** Hamstring injuries in sprinters. The role of concentric and eccentric hamstring muscle strength and flexibility. *Am. J. Sports Med.*, 1994., 22: 262–266.

147. **Kibler, W.B., Chandler, T.J., Uhl, T. et al.** A musculoskeletal approach to the preparticipation physical examination. *Am. J. Sports Med.*, 1989; 17: 525–531.

148. **Kujala, U.M. and Orava, S.** Ischial apophysis injuries in athletes. *Sports Med.*, 1993; 16: 290–294.

149. **Kujala, U.M., Orava, S., and Jarvinen, M.** Hamstring injuries. Current trends in treatment and prevention. *Sports Med.*, 1997; 23: 397–404.

150. **Kulund, D.N.** *The Injured Athlete,* 2nd ed. Philadelphia: J.B. Lippincott, 1988.

151. **Kurosawa, H. et al.** Complete avulsion of the hamstring tendon from the ischial tuberosity. A report of two cases sustained in judo. *Br. J. Sports Med.*, 1996; 30: 72–74.

152. **Levine, W.N. et al.** Intramuscular corticosteroid injection for hamstring injuries. A 13-year experience in the National Football League. *Am. J. Sports Med.*, 2000; 28: 297–300.

153. **Matasović, T. et al.** *Diagnostic Ultrasound of the Locomotor System.* Zagreb: Skolska Knjiga, 1990.

154. **Mattalino, A.J., Deese, J.M., Jr., and Campbell, E.D., Jr.** Office evaluation and treatment of lower extremity injuries in the runner. *Clin. Sports Med.*, 1989; 3: 461–475.

155. **Mellerowicz, H., Stelling E., and Kefenbaum, A.** Diagnostic ultrasound in the athlete's locomotor system. *Br. J. Sport Med.*, 1990; 24: 31–39.

156. **Orava, S. and Kujala, U.M.** Rupture of the ischial origin of the hamstring muscles. *Am. J. Sports Med.*, 1995; 23: 702–705.

157. **Orchard, J.W.** Intrinsic and extrinsic risk factors for muscle strain in Australian football. *Am. J. Sports Med.*, 2001; 29: 300–303.

158. **Orchard, J. et al.** Preseason hamstring muscle weakness associated with hamstring muscle injury in Australian footballers. *Am. J. Sports Med.*, 1997; 25: 81–85.

159. **Pećina, M.** Contribution to the etiological explanation of the piriformis syndrome. *Acta Anat.* (Basel), 1979; 105:181–187.

160. **Pećina, M., Krmpotić-Nemanić, J., and Markiewitz, A.D.** *Tunnel Syndromes. Peripheral Nerve Compression Syndromes,* 3rd ed. Boca Raton, FL: CRC Press, 2001.

161. **Pećina, M. and Bojanić, I.** Overuse injuries in track and field athletes. *Croat. Sports Med. J.,* 1991; 6: 24–37.

162. **Pilardeau, P. et al.** Le syndrome de Lucy. *J. Traumatol. Sport.*, 1990; 7: 171–175.

163. **Pilardeau, P. et al.** L'appareil extenseur de la jambe dans le syndrome de Lucy. *Actual. Sport Med.,* 1991; 12: 45–47.

164. **Pomeranz, S.J. and Heidt, R.S., Jr.** MR imaging in the prognostication of hamstring injury. Work in progress. *Radiology*, 1993; 189: 897–900.

165. **Puranen, J. and Orava, S.** The hamstring syndrome. *Am. J. Sports Med.*, 1988; 16: 517–521.

166. **Puranen, J. and Orava, S.** The hamstring syndrome — a new gluteal sciatica. *Ann. Chir. Gynaecol.,* 1991; 80: 212–214.

167. **Reynolds, J.F. et al.** Non-steroidal anti-inflammatory drugs fail to enhance healing of acute hamstring injuries treated with physiotherapy. *S. Afr. Med. J.*, 1995; 85: 517–522.

168. **Sallay, P.I. et al.** Hamstring muscle injuries among water skiers. Functional outcome and prevention. *Am. J. Sports Med.*, 1996; 24: 130–136.

169. **Samson, M. and Lequesne, M.** Tendinitis of the hip region. *Rev. Prat.*, 1991; 41: 1667–1671.

170. **Soldmonow, M., Baratta, R., and D'Ambrosia, R.** The role of the hamstrings in the rehabilitation of the ACL deficient knee in athletes. *Sports Med.,* 1989; 7: 42–48.

171. **Street, C.C. and Burks, R.T.** Chronic complete hamstring avulsion causing foot drop. A case report. *Am. J. Sports Med.,* 2000; 28: 574–576.

172. **Sutton, G.** Hamstring by hamstring strains. A review of the literature. *J. Orthop. Sports Phys. Ther.,* 1984; 5: 184–195.

173. **Taylor, B.F., Waring, C.A., and Brashear, T.A.** The effects of therapeutic application of heat or cold followed by static stretch on hamstring muscle length. *J. Orthop. Sports Phys. Ther.,* 1995; 21: 283–286.

174. **Torg, J.S., Vegso, J.J., and Torg, E.** *Rehabilitation of Athletic Injuries: An Atlas of Therapeutic Exercise.* Chicago: Year Book Medical Publishers, 1987; 107–110.

175. **Upton, P.A., Noakes, T.D., and Juritz, J.M.** Thermal pants may reduce the risk of recurrent hamstring injuries in rugby players. *Br. J. Sports Med.,* 1996; 30: 57–60.

176. **Varela, J.R. et al.** Complete rupture of the distal semimebranosus tendon with secondary hamstring muscles atrophy: MR findings in two cases. *Skel. Radiol.,* 2000; 29: 362–364.

177. **Yamamoto, T.** Relationship between hamstring strains and leg muscle strength. A follow-up study of collegiate track and field athletes. *J. Sports Med. Phys. Fitness,* 1993; 33: 194–199.

178. **Williford, H.N. et al.** Evaluation of warm-up for improvement in flexibility. *Am. J. Sports Med.,* 1986; 14: 316–319.

179. **Worrell, T.W.** Factors associated with hamstring injuries. An approach to treatment and preventative measures. *Sports Med.,* 1994; 17: 338–345.

Knee

8

I. OVERUSE INJURIES OF THE KNEE JOINT

The knee is a frequently injured joint in athletic and recreational activities. According to some statistics, one half, or possibly even more, of all sports-related injuries are incurred in the knee joint. The precise statistics differ between various athletic activities and depend on the specific movements habitually performed in these activities. Overuse injuries are also frequent in the knee joint; the reasons for this are that the knee joint participates in all sports activities (running, jumping, kicking, etc.) and that its joint area is characterized by numerous attachment sites for muscles and their tendons as well as by numerous bursae. It is also because of the nature of the specific joint between the patella and the femur (articulatio femoropatellaris) that constitutes a part of the knee joint.

These reasons amply explain why as much as 40% of all overuse injuries occurring in runners develop in the knee joint area. Overuse injuries in runners develop significantly less frequently in the Achilles tendon (15%), in the medial area of the lower leg (15%), in the hip and groin (15%), in the foot (10%), and in the lower back (5%). The impressive frequency of overuse injuries in the knee explains the existence of a special term to describe them, *runner's knee*. The term runner's knee, however, is used to describe two different localizations of overuse injuries in the knee. Recently, this term has been used to describe friction of the iliotibial band over the lateral femoral epicondyle, whereas today it is applied to the painful patellofemoral syndrome. This syndrome is also frequently described as chondromalacia, because of the pathological changes in the cartilage of the joint surfaces of the patella, or as malalignment of the extensor system of the knee (malalignment of the patella). Speaking in general terms, all overuse injuries in the knee can be differentiated, depending on their anatomical localization, into four groups (Table 8.1).

As Table 8.1 shows, there are numerous possible reasons for anterior knee pain. Note, however, that Table 8.1 primarily consists of chronic causes that lead to the development of anterior knee pain. The reason for this is that anterior knee pain caused by acute reasons (i.e., meniscus injury) completely disappears after a certain period of time if correct therapy is applied.

Irregularities in the course of the patella and malalignment of the extensor system of the knee are all described when discussing pain in the patellofemoral syndrome. Therefore, we feel it is imperative to clearly define the terms *patellar malalignment, chondromalacia of the patella,* and *anterior knee pain.*

II. PATELLOFEMORAL JOINT

A. PATELLAR MALALIGNMENT

Malalignment of the extensor system of the knee is difficult to define, which is not surprising because it is equally difficult to define a well-aligned extensor system of the knee. Perhaps the easiest way to define it is to say that malalignment of the extensor system of the knee entails changes in the architecture of the patellofemoral joint, which in turn change the relationship between the patellar stabilizers, leading to excessive tightness in some and insufficiency in others. Malalignment of the extensor system of the knee also leads to an incorrect distribution of strain in the patellofemoral joint, resulting in increased pressure in certain areas of patellofemoral contact (Scheme 8.1). According to Grelsamer[64] patellar malalignment is a translational or rotational

TABLE 8.1
Overuse Injuries of the Knee Joint

Anterior Aspect
Patellofemoral pain syndrome
Jumper's knee
Osgood-Schlatter disease
Sinding-Larsen-Johansson disease
Stress fracture of the patella
Fat pad syndrome

Medial Aspect
Plica syndrome
Semimembranosus tendinitis
Pes anserinus tendinitis/bursitis
Breaststroker's knee
Medial retinaculitis

Lateral Aspect
Iliotibial band friction syndrome
Popliteal tendinitis
Bicipital tendinitis

Posterior
Fabellitis
Gastrocnemius strain

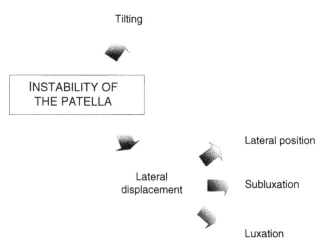

SCHEME 8.1 Classification of patellar instability.

deviation of the patella relative to any axis, and it can be a major component of patellar pain in adults. Currently, there are two theories to explain the origin of pain in patients with patellofemoral malalignment: the neural theory and the mechanical theory. Both theories are not exclusive, but complementary. Sanchis-Alfonso et al.[136] believe it is the neural factor that precipitates symptoms in patients with certain mechanical anomalies who also subject the knee to overuse. Before the 1980s, malalignment of the knee extensor system was nondynamically investigated, and the relationship between the patella and the femoral trochlea was studied solely by means of axial radiographic imaging of the patella.

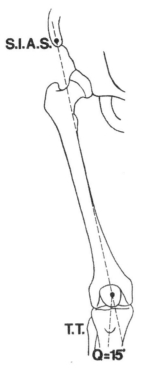

FIGURE 8.1 Schematic representation of the Q angle.

The first significant contribution to solving the problem of malalignment of the knee extensor system was made in 1979 by Larson.[24] His research indicated that in evaluating the orientation of the extensor system of the knee, special emphasis must be placed on the patellar stabilizers and their function, as well as on the orientation of the lower extremity, i.e., anatomical deviations of the lower extremity. Larson[24] differentiated between three groups of causative factors that resulted in malalignment of the knee extensor system: (1) changed (disturbed) relationships in the patellofemoral joint, (2) irregularities in the patellar stabilizers, and (3) malalignment of the lower extremity that affects the function of the patellofemoral joint. In the first group of causative factors resulting in malalignment of the knee extensor system, Larson lists abnormal tilting and/or displacement of the patella in the mediolateral direction, dysplasia and hypoplasia of the femoral trochlea, and displacement of the patella in the proximodistal direction — patella alta and patella infera. The second group consists of atrophy and/or high insertion site of the vastus medialis muscle ("dimple sign"[71]), excessive looseness of the medial stabilizers of the patella, which can result from trauma or a generalized laxity of the joints, and excessive tightness of the lateral stabilizers of the patella (vastus lateralis muscle, lateral patellar retinacul, and patellofemoral ligament). Anatomical deviations of the lower extremity that, according to Larson,[24] have an adverse effect on the function of the patellofemoral joint include excessive anteversion of the femoral head and neck, internal rotation of the femoral body, external rotation of the tibia, genu valgum, and lateral insertion of the patellar ligament. These causative factors can be determined clinically by the presence of an increased Q angle (Figure 8.1). Larson points out that in the vast majority of cases, a combination of the previously mentioned causes is present and that malalignment of the knee extensor system is not always accompanied by pain or other disturbances in the patellofemoral joint. It is also stressed that during clinical examination of a patient who exhibits the symptomatology characteristic of patellofemoral joint, the physician should direct attention to defining the underlying causative factors that have led to the development of malalignment of the extensor system. The basic principle of therapy consists of correcting these underlying causative factors.

Based on the preceding differentiation of causative factors, Gecha and Torg[59] reported on deviations of the knee extensor system most frequently encountered in patients with patellofemoral pain:

A. Changed relationships in the patellofemoral joint:
   1. Shallow femoral trochlea
   2. Hypoplastic lateral femoral condyle
   3. Deficient medial patellar facet
   4. Chondromalacia of the patella and/or of the femoral trochlea
   5. Osteochondral defect of the patella and/or the femoral trochlea
B. Parapatellar soft-tissue support abnormalities:
   1. Tight lateral parapatellar soft tissue
      a. Tight lateral retinaculum
      b. Tight lateral patellofemoral or patellotibial bands
      c. Presence of a band between patella and iliotibial or the vastus lateralis muscle
   2. Vastus medialis obliquus muscle deficiency
   3. Attenuated medial parapatellar soft-tissue structures
   4. Hypermobility of the patella
      a. Isolated patellar hypermobility
      b. Associated with generalized ligamentous laxity
      c. Associated with patella alta
      d. Associated with genu recurvatum
C. Lower extremity malalignment:
   1. Increased Q angle (greater than 15°)
   2. Increased femoral anteversion
   3. Increased external rotation of the tibia
   4. Increased genu valgum
   5. Foot hyperpronation

In 1988, Teitge[149] pointed out a number of mistakes made during evaluation of the orientation of the knee extensor system. His investigation showed that the orientation should be evaluated in all three planes — both in rest and during active movement. According to Teitge, this is necessary because the characteristics of some factors that determine the orientation of the knee extensor system change when placed under stress, when the knee is in a bent position, when changes occur in the rotation of the femur and/or tibia, and so forth. Teitge reported that in the frontal plane, the physician should take into consideration the value of the Q angle, the rotation of the patella (clockwise or counterclockwise), and the orientation of the tibiofemoral joint — genu valgum or genu varum. An evaluation of the orientation in the sagittal plane should consider the position of the patella: its height (patella alta or infera), inclination (proximal or distal), and displacement (anterior or posterior). In addition, a detailed investigation should define the possible presence of flexion or extension contracture of the knee, which can develop either as a consequence of bony changes or, more frequently, as a consequence of soft-tissue changes. Excessive tightness, i.e., shortening of some tissues such as the hamstrings, iliotibial band, and/or rotators of the hip, causes excessive strain to the patellofemoral joint. In the horizontal plane, special emphasis must be placed on identifying the possible presence of anatomical deviations of the femur, tibia, and the upper and lower foot joints, such as excessive anteversion of the femoral head and neck; internal torsion of the femur; excessive external rotation of the lower leg; and hyperpronation of the foot. Consideration should also be placed on the position of the patella, its possible displacement (either medially or laterally), and the tilt of the patella (medial or lateral) (Figure 8.2). If patellar malalignment can be detected by clinical examination, then condition-specific treatment interventions may be implemented in patients with patellofemoral pain syndrome.

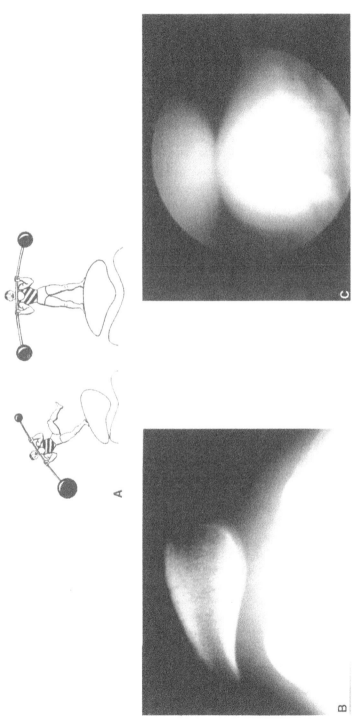

FIGURE 8.2 (A) Schematic representation of the tilt of the patella. (B) Axial roentgenogram of 30° knee flexion demonstrating tilt of the patella. (C) Arthroscopic view of the lateral displacement of the patella.

However, several clinical tests used to assess patellar mobility have recently been shown to have poor to fair reliability. Because the lateral pull test and the patellar tilt test, which are widely used clinically as diagnostic tests for patellofemoral pain syndrome, had not been previously tested for reliability, Watson et al.[157] examined these tests. Repeated lateral pull tests and patellar tilt tests had fair intrarater and poor interrater reliability. The results suggest that care must be taken in placing too much emphasis on these tests when making clinical decisions. According to Fulkerson,[51] standardized office radiographs are sufficient in most cases. Murray et al.[110] recommend an axial view at 30° of knee flexion and lateral radiographs at 30° of knee flexion in evaluating patellofemoral malalignment. Computerized tomography (CT) of the patellofemoral joint (precise midpatellar transverse images through the posterior femoral condyles with the knee at 15°, 30°, and 45° of knee flexion) will provide valuable objective information regarding subtle abnormalities of patellar alignment. Dong and Zheng[40] recommend CT scanning with and without quadriceps contraction to differentiate between static and dynamic abnormalities. Delgado-Martinez et al.[39] suggest that parameters for measuring lateral patellar tilt should be used from CT scanning only when planning treatment for patellofemoral malalignment. Biedert and Warnke[16] performed clinical and axial CT evaluation of correlation between the Q angle and the patella position. They concluded that there is no significance between the Q angle and the position of patella. The diagnostic relevance of the Q angle could not be established.

Magnetic resonance (MR) imaging, as a noninvasive and non-ionizing modality, has made a significant contribution to the understanding of musculoskeletal disorders including patellofemoral malalignment.[162] Static images through the patellofemoral joint in different degrees of flexion reveal only the degree of patellar tilt or subluxation, parameters that can be measured also on the axial view of conventional radiography. The accuracy of patellar position on static axial MR images is limited by the absence of muscle contraction, movement, and loading. Dynamic axial images of patellofemoral articulation can demonstrate the degree of flexion where patellar malalignment is maximal and assess whether or not it reduces. In cases of suspected patellofemoral malalignment with symptoms that mimic other types of internal derangement of the knee joint, dynamic MR imaging can be the procedure of choice for detection of transient patellar dislocation, which a single clinical examination cannot differentiate from other internal knee pathologies. Harman et al.[65] recommend kinematic MR fluoroscopy as an effective method in evaluating patellofemoral incongruency. Short time duration of investigation, ability to obtain nearly real-time images, suitable temporal contrast resolution, and investigation from very different angles of knee flexion are important advantages of the method. Shellock et al.[143] performed evaluation of patients with persistent symptoms after lateral retinacular release by kinematic MR imaging of the patellofemoral joint and 63% of patients had medial subluxation of the patella. Shellock[145] investigated the effect of a special patella brace on patients with lateral subluxation of the patella using kinematic MR imaging. This study provided objective findings that application of the brace improved or corrected lateral subluxation of the patella in the majority of patients. Shellock et al.[144] consider that the kinematic MR imaging technique may be used to determine the presence and severity of patellar malalignment and abnormal tracking patterns. In Witonski and Goraj's[161] opinion, patellar motion in the first 30° of knee flexion with thigh muscle contraction, analyzed by kinematic and dynamic axial MR imaging, is necessary for correct diagnosis in patients with anterior knee pain syndrome. Fulkerson[51–53] considers that by differentiating between rotational (tilt) and translational (subluxation) components of patellar malalignment, the clinician will be better able to prescribe appropriate treatment.

B. CHONDROMALACIA OF THE PATELLA

The term *chondromalacia patellae* (chondromalacia of the patella) was introduced into the medical literature by Konig in 1924.[62] Dugdale and Barnett,[44] however, offer the view that the term was first used by Aleman[6] and that the term chondromalacia of the patella became generally known and used only after publication of Aleman's paper in 1928. Shortly after, in 1933, Kulowski[44] introduced this term into English-language medical literature.

Budinger[55] was the first (in 1906) to notice changes in the patellar cartilage. Budinger, as well as Ludloff and Axhusen,[55] attributed these changes to the effects of trauma. Chondromalacia, the word that has defined the field of patellar pain during the last century, is now mostly a source of confusion and should be abandoned.[19] The presence of soft cartilage (the literal translation of the term chondromalacia) is not strongly correlated with patellar pain.[1,25,148] Moreover, surgeons often refer to cartilage changes anywhere in the knee as chondromalacia. The confusion is further compounded by the use of poorly defined grades (for example, grade III chondromalacia). Grelsamer[64] recommends: "Lesions are best called chondral or cartilage lesions, and they should be described qualitatively (for example, as blistering or fissuring) and quantitatively (in terms of size, location, and depth)." Kelly and Insall.[87] consider that the term chondromalacia patellae should not be used to diagnose patellofemoral pain but, rather, to describe lesions of articular cartilage. The term chondromalacia patellae, although once used as an all-inclusive term for anterior knee pain, is now widely accepted as a term used to describe pathological lesions of the patellar articular cartilage found at arthroscopy or arthrotomy.[67]

Numerous authors have investigated the causes leading to the development of chondromalacia of the patella.[12,81,108,112,129] In our opinion, the most concise report is one submitted by Morscher,[109] according to whom the etiology of chondromalacia of the patella can be classified into six groups:

1. Trauma and mechanical overloading
2. Anatomical variations (Wiberg types 3 and 4 and "Hunter's hat" form; Outerbridge ridge, bipartite patella, high riding patella, etc.)
3. Disturbance in alignment of the patella
4. Alteration of the gliding path of the patella
5. Nutritional disturbance of cartilage
6. Hormonal factors

Because changes in the patellofemoral joint cartilage are not always clinically visible, it is difficult to establish the incidence of these changes. Aleman,[6] based on 220 arthrotomies of the knee in a population of soldiers, reported a 33% incidence rate. In 1926, Heine[44] reported an 80% frequency of patellar cartilage change in his sample of patients between the ages of 50 and 59 years. Owen[44] noted an even greater frequency of patellar cartilage change in his sample of patients belonging to the same age group, and also reported a small incidence of patellar cartilage change in adolescents. Wiles et al.[44] pointed out that patellar cartilage change was, to some degree, present in all of the adult knees they examined. Contrary to the results obtained by Wiles et al., Outerbridge[117] has found patellar cartilage change in only 56 of 133 patients who have undergone open medial meniscectomy. Analysis of the patellofemoral joint of the knee after meniscectomy showed a decrease of contact surfaces, and altered distribution and magnitude of stresses on the side of meniscectomy.[46] An investigation carried out by Marrara and Pillay, which also deserves to be mentioned, indicated only a 50% frequency of patellar cartilage change in their group of patients with a mean age of 68 years.[44] Similar results were obtained by Casscells in 1978,[25] who noticed significant patellar cartilage changes in 37% of his patients and slight patellar cartilage changes in 25% of his patients. The analyzed sample consisted of elderly patients with a mean age of 70 years.

Numerous different categorization systems of chondromalacia of the patella are found in the medical literature, depending on the state and characteristics of the change in the cartilage of the patellofemoral joint and the size and localization of these changes.[73] Table 8.2 shows the most frequent classification systems encountered today. Outerbridge's classification is most frequently used.[117] The categorizations of Fulkerson and Hungerford[55] and Noyes and Stabler[115] should also be mentioned. The arthroscopic categorization, from Johnson,[84] is shown in Figure 8.3. Fulkerson

TABLE 8.2
Review of Classification Symptoms of Articular Cartilage Lesions

Author		Surface Descriptions of Articular Cartilage		Diameter	Location
Outerbridge	I:	Softening and swelling	I:	None	Starts most frequently on medial
	II:	Fragmentation and fissuring	II:	<½ in.	facet of patella; later extends to
	III:	Fragmentation and fissuring	III:	>½ in.	lateral facet "minor" lesion on
	IV:	Erosion of cartilage down to bone	IV:	None	intercondylar area of femoral
					condyles; upper border medial
					femoral condyle
Bentley	I:	Fibrillation or fissuring	I:	<5 cm	Most common at junction of medial
	II:	Fibrillation or fissuring	II:	5–1.0 cm	and odd facets of patella
	III:	Fibrillation or fissuring	III:	1.0–2.0 cm	
	IV:	Fibrillation with or without exposure of subchondral bone	IV:	>2.0 cm	
Casscells	I:	Superficial area of erosion	I:	≤1 cm	Patella and anterior femoral surfaces
	II:	Deeper layers of cartilage involved	II:	1–2 cm	
	III:	Cartilage is completely eroded and bone is exposed	III:	2–4 cm	
	IV:	Articular cartilage completely destroyed	IV:	"Wide area"	
Insall	I:	Swelling and softening of cartilage (closed chondromalacia)		None	I–IV: Midpoint of patellar crest with extension equally onto medial and lateral patellar facets
	II:	Deep fissures extending to subchondral bone			
	III:	Fibrillation			
	IV:	Erosive changes and exposures of subchondral bone (osteoarthrosis)			IV: Also involves opposite or mirror surface of femur
					Upper and lower ⅓ nearly always spared (patella); femur never severe

and Hungerford[55] differentiate among closed chondromalacia, open chondromalacia, chondrosclerosis, surface changes in the cartilage, and development of tufts.

1. **Closed Chondromalacia.** This change is characterized by a slight softening of the joint cartilage, which begins development in a localized area (usually consisting of a 1-cm area), and later radiates equally in all directions. The surface area remains intact. In some cases, small "blisters" appear and represent the first changes. Closed chondromalacia is, in most cases, localized on the lateral facet of the patella.
2. **Open Chondromalacia.** This change is characterized by having two basic types:
   Fissure — One or more fissures are encountered, usually on the surface but in some cases penetrating deep into the cartilage, all the way to the subchondral bone. These fissures are usually accompanied by greater or smaller areas of softened cartilage.
   Ulceration — A term used to describe a loss of cartilage that can be of greater or lesser degree. In cases of greater cartilage loss, the subchondral bone is usually visible and has a polished appearance (eburnated).
   Open chondromalacia is usually localized on the medial facet of the patella.
3. **Chondrosclerosis.** Chondrosclerosis is characterized by the presence of hard cartilage. This hard cartilage develops in the whole contact area of the joint and is so hard that it

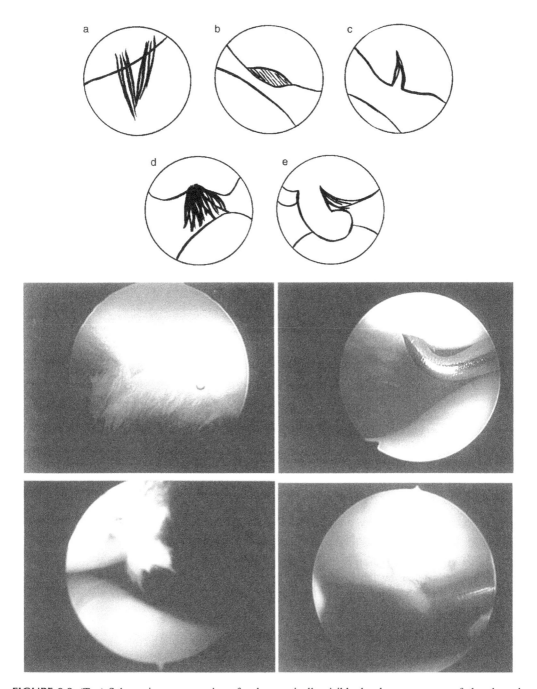

FIGURE 8.3 (Top) Schematic representation of arthroscopically visible development stages of chondromal-acia of the patella. (a) Bacon strip changes; (b) "bubble" defect; (c) fissuring; (d) fragmentation; (e) chondronecrosis. (Bottom) Arthroscopic representation of the same changes.

cannot be indented with a surgical probe. In appearance, the cartilage is yellow, translucent, and shiny.

4. **Superficial Surface Changes.** Superficial surface changes are characterized by a furrowed appearance of the joint surface of the patella; the furrows are oriented in a longitudinal direction.

TABLE 8.3
Noyes and Stabler's Classification of Articular Cartilage Lesions[115]

Surface Description	Extent of Inolvement	Diameter (mm)	Location	Degree of Knee Flexion
Cartilage surface intact	Definite softening with some resilience remaining	<10 ≥15 ≤20	Patella Proximal ¹/₃ Middle ¹/₃	Degree of knee flexion where the lesion is in weight-bearing contact
	Extensive softening with loss of resilience (deformation)	≤25 >25	Distal ¹/₃ Odd facet Middle facet Lateral facet	(e.g., 20–45°)
Cartilage surface damaged: cracks, fissures, condyle fibrillation, or fragmentation	<¹/₂ thickness ≥¹/₂ thickness		Trochlea Medial femoral condyle Anterior ¹/₃ Middle ¹/₃ Posterior ¹/₃ Lateral femoral condyle	
Bone exposed	Bone surface intact Bone surface cavitation		Anterior ¹/₃ Middle ¹/₃ Posterior ¹/₃ Medial tibial condyle Anterior ¹/₃ Middle ¹/₃ Posterior ¹/₃ Lateral tibial condyle Anterior ¹/₃ Middle ¹/₃ Posterior ¹/₃	

---

5. **Tuft Formation.** Tuft formation is characterized by the appearance of numerous "projections" of the patellar cartilage, which usually develop on the "odd" border and the medial facet of the patella; this takes the form of tufts. These tufts leave cracks of varying length and depth on the joint surface of the patella.

Lindberg et al.[94] have shown the need for a more precise and more reproducible classification system for joint cartilage injury. At present, in our opinion, the best existing classification system that meets both these criteria and the practical considerations encountered in everyday clinical examinations, i.e., routine arthroscopy, was devised in 1989 by Noyes and Stabler[115] (Table 8.3).

C. ANTERIOR KNEE PAIN

After the first reports of chondromalacia of the patella, which were all based on intraoperatively visible changes in the patellar cartilage, this principal criterion was gradually abandoned and more authors diagnosed chondromalacia of the patella clinically, on the basis of some very unreliable indicators, e.g., Freund's sign (percussion of the patella). During the mid-1970s interest renewed concerning the patellofemoral joint, while proof of cessation of pain solely after cutting through the lateral retinaculum, with the patellar cartilage injured, provoked further investigations concerning the precise localization of the pain. Numerous authors, among them Blazina et al.,[18] Goodfellow et al.,[61] Radin,[128] Fulkerson et al.,[57] and Dandy,[33] noticed other localizations of the pain, resulting in a new clinical syndrome — anterior knee pain, or dolor peri(para)patellaris. One of the most influential papers concerning this problem was published in 1985 by Radin.[128] The term *anterior knee pain* is suggested to encompass all pain-related problems, excluding anterior knee pain due to intra-articular pathology.[152] Anterior knee pain is a common complaint in the orthopedic clinic.

The differential diagnosis is wide and the principal goal of initial assessment is to detect remediable causes.[102] A clear understanding of the pathophysiology of anterior knee pain is inhibited by the use of imprecise, poorly defined, and often interchanged words, such as malalignment, patellar alignment, maltracking, subluxation, dislocation, and congruence.[124,125] Although some physicians compare the diagnosis of anterior knee pain to a "large wastepaper basket," these physicians still agree that it is better to begin treatment, even with this "provisory" diagnosis, and try to determine the precise localization of the injury and/or damaged area while monitoring the development of the syndrome. The leading symptom of this injury, pain in the anterior knee area, is included in the term used to describe this syndrome. The term does not, however, answer two important questions, namely, (1) the precise localization of the pain and (2) the etiology of the injury. For this reason, different authors use this term to describe numerous and different injuries within this clinical syndrome. To illustrate the large number of different injuries that "hide" under the name "anterior knee pain," we describe a number of classifications currently available in medical literature.

According to the classification proposed by Ireland,[77] when defining anterior knee pain, one should take into consideration the etiology of the pain. Ireland recognizes mechanical, inflammatory, and mixed causes of pain (Table 8.4). Contrary to this classification, Dandy[33–35] recommends a classification based on the localization of the injured area that leads to the development of pain and discomfort. According to Dandy,[34] the synovial membrane can be the cause of pain in cases of traumatic synovitis, while a much more frequent cause of pain is the synovial shelf syndrome, primarily the medial synovial shelf syndrome (medial plica syndrome). Pain can also be caused by changes on the patella, principally on the patellar cartilage — chondromalacia, arthrotic changes (Figure 8.4), osteochondral fractures, chondral flaps, osteochondritis dissecans patellae (Figure 8.5), and divided patella (patella partita; Figure 8.6). Dandy states that within this group of causative factors, the most frequent cause of anterior knee pain is the excessive lateral pressure syndrome. Certain tendon injuries can also cause anterior knee pain, the most frequent, according to Dandy,[33–35] is injury to the patellar ligament (jumper's knee). Reflex sympathic dystrophy is another common cause of anterior knee pain, and according to Dandy it represents an exceedingly complex diagnostic and therapeutic problem. In this group, in which pain results from changes in or on the bone, Dandy also includes Osgood-Schlatter disease, Sinding-Larsen-Johansson disease, and stress fractures of the patella. Possible causative factors are also so-called internal injuries of the knee, i.e., injuries of cruciate ligaments and meniscuses. A special group of causative factors consists of less frequently encountered causes of anterior knee pain such as inflammation or injury of the infrapatellar bursa and some tumors that develop in the knee area: ganglion, hemangiom, neurinom, etc.

Jacobson and Flandry[80] propose a different classification and recommend that, when evaluating patients with anterior knee pain, the physician should always bear in mind all possible causative factors. These authors include instability of the patellofemoral joint, synovial shelf syndromes,[119] inflammatory changes of the peripatellar tissue, injury to the patellofemoral cartilage, arthrotic changes in the cartilage of the patellofemoral joint, and trauma.

Anterior knee pain caused by overactivity in an athletic or military population is described by many authors.[2,29,41,43,105,151,164] There are clear differences between men and women regarding anterior knee pain. Anatomic factors including increased pelvic width and resulting excessive lateral thrust on the patella are primary factors that predispose females to anterior knee pain.[54] Effects of estrogen on connective tissue synthesis have been reported, but no clear mechanism has been

TABLE 8.4
Differential Diagnosis of Anterior Knee Pain[77]

Inflammatory
Bursitis
  Prepatellar
  Retropatellar
  Pes anserinus
Tendonitis
  Pes anserinus
  Semimembranosus
  Patellar
Synovitis

Mechanical
Hypermobility
Subluxation
Dislocation
Patellofemoral stress syndrome
Pathological plica syndrome
Osteochondral fracture
Arthrosis

Miscellaneous
Reflex sympathetic dystrophy
Osteochondritis dissecans
Fat pad syndrome
Systematic arthritis
Muscle strain
Stress fracture
Meniscal tear
Iliotibial band syndrome

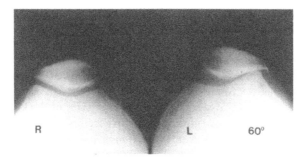

FIGURE 8.4 Axial view showing patellofemoral arthrosis.

demonstrated by which this would affect anterior knee pain. Postural and sociological factors such as wearing high heels and sitting with legs adducted can influence the incidence and severity of anterior knee pain in women.

Macnicol[96] has reported numerous causes of anterior knee pain with regard to the localization of the injury (Table 8.5). Fulkerson[57] has shown that patients with anterior knee pain frequently localize the area of greatest tenderness in the lateral retinaculum area and at the insertion site of the vascus lateralis muscle. This phenomenon, according to Fulkerson, results from injury to the

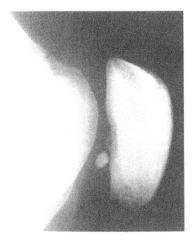

FIGURE 8.5 Osteochondritis dissecans of the patella.

FIGURE 8.6 Bipartite patella.

nerve endings in the retinaculum caused by malalignment of the extensor system of the knee. Johnson[84] also considers "retinacular pain" to be a possible causative factor of anterior knee pain. Fulkerson and Hungerford[55] stress that it is equally important, when dealing with patients suffering from anterior knee pain, to keep in mind other possible localizations of the injury and/or damaged area, which can manifest as anterior knee pain. These consist primarily of injury or damage to the hips or spine such as Legg-Calve-Perthes syndrome, epiphysiolysis of the femoral head, idiopathic aseptic necrosis of the femoral head, osteoarthritis of the hip, protrusion or prolapse of the intervertebral disk, and lumbosichialgia of various etiologies. The etiology of pain in anterior knee pain syndrome is a matter of controversy.[15,32,83,159–161] Witonski[159] suggests that anterior knee pain might be a psychosomatic syndrome associated with subclinical patellar instability and with little if any relation to levels of physical activity. Witonski et al.[160] describe the distribution of substance-P nerve fibers in the knee joint in patients with anterior knee pain syndrome. The results of this study provide immunohistochemical evidence suggesting that pain may originate in the fat pad and medial retinaculum of many patients with anterior knee pain syndrome.

As we pointed out in the beginning of this chapter, a synergistic effect and definite correlation exist among malalignment of the knee extensor system, instability of the patella, chondromalacia of the patella, and anterior knee pain; this explains why the terms used to describe these syndromes are often incorrectly applied (Scheme 8.2). Malalignment of the knee extensor system does not, for example, necessarily mean that instability of the patella, anterior knee pain, and chondromalacia of the patella are also present. Malalignment of the knee extensor system, can, however, contribute to the development of instability of the patella, principally because of the changed relationship

TABLE 8.5
Different Pathological Conditions Producing Anterior Knee Pain[96]

Site	Pathology
Patellar	Trauma (osteochondral fracture)
	Abnormal pressure or stress
	Increased or decreased
	With or without patellofemoral instability
	With or without patellar tilting
	Osteodystrophy
	Absnormal ossification center
	Sinding-Larson-Johansson's disease
	Patellofemoral arthropaty
	"True" chondromalacia patellae
	Osteoarthritis
Prepatellar	Synovial finge lesion
	Medial fat padsyndrome
	Synovitis
	Loose body
	Plica syndrome
Quadriceps mechanism	Chronic quadriceps weakness
	Quadriceps tendon partial rupture
	Patellar tendinitis
	Ligament laxity
Superficial	Prepatellar, infrapatellar, or suprapatellar bursitis
	Neuroma (especially of the infrapatellar branch of the saphenous nerve)
	Scarring
	Skin conditions
Other	Referred pain (meniscal tear, ligament rupture, hip pathology, lumbar disk herniation)
	Psychosomatic
	Idiopathic

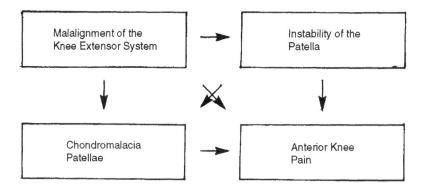

SCHEME 8.2 Synergistic effect and definite correlation between different etiological factors of anterior knee pain.

between the patellar stabilizers characterized in most cases by insufficiency in the medial stabilizers of the patella. In cases of malalignment of the knee extensor system, the architecture of the patellofemoral joint is also changed, which results in an incorrect distribution of the strain, increased pressure in certain areas of patellofemoral contact, and the consequent development of chondromalacia in these areas. The synergistic effects of malalignment of the knee extensor system therefore lead to pain in the anterior knee area. The point we are stressing here, however, is that neither instability of the patella, nor chondromalacia of the patella, nor anterior knee pain can be considered to be causes leading to the development of malalignment of the knee extensor system. Malalignment of the extensor system of the knee results exclusively as a result of anatomical deviations. Instability of the patella causes pain in the anterior area of the knee due to overuse and excessive strain to the surrounding tissue. Likewise, it leads to chondromalacia of the patella due to injury to the cartilage of the patellofemoral joint. Chondromalacia of the patella leads to pain in the anterior knee area due to the development of secondary synovitis. We also point out that currently a definite diagnosis of chondromalacia of the patella can only be reached intraoperatively (today, usually arthroscopically). Direct trauma can also cause pain in the anterior knee area. Anterior knee pain is primarily a clinical symptom and cannot be a cause of malalignment of the knee extensor system, or instability of the patella, or chondromalacia of the patella. The reverse, however, is quite possible.

From the material presented thus far, it is obvious that, after a provisory, symptomatic diagnosis of anterior knee pain, the physician should attempt to diagnose the cause leading to the development of this syndrome. In diagnosing the cause leading to the development of anterior knee pain, a detailed and targeted clinical examination is of the utmost importance.[22] Specific clinical signs must also be examined to establish the possible presence of instability of the patella, malalignment of the knee extensor system, chondromalacia of the patella, patellar tendinitis (jumper's knee, Osgood-Schlatter disease), and other syndromes.

Radiological examinations are of great assistance[9,17,20,24,26,36,37,42,48,72,76,93,104,106,123] in discovering anatomical deviations and irregularities in the patellofemoral joint — excessively high or low placed patella, inclination of the patella, Wiberg's angle (Figure 8.7), angle of the femoral trochlea, etc. A CT examination of the lower extremity is of immeasurable help when evaluating and assessing rotation deformations in the hip and knee area and the related changed kinematic relations in the patellofemoral joint[38,56,100,140] (Figure 8.8). The usefulness of kinematic analysis in the study of motion of the patellofemoral joint *in vivo* is proved by Matijasevic et al.[99] The future of functional examinations of the patellofemoral joint is closely related to the use of MR imaging techniques. This method allows examination of the femoropatellar joint during movements from 0 to 140° (Figure 8.9) and also allows analysis of the state of the joint facet patellar cartilage.[79,89,141,142] According to McCauley et al.[101] most patients with chondromalacia patellae have focal signal or focal contour defects in the patellar cartilage on T2-weighted MR images. These findings are absent in most patients with arthroscopically normal cartilage. In an *in vitro* study of van Leersum et al.[155] a total of 1000 MR, 200 histological, and 200 surface locations were graded for chondromalacia and statistically compared. The study demonstrates that fat-suppressed routine T2-weighted and fast spin echo T2-weighted sequences seem to be more accurate than proton density, T1-weighted, and gradient echo sequences in grading chondromalacia. Good histological and macroscopic correlation was seen in more severe grades of chondromalacia, but problems remain for the early grades in all sequences studied. Scintigraphic analysis can also be used in the diagnosis of anterior knee pain, i.e., in cases of reflex sympathetic dystrophy of the patella.[23] Bahk et al.[8] describe a pinhole scintigraphic sign of chondromalacia patellae in older subjects; that is, the spotty tracer uptake occurring exclusively in the central retropatellar facet without other knee joint alteration appears pathognomonic for chondromalacia patellae in older patients. Sympathic reflex dystrophy of the patella can also be diagnosed with the computerized telethermography method. This method can objectively determine the presence of anterior knee pain and can also enable the monitoring of the course of the disease and the results of the applied treatment.[156] Arthroscopy of the knee is, of course, of utmost importance and is basically an unavoidable examination

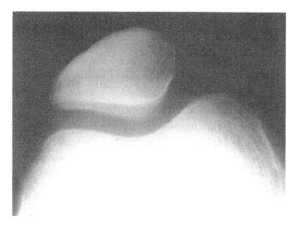

FIGURE 8.7 Wiberg type 4: Alpine hunter's cap deformity.

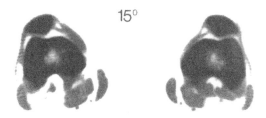

FIGURE 8.8 CT image of the patellofemoral joint at 15° of knee flexion.

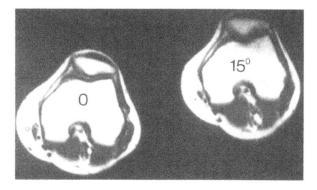

FIGURE 8.9 MR image of the patellofemoral joint at 0° (left) and 15° (right) of the knee flexion.

method.[13,33,34,84,94,97,115,134,147] Arthroscopy is also, at present, the only sure way to confirm the existence of suspected chondromalacia of the patella and other intra-articular causes of anterior knee pain, such as plica synovialis medialis.

A definite decision about the causes leading to the development of anterior knee pain, despite the auxiliary input of numerous diagnostic examination methods, can only be reached on the basis of history and a detailed physical examination.[130] A diagnosis of, for example, plicae synovialis medialis does not as yet mean that we have precisely defined the cause leading to the development of pain. Similarly, a diagnosis that confirms the presence of pathological changes on the patellar cartilage does not necessarily mean that these changes are the cause of pain. It is quite possible that these changes are a side effect and that the real cause of pain is, for example, Hoffa disease or patellar tendinitis (jumper's knee). LaBrier and O'Neill[92] have described patellofemoral stress

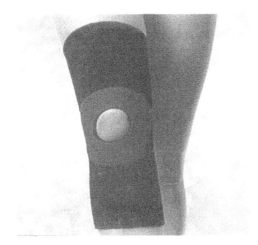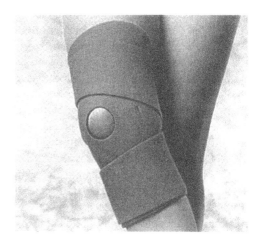

FIGURE 8.10 Two different types of knee braces for patellar instability.

syndrome, a condition of peripatellar pain without anatomic malalignment, history of trauma, patellar instability, or clinical evidence of patellofemoral crepitus. These patients demonstrate lateral retinacular and iliotibial band tightness. Frequently, the patient's pain occurs when sitting for prolonged periods of time with the knee flexed, and most commonly with sporting events. A lateral retinacular release is the surgical procedure recommended as a reliable solution in the majority of patients.

The preceding parts of this chapter illustrate the complexity related to the anterior knee pain syndrome and likewise explain the complexity present when treating this syndrome.[10,35,62,68,70,72,98] After a precise diagnosis, the physician should prescribe treatment of the cause of the pain, which can be either non-operative or operative. If, for example, the primary cause of pain is excessive pressure on the lateral part of the patella (the lateral patellar joint facet) caused by malalignment of the knee extensor system, then the physician can attempt to correct this malalignment with non-operative treatment such as electrostimulation of the vastus medialis muscle or by having the patient wear a brace designed for stabilizing the patella (Figure 8.10). The goal of conservative treatment is pain relief.[45] Proprioceptive muscle stretching and strengthening is recommended by Clark et al.,[28] and Alaca et al.[5] consider that an isokinetic exercise treatment program prevents extensor power loss due to patellofemoral pain syndrome. It seems clinically important to begin the treatment program before the anterior knee pain becomes chronic and treatment becomes less effective.[164] There is inconclusive evidence to support superiority of one physiotherapy intervention over others.[30,138,139] The study of Naslund et al.[111] shows that patients with idiopathic anterior knee pain benefit from both electroacupuncture treatment and subcutaneous needling. Central pain inhibition, caused either by afferent stimulation or by nonspecific therapeutic (placebo) effects, is a plausible explanation for the treatment effects. In a randomized, double-blind study of low laser treatment of chondromalacia of the patella in 40 patients, no statistical difference was found between real and sham use of low laser for the symptoms of chondromalacia of the patella.[133] Patellar taping and/or bracing can reduce pain in people with patellofemoral pain syndrome, but it does not do so by medializing the patella.[31,60,113,127]

If non-operative treatment does not lead to any appreciable results, the physician can attempt to resolve the problem of malalignment of the knee extensor system and the syndrome of lateral hyperpressure of the patella operatively. Today, this usually entails arthroscopic release of the lateral retinaculum of the patella.[19,27,116,153,154] When the pain is caused by plicae synovialis medialis, the latter can be arthroscopically resected while softened patellar cartilage can be arthroscopically shaved (shaving of the patella). In patients with normal patellar alignment and isolated chondromalacia patellae noted during arthroscopic examination, isolated patellar debridement is recommended.[47] Kasim and Fulkerson[86] reviewed the long-term results of 25 patients who had localized soft-tissue resections for refractory anterior retinacular knee pain. Their results show that specific soft-tissue excision of painful tissue can often lead to successful clinical outcomes.

In the beginning stages, when the precise etiology of anterior knee pain is not yet known, immediate treatment consists of ceasing all physical activities that cause pain. This, however, does not necessarily entail a complete cessation of all athletic activities. If, and when, the symptoms grow in intensity, which usually occurs when the athlete persists in his or her athletic activities despite the pain, a complete unburdening and relaxation of the knee, including walking with crutches for a short period of time, can be recommended. Complete immobilization of the affected knee with a plaster of Paris cast is rarely necessary. Classical treatment, in the sense of recommending cryotherapy (ice), nonsteroidal anti-inflammatory drugs, and isometric exercises for the quadriceps muscle, is a necessary part of any treatment for anterior knee pain. When performing exercises for the quadriceps muscle, the patient's knee should be in a position of flexion that is comfortable, i.e., in a position where contraction of the quadriceps muscle is painless. Electrotherapy, either for the purposes of stimulation or for its analgesic effect, is another non-operative treatment method that can be prescribed. Special knee braces that stabilize the patella and prevent its lateral displacement, as well as special bands used when treating patellar tendinitis, are other methods that fall within the domain of non-operative treatment. Another important step in the treatment of anterior knee pain is a slow and gradual return to sports activities, beginning at first with fast walking and progressing gradually to jogging, sprinting, running with sudden changes of direction, and finally jumping. However, some exercises and procedures routinely carried out during training will have to be permanently banned. These include lifting weights from a crouched position, performing deep knee bends, and running up and down a hill. In the treatment of anterior knee pain syndrome, an important place is reserved for stretching exercises, especially for the quadriceps muscle and hamstrings. The latter enables complete extension of the knee, which has the effect of decreasing the pressure in the patellofemoral joint. When all of the aforementioned methods fail to produce significant results, in the sense of lessening the intensity or alleviating the painful symptoms, surgical treatment is, perforce, the only remaining option.

Surgical treatment can be complex, and during the course of one intervention, a number of surgical procedures can be performed. It is not uncommon to perform procedures to release the lateral patellar retinaculum, to shave the patellar cartilage, to transpose the tibial tuberosity and its ventralization,[121] as well as an apicotomy of the patella, all during one surgical intervention. There are several surgical techniques for anteromedial tibial tubercle transfer in patients with chronic anterior knee pain and a subluxation-type patellar malalignment (Maquet-Bandi, Blauth-Mann, Elmslie-Trillat, modified Elmslie-Trillat procedure, and Fulkerson's modified Elmslie-Trillat procedure).[4,11,82,131,132] A cadaveric study of articular cartilage contact pressure after tibial tuberosity transfer documented that medialization of the tibial tuberosity significantly increased the patellofemoral contact pressure and, also, significantly increased the average contact pressure of the medial tibiofemoral compartment; thus, overmedialization of the tibial tuberosity should be avoided.[91] Lateral patellar subluxation associated with malalignment can be corrected by a distal realignment procedure such as the anteromedial tibial tubercle transfer, but repair of the medial patellofemoral ligament in cases of patellar dislocation has considerably lowered the incidence of recurrent instability.[7,66,146,165]

Hašpl et al.[66] present a new, fully arthroscopic technique for treatment of patellofemoral instability consisting of plication of the medial patellar retinaculum and release of the lateral patellar retinaculum (Figure 8.11). The procedure has been performed on 17 patients; 3 patients with patellar instability, acute patellar luxation in 4, and recurrent patellar luxation in 10 patients. Postoperative results after follow-up of more than 2 years have been good with no recurrence of subluxation or luxation. Another valuable contribution to the field of surgical treatment for anterior knee pain syndrome has been made by Morscher,[109] who introduced longitudinal (sagittal) osteotomy of the patella into clinical practice. In 1987, Lippert and Paar[95] published an experimental study of sagittal

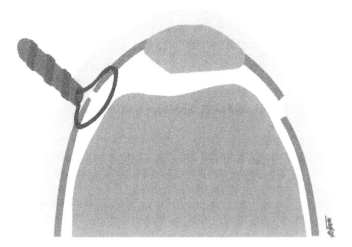

FIGURE 8.11 Schematic representation of the full arthroscopic realignment of the patella (release of the lateral retinaculum and raphia of the medial retinaculum).

patella osteotomy. We have successfully applied longitudinal (sagittal) osteotomy of the patella since 1980.[120,122] As of 1991, we had performed 89 longitudinal osteotomies of the patella, of which 16 were performed on top-level athletes or ballet dancers.[122] The mean value of Wiberg's patellar angle was 112° preoperatively, and 142° postoperatively. The results, judged on the basis of criteria evaluation compiled by Bandi[10] and Ficat,[48] were excellent. Our successful application of longitudinal osteotomy of the patella is confirmed by the fact that all of the operated athletes, except one (karate), returned to competitive sports, and that three ballerinas returned to professional dancing.

The experimental results of Graf et al.[63] show, that patients with chondromalacia have increased intramedullary pressure. Schneider et al.[138] after measurement of intraosseous pressure of the patella treated 69 patients (136 knees) with a new method of intraosseous drilling and decompression and 90% of treated patients experienced pain relief. Owens et al.[118] present prospective analysis of radiofrequency vs. mechanical debridement of isolated patellar chondral lesions. This study presents clear evidence of superior clinical outcome of debridement of patellar grade 2 and 3 chondral lesions with the use of bipolar radiofrequency vs. a mechanical shaver. According to Bentley and Dowd[14] operative treatment of chondromalacia patellae is indicated for patients with persistent pain and macroscopic involvement of more than half a centimeter of the articular cartilage surface.

Fulkerson[53] concludes that current thinking of diagnosis and treatment of patients with patellofemoral pain emphasizes precise diagnosis, rehabilitation involving the entire kinetic chain, restoration of patella homeostasis, minimal surgical intervention, and precise indications for more definitive corrective surgery. After every surgical intervention, an adequate postoperative rehabilitation program, including a slow and gradual return to sports activities, must be carried out. In some cases, however, a complete return to the normal state before the injury (restitutio ad integrum) will not be obtainable.

According to Jackson[78] no discussion of anterior knee pain is complete without alerting the reader to the existence of the "genupath." The entire life and being of these unusual individuals center around their knee symptoms, which become chronic and are blamed for failure both at work and in their private lives. With consummate skill and patience they can manipulate a succession of orthopedic surgeons to perform a series of procedures, each more drastic than the last. The disruptive chain of events invariably commences as "anterior knee pain of unknown cause" in adolescence and this progresses in stages, which include patellectomy, knee replacement, arthrosdesis, and even above-knee amputation in just 10 to 15 years. Orthopedic surgeons must be on their guard because these patients are deliberately misleading; they need psychiatric help, not surgery. With the exception of diagnostic arthroscopy, it is wise to make a rule never to operate on the basis of subjective symptoms alone and to adhere to it.

III. PATELLAR TENDINITIS/TENDINOSIS
(JUMPER'S KNEE)

Patellar tendinitis (jumper's knee) is an overuse injury characterized by pathological changes in the distal parts of the extensor system of the knee joint: the quadriceps tendon and its insertion to the proximal pole of the patella, and the patellar tendon (patellar ligament) and its proximal insertion to the apex of the patella or distal insertion to the tibial tubercle. Other terms are also found in the medical literature that apply to the same syndrome: patellar or quadriceps tendinitis, patellar apicitis, and enthesitis apicis patellae, volleyball's knee, basketball's knee.[169,170,175] The first description of patellar tendinitis dates from 1921 when Sinding-Larsen and Johansson first described pathological changes on the proximal insertion of the patellar tendon. However, only in 1962 did Smillie describe this clinical entity in adults.[169] In 1973, a detailed description of the clinical picture and a form of therapy were published by Blazina,[169] who, at the same time, also introduced in the medical literature the term *jumper's knee*.

Jumper's knee is a clinical entity most commonly found in athletes who, during their athletic activities, habitually place excessive strain on the extensory system of their knees with numerous jumps or long periods of running.[187,192,198,271] The high frequency of patellar tendinitis in volleyball players was first noticed by Maurizio in 1963.[192] Ferretti,[189] who was himself a volleyball player, conducted an epidemiological study, the results of which showed that jumper's knee accounted for 28% of all sports-related injuries in volleyball and that fully 40% of top-level volleyball players suffer from this syndrome at least once during their athletic career. Volleyball has become an extremely popular participation sport worldwide and patellar tendinitis represents the most common overuse injury, although shoulder tendinitis secondary to the overhead activities of spiking and serving is also commonly seen.[172] A high incidence of jumper's knee was also noticed in other athletic activities, primarily in the so-called jumping sports, such as the high jump, the long jump, the triple jump, and basketball.[205,207,220,235] Hickey et al.[206] found patellar tendinitis in 6.7% of young elite female basketball players over a 6-year period. Linenger and West[225] determined the incidence of patellar tendinitis as 15.1% among U.S. Marine recruits undergoing basic training. In other athletic activities, this syndrome is noted in lesser frequencies but is encountered occasionally in soccer players, weight lifters, and bicyclists.[34] Dubravćić-Šimunjak et al.[183,184] reported that jumper's knee is also found in top-level figure skaters because of the numerous jumps now being performed in this athletic activity. Jumper's knee can also develop in athletes who habitually run for long periods of time and in hockey players.[222] Painful symptoms very similar to patellar tendinitis can be present during the postoperative treatment of patients who have had various surgical procedures performed on their knee joints. With these patients, however, the clinical symptoms disappear as soon as the quadriceps femoris muscle regains its initial strength. Kujala et al.[222] reported in their retrospective study that during a 5-year interval in a test sample of 2672 ambulatory patients with various knee injuries, fully 26.4% suffered from complications related to jumper's knee. These findings led them to believe that jumper's knee is the most common athletic injury to the knee joint and that it is encountered in higher frequencies than either meniscal or anterior cruciate ligament injuries.

A. ETIOPATHOGENESIS

Jumper's knee is usually diagnosed in athletes who have taken part in strenuous athletic activities that place strong and repeated mechanical strain on the extensory system of their knees. Repeated mechanical excessive strain is, without doubt, the basic prerequisite for the development of this syndrome. However, it should be noted that, of different athletes who participate in the same sport, play in the same position on the team, and are placed under the same repeated mechanical stresses, some develop jumper's knee while others remain free from any symptoms.[187,189,221] Thus, it is necessary to discover the factors that predispose some athletes to develop this syndrome.

The main athletic activity that substantially increases the amount of mechanical strain placed on the knee extensory system is various types of jumps. These consist of both sudden and strongly performed jumps from a stationary position (e.g., when performing a block in volleyball), and jumps taken while running (e.g., in the high or long jump). Both types of jumps are performed with one or with both feet stationary during take-off. It is important to note that the maximal amount of mechanical strain is placed on the tendon during the deceleration phase of the landing — on the landing knee(s) — during the time the quadriceps femoris muscle is overcoming the force of gravity with eccentric contraction.[263,272] In fact, these contractions of the quadriceps femoris muscle are one of the basic causative factors in the development of jumper's knee.[191] In practice, these contractions are present, for example, when performing exercises in which the athlete jumps on a barrier 1 to 2 m in height and then lands from that height on the floor to immediately take off from the floor in a new jump. It is possible that stress shielding is a more important etiological factor in insertional tendinopathy as opposed to repetitive tensile loads.[166]

The development of jumper's knee is significantly correlated with the weekly amount of strain placed on the knee during training. The results of a study carried out by Ferretti et al.[189,191,192] confirm this: 40% of the top-level volleyball players they have treated who train at least four times a week develop clinical symptoms due to overstrain of the patellar tendon. At the same time, it was noted that athletes who train on hard surfaces (e.g., concrete) develop clinical symptoms in 37.5% of the cases, whereas those athletes who train on a floor develop jumper's knee in only 4.7% of the cases.[191] This difference is attributed to the poor absorptive qualities of hard surfaces, which place increased strain on the muscle–tendon unit of the knee extensory system. Another characteristic of jumper's knee is that it develops with equal frequency in adolescents (beginner athletes) and in mature athletes.[192] Thus, it is believed that the length of time the athlete has been engaged in a particular athletic activity has little to do with the potential development of this syndrome. There are, however, some indications that the syndrome has a tendency to develop in the third year of intensive training.[192]

An analysis of training methods and procedures has indicated that the type of training method used has no significant bearing on the development of jumper's knee. A much more important causative factor was found to be the amount of training (both the amount of time and the amount of mechanical strain placed on the knee) that the athlete habitually carries out.[190] An interesting fact noted with regard to the development of jumper's knee was that the syndrome has a tendency to develop after relatively longer breaks in the training process, e.g., when renewing intensive physical activities after the summer holidays. Jumper's knee has an equal propensity for developing in both sexes and to develop in ages older than 15 years — in other words, when growth and development are finished.[192] In the younger age groups (younger than 15 years), mechanical overstrain is more often followed by the appearance of juvenile osteochondrosis of the knee joint. This is because in those age groups, the bony centers of growth are delicate and therefore prone to injury through excessive mechanical strain.[192]

The development of jumper's knee, to a large degree, also depends on the somatic characteristics of the athlete, of which the best known and most intensively studied are the anatomic features of the lower extremities.[221] Studies conducted with this in mind have shown that athletes suffering from patellar tendinitis sometimes also have concomitant genu valga, genu vara, and a varus position of the proximal tibia.[168,190] In a small number of patients, increased anteversion of the femoral neck and a prominent tibial tuberosity were also noted.[192] According to Richards et al.[247] the external tibial torsional moment (during the take-off for the right knee with the spike jump and for the left knee with the block jump) was a significant predictor of patellar tendinitis. Martens et al.[229] have shown, by studying the physical height of athletes afflicted with jumper's knee, that physical height is not a factor and that there is no physical constitution of the organism that predisposes an athlete to develop this syndrome. However, Kujala et al.[221] report that an unequal length (inegality) of the lower extremities and patella alta can significantly increase the likelihood of developing patellar tendinitis. They believe that in these cases, the patella is unable to fully perform its function as a movable center of force between the quadriceps femoris tendon and the patellar tendon, which leads to increased mechanical strain on the extensor system of the knee joint. A frequently analyzed possible causative factor of patellar tendinitis is the orientation of the extensor system of the knee.[187,189,191,234–236] On radiological examination of the knee joint in 30°, 45°, 60°, and 90° flexion in the axial projection, it is possible to analyze the orientation of this system based on the position tilting or lateralization of the patella and the congruence of the patella and the femoral trochlea.[217] From a clinical standpoint, the orientation of this system is determined by the value of the angle of the quadriceps femoris muscle, or the Q angle. The normal value of this angle is up to 10° to 15° in males and no more than 15° to 20° in females. The Q angle is slightly greater in females because of the width of the female pelvis. Pećina et al.[235] reported a significant correlation between a pathological Q angle and the development of jumper's knee, while Ferretti et al.[191] reported a 50% presence of pathological values for the Q angle in their total sample. Another clinical indication of a badly oriented extensor knee system is the so-called bayonet symptom. Pećina et al.[235] reported a 70% presence of this symptom in athletes suffering from patellar tendinitis. Tyler et al.[266] consider that an abnormal anteroposterior patellar tilt angle may be a contributing factor to pathological conditions of the knee. The results of their study demonstrate that patients with patellar tendinitis have abnormal patellar tilt in the sagittal plane. Although a pathological value of the Q angle and the bayonet symptom are generally present in athletes afflicted with jumper's knee, Ferretti et al.[192] reported that a badly oriented knee extensor system need not be a risk factor because an athlete should be encouraged to take up other, nonjumping sports. A badly oriented extensor system is, however, without doubt an important factor that should be taken into account when prescribing treatment for this syndrome. Chronic overload is considered the main cause of patellar tendinitis, but it has been postulated that impingement of the inferior patellar pole against the patellar tendon during knee flexion could be responsible (Figure 8.12).[211] Schmid et al.[255] present dynamic and static MR imaging of patellar tendinitis in an open-configuration system. They compared 19 knees with patellar tendinitis and 32 asymptomatic knees and the relationship between the patella and the patellar tendon was identical in both groups. They conclude that chronic overload seems to be a major cause of patellar tendinitis.

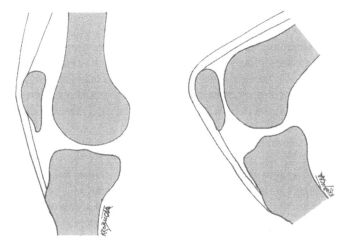

FIGURE 8.12 The impingement of the inferior patellar pole against the patellar tendon during knee flexion.

The functional imbalance of the muscles that stabilize the pelvis and the lower extremity is another factor that should be analyzed in the context of predisposing an athlete to developing jumper's knee. It is well known that strong and shortened muscles of the posterior part of the thigh (hamstring muscles) cause significant mechanical overstrain to the extensor system of the knee joint. A biomechanical and kinematographical analysis of a typical jump performed by a basketball player[260] showed that a weak iliopsoas, gluteus maximus, and rectus abdominis muscle contribute to increased strain of the extensor musculature of the knee, caused by an inadequate distribution of force during the jump. Thus, Sommer[260] recommends strengthening the abdominal muscles and stabilizing the muscles of the pelvis in patients suffering from this syndrome. A 2-year prospective study of Witvrouw et al.[274] examining intrinsic risk factors for the development of patellar tendinitis in an athletic population revealed that the only significant determining factor was muscular flexibility, with the patellar tendinitis patients less flexible in the quadriceps and hamstring muscles.

In the study of Sanchis-Alfonso et al.[253] pathological neural changes were observed in 17 pathological specimens retrieved during surgery for jumper's knee. In 8 cases, free nerve endings showed a histological pattern of "nerve sprouting" in the patellar tendon–bone junction. Vascular innervation was seen in 7 cases. S-100 positive fibers were observed within the muscular layer of medium and small arteries. These findings show an increase in vascular innervation. Last, neuromatous changes were observed in 4 cases, demonstrating a clear relationship with pain. These observations provide a neuroanatomic basis for pain in active, young patients with jumper's knee.

Based on what is reported in the medical literature, we feel confident in concluding the following. Although most of the studies carried out to date have been less interested in the external factors causing jumper's knee, it is quite certain that excessive strain caused by training and exercising on hard surfaces contributes significantly to the development of this syndrome. With regard to the group of anatomical changes of the lower extremity, the inegality of the lower extremities and patella alta are causative factors for the development of jumper's knee. In spite of this, it seems that the underlying causes of patellar tendinitis are based not on anatomical or biomechanical changes in the knee joint, but on the mechanical characteristics of the tendon and the area of insertion of the tendon into the bone (its elasticity and its ability to stretch). Therefore, the basic etiopathogenetic course of events leading to the development of overuse syndrome of the quadriceps tendon and the patellar tendon, i.e., jumper's knee, can be defined as the state that arises when mechanical overstrain overcomes the adaptive ability of the excessively strained tissue.

B. CLINICAL PICTURE AND DIAGNOSTICS

The clinical picture of jumper's knee is characterized by the presence of pain as the basic symptom, and a decreased functional ability of the afflicted lower extremity.[233,234,252] Patellar tendinitis/tendinosis, or jumper's knee, is an important cause of anterior knee pain.[185] The pain can appear either in the area of the upper or lower pole of the patella, or in the area of the tibial tuberosity. Pećina et al.[234–241] reported the appearance of pain at the junction of the quadriceps tendon to the base of the patella present in about 10% of their patients, at the insertion of the patellar tendon to the tibial tuberosity in 10% of their patients, and at the insertion site of the patellar tendon at the tip of the patella in 80% of athletes suffering from jumper's knee (Figure 8.13). The main features of this pain consist of sharpness of varying intensity that gradually evolves and whose appearance is not connected with evident trauma.

In the beginning stages of the disease, the pain occurs only after training/competition or after running down an incline[169,207] and disappears after a short period of complete rest (a couple of hours or 1 day).[267,268] In later stages, pain felt at the insertion areas of the quadriceps tendon and the patellar tendon becomes continuous and is present before, during, and long after athletic activities. The appearance of pain is quite frequent after long periods of sitting with the knees in a flexed position, e.g., when driving a car for long periods of time or when watching a movie at the theater. The appearance of this pain is sometimes called the *movie sign*[169,192,235] and can usually be relieved by rubbing the painful area and stretching the leg in the knee with the sole of the foot in supination. Some patients complain of a feeling of weakness and feebleness in the knee when this joint is subjected to stronger mechanical strain.[222] The functional inability of the afflicted lower extremity is accompanied by intense pain and shows a range from slight to complete inability to participate in athletic activities.

In very rare cases, continuation of intensive athletic activities, despite the presence of evident symptoms of the disease, leads to a complete break (rupture) of the patellar ligament.[251,254,258] Ferretti et al.[192] describe this state in 3 of 110 patients (2.7%) suffering from jumper's knee. Although considerably less frequent, a complete rupture can sometimes be seen at the junction of the quadriceps tendon to the base of the patella. Kelly et al.[216] describe one-sided ruptures of the quadriceps tendon in 3 patients, and a complete break of the patellar tendon in 11 patients with jumper's knee. They also report that, in their opinion, important causative factors leading to the development of this rupture are the degeneration of the tendon caused by mechanical overstrain, as well as structural changes in the tendon tissue caused by aging. Tarsney[264] reported the appearance of sudden, bilateral ruptures of the quadriceps tendon and the patellar tendon in athletes while they were playing basketball. These bilateral ruptures should be diagnostically differentiated from complete tendon breaks, which develop during the course of rheumatic diseases.[226] It has also been noted that a complete tendon break is very frequently preceded by the local application of corticosteroid medication.[216,264]

Based on histological analysis of tendon tissue of the knee extensor system performed during the course of the overuse syndrome, Ferretti et al.[188] note that the basic pathological changes develop on the insertion sites of the quadriceps tendon and patellar tendon to the patella and tibial tuberosity. The changes consist of a thickening of the transition cartilage between the tendon and the bone, the appearance of cystic cavities, and the loss of the border between the two transition cartilage (the blue line). Further research has shown that histopathological changes are also evident in the tendon structure.[242] Thus, it is today believed that there exists, during the course of jumper's knee, an enthesitis (insertion tendinopathy) as well as a change in the tendon structure (tendinosis) of varying intensity.

We performed an investigation to document pathological changes in bone, the bone–tendon junction, and in the patellar ligament in 34 athletes treated surgically because of jumper's knee.[239] In all patients apicotomia of the patella and partial excision of the patellar ligament were performed (half-open arthroscopic-assisted procedure). Pathological changes in the bone were found in one third of operated patients and included foci of necrosis, fat-changed cancellous bone, bone marrow replaced by highly vascularized granulation tissue with scattered mononuclear inflammatory cells. Abnormality of the bone–tendon junction was found in 75% of the patients and included microtears of the tendinous tissues, destruction of bone architecture, foci of ossification, chronic inflammatory cell infiltration, exaggerated fibrocartilaginous metaplasia, and mucoid degeneration. Changes in patellar tendon were found in all operated patients and included cellular proliferation within the tendinous tissue accompanied by prominence of capillary proliferation, chronic inflammatory cell infiltration, hyaline degeneration, mucoid degeneration, microtears of the tendinous tissue, neovascularization, and tenocyte infiltration, etc. Polarization microscopy showed loss of clear demarcation of collagen bundles accompanied by a loss of the normal dense, homogeneous polarization pattern.

The main clinical symptom of jumper's knee is the presence of a very intense, palpatory pain in the lower or upper pole of the patella or on the tibial tuberosity. In some cases, a cystic fluctuation is present in one of three predilected areas.[169,220,249,270] Intense pain can be produced by extending the lower leg against pressure.[169] Jumper's knee is also characterized by the presence of concomitant ligament or meniscus lesions, but chondromalacia of the patella is very rarely seen.[192] Blazina,[169]

TABLE 8.6
Classification of the Patellar Tendinitis According to Incidence and Progression of Symptoms

Stage	Symptoms	Ref.
Stage 1:	Pain after activity only	169
	No undue functional impairment	
Stage 2:	Pain during and after activity	
	Still able to perform at a satisfactory level	
Stage 3:	Pain during and after activity and more prolonged	
	Patient has progressively increasing difficulty in performing at satisfactory level	
Stage 1:	Pain only after sports activity	249
Stage 2:	Pain at the onset of sports activity, disappearing after warm-up and reappearing at fatigue	
Stage 3:	Constant pain at rest and during activity	
	Inability to participate in sports at previous level	
Stage 4:	Complete rupture of patellar tendon	
Stage 1:	Pain only after sports activity	220
Stage 2:	Pain at the beginning of sports activity, disappearing after warm-up and reappearing after activity	
Stage 3:	Pain at the beginning, during, and after sports activity	
Stage 4:	Constant pain at rest and during activity	
	Inability to participate in sports	
Stage 5:	Complete rupture of patellar tendon	

Krahl,[220] and Roels[249] have suggested the categorization of jumper's knee into different stages, based on the prevalence of the main clinical symptoms — pain and loss of function in the extremity (Table 8.6). This categorization is, however, based on subjective evaluation and as such does not represent a sure base on which a definite decision regarding the type and method of therapy to be employed can be made.

Radiographic analysis of patients suffering from jumper's knee can reveal bony changes on the poles of the patella and the tibial tuberosity, as well as ossification in the tendon structure[203] (Figure 8.13). The range of possible pathological changes seen in radiographic analysis is described by Blazina et al.[169] and Kelly et al.[216] (Table 8.7). The most characteristic radiological indications of jumper's knee are elongation of the poles of the patella,[202] irregular centers of ossification seen in the patellas of adolescents, stress fractures of the lower patellar pole, and a marked spiking of the anterior surface of the patella. Elongation of the lower pole of the patella is referred to as the "beak" of the patella, and the spiky anterior surface of the patella, which can be seen in axial radiographic pictures, is called the *tooth sign*.[200]

Scintigraphic analysis of patients suffering from jumper's knee can reveal pathological changes at the insertion sites of the tendon into the bone, in which there exists increased vascularization and an accumulation of radionuclides.[213] This accumulation of radionuclides is not, however, unique in jumper's knee, a fact that should be kept in mind when interpreting the results of the scintigraphic analysis. In the study of Green et al.[199] on 34 patients with intractable symptoms of patellar tendinitis, bone scintigraphy showed 71% of patients to have abnormalities on the delayed images, 8 with diffusely increased activity in the patella and 16 with increased activity localized to the lower pole.

There have been reports in the medical literature about the use of CT with the aim of achieving an objective diagnosis of jumper's knee.[226,229,231] King et al.[219] reported that by using this method,

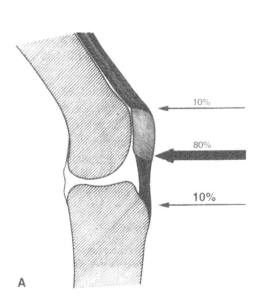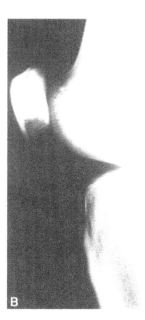

FIGURE 8.13 (A) Distribution of the pain and tenderness localization in patients with patellar tendonitis (jumper's knee); (B) changes (radiolucency) of the lower pole of the patella in patellar tendonitis (jumper's knee).

TABLE 8.7
Radiological Signs of the Patellar Tendinitis

	Ref.
1. Radiolucency at the involved pole	77
2. Irregular centers of ossification	
3. Periosteal reaction at the anterior surface	
4. Elongation of the involved pole with an occasional fracture at the junction of the elongation with the main portion of the patella	
5. Stress fracture of the inferior pole of the patella	
6. Calcification of the involved tendon	
1. Calcification in the quadriceps tendon	106
2. Elongation of the proximal pole of the patella	
3. Tooth sign (anterior surface of the patella)	
4. Elongation of the distal pole of the patella	
5. Calcification in the patellar tendon	
6. Osteophytes in the area of the tibial tubercule	

---

they were able to see pathological changes of the real tendon structure such as localized thickening of the tendon and the presence of cystic cavities within the tendon.

The diagnosis of jumper's knee is facilitated by the use of ultrasound examination of the quadriceps tendon and the patellar ligament.[177–179,180,193–195,204,209,210,212,223,232,245,248,262,265] Fritschy et al.[196] have used ultrasound examination to analyze the patellar ligament of patients in whom jumper's knee was clinically diagnosed. They note that in the beginning stages of this syndrome, there is swelling of the tendon, usually found in the area of the proximal insertion site of the patellar tendon. The later stages in the tendon take the form of a heterogeneous tendon structure

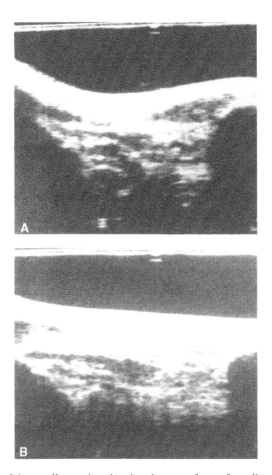

FIGURE 8.14 Sonogram of the patellar tendon showing the acute form of patellar tendinitis (jumper's knee). (A) Relaxation; (B) contraction.

accompanied by an unclear definition of the tendon sheath. Concomitant ultrasound examination of the knee patellar bursae, which are clearly defined using this technique, is also performed. Ultrasound examination also enables examination of the tendon structure during contraction of the muscle, which allows dynamic examination of the knee extensor system.[196] The thickening of the tendon in the area of its insertion, which remains present during muscle contraction, is called a *vacuola* and is a characteristic sign of the acute stage of jumper's knee (Figure 8.14). According to Kalebo et al.,[212] a cone-shaped poorly echogenic area exceeding 0.5 cm in length in the center of the patellar tendon in combination with its localized thickening has proved to be a reliable indicator of jumper's knee. In the tendon, hematoma, degenerative changes, and the beginnings of ossification (Figure 8.15) can be seen. At this stage of the disease, these changes are not visible by radiographic examination. For a detailed analysis of the extensor system of the knee, a comprehensive knowledge of the clinical picture and the anatomy of the afflicted area is mandatory. Fritschy et al.[196] and Jerosch et al.[210] have recommended an ultrasound classification of jumper's knee with the aim of facilitating diagnosis and making it more objective and reproducible (Table 8.8). Mahlfeld et al.[228] analyzed the sonograms of 87 patients with jumper's knee and concluded that visualization of pathological findings of the patellar tendon, such as focal or generalized thickenings, calcifications, and partial or total ruptures, was possible with ultrasound. They could classify six different sonopathological stages of the jumper's knee syndrome. Ultrasound diagnostics is becoming an important and invaluable tool in diagnosing jumper's knee because it is noninvasive, inexpensive, safe, and has a wide range of application.[223] However, according to Cook et al.[177–179]

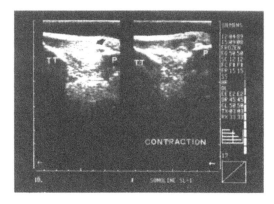

FIGURE 8.15 Sonogram of the patellar tendon showing chronic form of patellar tendinitis (jumper's knee). P = patella; TT = tibial tubercle.

TABLE 8.8
Ultrasound Classification of the Patellar Tendinitis

		Ref.
1. Pure inflammatory stage	Initial stage characterized by edema of the tendon fibers; tendon is swollen and thickened but still presents a homogeneous appearance	196
2. Stage with irreversible anatomical lesions	Tendon has a heterogeneous appearance; there are hypoechoic and hyperechoic images with or without edema; tendinous envelope is more or less well defined but may have a variable appearance	
3. Final stage of lesion	Tendinous envelope is irregular and thickened and the tendon fibers appear heterogeneous, but the swelling has disappeared	
Stage 1: Normal tendon		210
Stage 2: Edema of the tendon at the distal patellar pole		
Stage 3: Edema of the whole tendon; normal echogenicity; tendon sheath smooth		
Stage 4: a. Edema of the whole tendon; hyperechogenicity; tendon sheath smooth		
b. Edema of the whole tendon; hyperechogenicity; irregular tendon sheath		
Stage 5: Rupture of the tendon		

there is no statistically significant relationship between ultrasonographic patellar tendon abnormalities and clinical outcome in elite male athletes. In our study in a group of 61 athletes with a clinical diagnosis of jumper's knee, radiographic findings confirmed diagnosis in 13.1% of patients and ultrasound examination confirmed the clinical diagnosis in 90.2% of patients.[245] Management of jumper's knee should not be solely based on ultrasonographic appearance, clinical assessment remains the cornerstone of appropriate management.

Diagnosis of overuse injury of the knee extensor system can also be achieved by thermography.[238] Thermographic analysis distinguishes the temperature difference between the affected and healthy part of the knee (see Figure 1.19 in Chapter 1). This enables the physician to evaluate the severity of the symptoms and also affords the opportunity to monitor the course and success of the prescribed treatment.

To date, there have been a number of reports concerning the success of MR imaging diagnostics of jumper's knee.[171,186,214,230,243,246,256,275] Bodne et al.[171] claim that they are able to differentiate pathological changes, both in the bony and tendinous part of the knee extensor system, by using this diagnostic method. They feel that based on these results they are better able to objectively prescribe the most suitable therapy. In the study of Shalaby and Almekinders,[256] only Blazina stage 3 lesions were associated with abnormal findings on MR images. In younger patients with relatively mild symptoms, MR imaging did not show significant changes; in older, active patients changes may be present in asymptomatic knees. Yu et al.[275] concluded that in athletes with chronic patellar tendinitis areas of abnormal signal intensity on MR imaging corresponded to degenerative patho-logical changes consistent with angioblastic tendinosis. In nearly all patients, the tendon thickening occurred eccentrically. Disproportionate medial tendon thickening may be related to unequal tensile forces across the knee joint, resulting in greater stress on the medial portion of the extensor mechanism of the knee. Patellar tendinitis demonstrates a consistent spectrum of changes at MR imaging that can aid understanding of the origin and treatment of damage.[230]

Davies et al.[181] describe the ultrasound, CT, and MR imaging findings in 16 cases of patellar tendinitis. In all cases tendon enlargement and reduced echogenicity were visible on ultrasound. CT demonstrated enlargement of the tendon with reduced attenuation of the central portion. MR imaging showed focal tendon enlargement in all patients with high-signal lesions in 88% of cases. This study has shown that patellar tendinitis may be identified with all three modalities. Ultrasound is recommended as the initial investigation in the assessment of patients with this condition.

C. TREATMENT

The basic principles of treating jumper's knee consist of reducing the local inflammatory process, encouraging and facilitating tissue healing, and completely rehabilitating the afflicted extremity with the aim of returning the athlete as soon as possible to normal athletic activities.[168,173] In acute stages of the disease, the physician generally recommends cessation of sporting activities that place strain on the afflicted extremity. In the first 72 h after injury, cryotherapy is applied, along with a compressive bandage, and the afflicted extremity is placed in an elevated position. The inflammatory process facilitates healing during the first 3 days. This time interval is therefore the optimal time span during which the inflammatory process should be cured.

Inflammatory edemas, which last for longer periods of time, cause hypoxic changes, diminish tissue vascularity, lower the local pH, and lead to damage of the surrounding healthy tissue. It is believed that application of cryotherapy reduces the inflammation by diminishing the edema and hematoma and eliminating pain. There are many different methods of applying cryotherapy. The safest and most effective method is crushed ice in a damp towel. However, ice-cold bandages, ice massage of the involved area, immersion in ice water, and application of ethyl chloride are also very effective. Ice should be applied for a limited time (less than 20 min) and repeated every 1 to 2 h in acute cases because continuous treatment may damage the surface tissue and result in unwanted consequences.

We have mentioned both the importance of the inflammatory reaction in initiating healing and the desirability of limiting this reaction if it is prolonged more than necessary. Oral nonsteroidal anti-inflammatory drugs are prescribed to decrease inflammation. Although local application of corticosteroids combined with prolonged-effect anesthetics is also recommended in the treatment of overuse syndrome of the soft tissues of the locomotor system, it is counterproductive when treating jumper's knee syndrome. Corticosteroids are not recommended because of the increased risk of total rupture of the patellar tendon. After the initial treatment to quickly soothe the inflam-mation, on the fourth day heat therapy or contrast heat–cold therapy, in a ratio of 3:1 or 1:1, is applied to the knee. Heating facilitates vascularization and increases the speed of the healing process. The heating effect is produced by different methods, including the application of ointments, ultrasound, laser, electric stimulation, and many others. When inflammation and pain have been reduced, a rehabilitation program is introduced. The program consists of stretching exercises and strengthening of the extensor muscle system of the knee. Smith et al.[259] stress the importance of stretching exercises and the increased flexibility of the posterior area of the upper leg in successful non-operative treatment. Apple[167] presents a detailed description of a stretching exercise program for gradual strengthening of the afflicted limb. Exercises are conducted in such a fashion that the patient repeatedly performs one exercise (150 to 300 times), but with very light weights (1 to 5 kg). This promotes vascularization and the healing process and does not damage the tissue any further. The exercise program is called Progressive Resistance Exercise (PRE) and is characterized by fully extending the lower extremity in an elevated position, while burdened with a light weight (straight leg raising technique). There is also another approach to the strengthening of the extensor system of the knee joint — concentric and eccentric exercises.[208,209] When performing concentric contraction of the quadriceps femoris muscle, the force performed is antiparallel to the ground force, and the muscle fibers contract. This causes the muscle tissue to strengthen. An example of these exercises is when the body, appropriately loaded, is lifted from a semisquatting position to a standing position. Eccentric contraction, on the other hand, causes the extension of the muscle fibers as the force is parallel to the ground force. An example of this is when the body slowly descends from a standing to a semisquatting position. Apple[167] and Jensen and Di Fabrio[208] reported that eccentric exercises cause the greatest stress to the tendon tissue, thus preparing it to withstand further heavy mechanical loads. They concluded that eccentric exercise may be an effective treatment for patellar tendinitis, but that knee pain may limit optimal gains in strength. Proprioceptive exercises (balance board) are included, depending on the progress of the rehabilitation program. These exercises stimulate the interaction of the nervous system, sensory receptors, muscles, tendons, and ligaments.[168] Wearing a patellar brace knee strap (Figure 8.16) is also highly recommended.[261]

To conclude the description of non-operative treatment for jumper's knee, we must point out the importance of alternative training constantly performed during the treatment. Alternative training consists of workouts for uninjured body parts and is critical to maintain cardiovascular abilities, stamina, and fitness of the body. The exercises include swimming, strengthening, and increasing the flexibility of the upper body. Non-operative treatment of jumper's knee syndrome calls for persistence and commitment and is performed for several months.

Although tendinitis of the knee is relatively easy to diagnose, its treatment is more difficult.[182] Of the numerous treatments available, specific physiotherapy and correction of technical errors are often efficient.

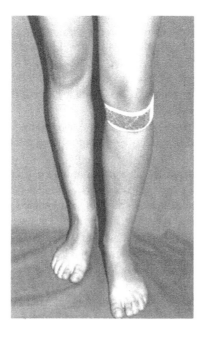

FIGURE 8.16 Knee strap.

Surgical treatment is indicated only if a prolonged and well-supervised conservative treatment program fails.[176,215] Surgical treatment is needed in cases of irreversible pathological changes of the knee extensor system appearing in the later stages of patellar tendinitis/tendinosis, but also in cases of total rupture of the quadriceps tendon and the patellar tendon. The general principle of surgical treatment consists of removing the devitalized tissue, initiating the healing process, and correcting the wrongly oriented knee extensor system. Surgical excision of irreversible lesions, demonstrated on ultrasonography, is a logical procedure, which provides good results.[197] Patients encouraged to undergo surgery are usually highly motivated professional top athletes who will not give up their athletic careers.

There are numerous different operative approaches. One is reported by Smillie and consists of drilling the affected patellar apex to improve vascularization and healing of the damaged area.[237] Basset describes excision of the degenerate part of the patella tendon, followed by restoration of the defect.[237] Blazina[169] outlines an operative technique involving resection of the affected patellar apex (apicotomy), patellar inspection, relegation of the patellar tendon, and retinacular strengthening. Ferretti et al.[190] suggest the following operative procedure based on their own experience: releasing the deep tendon fibers, drilling and "cleansing" the tendon insertion, and scarifying and excising the degenerate tendon tissue. According to Martens et al.[229] surgery directed at the tendon, rather than a bony procedure, yielded favorable results in 27 of 29 patients.

It is necessary to reorient the knee extensor system (if it is incorrectly oriented) by proximal realignment, lateral retinacular release, and advancement of the vastus medialis obliques muscle. According to Whitaker,[236] total disjunction of the quadriceps tendon and patellar tendon is treated surgically by nonresorptive tendon stitches, taking care to adequately correct the proximodistal position of the patella. Shelbourne[257] uses the resection of the middle third of the patellar ligament with a small piece of bone on the apex of the patella; this is similar to the method of ACL reconstruction (bone–tendon–bone graft).

Verheyden et al.[269] present the clinical results of 31 knees in 29 patients treated surgically for patellar tendinitis. A longitudinal strip of patellar tendon containing the pathological tissue was resected in all cases without bony procedure. Minimum follow-up time was 3 years. The results were very good in 26 knees, good in 1 knee, and poor in 4 knees. Persistent patellofemoral pain was considered the most important cause leading to a poor result. When patellofemoral pain due to maltracking is associated with patellar tendinitis, it seems logical that both pathologies should be addressed during surgical treatment. Griffiths and Selesnick[201] recommend operative intervention in patients with chronic patellar tendinitis who do not improve with well-supervised, comprehensive conservative treatment.

Maffulli et al.[227] report the results of surgery in 28 patients reviewed at an average follow-up of 42 months from surgery for tendinopathy of the main body of the patellar tendon after failed conservative treatment. Intervention consists of exploration of the affected patellar tendon, stripping of the paratendon, excision of pathological areas, and multiple longitudinal tenotomies. At follow-up, 23 patients were completely free of pain and had resumed full sporting activity at the same preoperative level. In fact, 3 patients were improved enough to have returned to their preoperative sporting level or just below it. In 2 patients, the initial operation failed. In the patients who resumed sport, the average time from surgery to resuming full sporting activity was 7 months (range 6 weeks to 12 months).

Romeo and Larson[250] describe the technique and two case reports of the arthroscopic treatment of infrapatellar tendonitis. A routine arthroscopic examination of the knee is conducted and soft tissue is debrided from the retropatellar tendon surface for direct visualization of the patellar tendon as it inserts on the inferior pole of the patella. An 18-gauge needle is advanced through the site of maximum discomfort as defined clinically and supported by ultrasound and MR imaging studies. The tip of the needle is visualized arthroscopically to define the proper position of the direct inferior patellar portal. The portal is made in a position that will allow advancement of the shaver perpendicular to the inferior pole of the patella. The shaver is placed into direct inferior patellar portal and the cutting surface of the blade is oriented toward the inferior pole of the patella. The shaver is then slowly advanced out of the knee joint, removing the soft tissue attachment at the inferior pole of the patella. An area of approximately 8 to 10 mm is resected. At the completion of the procedure, the patient is placed into a soft dressing without immobilization.

Coleman et al.[174] compared the outcomes in 25 subjects (29 tendons) who had had open patellar tenotomy and 23 subjects (25 tendons) who had had arthroscopic patellar tenotomy at a mean follow-up of 3.8 and 4.3 years, respectively. During the arthroscopic patellar tenotomy after the diagnostic procedure, the arthroscope was transferred to a superolateral portal and the power shaver was introduced through the anterolateral portal. Part of the infrapatellar fat pad was excised to reveal normal patellar tendon fibers that were then traced proximally to locate the abnormal disorganized area of tendinosis. All macroscopically abnormal tissue was debrided. No bone procedure was performed. At follow-up, outcomes in the open and arthroscopic groups were as follows: (1) symptomatic benefit was seen in 81% of open and 96% of arthroscopic tenotomy patients, (2) sporting success was seen in 54% of open and 46% of arthroscopic tenotomy patients, (3) median time to return to preinjury level of activity was 10 months for open and 6 months for arthroscopic tenotomy patients, and (4) median Victorian Institute of Sport Assessment score at follow-up was 88 for open and 77 for arthroscopic tenotomy patients. Both procedures provided virtually all subjects with symptomatic benefit, but only about half the subjects who underwent either open or arthroscopic patellar tenotomy were competing at their former sporting level at follow-up.

The method of surgical intervention we use is determined individually, taking into consideration the localization of the pain, knee extensor mechanism alignment, ultrasound, MR imaging, and arthroscopic intraoperative findings. In the past, when the pain was localized at the inferior pole of the patella, the resection of the nonarticular part of the apex (open apicotomy) was made without further reinforcement of the ligament fibers (Figure 8.17). On resection (always by saw), we proceeded with the drilling of the subcortical pole of the patella, depending on the changes of the patellar cartilage. In cases in which the pain is localized at the superior pole of the patella, multiple drilling of the affected pole combined with the excision of the degenerated tendon tissue and sometimes a lateral retinacular release is performed. When extensor mechanism malalignment is

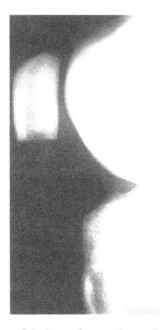

FIGURE 8.17 Lateral roentgenogram of the knee after patellar tendinitis surgery (open apicotomy).

evident, the proximal (lateral retinacular release and vastus medialis obligmus (VMO) advancement) or distal realignment (anterior and medial displacement of the tibial tuberosity) of the patella is attempted. If degenerative changes of the tendon are diagnosed by ultrasonography or during surgery, the altered part is excised completely. In cases where a totally enlarged and edematose patellar ligament is discovered, we use the method of longitudinal incision, i.e., decompression of the patellar ligament. If cartilage of the patella is changed, the damaged area of cartilage is shaved; when necessary, additional surgical procedures are attempted. Thus, in the case of a patient with obvious dysplasia of the patella, we effect longitudinal osteotomy of the patella.

Postoperatively, when apical osteotomy is performed, we do not permit any active extension of the knee during the first 6 weeks following surgery. At 3 months after surgery, the patient starts with gradual sports training; full sports activity is allowed 6 to 9 months after surgery. The ability of the athlete to return to sports varies considerably. We analyzed the results of such complex treatments on 15 top-level athletes surgically treated in our department from 1983 to 1989 for third stage jumper's knee.[121] The postoperative results were graded according to Ferretti et al.[188] criteria: 11 patients' results were very good, 3 good, and 1 poor, on an average follow-up time of 35 months (12 to 81 months).

Since 1989, we have preferred the surgical procedure known as arthroscopically assisted apicotomy of the patella or the so-called half-open method of arthroscopically assisted apicotomy of the patella. The procedure involves removal of the tip of the patella similar to the Kenneth Jones method of loose transplantation taken for the reconstruction of the ACL (Figure 8.18). From 1989 to 1997, 36 patients were surgically treated and we present the results of this treatment with a postoperative follow-up period from 1 to 8 years (mean of 4.7 years). Among the athletes, 11 were basketball players, 5 were soccer players, 4 track-and-field athletes, 4 handball players, 2 volleyball players, and 1 hockey player; 6 dancers, 2 soldiers, and 1 policeman complete the group. Postoperative results were classified as very good if the athlete returned to sports activity without any side effects, good if the athlete resumed his or her sports activities with painful sensations present only at maximum levels of physical exertion, and poor if any reduction of athletic activity was present. On the basis of this evaluation scale very good results were achieved in 21 patients, good

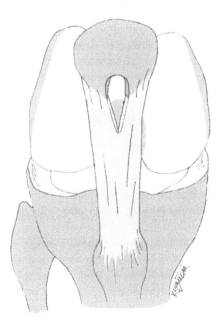

FIGURE 8.18 The half-open method of arthroscopically assisted apicotomy of the patella and excision of degenerated tissue from patellar tendon.

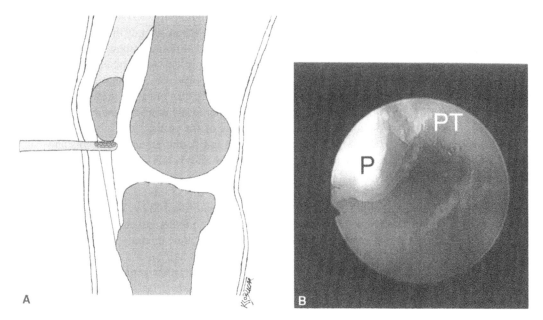

FIGURE 8.19 (A) Schematic representation of full arthroscopic technique of patellar apicotomy. (B) Arthroscopic view after abrasion of the nonarticular part of the patellar apex (P) and debridement of patellar tendon (PT).

results in 12, and poor results in 3 patients. Since 1999, our surgical treatment of jumper's knee has been a modified full arthroscopic technique described by Romeo and Larson[250] with abrasion of the non-articular part of the apex of the patella (Figure 8.19). Early results with this technique are encouraging.

The results of surgical treatment of jumper's knee are more than satisfactory,[237,238] and we conclude that surgical treatment of jumper's knee should not be unnecessarily postponed, as over 90% of the our analyzed samples show good results after surgery, which enabled the athletes to return to their athletic or professional activities. Nevertheless, let us not forget that the fundamental strategy is concentrating on intensive non-operative treatment. Stretching exercises are important as an overuse preventive measure. Surgical intervention is always the last choice of treatment.

IV. ILIOTIBIAL BAND FRICTION SYNDROME

Iliotibial band friction syndrome (ITBFS) results from activity comprising many repetitive flexion and extension movements of the knee, during which rubbing of the band against the lateral femoral epicondyle occurs; this produces irritation and inflammatory reactions within the iliotibial band or the underlying bursa. ITBFS is one of the most common overuse injuries in runners, not only professional athletes, but also in recreational joggers and in other athletes whose activities entail a lot of running.

Staff and Nilsson[317] were among the first to describe the symptoms of ITBFS in their paper published in 1971. The term *iliotibial band friction syndrome* was introduced by Renne in 1975.[314] Orava[309] diagnosed ITBFS in 6.4% of 1311 athletes with overuse injuries. Sutker et al.[318] found a 4.7% frequency of ITBFS in 4173 injured runners, as well as a higher incidence of ITBFS in long-distance runners than in middle-distance runners and sprinters. In a retrospective case-control analysis of 2002 running injuries, patellofemoral pain syndrome was the most common injury followed by ITBFS, plantar fasciitis, meniscal injuries of the knee, and tibial stress syndrome.[320] Jordaan and Schwellnus[289] have undertaken a study to document the incidence of overuse injuries sustained during basic military training. The highest incidence (injuries/1000 training hours) of specific overuse injuries were tibial bone stress reaction (0.33), patellofemoral pain (0.22), and ITBFS (0.08). The exact incidence of the syndrome has been estimated to range from 1.6 to 52.0% depending on the population studied.[291] In a series of 200 knee injuries in long-distance runners, Noble[307,308] found that 52% of the injuries were secondary to ITBFS. ITBFS is not unique to distance runners; it has been reported in cyclists, football players, skiers, hammer throwers, racket sports participants, and ballet dancers.[286,292,298,301,309,311–313,315,322]

A. ETIOPATHOGENESIS

The iliotibial band or tract is a thickened band of fascia extending from the iliac crest down the lateral side of the thigh to its attachment on the lateral tibial condyle (Gerdy's tubercle).[290,321] At the level of the greater trochanter, the iliotibial band receives the insertions of the tensor fasciae latae muscle anteriorly and superficial tendinous layer of the gluteus maximus muscle posteriorly. It then attaches to the linea aspera of the femur through the lateral intermuscular septum, while its distal segment moves freely over the lateral femoral condyle. With the knee in the extended position, the iliotibial band lies anterior to the lateral femoral epicondyle; in knee flexion of 30° it lies behind the lateral femoral epicondyle (Figure 8.20A). According to Orchard et al.[310] friction (or impingement) occurs near footstrike, predominantly in the foot contact phase at or slightly below 30° of flexion, between the posterior edge of the iliotibial band and the underlying lateral femoral epicondyle. Because of its mobility, activities entailing many repetitive flexion and extension movements of the knee cause the band to rub against the lateral femoral epicondyle. This produces irritation and subsequent inflammatory reactions within the iliotibial band or formation of underlying bursae and secondary inflammation.

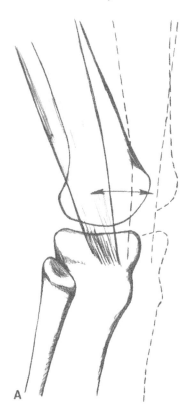
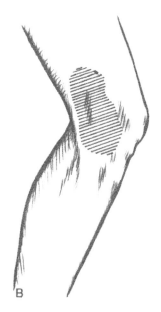

FIGURE 8.20 Iliotibial band friction syndrome. (A) Mechanism of development; (B) area of pain.

TABLE 8.9
Predisposing Factors Leading to Overuse Injuries of the Musculoskeletal System in Runners

Training Errors
Abrupt changes in intensity, duration, and/or frequency of training
Poorly trained and unskilled athlete

Muscle-Tendon Imbalance of
Flexibility
Strength

Anatomical Malalignment
Leg-length discrepancy
Excessive femoral anteversion
Knee alignment abnormalities (genu valgum, varum, or recurvatum)
Position of the patella (patella alta or infera)
Excessive Q angle
Excessive external tibial rotation
Flat foot

Footwear
Inappropriate running shoes
Worn-out running shoes

Surface
Hard
Uneven

Other
Growth
Disturbances of the menstrual cycle

The etiology of ITBFS, similar to other overuse injuries, is a multifactorial process, i.e., there are many interacting agents that contribute to the development of ITBFS (Table 8.9). Most commonly, the ITBFS is a result of training errors and anatomical malalignment of the lower extremity.[277,279,303] According to Taunton et al.,[319] training errors and abrupt changes in intensity, duration, and/or frequency of training cause ITBFS in 42%, and according to Grana and Coniglione,[284] in 35%. Malalignment conditions of forefoot varus and/or subtalar varus, tibia vara, and genu varum lead to excessive and/or prolonged forefoot pronation during the support phase of a running cycle; this, as research results show, seems to cause ITBFS in more than 50% of cases.[280,288,293,300,302,318,319] During forefoot pronation, the tibia rotates inwardly. In the case of excessive and/or prolonged forefoot pronation, an excessive and prolonged internal rotation of the tibia occurs, producing excessive irritation to the iliotibial band. Other predisposing factors to ITBFS have been cited: poor iliotibial band flexibility, leg length discrepancies, increased prominence of the lateral femoral epicondyle, hard and/or uneven running surface, and inadequate workout running shoes.[277,301,307,308,317,318]

B. CLINICAL PICTURE AND DIAGNOSTICS

The patient with ITBFS experiences pain at the lateral side of the knee. Pain is stinging in nature, and is located at the lateral femoral condyle 2 cm above the joint line. In some cases, however, the pain may radiate downward along the iliotibial band, or upward along the lateral side of the thigh. As with other overuse injuries, there is characteristic onset and progression of symptoms. Initially, the pain appears immediately after engagement in activity necessitating repetitive flexion and

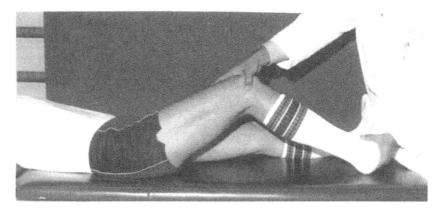

FIGURE 8.21 Provocation of pain in ITBFS (Noble's test).

extension movements of the knee (i.e., after running, bicycle riding, skiing) and usually disappears following a few hours of rest. The next phase is characterized by pain at the very beginning of the activity, its disappearance after warming up, and appearance again on completion of the activity. It is common that the athletes do not seek medical attention in that time, but rather continue their activity at an unchanged intensity. This results in progressive development of the syndrome so that the pain appearing at the beginning of activity persists throughout the activity and intensifies on completion. In the final stage, the pain impairs even normal walking.

Lindenberg et al.[294] have proposed the following classification of injury grade according to symptoms in ITBFS:

Grade 1: Pain comes on after the run but does not restrict distance or speed.
Grade 2: Pain comes on during the run but does not restrict distance or speed.
Grade 3: Pain comes on during the run and restricts distance or speed.
Grade 4: Pain is so severe that it prevents running.

The clinical history data are of great importance in the diagnosis of ITBFS, especially those concerned with the initiation of pain either during or after athletic activity consisting of many flexion and extension movements of the knee without previous knee injury, and disappearance of the pain during walking with a stiff knee in extension.

The most frequent sign is tenderness over the lateral femoral epicondyle of the injured leg (Figure 8.20B). Various provocative tests for ITBFS have been described. In the Renne test, pain is provoked by having the patient support all of the weight on the affected leg with the knee in 30° or 40° flexion.[314] A compression test was described by Noble in 1979.[307] In this test, the patient lies in a supine position and the knee is flexed to 90°. The examiner holds the ankle of the affected leg in one hand and presses on the lateral epicondyle with the thumb of the other hand. While maintaining constant pressure, the examiner slowly extends the leg (Figure 8.21). Pain appears when the knee is flexed to 30°, and the patient usually reports that it is the kind of pain experienced when running. The test modification according to Pećina consists of putting the lower leg in varus position when performing extension.[311]

In clinical examination, Ober's test is used to diagnose flexibility of the iliotibial band (Figure 8.22). During the test, the patient lies on the uninjured side with that hip flexed to obliterate any lumbar lordosis. The affected knee is then flexed to 90°, and the leg is held with one hand, while the pelvis is stabilized with the other. The hip is then passively abducted and extended so that the thigh is in line with the body and will catch the iliotibial band on the greater trochanter, maximizing its excursion. The leg is brought toward the table in adduction, and if iliotibial band shortening is present, the knee cannot reach the table. According to many reports and on the basis of our own

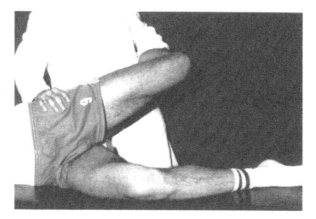

FIGURE 8.22 Ober's test; used for assessing the flexibility of the iliotibial band.

experience, in practically all patients with ITBFS, tightness of the iliotibial band takes place, although in varying degrees.[277,294,299,301,308,309,317,318] All patients exhibit normal range of motion of the affected knee; in some, during extension and flexion movements of the knee and simultaneous pressure on the lateral condyle, excursion of the band over the lateral femoral epicondyle may be felt and sometimes even heard.

Bonaldi et al.[278] describe sonographic findings in ITBFS, and Ekman et al.,[282] Nishimura et al.,[306] and Muhle et al.[304] present MR findings in ITBFS. According to Nishimura et al.[306] MR signal alteration predominant in the region beneath the posterior fibers of the iliotibial band supports the current opinion that the posterior fibers of the iliotibial band are tighter against the lateral femoral epicondyle than the anterior fibers. MR imaging accurately depicts the compartment-like distribution of signal intensity abnormalities in patients with ITBFS.[304]

As part of the differential diagnosis, other injuries of the knee joint and its structures should be taken into consideration, especially those primarily manifested by pain at the lateral side of the knee. These are popliteal tendinitis, rupture of the lateral knee joint capsule and/or lateral meniscus, meniscal degeneration, cyst of the lateral meniscus, lesion of the lateral collateral ligament, patellar chondromalacia, lateral patellar compression syndrome, patellar subluxation and/or dislocation, and arthritic changes of the knee joint. However, most often the differential diagnosis should be made between the ITBFS and popliteal tendinitis.[277,288,292]

C. TREATMENT

The treatment of ITBFS is usually non-operative, although in some cases surgery may be required.

1. Non-Operative Treatment

Based on the most recent knowledge regarding the etiology of overuse injury syndromes and evaluation of the applied treatment, a program of non-operative treatment of ITBFS has been conceived as follows:

- Short-term cessation or modification of athletic activities
- Iliotibial band stretching exercises
- Ice massage of the painful area
- Analgesics/nonsteroidal anti-inflammatory drugs
- Correction of predisposing factors — training errors, anatomical malalignment of the lower extremity, running shoes, etc.

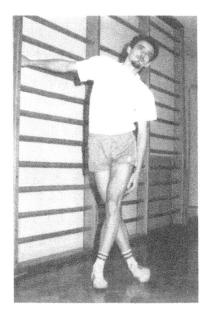 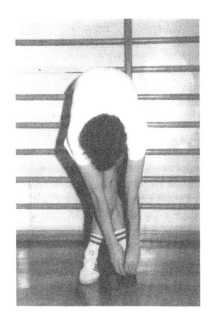

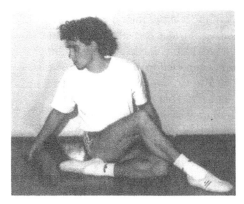 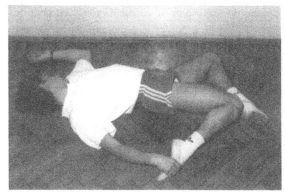

FIGURE 8.23 Stretching exercises for the iliotibial band.

Some authors[276,305,314,317] suggest complete rest from athletic activities for 3 weeks; others[277,284,288,294,301,307,309,311,318] consider the period of rest to be from 1 week to 2 months, depending on the severity of the condition. Our experience has shown that in the initial stages (grades 1 and 2), it is not necessary to completely refrain from athletic activities but that, in addition to other non-operative treatment methods, it is sufficient to decrease training intensity, especially painful activities, e.g., running. In more advanced cases (grades 3 and 4), complete rest from athletic activities is needed for 3 to 4 weeks. Only alternative training activities are allowed to maintain functional abilities of the athlete — pool running and treading water in the deep end of the pool with or without a flotation device.

Stretching exercises, especially passive or static exercises, are the basis of ITBFS treatment (Figure 8.23). Passive stretching exercises necessitate a strictly defined position for each exercise to be performed, slow movement until the sensation of stretching appears, and maintenance of the position for a given period of time. In doing these exercises, the idea of "no pain, no gain" should be disregarded. Prolonged stretching in a painful position decreases the possibility of longer maintenance of stretching, increases the possibility of reflex muscle contraction, and may sometimes cause damage of these muscles. On the other hand, remaining at the point of "initial" stretching enables complete relaxation of these muscles and maintenance of the position for a longer period of time. The athlete who is beginning to do the stretching exercises should keep stretching at the point of initial stretching for 15 s, gradually increasing the time to a maximum of 25 s. According to the clinical trial of Schwellnus et al.,[316] physiotherapy in combination with analgesic/anti-inflammatory medication is effective early treatment of ITBFS.

In both treatment and prevention of ITBFS, identifying and correcting predisposing factors play a significant role. It should be pointed out again that the most common predisposing factors to ITBFS are the following: excessive and/or prolonged pronation of the foot during running, training errors, genu varum, excessive tightness of iliotibial band, and uneven and hard running surfaces. Although infiltration of steroids combined with local anesthetic into the site of most intense pain is recommended as a method of choice by some authors,[297,307,318] it is our opinion that this method should be utilized only in advanced stages. However, it should not be considered as the last resort, but rather as part of a non-operative treatment program. When formation of a bursa has been confirmed, the application of steroid injections is also indicated.

2. Surgical Treatment

Surgery is recommended in resistant cases, i.e., when, following a long-term adequate non-operative treatment, the ITBFS symptoms do not disappear. Only a few authors have reported on surgical treatment for ITBFS: Noble,[307,308] Pećina et al.,[277,311] Firer,[283] Martens et al.,[297] and Drogest et al.[281]

As a method of choice, Noble[307,308] suggests surgery during which a transverse cut is made in the 2-cm-long posterior portion of the iliotibial band at the level of the lateral femoral epicondyle. In this way, a V-shaped defect is obtained, which decreases tension in that part of the iliotibial band, preventing friction between the iliotibial band and lateral femoral epicondyle at knee flexion of 30°. Noble has used this surgical method in five athletes and has reported excellent results. All of the operated patients resumed training activities (running) 2 to 5 weeks following surgery; one patient completed a 32-km race without pain 3 weeks after surgery. This procedure has been effective in James'[287] experience and usually allows a return to running within 4 weeks.

Firer[283] used the same method in 64 athletes. He has also reported excellent results — disappearance of pain during running and the possibility of running an equally long or even longer race than before ITBFS signs appeared. These positive results were observed in 57 (89.5%) operated patients; 3 patients (4.70%) reported temporary difficulties when running; and 4 patients (6.25%) could not continue with athletic activities. Our patients treated by this method (optionally, the underlying bursa is removed) have also shown excellent results.[277,311]

Martens et al.[297] used a similar (modified) method of surgical treatment in 23 athletes and have reported excellent results in 19 regularly followed patients. Surgery was done with the knee held in 60° of flexion and consisted of a limited resection of a small triangular piece at the posterior part of the iliotibial band covering the lateral femoral epicondyle. The resected part concerns the iliotibial band fibers, measuring about 2 cm at the base and 1.5 cm in length toward the top of the triangle.

Drogest et al.[281] present the results of a retrospective study of 45 patients operated on in Trondheim. Of the patients, 22 had excellent results, 16 had good results, 6 had fair results, and 1 patient had a poor result.

V. BREASTSTROKER'S KNEE

In 1974, conducting a survey on the incidence of injuries to various parts of the musculoskeletal system of swimmers, Kennedy and Hawkins[327] noticed that a high percentage of breaststroke swimmers complained of pain in the medial knee. This condition has been termed breaststroker's knee, although further studies by Vizsoly et al.[334] on a population of 391 competitive swimmers showed that breaststroker's knee was diagnosed in 56 of 77 breaststroke swimmers (73%), but also in 153 of 314 (48%) swimmers who used the freestyle, backstroke, or butterfly stroke. Knee pain ranks second to shoulder pain as a common complaint in competitive swimmers.[330]

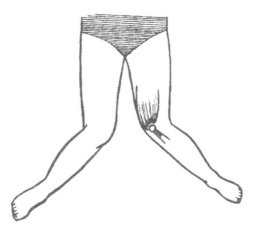

FIGURE 8.24 Biomechanical explanation of the causes leading to the development of the breaststroker's knee.

Kennedy and Hawkins[327] believed that a tibial collateral ligament strain on the proximal femoral origin of the ligament, resulting from repeated stretching of the origin during breaststroke swimming, was the primary disorder leading to breaststroker's knee (Figure 8.24). In their opinion, the stretching of the ligament origin was caused by the extension of the knee during the "whip kick" phase of breaststroke swimming, accompanied by an excessive valgus stress on the knee joint and the outward rotation of the leg in the final phase of the stroke. Stulberg and co-workers[332] reported that, in most cases, the pain was localized in the lower area of the medial facet of the patella. The areas of the medial facet of the patella and the medial collateral ligament were indicated as the areas of greatest tenderness in 25% of the cases.[323] Rovere and Nichols[331] cite inflammation, thickening, and fibrosis of the medial parapatellar plica as potential causes of breaststroke knee pain.

Arthroscopic findings range from localized medial synovitis of the knee[328,335] to generalized synovitis and chondromalacic changes on the medial facet of the patella.[332]

Slow-motion analysis of the mechanics of the breaststroke showed that the primary cause of breaststroker's knee was the incorrect technique used in performing the "whip kick."[324,333] One group of authors believes that breaststroker's knee develops as a consequence of the amount of abduction in the hip joint in the beginning phase of the kick; both insufficient and excessive abduction lead to a strong valgus stress and excessive rotation of the lower leg in the final phase of the kick. Another group of authors is of the opinion that the final phase of the kick, characterized by extension of the lower leg with abducted legs, after which a sudden and strong abduction with excessive outward rotation follows, is the primary cause of breaststroker's knee.

Breaststroker's knee symptoms usually appear after 3 years of competitive breaststroke swimming. In most cases, both knees are affected. In the beginning stages, pain occurs only when performing the breaststroke. The area of greatest tenderness is localized in the proximal origin of the medial collateral ligament. The later phase is characterized by pain in the lower medial patellar facet area; this occurs regardless of swimming and inhibits other athletic and everyday activities, such as walking up steps and rising from a chair.

As with other overuse injuries, the ideal treatment of breaststroker's knee is prevention. Many injuries originate from faulty techniques or mechanisms, and an assessment must be made of the swimming biomechanics of any injured athlete to identify faults that may contribute to injury.[329] According to Jones[325] identifying the mechanism of injury and prescribing appropriate management is not easy unless one has a thorough understanding of proper technique of the four competitive strokes. Abnormal kick mechanics should be corrected as soon as possible. Proper warm-up exercises, local applications of ice, and ultrasound can be helpful. The symptomatic breaststroke swimmer should train infrequently with the "whip kick" and should use other kicks during workouts. In the early stages, stretching exercises of the hamstring muscles and strengthening exercises for the medial vastus muscle should also be performed.[326] In more advanced stages of breaststroker's knee, breaststroke swimming should be stopped. Cryotherapy and nonsteroidal anti-inflammatory drugs can be prescribed. Surgical treatment is rarely indicated.

VI. OSGOOD-SCHLATTER DISEASE

The most often encountered overuse injuries in children and adolescents are the traction apophysitises, among which the most common and best known is Osgood-Schlatter disease,[347,392] that is, traction apophysitis of the tibial tubercle. Often throughout history, the simultaneous discovery of a disorder is described by two independent researchers, resulting in a hyphenated eponym.[398] Such is the case in the observations made by two physicians, Robert Bayley Osgood[402] and Carl Schlatter,[409] concerning overuse injuries of the tibial tubercle in adolescents. This disorder subsequently became known as Osgood-Schlatter disease.

Osgood-Schlatter disease is a traction apophysitis that develops during the adolescent growth spurt, most often at around 11 years of age in girls (because of their earlier bone growth development) and at about 13 years of age in boys.[336,339,352,379–381,386,392,399] It occurs slightly more often in boys; in large series, the ratio is 3:2. Segawa et al.[412] report an active 12-year-old boy with a combination of multiple osteochondroses of bilateral knee joints, including Osgood-Schlatter disease on one knee and Sinding-Larsen-Johansson disease on the other knee.

The clinical picture consists of pain localized to the area of the tibial tubercle. In some cases, the tubercle may be swollen and hypertrophied. Most authors agree that rapid adolescent skeletal growth leads to relative "tightness" of the soft tissues, as skeletal growth is faster than the elongation of the muscle–tendon units. This in turn creates increased tensile forces on the muscles, tendons, and their attachment sites (the apophyses), which cause avulsion fractures of the bony part of the traction apophysis on the tibial tubercle.[345,379,380,392,399,410,414]

Physical examination reveals pain during palpation of the tibial tubercle. Resisted extension of the knee from the 90° flexed position will usually reproduce pain, but resisted straight-leg raising is usually painless. The Ely test, which proves excessive tightness of the quadriceps femoris muscle, is positive in all cases. Radiographic examinations of both knees should always be performed, in both the anterior-posterior (AP) and lateral (LL) projections, to rule out the possibility of tumors, fractures, or infections. The lateral radiograph generally shows the characteristic picture of prominent tibial tubercle with irregularly fragmented ossific nucleus, or a free bony fragment proximal to the tubercle (Figure 8.25).

Non-operative treatment of Osgood-Schlatter disease, as with other traction apophysitises, is based on the same principles that apply to all overuse injuries.[336,339,345,347,348,380,392,415] Today, there is no need, in fact there is no excuse, for total immobilization, or for totally refraining from athletic activities. Corticosteroid injections are not indicated because the condition is not primarily inflammatory and because of their numerous unwanted side effects. Of vital importance is that the physician inform the parents, the coach, and the child athlete of the natural course of Osgood-Schlatter disease. The child, who is an active athlete, should be allowed to continue with normal athletic activities, to the limit that the pain allows it, but the child should also be advised to take up, as secondary athletic activities, other sports that do not cause any discomfort, i.e., swimming. In addition to other non-operative methods of treatment, wearing knee braces is recommended.[379,392] The symptoms of Osgood-Schlatter disease will generally decline and disappear in most patients if non-operative treatment is carried out long enough, especially after bone growth is terminated. Persistent symptoms are followed by development of loose fragments above the tibial tubercle, or within the patellar ligaments. In these cases, the symptoms will disappear only after these fragments are excised.[339,340,355,360,393,401,416,426]

Orava et al.[401] present their experience with surgical treatment of unresolved, painful, late Osgood-Schlatter disease. In 70 operations performed in 67 patients an ossicle under the distal patellar tendon was removed in 62 cases. In 8 cases, excision of the prominent tibial tubercle and

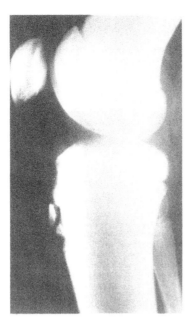

FIGURE 8.25 Roentgenogram of Osgood-Schlatter disease in a young gymnast.

or drilling of the epiphysis was performed. Additional procedures, such as rasping of the uneven anterior tibial surface, excision of inflamed bursa, and the devitalized portion of the tendon, were done in 21 cases. The final results were excellent or good in 56, moderate in 9, poor in 3, and unknown in 2 cases. In our experience in athletes or physically active young people surgical treatment gives good results in chronic unresolved cases.

VII. SINDING-LARSEN-JOHANSSON DISEASE

Sinding-Larsen-Johansson disease is a traction apophysitis of the inferior pole of the patella (in rare cases it affects the superior pole, as well), which is in most respects similar to Osgood-Schlatter disease.[345,389,390,392,399] The coexistence of Osgood-Schlatter disease with Sinding-Larsen-Johansson disease in an adolescent soccer player has been reported.[417] Two cases of osteochondrosis of the superior pole of the patella are reported with histological findings.[418] The histological features of these two cases showed osteonecrosis with reparative changes. These findings support that this entity is similar to other osteochondroses of the quadriceps mechanism: Osgood-Schlatter disease and Sinding-Larsen-Johansson disease. Sinding-Larsen-Johansson disease is more common in boys, generally between the ages of 10 to 15 years, and is characterized by tenderness of the knee and limping.[390] Although it is basically an overuse syndrome, in most cases, some sort of trauma, e.g., falling on the knees, provokes the onset of the disease or intensifies the symptoms in cases in which the disease is already present.

Clinical examination reveals localized tenderness and swelling over the distal pole of the patella. Lateral radiograph reveals delayed ossification of the inferior pole of the patella (Figure 8.26). Barbuti et al.[338] analyzed three patients with Sinding-Larsen-Johansson disease. Ultrasound gave complete information about the involvement of bone, cartilage, and patellar tendon. In these patients the lower pole of the patella appeared irregular, fragmented, with swelling of the cartilage and thickening at the insertion of the patellar tendon. Ultrasonography is also suitable for periodic follow-up of the course of the disease. Treatment is the same as with Osgood-Schlatter disease.[336,390,392]

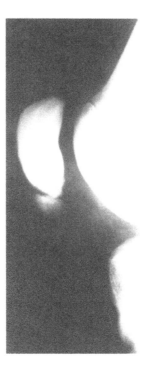

FIGURE 8.26 Roentgenogram of Sinding-Larsen-Johansson disease in a young athlete.

VIII. FAT PAD SYNDROME (HOFFA DISEASE)

Although the etiology of fat pad syndrome (Hoffa disease) is not yet completely understood, most authors believe that the primary cause of fat pad syndrome is repeated traumatization of the infrapatellar fatty pad during activities that require constant repetition of maximal extension in the knee.[342,361,368,381,384,397,411] This disease, first described by Hoffa in 1904, has always been fairly obscure, and it is necessary to distinguish two phases, acute and chronic.[385] Duri et al.[351] conclude that fat pad pathology is usually secondary to other knee joint pathology, and its primary involvement is rare.

Diagnosis is usually made by exclusion because there are no specific symptoms characterizing this disease. Unlike the asymptomatic projecting infrapatellar fatty pad at the patella alta ("camel back sign"), fat pad syndrome is characterized by contact tenderness of the fatty pad, as well as during palpation along the edge of the patellar ligament. Fat pad syndrome is further characterized by the appearance of pain during hyperextension of the knee — in other words, by a positive Smillie's sign (appearance of pain during sudden passive hyperextension of the knee), by the appearance of blockades that are hard to differentiate from meniscal blockades, and by a normal radiograph. According to many authors[337,367,369,394,404,413,420] MR imaging is a useful tool in the study of Hoffa's fat pad, whose local and systematic involvement is an often ignored cause of anterior knee pain. Tang et al.[413] describe the MR appearance of fibrous scars in the infrapatellar fat pad after arthroscopy. Post-traumatic change in Hoffa's fat pad is a constant secondary MR feature that can be added to the spectrum of indirect findings in cases of occult patellar dislocation.[337] It is important to be familiar with the various pathological entities that may occur in the area of the infrapatellar fat pad of Hoffa. Abnormalities that are intrinsic to this fat pad include Hoffa disease, intracapsular chondroma, localized nodular synovitis, postarthroscopy and postsurgery fibrosis, and shear injury. In addition, the infrapatellar fat pad may be involved secondarily from extrinsic processes, including articular disorders (joint effusion, intra-articular bodies, meniscal cyst, ganglion cyst, cyclops lesion), synovial abnormalities (pigmented villonodular synovitis, hemophilia, synovial hemangioma, primary synovial chondromatosis, chondrosarcoma, lipoma arborescens, rheumatoid synovitis associated with primary arthritis), and anterior extracapsular abnormalities.

In most cases, treatment is non-operative; it involves rest, cryotherapy, nonsteroidal anti-inflammatory drugs, and elevation of the heels of the shoes, which reduces, and in some cases, completely disables hyperextension of the knee. In persistent cases, surgical treatment is indicated — resection of the fatty pad.[405] That is, arthroscopic resection of the fat pad is performed, but different fat pad injuries may require an arthroscopic approach different from the classic approaches.[378,385,394,400]

IX. PLICA SYNDROME

Fatty tissue pads located on the anterior wall of the joint capsule of the knee, between the fibrous and synovial membrane, project from the synovial membrane into the cavity of the joint, forming plicae, the so-called plicae synovialis (Figure 8.27). Plicae are some of the normal synovial structures of the knee joint cavity. They are remnants of the mesenchymal tissue that occupies the space between the distal femoral and proximal tibial epiphyses in the 8-week embryo. Incomplete resorption leaves synovial pleats in most of the knee.[350] The infrapatellar plica is the most constant of these plicae. It projects from the infrapatellar fatty pad to the intertrochlear fossa and is also called the *mucosum ligament*. The suprapatellar plica partially divides the suprapatellar recessus from the knee joint and is found in about 60 to 80% of cases reported.[403] The medial plica, which can in some cases be joined to the suprapatellar plica, projects along the anteromedial part of the knee joint to the infrapatellar fatty pad and is found in 18 to 55% of cases reported.[403] The medial plica is present at autopsies in one of every three or four knees.

Arthrography, ultrasonography, CT scan with arthrography, and MR imaging can demonstrate their presence and measure their size with good accuracy.[358,370,396] In the study of Jee et al.[370] whose goal was to evaluate the diagnostic value of MR imaging in plica syndrome, sensitivity and specificity were 73 and 78% on axial multiplanar gradient, axial T1-weighted, and sagittal T2-weighted MR images. Kobayashi et al.[376] consider that direct MR arthrography enables accurate diagnosis of plica synovialis medialis and could replace diagnostic arthroscopy. Kosarek and Helms[377] described the MR appearance of the infrapatellar plica as a low-signal-intensity structure

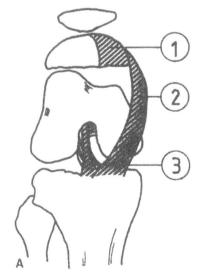
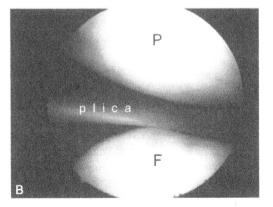

FIGURE 8.27 (A) Schematic representation of plicae synovialis of the knee: (1) suprapatellar; (2) medial; (3) infrapatellar. (B) Arthroscopic view of the symptomatic plica synovialis medialis. P = patella; F = femur.

in the intercondylar notch just anterior to the anterior cruciate ligament. The infrapatellar plica is important to recognize for the following reasons: it can be confused with an intact ACL, it may pose a problem to the arthroscopist when attempting to move instruments from the medial to lateral compartments of the knee; it can block clear visualization of the ACL during arthroscopy; and it can impair retrieval of loose bodies in the intercondylar notch. The infrapatellar plica was found to be thickened and fibrotic and to have lost its normal elasticity. The pathological plica was impinged at the intercondylar notch and trochlea, blocking further extension beyond 25° of knee flexion.[375] Arthroscopy allows a very precise assessment of the plica, including dynamic examination. Arthroscopic findings of the synovial plicae of the knee on 400 knees in 363 patients showed the following incidences: suprapatellar plica, 86.0%; mediopatellar plica, 72.0%; infrapatellar plica, 86.0%; and lateral patellar plica, 1.3%.[374]

The symptoms are, in most cases, caused by a chronically changed (fibrotic, enlarged, and sometimes calcified) medial plica, and only rarely by chronic changes of the suprapatellar plica.[348,363,403,411] While bending the knee, the affected plica strikes the medial facet of the patella; while extending the knee, it is in contact with the anteromedial part of the femoral condyle. Malacia, clinically manifested as chondromalacia, develops at the contact points. Anamnestic data of repeated audible effects described as explosive snaps and occasional blockades help in diagnosing the plica syndrome. The clinical picture mimics a torn medial meniscus or a maltracking patella. Clinical examination is extremely helpful if the snapping plica is palpated at the medial edge of the patella, reproducing the patient's symptoms. Gerbino and Micheli[359] describe a bucket-handle tear of the medial plica in two patients with medial knee pain and pseudolocking. These cases show that a medial plica with a longitudinal split can behave in a manner that can be mistaken for locking. Atraumatic hemarthrosis caused by a large mediopatellar plica has also been described.[429] Clinical examination sometimes reveals the plica during palpation, but in most cases the only symptom is tenderness to palpation of the medial facet of the patella and medial femoral condyle.

Non-operative treatment consisting of rest, use of nonsteroidal anti-inflammatory drugs, stretching exercises for the hamstrings, strengthening exercises for the quadriceps, and wearing of special knee braces, generally produces good results. In resistant cases, surgical treatment is indicated — arthroscopic excision of the plica.[344,348,349,354,363,371,381,403] Arthroscopic excision of a painful medial plica can provide lasting and satisfactory relief of symptoms.[354] Calpur et al.[344] recommend arthroscopic mediopatellar plicaectomy and lateral retinacular release in mechanical patellofemoral disorders.

X. SEMIMEMBRANOSUS TENDINITIS

Semimembranosus tendinitis is not an uncommon entity and is often an overlooked cause of posteromedial knee pain. This entity is usually associated with other knee disorders caused by overuse, mostly chondromalacia of the patella, but may occur as an isolated syndrome. The main symptom is pain located at the very posteromedial corner of the knee just immediately below the joint line.[406] During physical examination, pain is produced by applying pressure to the anterior medial tendon of the semimembranosus muscle, immediately below the knee joint, and at the insertion of the posterior medial tendon on the posterior part of the tibial medial condyle (Figure 8.28). Tenderness is amplified if the knee is in 90° flexion and the lower leg in maximum outward rotation.

Semimembranosus tendinitis is often confused with injury of the medial meniscus. A proper diagnosis is reached by taking a detailed history and by the absence of pain during clinical tests for medial meniscus injuries.[341] Differential diagnosis includes ruling out the possibility of medial collateral ligament bursitis, which is characterized by pain and a slight swelling above the medial collateral ligament immediately below the knee joint.[373] According to Rothstein et al.,[408] semimembranosus-tibial collateral ligament bursitis has a characteristic MR imaging appearance of fluid draped over the semimembranosus tendon in the shape of an inverted U. This entity can clinically

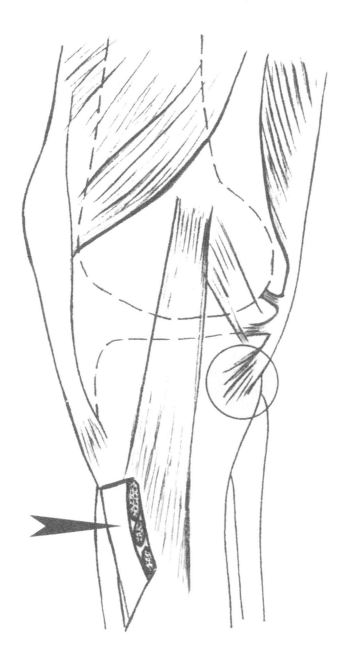

FIGURE 8.28 Insertion of the semimembranosus tendon to the posteromedial aspect of the tibia (circle) and insertion of the sartorius, semitendinosus, and gracilis muscles (pes anserinus) on the medial plane of the tibia (arrowhead).

mimic internal derangement of the knee, typically causing pain more superior and posterior to that of pes anserinus bursitis. MR imaging is useful in diagnosis of semimembranosus-tibial collateral ligament bursitis and avoiding unnecessary knee arthroscopy. The pes anserinus tendons should also be palpated to rule out the possibility of enthesitis of those tendons and, in some cases, the inflammation of the pes anserinus bursae.

In most cases, treatment is non-operative and surgical intervention is rarely indicated. Of 115 patients diagnosed and treated for semimembranosus tendinitis by Ray et al.[406] over a 5-year period,

10 patients were refractory to conservative treatment, and in these 10 patients surgical exploration, drilling of the insertion site, and semitendinosus tendon transfer were performed.

XI. PES ANSERINUS TENDINITIS AND BURSITIS

The tendons of the sartorius, semitendinosus, and gracilis muscles insert on the medial plane of the tibia, just below the condyle, forming the pes anserinus (goose foot) (Figure 8.28). Pes anserinus syndrome is frequently found in long-distance runners. Predisposing factors for the development of this syndrome include incorrect training techniques, excessive tightness of the hamstring muscles, valgus alignment of the knee, and excessive rotation of the lower leg in the outward direction.[361,381,388,397]

Bursitis is more frequent and presents fewer problems, both in diagnosis and treatment. During physical examination, a slight swelling is usually found on the medial side of the knee joint at the level of the tibial tubercle. Ultrasound examination facilitates correct diagnosis of bursitis.[419,421] Pes anserine bursitis has a characteristic MR appearance of fluid beneath the tendons of the pes anserinus at the medial aspect of the tibia near the joint line.[356]

Diagnosing enthesitis presents more problems. In older athletes, medial meniscus injury must be ruled out as must arthrosis of the medial compartment of the knee.[362,372] Pes anserine bursitis can clinically mimic an internal derangement of the knee, which can result in the performance of unnecessary arthroscopy. MR imaging can be useful in diagnosing pes anserine bursitis and obviating surgery. In some cases, scintigraphy is performed to rule out the possibility of stress fractures, which typically appear on the posteromedial part of the proximal tibia.[366]

Treatment is usually non-operative.[361,405] Kang and Han[372] consider that local injection of methylprednisolone plus lidocaine at the anserine bursa is more effective than noninjection therapy.

XII. POPLITEAL TENDINITIS

Popliteal tendinitis is characterized by localized tenderness in the area above the origin of the popliteal muscle on the lateral part of the lateral femoral condyle.[343] Excessive and/or extended pronation of the foot during running is considered to be a predisposing factor in developing this syndrome.[381,414] Popliteal tendinitis is one of the many injuries to the knee joint that is characterized by tenderness in the lateral area of the knee. Meier[391] describes popliteal tenosynovitis in 12 athletes. Werlich[425] presents a case of calcific tendinitis of the popliteal tendon. In the course of treatment the calcium deposit drained spontaneously into the knee joint. Weber et al.[422] present one patient with posterolateral knee pain after a minor contusion. MR imaging revealed a degenerative posterior horn of the lateral meniscus and a somewhat unclear polypoid structure in the intercondylar region. As the posterior component of the pain persisted even after an arthroscopic partial meniscectomy, an operative revision was performed. A small ganglion of the sheath of the popliteal tendon was found and excised. Knee impingement syndromes in terms of the site of symptom onset were classified in a study by Faletti et al.[353] into medial, lateral, anterior, and posterior. Regarding the lateral syndromes, the phlogistic involvement of the distal insertional tract of the broad fascia tensor tendon with bursa reaction is very frequently reported, while the inflammation of the popliteal tendon and the femoral bicipital tendon is less common. To localize the exact area of greatest tenderness, the afflicted leg is placed in the so-called figure four position (Figure 8.29), where the popliteus muscle tendon and the lateral collateral ligament are extended and thus accessible to palpation (Figure 8.30). Pain is produced by applying pressure with a finger to the area of the insertion of the popliteus muscle located slightly anteriorly and distally from the origin of the lateral collateral ligament.

Treatment is usually non-operative and carried out according to the principles set down for treating enthesitis. Surgical treatment is rarely performed.[405]

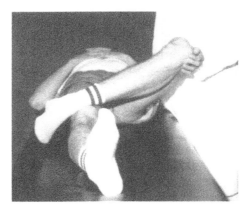

FIGURE 8.29 Figure four diagnostic test for popliteal tendinitis.

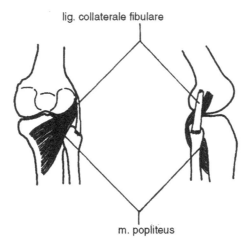

lig. collaterale fibulare

m. popliteus

FIGURE 8.30 Relationship of the lateral collateral ligament to the popliteal tendon.

XIII. FABELLA SYNDROME (FABELLITIS)

The fabella is a sesamoid bone located on the posterior side of the lateral femoral condyle in the lateral head of the gastrocnemius muscle (Figure 8.31). It is present in 10 to 18% of the population.[395] According to the study of Houghton-Allen[365] the fabella was bilateral in 63% of people, although this percentage is lower than that reported elsewhere (81 to 85%). The fabella serves as an attachment site for strands from the popliteum arcuatum and popliteum obliquum ligaments. The anterior side of the fabella is covered in cartilage, which forms a joint with the lateral femoral condyle.

The presence of the fabella and, more specifically, injuries to the fabella can cause tenderness and sensations of radiating pain in the lower leg. The causes of this pain are multiple and include direct trauma to the fabella, overuse syndrome, changes on the fabellar cartilage,[383] and arthritic changes in the fabella. Fracture of the fabella was been described by several authors[346,387,428] and Frey et al.[357] have described knee dysfunction secondary to dislocation of the fabella. In athletes, fabella syndrome is mostly the direct result of long-lasting microtraumas. Moyen et al.[395] reported that fabella syndrome constitutes 1.7% of the pathological changes in athletes' knees. Excessive functioning of the lateral head of the gastrocnemius muscle, especially during the beginning stages of flexion in the knee and during outward rotation of the lower leg immediately before full extension,

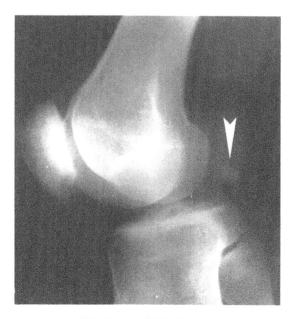

FIGURE 8.31 Lateral roentgenogram of the knee with fabella (arrowhead).

are thought to be related to the etiopathogenesis of fabella syndrome. Predisposing factors for developing fabella syndrome include existence of genu recurvatum accompanied by hypermobility of the lateral compartment of the knee.

Clinical manifestations are characterized by the gradual onset of pain that radiates into the lower leg, specifically the peroneus communis nerve dermatoma. The pain is usually moderate in intensity and associated with knee movements, either due to extension of the muscles during hyperextension of the knee or due to direct pressure on the fabella, e.g., when sitting with legs crossed. Weiner and Macnab[424] consider that the fabella syndrome is recognized by a sharp pain, local tenderness, and intensification of pain in the area of the fabella by full extension of the knee. Pain can be provoked by transverse movement of the fabella when the knee is extended or slightly flexed. Both the localized tenderness and the radiating pain can be amplified or provoked by applying pressure to the fabella, in the area posterior to the lateral femoral condyle and above the joint line. The fabella syndrome appears to be unique to late adolescence, that is 15 to 17 years of age.[424] According to Rettori and Boespflug[407] in sports pathology one must be able to recognize the painful fabella syndrome, so that vascular disease is not mistakenly implicated. Radiographic examination usually does not help, whereas arthroscopy, using the complicated posteroexternal approach, generally does.

Differential diagnosis must rule out the possibility of rupture of the posterior horn of the lateral meniscus and also tendinitis of the lateral head of the gastrocnemius muscle, the biceps femoris, and the popliteus muscle. Hypertrophic and arthritic fabellas that press the peroneus communis nerve are rarely seen.

If the usual non-operative treatment, including infiltration of anesthetics with corticosteroids, does not produce improvement, surgical treatment, consisting of extirpation of the fabella (fabellectomy), is indicated.[382] Weiner and Macnab[424] described 16 adolescents with fabella syndrome: 5 patients responded to conservative measures; 11 patients required surgery, all of whom obtained immediate relief of symptoms. Extirpation of the fabella must be accompanied by reconstruction of the posterior wall of the joint capsule.[426]

REFERENCES

Patellofemoral Joint

1. **Abernethy, P.J., Townesend, P.R., Rose, R.M., and Radin, E.L.** Is chondromalacia patellae a separate clinical entity? *J. Bone Joint Surg. (Br.).*, 1978; 60: 205–210.
2. **Adirim, T.A. and Cheng, T.L.** Overview of injuries in the young athlete. *Sports Med.*, 2003; 33: 75–81.
3. **Aglietti, P., Insall, J.N., and Cerulli, G.** Patellar pain and incongruence. I: Measurements of incongruence. *Clin. Orthop.*, 1983; 176: 217–224.
4. **Aglietti, P., Pisaneschi, A. and De Biase, P.** Recurrent dislocation of patella: three kinds of surgical treatment. *Ital. J. Orthop. Traumatol.*, 1992; 18: 25–36.
5. **Alaca, R., Yilmaz, B., Goktepe, A.S. et al.** Efficacy of isokinetic exercise on functional capacity and pain in patellofemoral pain syndrome. *Am. J. Phys. Med. Rehabil.*, 2002; 81: 807–813.
6. **Aleman, O.** Chondromalacia post traumatica patellae. *Acta Orthop. Scand.*, 1928; 63: 149–189.
7. **Arendt, E.A., Fithian, D.C., and Cohen, E.** Current concepts of lateral patella dislocation. *Clin. Sports Med.*, 2002; 21: 499–519.
8. **Bahk, Y.W., Park, Y.H., Chung, S.K. et al.** Pinhole scintigraphic sign of chondromalacia patellae in old subjects: a prospective assessment with differential diagnosis. *J. Nucl. Med.*, 1994; 35: 855–862.
9. **Bajraktarevic-Cicin-Sain, T. and Pećina, M.** Radioloska istrazivanja nestabilnosti patele. *Rad. Med. Fak. Zagrebu*, 1989; 30: 41–50.
10. **Bandi, W.** Chondromalacia patellae und femoro-patellare Arthrose. *Helv. Chir. Acta Suppl.*, 1972; 1: 3–70.
11. **Bellemans, J., Cauwenberghs, F., Witvrow, E., Brys, P., and Victor, J.** Anteromedial tibial tubercle transfer in patients with chronic anterior knee pain and subluxation-type patellar malalignment. *Am. J. Sports Med.*, 1997; 25: 375–381.
12. **Bentley, G.** Articular cartilage changes in chondromalacia patellae. *J. Bone Joint Surg. (Br.).*, 1985; 67: 769–774.
13. **Bentley, G.** Anterior knee pain: diagnosis and management. *J. R. Coll. Surg. Edinb.*, 1989; 34(Suppl. 6): 2–3.
14. **Bentley, G. and Dowd, G.** Current concepts of etiology and treatment of chondromalacia patellae. *Clin. Orthop.*, 1984; 189: 209–228.
15. **Biedert, R.M. and Sanchis-Alfonso, V.** Sources of anterior knee pain. *Clin. Sports Med.*, 2002; 21: 335–347.
16. **Biedert, R.M. and Warnke, K.** Correlation between the Q angle and the patella position: a clinical and axial computed tomography evaluation. *Arch. Orthop. Trauma Surg.*, 2001; 121: 346–349.
17. **Blackburne, J.S. and Peel, T.E.** A new method of measuring patellar height. *J. Bone Joint Surg.*, 1977; 59(B): 241–242.
18. **Blazina, M.E., Kerlan, R.K., Jobe, F.W., Carter, V.S., and Carlson, J.G.** Jumper's knee. *Orthop. Clin. North Am.*, 1973; 4: 665–678.
19. **Boden, B.P., Pearsall, A.W., Garret, W.E., Jr., and Feagin, J.A., Jr.** Patellofemoral instability: evaluation and management. *J. Am. Acad. Orthop. Surg.*, 1997; 5: 47–57.
20. **Bojanić, I. and Pećina, M.** Axial stress x-rays in diagnosing patellar instability. *Period. Biol.*, 1993; 95: 175–178.
21. **Bourne, M.H., Hazel, W.A., Jr., Scott, S.G., and Sim, F.H.** Anterior knee pain. *Mayo Clin. Proc.*, 1988; 63: 482–491.
22. **Burgess, R.C.** A new method of determining patellar position. *J. Sports Med.*, 1989; 29: 398–399.
23. **Butler-Manuel, P.A., Guy, R.L., Heatley, F.W., and Nunan, T.O.** Scintigraphy in the assessment of anterior knee pain. *Acta Orthop. Scand.*, 1990; 61: 438–442.
24. **Carson, W.G., Jr., James, S.L., Larson, R.L. et al.** Patellofemoral disorders: physical and radiographic evaluation. Part I and II. *Clin. Orthop.*, 1984; 185: 165–186.
25. **Casscells, S.W.** Gross pathological changes in the knee joint of the aged individual: a study of 300 cases. *Clin. Orthop.*, 1978; 132: 225–232.
26. **Caton, J., Deschamps, G., Chambat, P. et al.** Les rotules basses. A propos de 128 observations. *Rev. Chir. Orthop.*, 1982; 68: 317–325.

27. **Christensen, F., Soballe, K., and Snerum, L.** Treatment of chondromalacia patellae by lateral retinacular release of the patella. *Clin. Orthop.*, 1988; 234: 145–147.

28. **Clark, D.I., Downing, N., Mitschell, J. et al.**. Physiotherapy for anterior knee pain: a randomised controlled trial. *Ann. Rheum. Dis.*, 2000; 59: 700–704.

29. **Cook, J.L., Khan, K.M., Kiss, Z.S., and Griffiths, L.** Patellar tendinopathy in junior basketball players: a controlled clinical and ultrasonographic study of 268 patella tendons in players aged 14–18 years. *Scand. J. Med. Sci. Sports*, 2000; 10: 216–220.

30. **Crossley, K., Crowan, S.M., Bennell, K.L., and McConnell, J.** Patellar taping: is clinical success supported by scientific evidence? *Man. Ther.*, 2000; 5: 142–150.

31. **Crossley, K., Bennell, K., Green, S., and McConnell, J.** A systematic review of physical interventions for patellofemoral pain syndrome. *Clin. J. Sports Med.*, 2001; 11: 103–110.

32. **Csintalan, R.P., Schulz, M.M., Woo, J. et al.** Gender differences in patellofemoral joint biomechanics. *Clin. Orthop.*, 2002; 402: 260–269.

33. **Dandy, D.J.** Arthroscopy in the treatment of young patients with anterior knee pain. *Orthop. Clin. North Am.*, 1986; 17: 221–229.

34. **Dandy, D.J.** *Arthroscopic Management of the Knee*, 2nd ed. Edinburgh: Churchill Livingstone, 1987.

35. **Dandy, D.J. and Griffiths, D.** Lateral release for recurrent dislocation of the patella. *J. Bone Joint Surg.*, 1989; 71(B): 121–125.

36. **De Carvahlo, A., Andersen, A.H., Topp, S., and Jurik, A.G.** A method for assessing the height of the patella. *Int. Orthop. (SICOT)*, 1985; 9: 195–197.

37. **Dejour, H., Walch, G., Neyret, P., and Adeleine, P.** La dysplasie de la trochlee femorale. *Rev. Chir. Orthop.*, 1990; 76: 45–54.

38. **Delgado-Martinez, H.** A study of the position of the patella using computerized tomography. *J. Bone Joint Surg.*, 1979; 61(B): 443–444.

39. **Delgado-Martinez, A.D., Rodriguez-Merchan, E.C., Ballesteros, R., and Luna, J.D.** Reproducibility of patellofemoral CT scan measurements. *Int. Orthop.*, 2000; 24: 5–8.

40. **Dong, Q. and Zheng, Z.** CT scanning and arthroscopic evaluation of patellofemoral malalignment. *Chin. Med. J.*, 2000; 113: 133–135.

41. **Dorotka, R., Boj, E.J., Kypta, A., and Kollar, B.** Patellofemoral pain syndrome in young men compared to a normal population exposed to the same physical strain. *Z. Orthop. Ihre Grenzgeb.*, 2002; 140: 48–51.

42. **Dowd, G.S. and Bentley, G.** Radiographic assessment in patellar instability and chondromalacia patellae. *J. Bone Joint Surg. Br. Vol.*, 68: 297–300.

43. **Duffey, M.J., Martin, D.F., Cannon, D.W. et al.** Etiologic factors associated with anterior knee pain in distance runners. *Med. Sci. Sports Exerc.*, 2000; 32: 1825–1832.

44. **Dugdale, T.W. and Barnett, P.R.** Historical background: patellofemoral pain in young people. *Orthop. Clin. North Am.*, 1986; 17: 211–219.

45. **Dupont, J.Y.** Patellofemoral pain. *Rev. Prat.*, 1998; 48: 1781–1786.

46. **Dzolev, G., Simoncev, V., Pećina, M., and Serafimov, L.** Finite elements method in the biomechanical analysis of the knee following meniscectomy. *Orthop. Trauma*, 1992; 23: 27–33.

47. **Federico, D.J. and Reider, B.** Results of isolated patellar debridement for patellofemoral pain in patients with normal patellar alignment. *Am. J. Sports Med.*, 1997; 25: 663–669.

48. **Ficat, P. and Hungerford, D.S.** *Disorders of the Patellofemoral Joint.* Baltimore: Williams & Wilkins, 1977.

49. **Ficat, R.P. and Hungerford, D.S.** *Disorders of Patello-Femoral Joint.* Paris: Masson, 1997.

50. **Ficat, R.P., Philippe, J., and Hungerford, D.S.** Chondromalacia patellae: a system of classification. *Clin. Orthop.*, 1979; 144: 55–62.

51. **Fulkerson, J.P.** Patellofemoral pain disorders: evaluation and management. *J. Am. Acad. Orthop. Surg.*, 1994; 2: 124–132.

52. **Fulkerson, J.P.** *Disorders of the Patellofemoral Joint*, 3rd ed. Baltimore: Williams & Wilkins, 1997.

53. **Fulkerson, J.P.** Diagnosis and treatment of patients with patellofemoral pain. *Am. J. Sports Med.*, 2002; 30: 447–456.

54. **Fulkerson, J.P. and Arendt, E.A.** Anterior knee pain in females. *Clin. Orthop.*, 2000; 372: 69–73.

55. **Fulkerson, J.P. and Hungerford, D.S.** *Disorders of the Patellofemoral Joint.* Baltimore: Williams & Wilkins, 1990.

56. **Fulkerson, J.P., Schutzer, S.F., and Ramsby, G.R.** Computerized tomography of the patellofemoral joint before and after lateral release or realignment. *J. Arthrosc. Rel. Surg.*, 1987; 3: 19–24.

57. **Fulkerson, J.P. and Shea, K.P.** Disorders of patellofemoral alignment. *J. Bone Joint Surg.*, 1990; 72(A): 1424–1429.

58. **Garrick, J.G.** Anterior knee pain (chondromalacia patellae). *Phys. Sportsmed.*, 1989; 17: 75–84.

59. **Gecha, S.R. and Torg, E.** Knee injuries in tennis. *Clin. Sports Med.*, 1988; 7: 435–452.

60. **Gigante, A., Pasquinelli, F.M., Paladini, P. et al.** The effects of patellar taping on patellofemoral incongruence. A computed tomography study. *Am. J. Sports Med.*, 2001; 29: 88–92.

61. **Goodfellow, J., Hungerford, D.S., and Zindel, M.** Patello-femoral joint mechanics and pathology. I. Functional anatomy of the patellofemoral joint. *J. Bone Joint Surg.*, 1976; 58(B): 287–290.

62. **Graf, J., Neithard, F.U., and Cotta, H.** Zur Begriffsbestimmung von Chondropathia und Chondromalacia Patellae. *Z. Orthop.*, 1990; 128: 289–294.

63. **Graf, J., Christophers, R., Schneider, U., and Neithard, F.U.** Chondromalacia of the patella and intraosseous pressure. A study of 43 patients. *Z. Orthop. Ihre Grenzgeb.*, 1992; 130: 495–500.

64. **Grelsamer, R.P.** Patellar malalignment. *J. Bone Joint Surg. Am. Vol.*, 2000; 82: 1639–1650.

65. **Harman, M., Dogan, A., Arslan, H. et al.** Evaluation of the patellofemoral joint with kinematic MR fluoroscopy. *Clin. Imaging,* 2002; 26: 136–139.

66. **Hašpl, M., Čičak, N., Klobucar, H., and Pećina, M.** Full arthroscopic stabilization of the patella. *Arthroscopy,* 2002; 18/1: E2 (1–3).

67. **Hehne, H.J.** Biomechanics of the patellofemoral joint and its clinical relevance. *Clin. Orthop.,* 1990; 258: 73–85.

68. **Holmes, S.W., Jr., and Clancy, W.G., Jr.** Clinical classification of patellofemoral pain syndrome. *J. Orthop. Sports Phys. Ther.,* 1998; 28: 299–306.

69. **Holmes, S.W., Jr., and Clancy, W.G., Jr.** Clinical classification of patellofemoral pain and dysfunction. *J. Orthop. Sports Phys. Ther.,* 1998; 28: 299–305.

70. **Hughston, J.C.** Patellar subluxation. *Clin. Sports Med.,* 1989; 8: 153–162.

71. **Hughston, J.C. and Deese, M.** Medial subluxation of the patella as a complication of lateral retinacular release. *Am. J. Sports Med.,* 1988; 16: 383–388.

72. **Imai, N., Tomatsu, T., Takeuchi, H., and Noguchi, T.** Clinical and roentgenological studies on malalignment disorders of the patellofemoral joint. Part I. Classification of patellofemoral alignments using dynamic sky-line view arthrography with special consideration of the mechanism of the malalignment disorders. *J. Jpn. Orthop. Assoc.,* 1987; 61: 1–15.

73. **Imai, N. and Tomatsu, T.** Cartilage lesions in the knee of adolescents and young adults: arthroscopic analysis. *Arthroscopy,* 1991; 7: 198–203.

74. **Inoue, M., Shino, K., Hirose, H., Horibe, S., and Ono, K.** Subluxation of the patella. *J. Bone Joint Surg.,* 1988; 70(A): 1331–1337.

75. **Insall, J.** Patellar pain. *J. Bone Joint Surg.,* 1982; 64(A): 147–151.

76. **Insall, J.N. and Salvati, E.** Patella position in the normal knee joint. *Radiology,* 1971; 101: 101–104.

77. **Ireland, M.L.** Patellofemoral disorders in runners and bicyclists. *Ann. Sports Med.,* 1987; 3: 77–84.

78. **Jackson, A.M.** Anterior knee pain. *J. Bone Joint Surg. Br. Vol.,* 2001; 83: 937–948.

79. **Jackson, D.W., Jennings, L.D., Maywood, R.M., and Berger, P.E.** Magnetic resonance imaging of the knee. *Am. J. Sports Med.,* 1988; 16: 29–38.

80. **Jacobson, K.E. and Flandry, F.C.** Diagnosis of anterior knee pain. *Clin. Sports Med.,* 1989; 8: 179–195.

81. **Jensen, D.B. and Albrektsen, S.B.** The natural history of chondromalacia patellae. A 12-year follow-up. *Acta Orthop. Belg.,* 1990; 56: 503–506.

82. **Jenny, J.Y., Sader, Z., Henry, A. et al.** Elevation of the tibial tubercle for patellofemoral pain syndrome. An 8- to 15-year follow-up. *Knee Surg. Sports Traumatol. Arthrosc.,* 1996; 4: 92–96.

83. **Joensen, A.M., Hahn, T., Gelineck, J. et al.** Articular cartilage lesions and anterior knee pain. *Scand. J. Med. Sci. Sports,* 2001; 11: 115–119.

84. **Johnson, L.L.** *Arthroscopic Surgery: Principles and Practice.* St. Louis: C.V. Mosby, 1986.

85. **Karadimas, J.E., Piscopakis, N., and Syrmalis, L.** Patella alta and chondromalacia. *Int. Orthop. (SICOT),* 1981; 5: 247–249.

86. **Kasim, N. and Fulkerson, J.P.** Resection of clinically localized segments of painful retinaculum in the treatment of selected patients with anterior knee pain. *Am. J. Sports Med.,* 2000; 28: 811–814.

87. **Kelly, M.A. and Insall, J.N.** Historical perspectives of chondromalacia patellae. *Orthop. Clin. North Am.*, 1992; 23: 517–521.

88. **Kujala, U.M., Osterman, K., Kvist, M. et al.** Factors predisposing to patellar chondropathy and patellar apicitis in athletes. *Int. Orthop. (SICOT)*, 1986; 10: 195–200.

89. **Kujala, U.M., Osterman, K., Kormano, M. et al.** Patellar motion analyzed by magnetic resonance imaging. *Acta Orthop. Scand.*, 1989; 60: 13–16.

90. **Kujala, U.M., Osterman, K., Kormano, M. et al.** Patellofemoral relationships in recurrent patellar dislocations. *J. Bone Joint Surg.*, 1989; 71(B): 788–792.

91. **Kuroda, R., Kambic, H., Valdevit, A., and Andrish, J.T.** Articular cartilage contact pressure after tibial tuberosity transfer. A cadaveric study. *Am. J. Sports Med.*, 2001; 29: 403–409.

92. **LaBrier, K. and O'Neill, D.B.** Patellofemoral stress syndrome. Current concepts. *Sports Med.*, 1993; 16: 449–459.

93. **Laurin, C.A., Dussault, R., and Levesque, H.P.** The tangential x-ray investigation of the patellofemoral joint: x-ray technique, diagnostic criteria and their interpretation. *Clin. Orthop.*, 1979; 144: 16–26.

94. **Lindberg, U., Hamberg, P., Lysholm, J., and Gillquist, J.** Arthroscopic examination of the patellofemoral joint using a central, one-portal technique. *Orthop. Clin. North Am.*, 1986; 17: 263–268.

95. **Lippert, M.J. and Paar, O.** Patellofemoral pressure and contact surface measurement in the "hunter's hat patella." Experimental studies of sagittal patella osteotomy. *Z. Orthop. Ihre Grenzgeb.*, 1987; 125: 679–686.

96. **Macnicol, M.F.** *The Problem Knee. Diagnosis and Management in the Younger Patient.* London: William Heinemann Medical Books, 1986.

97. **Main, W.K. and Hershman, E.B.** Chronic knee pain in active adolescents. *Phys. Sportsmed.*, 1992; 20: 139–156.

98. **Maquet, P.** *Biomechanics of the Knee.* Berlin: Springer-Verlag, 1976.

99. **Matijasevic, B., Pećina, M., Jelic, M., and Bajraktarevic, T.** Kinematic analysis of the patellofemoral joint. *Orthop. Trauma*, 1992; 23: 7–13.

100. **Martines, S., Korobkin, M., Fondren, F.B. et al.** Computed tomography of the normal patellofemoral joint. *Invest. Radiol.*, 1983; 18: 249–252.

101. **McCauley, T.R., Kier, R., Lynch, K.J., and Jokl, P.** Chondromalacia patellae: diagnosis with MR imaging. *Am. J. Roentgenol.*, 1992; 158: 106–107.

102. **McNally, E.G.,** Imaging assessment of anterior knee pain and patellar maltracking. *Skel. Radiol.*, 2001; 30: 484–495.

103. **Merchant, A.C.** Classification of patellofemoral disorders. *Arthroscopy*, 1988; 4: 235–240.

104. **Merchant, A.C., Mercer, R.L., Jacobsen, R.H., and Cool, C.R.** Roentgenographic analysis of patellofemoral congruence. *J. Bone Joint Surg.*, 1974; 56(A): 1391–1396.

105. **Milgrom, C., Finestone, A., Shlamkowitsch, N. et al.** Anterior knee pain caused by overactivity: a long term prospective follow up. *Clin. Orthop.*, 1996; 33: 256–260.

106. **Minkoff, J. and Fein, L.** The role of radiography in the evaluation and treatment of common anathrotic disorders of the patellofemoral joint. *Clin. Sports Med.*, 1989; 8: 203–260.

107. **Moller, B.N., Krebs, B., and Jurik, A.G.** Patellofemoral incongruence in chondromalacia and instability of the patella. *Acta Orthop. Scand.*, 1986; 57: 232–234.

108. **Mori, Y., Kubo, M., Okumo, H., and Kuroki, Y.** Histological comparison of patellar cartilage degeneration between chondromalacia in youth and osteoarthritis in aging. *Knee Surg. Sports Traumatol. Arthrosc.*, 1995; 3: 167–172.

109. **Morscher, E.** Osteotomy of the patella in chondromalacia. Preliminary report. *Arch. Orthop. Trauma Surg.*, 1978; 92: 139–147.

110. **Murray, T.F., Dupont, J.Y., and Fulkerson, J.P.** Axial and lateral radiographs in evaluating patellofemoral malalignment. *Am. J. Sports Med.*, 1999; 27: 580–584.

111. **Naslund, J., Naslund, U.B., Odenbring, S., and Lundeberg, T.** Sensory stimulation (acupuncture) for the treatment of idiopathic anterior knee pain. *J. Rehabil. Med.*, 2002; 34: 231–238.

112. **Neusel, E. and Graf, J.** The influence of subchondral vascularisation on chondromalacia patellae. *Arch. Orthop. Trauma Surg.*, 1996; 115: 313–315.

113. **Ng, G.Y. and Cheng, J.M.** The effect of patellar taping on pain and neuromuscular performance in subjects with patellofemoral pain syndrome. *Clin. Rehabil.*, 2002; 16(8): 821–827.

114. **Nimon, G., Murray, D., Sandow, M., and Goodfellow, J.** Natural history of anterior knee pain: a 14 to 20 years follow-up of nonoperative management. *J. Pediatr. Orthop.*, 1998; 18: 118–122.

115. **Noyes, F.R. and Stabler, C.L.** A system for grading articular cartilage lesions at arthroscopy. *Am. J. Sports Med.*, 1989; 17: 505–513.

116. **Ogilvie-Harris, D.J. and Jackson, R.W.** The arthroscopic treatment of chondromalacia patellae. *J. Bone Joint Surg. Br. Vol.*, 1984; 66: 660–665.

117. **Outerbridge, R.E.** The etiology of chondromalacia patellae. *J. Bone Joint Surg.*, 1961; 43(B): 752–757.

118. **Owens, B.D., Stickles, B.J., Balikian, P., and Busconi, B.D.** Prospective analysis of radiofrequency versus mechanical debridement of isolated patellar chondral lesions. *Arthroscopy*, 2002; 18: 151–155.

119. **Patel, D.** Plica as a cause of anterior knee pain. *Orthop. Clin. North Am.*, 1986; 17: 273–277.

120. **Pećina, M.** Longitudinal osteotomy of the patella after Morscher, in *Surgery and Arthroscopy of the Knee*, Mueller, W. and Hackenbruch, W.H., Eds. Berlin: Springer-Verlag, 1988; 471–476.

121. **Pećina, M., Bilic, R., and Korzinek, K.** Ventralisation der Patella unsere zehnjahrige Erfahrung, in *Das Kniegelenk*, Chapchal, G., Ed. Stuttgart: Georg Thieme Verlag, 1989; 118–120.

122. **Pećina, M.** Longitudinal osteotomy of the patella in the treatment of chondromalacia in the top-level athletes. 1st World Cong. Sports Trauma, Palma de Mallorca, 1992, Abstracts Book, 205–206.

123. **Perrild, C., Hejgaard, N., and Rosenklint, A.** Chondromalacia patellae. A radiographic study of the femoropatellar joint. *Acta Orthop. Scand.*, 1982; 53: 131–134.

124. **Post, W.R. and Fulkerson, J.P.** Anterior knee pain — a symptom, not a diagnosis. *Bull. Rheum. Dis.*, 1993; 4: 5–7.

125. **Post, W.R. and Fulkerson, J.P.** Knee pain diagrams: correlation with physical examination findings in patients with anterior knee pain. *Arthroscopy*, 1994; 10: 618–623.

126. **Post, W.R., Tetige, R., and Amis, A.** Patellofemoral malalignment: looking beyond the viewbox. *Clin. Sports Med.*, 2002; 21: 521–546.

127. **Powers, C.M., Shellock, F.G., Beering, T.V. et al.** Effect of bracing on patellar kinematics in patients with patellofemoral joint pain. *Med. Sci. Sports Exerc.*, 1999; 31: 1714–1720.

128. **Radin, E.L.** Anterior knee pain. The need for a specific diagnosis: stop calling it chondromalacia! *Orthop. Rev.*, 1985; 14: 128–134.

129. **al-Rawi, Z. and Nessan, A.H.** Joint hypermobility in patients with chondromalacia patella. *Br. J. Rheumatol.*, 1997; 36: 1324–1327.

130. **Reider, B., Marshall, J.L., and Ring, B.** Patellar tracking. *Clin. Orthop.*, 1981; 157: 143–148.

131. **Rillmann, P., Dutly, A., Kieser, C., and Berbig, R.** Modified Elmslie-Trillat procedure for instability of the patella. *Knee Surg. Sports Traumatol. Arthrosc.*, 1998; 6: 31–35.

132. **Rillmann, P., Oswald, A., Holzach, P., and Ryf, C.** Fulkerson's modified Elmslie-Trillat procedure for objective patellar instability and patellofemoral pain syndrome. *Swiss Surg.*, 2000; 6: 328–334.

133. **Rogvi-Hansen, B., Ellitsgaard, N., Funch, M. et al.** Low level laser treatment of chondromalacia patellae. *Int. Orthop.*, 1991; 15: 359–361.

134. **Roland, G.C., Beagley, M.J., and Cawley, P.W.** Conservative treatment of inflamed knee bursae. *Phys. Sportsmed.*, 1992; 20: 67–77.

135. **Sallay, P.I., Poggy, J., Speer, K.P., and Garrett, W.E.** Acute dislocation of the patella. A correlative pathoanatomic study. *Am. J. Sports Med.*, 1996; 24: 52–60.

136. **Sanchis-Alfonso, V., Rosello-Sastre, E., and Martinez-Sanjuan, V.** Pathogenesis of anterior knee pain syndrome and functional patellofemoral instability in the active young. *Am. J. Knee Surg.*, 1999; 12: 29–40.

137. **Sandow, M.J. and Goodfellow, J.W.** The natural history of anterior knee pain in adolescents. *J. Bone Joint Surg.*, 1985; 67(B): 36–38.

138. **Schneider, U., Breusch, S.J., Thomsen, M. et al.** A new concept in the treatment of anterior knee pain: patellar hypertension syndrome. *Orthopedics*, 2000; 23: 581–586.

139. **Schneider, F., Labs, K., and Wagner, S.** Chronic patellofemoral pain syndrome: alternatives for cases of therapy resistance. *Knee Surg. Sports Traumatol. Arthrosc.*, 2001; 9: 290–295.

140. **Schutzer, S.F., Ramsby, G.R., and Fulkerson, J.P.** Computed tomographic classification of patellofemoral pain patients. *Orthop. Clin. North Am.*, 1986; 17: 235–248.

141. **Shellock, F.G., Mink, J.H., and Fox, J.M.** Patellofemoral joint: kinematic MR imaging to assess tracking abnormalities. *Radiology,* 1988; 168: 551–553.
142. **Shellock, F.G., Mink, J.H., Deutsch, A.L., and Fox, J.M.** Patellar tracking abnormalities: clinical experience with kinematic MR imaging in 130 patients. *Radiology,* 1989; 172: 799–804.
143. **Shellock, F.G., Mink, J.H., Deutsch, A., Fox, J.M., and Ferkel, R.D.** Evaluation of patients with persistent symptoms after lateral retinacular release by kinematic resonance imaging of the patellofemoral joint. *Arthroscopy,* 1990; 6: 226–234.
144. **Shellock, F.G., Stone, K.R., and Crues, J.V.** Development and clinical application of kinematic MRI of the patellofemoral joint using an extremity MR system. *Med. Sci. Sports Exerc.,* 1999; 31: 788–791.
145. **Shellock, F.G.** Effect of a patella-stabilizing brace on lateral subluxation of the patella: assessment using kinematic MRI. *Am. J. Knee Surg.,* 2000; 13: 137–142.
146. **Small, N.C., Glogau, A.I., and Berezin, M.A.** Arthroscopically assisted proximal extensor mechanism realignment of the knee. *Arthroscopy,* 1993; 9: 63–67.
147. **Soejbjerg, J.O., Lauritzen, J., Hvid, I., and Boe, S.** Arthroscopic determination of patellofemoral malalignment. *Clin. Orthop.,* 1987; 215: 243–247.
148. **Stougard, J.** Chondromalacia of the patellae. Physical signs in relation to operative findings. *Acta Orthop. Scand.,* 1975; 46: 685–694.
149. **Teitge, R.A.** Stress x-rays for patellofemoral instability. Monograph accompanying exhibit at the 3rd Eur. Cong. Knee Surgery (ESKA), Amsterdam, May 1988.
150. **Terry, G.C.** Office evaluation and management of the symptomatic knee. *Orthop. Clin. North Am.,* 1988; 19: 699–713.
151. **Thomee, R., Renstrom, P., Karlsson, J., and Grimby, G.** Patellofemoral pain syndrome in young women. I. A clinical analysis of alignment, pain parameters, common symptoms and functional activity level. *Scand. J. Med. Sci. Sports,* 1995; 5: 237–244.
152. **Thomee, R., Augustsson, J., and Karlson, J.** Patellofemoral pain syndrome: a review of current issues. *Sports Med.,* 1999; 28: 245–262.
153. **Vaatainen, U., Kiviranta, I., Jaroma, H., and Airaksinen, O.** Lateral release in chondromalacia patellae using clinical, radiologic, electromyographic, and muscle force testing evaluation. *Arch. Phys. Med. Rehabil.,* 1994; 75: 1127–1131.
154. **Vahasarja, V., Kinnunen, P., and Serlo, W.** Lateral release and proximal realignment for patellofemoral malalignment. A prospective study of 40 knees in 36 adolescents followed for 1–8 years. *Acta Orthop. Scand.,* 1998; 69: 159–162.
155. **van Leersum, M., Schweitzer, M.E., Gannon, F. et al.** Chondromalacia patellae: an *in vitro* study. Comparison of MR criteria with histological and macroscopic findings. *Skel. Radiol.,* 1996; 25: 727–732.
156. **Vujcic, M. and Nedelkovic, R.** Thermography in the detection and follow-up of chondromalacia patellae. *Ann. Rheum. Dis.,* 1991; 50: 921–925.
157. **Watson, C.J., Leddy, H.M., Dynjan, T.D., and Parham, J.L.** Reliability of the lateral pull test and tilt test to assess patellar alignment in subjects with symptomatic knees: student raters. *J. Orthop. Sports Phys. Ther.,* 2001; 31: 368–374.
158. **Wiberg, G.** Roentgenographic and anatomic studies of the patellofemoral joint. *Acta Orthop. Scand.,* 1941; 12: 319–410.
159. **Witonski, D.** Anterior knee pain syndrome. *Int. Orthop.,* 1999; 23: 341–344.
160. **Witonski, D. and Wagrowska-Danielewicz, M.** Distribution of substance-P nerve fibers in the knee joint in patients with anterior knee pain syndrome. A preliminary report. *Knee Surg. Sports Traumatol. Arthrosc.,* 1999; 7: 177–183.
161. **Witonski, D. and Goraj, B.** Patellar motion analyzed by kinematic and dynamic axial magnetic resonance imaging in patients with anterior knee pain syndrome. *Arch. Orthop. Trauma Surg.,* 1999; 119: 46–49.
162. **Witonski, D.** Dynamic magnetic resonance imaging. *Clin. Sports Med.,* 2002; 21: 403–415.
163. **Witvrouw, E., Lysen, R., Bellemans, J., Cambier, D., and Vanderstraeten, G.** Intrinsic risk factors for the development of anterior knee pain in an athletic population. A two-year prospective study. *Am. J. Sports Med.,* 2000; 28: 480–489.
164. **Witvrouw, E., Lysens, R., Bellemans, J. et al.** Which factors predict outcome in the treatment program of anterior knee pain? *Scand. J. Med. Sci. Sports,* 2002; 12: 40–46.

165. **Yamamoto, R.K.** Arthroscopic repair of the medial retinaculum and capsule in acute patellar dislocations. *Arthroscopy*, 1986; 2: 125–131.

Patellar Tendinitis/Tendinosis (Jumper's Knee)

166. **Almekinders, L.C., Vellema, J.H., and Weinhold, P.S.** Strain patterns in the patellar tendon and the implications for patellar tendinopathy. *Knee Surg. Sports Traumatol. Arthrosc.*, 2002; 10: 2–5.

167. **Apple, D.F., Jr.** Progressive quadriceps strengthening — best cure for jumper's knee. *J. Musculoskel. Med.*, 1987; 4: 11.

168. **Beckman, M., Craig, R., and Lehman, R.C.** Rehabilitation of patellofemoral dysfunction in the athlete. *Clin. Sports Med.*, 1989; 8: 841–861.

169. **Blazina, M.E., Kerlan, R.K., Jobe, F.W., Karter, V.S., and Carlson, G.J.** Jumper's knee. *Orthop. Clin. North Am.*, 1973; 4: 665–678.

170. **Black, J.E. and Alten, S.R.** How I manage infrapatellar tendinitis. *Phys. Sportsmed.*, 1983; 12: 86–92.

171. **Bodne, D., Quinn, S.F., Murray, W.T. et al.** Magnetic resonance images of chronic patellar tendinitis. *Skel. Radiol.*, 1988; 17: 24–28.

172. **Briner, W.W., Jr. and Kacmar, L.** Common injuries in volleyball. Mechanisms of injury, prevention and rehabilitation. *Sports Med.*, 1997; 24: 65–71.

173. **Brunet-Quedi, E. and Imbert, J.C.** Les tendinites du genou, in *Lesions Traumatiques des Tendons chez le Sportif*, Catonne, Y. and Saillant, G., Eds. Paris: Masson, 1992; 100–106.

174. **Coleman, B.D., Khan, K.M., Kiss, Z.S. et al.** Open and arthroscopic patellar tenotomy for chronic patellar tendinopathy. *Am. J. Sports Med.*, 2000; 28: 183–190.

175. **Colosimo, A.J. and Basset, F.H.** Jumper's knee. Diagnosis and treatment. *Orthop. Rev.*, 1990; 19: 139–149.

176. **Combelles, F. and Saillant, G.** Place de la chirurgie dans le traitement des tendinites rotuliennes du sportif. *Lett. Chir.*, 1989; 77: 28–30.

177. **Cook, J.L., Khan, K.M., Kiss, Z.S., Purdam, C.R., and Griffiths, L.** Prospective imaging study of asymptomatic patellar tendinopathy in elite junior basketball players. *J. Ultrasound Med.*, 2000; 19: 473–479.

178. **Cook, J.L., Khan, K.M., Kiss, Z.S., Coleman, B.D., and Griffiths, L.** Asymptomatic hypoechoic regions on patellar tendon ultrasound: A 4-year clinical and ultrasound follow-up of 46 tendons. *Scand. J. Med. Sci. Sports*, 2001; 11: 321–327.

179. **Cook, J.L., Khan, K.M., Harcourt, P.R. et al.** Patellar tendon ultrasonography in asymptomatic active athletes reveals hypoechoic regions: a study of 320 tendons. *Clin. J. Sport Med.*, 1998; 8: 73–77.

180. **Crass, J.R., Lucy van de Vegte, G., and Harkavy, L.A.** Tendon echogenicity: *ex vivo* study. *Radiology*, 1988; 167: 499–501.

181. **Davies, S.G., Baudouin, C.J., King, J.B., and Perry, J.D.** Ultrasound, computed tomography and magnetic resonance imaging in patellar tendinitis. *Clin. Radiol.*, 1991; 43: 52–56.

182. **de Lecluse, J.** Tendinitis of the knee. *Rev. Prat.*, 1998; 48: 1793–1797.

183. **Dubravčić-Šimunjak, S., Pećina, M., Hašpl, M., Šimunjak, B., and Bobinac, D.** Most common injuries in jumping sports and its rehabilitation, 2nd Mediterranean Congress of Physical Medicine and Rehabilitation, Valencia, 1998; Abstracts, p. 197.

184. **Dubravčić-Šimunjak, S., Pećina, M., Kuipers, H., Moran, J., and Hašpl, M.** The incidence of injuries in elite junior figure skaters. *Am. J. Sports Med.*, in press.

185. **Duri, Z.A., Aichroth, P.M., Wilkins, R., and Jones, J.** Patellar tendonitis and anterior knee pain. *Am. J. Knee Surg.*, 1999; 12: 99–108.

186. **el-Khoury, G.Y., Wira, R.L., Berbaum, K.S., Poppe, T.L., Jr., and Monu, J.U.** MR imaging of patellar tendinitis. *Radiology*, 1992; 184: 849–854.

187. **Ferretti, A., Nevi, M., Mariani, P.P., and Puddu, G.** Etiopathogenetic considerations on the jumper's knee. *Ital. J. Sports Trauma*, 1983; 5: 101–105.

188. **Ferretti, A., Ippolito, E., Mariani, P.P., and Puddu, G.** Jumper's knee. *Am. J. Sports Med.*, 1983; 11: 58–62.

189. **Ferretti, A., Puddu, G., Mariani, P.P., and Neri, M.** Jumper's knee. An epidemiological study of volleyball players. *Phys. Sportsmed.*, 1984; 12: 97–106.

190. **Ferretti, A., Puddu, G., Mariani, P.P., and Neri, M.** The natural history of jumper's knee. *Int. Orthop. (SICOT)*, 1985; 8: 239–242.

191. **Ferretti, A.** Epidemiology of jumper's knee. *Sports Med.*, 1986; 3: 289–295.

192. **Ferretti, A., Papandrea, P., and Conteduca, F.** Knee injuries in volleyball. *Sports Med.*, 1990; 10: 132–138.

193. **Fornage, B.D. and Rifkin, M.D.** Ultrasound examination of tendons. *Radiol. Clin. North Am.*, 1988; 26: 63–75.

194. **Fornage, B.D., Rifkin, M.D., Touche, D.H., and Segal, P.M.** Ultrasonography of the patellar tendon: preliminary observations. *AJR*, 1984; 143: 179–182.

195. **Friedl, E.W. and Glaser, F.** Dynamic sonography in the diagnosis of ligament and meniscal injuries of the knee. *Arch. Orthop. Trauma Surg.*, 1991; 110: 132–139.

196. **Fritschy, D. and Gautard, R.** Jumper's knee and ultrasonography. *Am. J. Sports Med.*, 1988; 16: 637–640.

197. **Fritschy, D. and Wallensten, R.** Surgical treatment of patellar tendinitis. *Knee Surg. Sports Traumatol. Arthrosc.*, 1993; 1: 131–133.

198. **Giacomelli, E., Grassi, W., and Zampa, A.M.** Le atlopatie nei pallavolisti. *Med. Sport.*, 1986; 39: 425–434.

199. **Green, J.S., Morgan, B., Lauder, I. et al.** The correlation of bone scintigraphy and histological findings in patellar tendinitis. *Nucl. Med. Commun.*, 1996; 17: 231–234.

200. **Greenspan, A., Norman, A., and Kia-Ming Tchang, F.** "Tooth" sign in patellar degenerative disease. *J. Bone Joint Surg.*, 1977; 59(B): 483–485.

201. **Griffiths, G.P. and Selesnick, F.H.** Operative treatment and arthroscopic findings in chronic patellar tendinitis. *Arthroscopy*, 1998; 14: 836–839.

202. **Grossfeld, S.L. and Engebretsen, L.** Patellar tendinitis — a case report of elongation and ossification of the inferior pole of the patella. *Scand. J. Med. Sci. Sports*, 1995; 5: 308–310.

203. **Haller, W. and Lehner, K.** Bildgebende Verfahren zur Diagnostic von Kniegelenksverletzungen und -Erkrankungen. *Roentgenpraxis*, 1989; 42: 198–204.

204. **Hannesschlager, G., Neumuller, H., Riedelberger, W., and Reschauer, R.** Sonographische Diagnostic von pathologischen Veränderungen des vorderen Kniegelenksbereiches. *Ultraschall*, 1990; 11: 33–39.

205. **Henry, J.H.** Jumper's knee. *Sport Med. Actual.*, 1988; 3: 10–13.

206. **Hickey, G.J., Fricker, P.A., and McDonald, W.A.** Injuries of young elite female basketball players over a six-year period. *Clin. J. Sport Med.*, 1997; 7: 252–256.

207. **Janssen, G.** Das Patellaspitzensyndrom. *Orthop. Praxis*, 1983; 19: 12–15.

208. **Jensen, K. and Di Fabrio, R.P.** Evaluation of eccentric exercises in treatment in patellar tendinitis. *Phys. Ther.*, 1989; 69: 211–216.

209. **Jerosch, J., Castro, W.H.M., Sons, H.U., and Winkelman, W.** Der Aussagewert der Sonographic bei Verletzungen des Kniegelenkes. *Ultraschall*, 1989; 10: 275–278.

210. **Jerosch, J., Castro, W.H.M., Sons, H.U., and Winkelman, W.** Möglichkeiten der Sonographic beim Patellaspitzen Syndrom. *Ultraschall*, 1990; 11: 44–47.

211. **Johnson, D.P., Wakeley, C.J., and Watt, I.** Magnetic resonance imaging of patellar tendonitis. *J. Bone Joint Surg (Br.).*, 1996; 78: 452–457.

212. **Kalebo, P., Sward, L., Karlssen, J., and Peterson, L.** Ultrasonography in the detection of partial patellar ligament ruptures (jumper's knee). *Skel. Radiol.*, 1991; 20: 285–289.

213. **Kahn, D. and Wilson, M.A.** Bone scintigraphic findings in patellar tendinitis. *J. Nucl. Med.*, 1987; 28: 1769.

214. **Karantanas, A.H., Zibis, A.H., and Papanikolaou, N.** Increased signal intensity on fat-suppressed three-dimensional T1-weighted pulse sequences in patellar tendon: magic angle effect? *Skel. Radiol.*, 2001; 30: 67–71.

215. **Karlsson, J., Lundin, O., Lassing, I.W., and Peterson, L.** Partial rupture of the patellar ligament. Results after operative treatment. *Am. J. Sports Med.*, 1991; 19: 403–408.

216. **Kelly, D.W., Carter, V.S., Jobe, F.W., and Kerlan, R.K.** Patellar and quadriceps tendon ruptures — jumper's knee. *Am. J. Sports Med.*, 1984; 12: 375–380.

217. **Kettelkamp, D.B.** Management of patellar malalignment. *J. Bone Joint Surg.*, 1981; 63(B): 1344–1347.

218. **Khan, M.K., Bonar, F., Desmond, M.P. et al.** Patellar tendinosis (jumper's knee): findings at histopathologic examination, US, and MR imaging. *Radiology*, 1996; 200: 821–827.

219. **King, J.B., Perry, D.J., Mowad, K., and Kumar, S.J.** Lesions of the patellar ligament. *J. Bone Joint Surg.*, 1990; 72(B): 46–48.

220. **Krahl, H.** "Jumper's knee." Atiologie, differential Diagnose und therapeutische Möglichkeiten. *Orthopade*, 1980; 9: 193–197.

221. **Kujala, M.H., Osterman, K., Kvist, M., Aalto, T., and Friberg, O.** Factors predisposing to patellar chondropathy and patellar apicitis in athletes. *Int. Orthop. (SICOT)*, 1986; 10: 195–200.

222. **Kujala, M.H., Kvist, M., and Osterman, K.** Knee injuries in athletes, review of exertion injuries and retrospective study of outpatient sports clinic material. *Sports Med.*, 1986; 3: 447–460.

223. **Laine, H.R., Harjube, A., and Peltokallio, P.** Ultrasound in the evaluation of the knee and patellar regions. *J. Ultrasound Med.*, 1987; 6: 33–36.

224. **Lian, O., Holen, K.J., Engebretsen, L., and Bahr, R.** Relationship between symptoms of jumper's knee and the ultrasound characteristics of the patellar tendon among high level male volleyball players. *Scand. J. Med. Sci. Sports*, 1996; 6: 291–296.

225. **Linenger, J.M. and West, L.A.** Epidemiology of soft-tissue/musculoskeletal injury among U.S. Marine recruits undergoing basic training. *Mil. Med.*, 1992; 157: 491–493.

226. **Maddox, P.A. and Garth, W.P.** Tendinitis of the patellar ligament and quadriceps (jumper's knee) as an initial presentation of hyperparathyroidism. A case report. *J. Bone Joint Surg.*, 1986; 68(A): 289–292.

227. **Maffulli, N., Binfield, P.M., Leach, W.J., and King, J.B.** Surgical management of tendinopathy of the main body of the patellar tendon in athletes. *Clin. J. Sport Med.*, 1999; 9: 58–62.

228. **Mahlfeld, K., Kayser, R., Mahlfeld, A., and Merk, H.** Ultrasound findings of the patellar tendon and its insertion sites. *Ultraschall Med.*, 1997; 18: 249–253.

229. **Martens, M., Wonkers, P., Bursens, A., and Mulier, J.C.** Patellar tendinitis. Pathology and result of treatment. *Acta Orthop. Scand.*, 1982; 53: 445–450.

230. **McLoughlin, R.F., Raber, E.L., Vellet, A.D., Wiley, J.P., and Bray, R.C.** Patellar tendinitis: MR imaging features, with suggested pathogenesis and proposed classification. *Radiology*, 1995; 197: 843–848.

231. **Mourad, K., King, J., and Guggina, P.** Computed tomography and ultrasound imaging of jumper's knee — patellar tendinitis. *Clin. Radiol.*, 1988; 39: 162–165.

232. **Mellerowicz, H., Stelling, E., Kafenbaum, A.** Diagnostic ultrasound in the athlete's locomotor system. *Br. J. Sports Med.*, 1990; 24: 32–39.

233. **Noesberger, B., Fernandez, D., and Meyer, R.P.** Das jumper's knee. *Helv. Chir. Acta*, 1976; 43: 447–450.

234. **Pećina, M. and Bilic, R.** Mogucnosti lijecenja "koljena skakaca." *SMO*, 1983; 20: 143–148.

235. **Pećina, M., Dubravčić, S., Smerdelj, M., and Ribarić, G.** Contribution to the etiological explanation of "basketball knee." *Sport Med. Actual.*, 1988; 3: 29–31.

236. **Pećina, M., Ribarić, G., Bojanić, I., and Dubravčić, S.** Jumper's knee. *KMV*, 1989; 4: 15–21.

237. **Pećina, M. and Bojanić, I.** Surgical treatment of jumper's knee in top level athletes, in *Sports, Medicine and Health*, Hermans, G.P.H., Ed. Amsterdam: Elsevier Science Publishers, 1990; 299–304.

238. **Pećina, M., Bojanić, I., Pećina, H.I., and Hašpl, M.** Surgical treatment of "jumper's knee." *Croat. Sports Med. J.*, 1997; 12: 92–100.

239. **Pećina, M., Manojlovi, S., Bojanić, I., Hašpl, M., and Seiwert, S.** Histopathologic examinations of bone and tendon in patellar tendinitis (jumper's knee), paper presented at 8th Congress of the ESSKA, Nice, 1998; Book of Abstracts, p. 148.

240. **Pećina, M.** Overuse injuries of the knee joint, paper presented at 10th SICOT trainees meeting, Portoroć, 1999; Abstracts Book, pp. 47–48.

241. **Pećina, M., Bojanić, I., and Hašpl, M.** Overuse injuries of the knee joint. *Arch. Indust. Hyg. Toxicol.*, 2001; 52: 429–440.

242. **Perrugia, L., Pastacchini, F., and Ippolito, E.** *The Tendons: Biology, Pathology, Clinical Aspects.* Milan: Editrice Kurtis, 1986.

243. **Popp, J.E., Yu, J.S., and Kaeding, C.C.** Recalcitrant patellar tendinitis. Magnetic resonance imaging, histologic evaluation, and surgical treatment. *Am. J. Sports Med.*, 1997; 25: 218–222.

244. **Powell, R.S., Wilson, J.S., and Shall, L.M.** Bilateral bony avulsion at the inferior patellar pole in a patient with jumper's knee. *Am. J. Knee Surg.*, 1998; 11: 189–191.

245. **Ribarić, G., Pećina, H.I., and Pećina, M.** Jumper's knee — comparison of clinical, radiological and sonographic findings. *Croat. J. Sport Med.*, 1996; 11: 67–75.

246. **Reiff, D.B., Heenan, S.D., and Heron, C.W.** MRI appearances of the asymptomatic patellar tendon on gradient echo imaging. *Skel. Radiol.*, 1995; 24: 123–126.

247. **Richards, D.P., Ajemian, S.V., Wiley, J.P., and Zernicke, R.F.** Knee joint dynamics predict patellar tendinitis in elite volleyball players. *Am. J. Sports Med.*, 1996; 24: 678–683.

248. **Richardson, M.I., Selby, B., Montana, M.A., and Mack, L.A.** Ultrasonography of the knee. *Radiol. Clin. North Am.*, 1988; 26: 63–75.

249. **Roels, J., Martens, M., Mulier, J.C., and Burssens, A.** Patellar tendinitis (jumper's knee). *Am. J. Sports Med.*, 1978; 6: 362–368.

250. **Romeo, A.A. and Larson, V.R.** Arthroscopic treatment of infrapatellar tendonitis. *Arthroscopy*, 1999; 15: 341–345.

251. **Rosenberg, J.M. and Whitaker, J.H.** Bilateral infrapatellar tendon rupture in a patient with jumper's knee. *Am. J. Sports Med.*, 1991; 19: 94–95.

252. **Sala, H.** Jumper's knee: diagnosis and treatment. *Acta Orthop. Scand.*, 1985; 56: 450.

253. **Sanchis-Alfonso, V., Rosello-Sastre, E., and Subias-Lopez, A.** Neuroanatomic basis for pain in patellar tendinosis ("jumper's knee"): a neuroimmunohistochemical study. *Am. J. Knee Surg.*, 2001; 14: 174–177.

254. **Schmidt, D.R. and Henry, J.H.** Stress injuries of the adolescent extensor mechanism. *Clin. Sports Med.*, 1989; 8: 343–357.

255. **Schmid, M.R., Hodler, J., Cathrein, P. et al.** Is impingement the cause of jumper's knee? Dynamic and static magnetic resonance imaging of patellar tendinitis in an open-configuration system. *Am. J. Sports Med.*, 2002; 30: 388–395.

256. **Shalaby, M. and Almekinders, L.C.** Patellar tendinitis: the significance of magnetic resonance imaging findings. *Am. J. Sports Med.*, 1999; 27: 345–349.

257. **Shelbourne, K.D.** Personal communication.

258. **Siwek, C.W. and Rac, P.Y.** Ruptures of the extensor mechanism of the knee joint. *J. Bone Joint Surg.*, 1981; 63(A): 932–937.

259. **Smith, A.D., Stround, L., and McQueen, C.** Flexibility and anterior knee pain in adolescent elite figure skaters. *J. Pediatr. Orthop.*, 1991; 11: 77–82.

260. **Sommer, H.** Patellar chondropathy and apicitis and muscle imbalances of the lower extremities in competitive sports. *Sports Med.*, 1988; 5: 386–394.

261. **Stanish, W.D., Rubinovich, R.M., and Curwin, S.** Eccentric exercise in chronic tendinitis. *Clin. Orthop.*, 1986; 208: 65–68.

262. **Teitz, C.C.** Ultrasonography in the knee. Clinical aspects. *Radiol. Clin. North Am.*, 1988; 26: 55–62.

263. **Terry, G.C.** The anatomy of the extensor mechanism. *Clin. Sports Med.*, 1989; 8: 163–179.

264. **Tarsney, F.F.** Catastrophic jumper's knee. A case report. *Am. J. Sports Med.*, 1981; 9: 60–61.

265. **Terslev, L., Qvistgaard, E., Torp-Pedersen, S. et al.** Ultrasound and power Doppler findings in jumper's knee — preliminary observations. *Eur. J. Ultrasound*, 2001; 13: 183–189.

266. **Tyler, T.F., Hershman, E.B., Nicholas, S.J., Berg, J.H., and McHugh, M.P.** Evidence of abnormal anteroposterior patellar tilt in patients with patellar tendinitis with use of a new radiographic measurement. *Am. J. Sports Med.*, 2002; 30: 396–401.

267. **Urban, K. and Michalek, J.,** Moznosti Diagnostiky a Leceni Skokanskeno Koleno. *Suppl. Sb. Ved. Pr. Lek. Fak. Karlovy Univ. Hradci Kralove*, 1989; 32: 201–208.

268. **Van der Ent, A. and De Baere, A.J.** Jumper's knee: results of operative therapy. *Acta Orthop. Scand.*, 1985; 56: 450.

269. **Verheyden, F., Geens, G., and Nelen, G.** Jumper's knee: results of surgical treatment. *Acta Orthop. Belg.*, 1997; 63: 102–105.

270. **Voto, S.J. and Ewing, J.W.** Retrotendinous calcification of the infrapatellar tendon: unusual cause of anterior knee pain syndrome. *Arthroscopy*, 1988; 4: 81–84.

271. **Walsh, W.M., Hunrman, W.W., and Shelton, G.L.** Overuse injuries of the knee and spine in girls gymnastics. *Orthop. Clin. North Am.*, 1985; 16: 329–334.

272. **Weinstabl, R., Scharf, W., and Firbas, W.** The extensor apparatus of the knee joint and its peripheral vasti: anatomic investigation and clinical relevance. *Surg. Radiol. Anat.*, 1989; 11: 17–22.

273. **Wirth, M.A. and De Lee, J.C.** The history and classification of knee braces. *Clin. Sports Med.,* 1990; 9: 731–741.
274. **Witvrouw, E., Bellemans, J., Lysens, R., Danneels, L., and Cambier, D.** Intrinsic risk factors for the development of patellar tendinitis in an athletic population. A two-year prospective study. *Am. J. Sports Med.,* 2001; 29: 190–195.
275. **Yu, J.S., Popp, J.E., Kaeding, C.C., and Lucas, J.** Correlation of MR imaging and pathologic findings in athletes undergoing surgery for chronic patellar tendinitis. *Am. J. Roentgenol.,* 1995; 165: 115–118.

Iliotibial Band Friction Syndrome

276. **Andrews, J.R.** Overuse syndromes of the lower extremity. *Clin. Sports Med.,* 1983; 2: 137–148.
277. **Bojanić, I., Pećina, M., and Ribarić, G.** Sindrom trenja iliotibijalnog traktusa. *Acta Orthop. Lugosl.,* 1989; 20: 68–75.
278. **Bonaldi, V.M., Chhem, R.K., Drolet, R. et al.** Iliotibial band friction syndrome: sonographic findings. *J. Ultrasound Med.,* 1998; 17: 257–260.
279. **Brody, D.M.** Running injuries. *Clin. Symp.,* 1987; 39: 1–36.
280. **Cook, S.D., Brinker, M.R., and Pocke, M.** Running shoes: their relationship to running injuries. *Sports Med.,* 1990; 10: 1–8.
281. **Drogest, J.O., Rossvoll, I., and Grontvedt, T.** Surgical treatment of iliotibial band friction syndrome. A retrospective study of 45 patients. *Scand. J. Med. Sci. Sports,* 1999; 9: 296–298.
282. **Ekman, E.F., Pope, T., Martin, D.F., and Curl, W.W.** Magnetic resonance imaging of iliotibial band syndrome. *Am. J. Sports Med.,* 1994; 22: 851–854.
283. **Firer, P.** Aetiology and results of treatment of iliotibial band friction syndrome, paper presented at 6th Cong. Int. Soc. Knee, Rome, 1989.
284. **Grana, W.A. and Coniglione, T.C.** Knee disorders in runners. *Phys. Sportsmed.,* 1985; 13: 127–133.
285. **Hodge, J.C.** Clinics in diagnostic imaging. Iliotibial band syndrome. *Singapore Med. J.,* 1999; 40: 547–549.
286. **Holmes, J.C., Pruitt, A.L., and Whalen, N.J.** Iliotibial band syndrome in cyclists. *Am. J. Sports Med.,* 1993; 21: 419–424.
287. **James, S.L.** Running injuries to the knee. *J. Am. Acad. Orthop. Surg.,* 1995; 3: 309–318.
288. **Jones, D.C. and James, S.L.** Overuse injuries of the lower extremity. *Clin. Sports. Med.,* 1987; 6: 273–290.
289. **Jordaan, G. and Schwellnus, M.P.** The incidence of overuse injuries in military recruits during basic military training. *Mil. Med.,* 1994; 159: 421–426.
290. **Kaplan, E.B.** The iliotibial tract. *J. Bone Joint Surg.,* 1958; 40(A): 817–832.
291. **Kirk, K.L., Kuklo, T., and Klemme, W.** Iliotibial band friction syndrome. *Orthopaedics,* 2000; 23: 1209–1214.
292. **Kujala, U.M., Kvist, M., and Osterman, K.** Knee injuries in athletes. *Sports Med.,* 1986; 3: 447–460.
293. **Lehman, W.L.** Overuse syndromes in runners. *AFP,* 1984; 29: 157–161.
294. **Lindenberg, G., Pinshaw, R., and Noakes, T.D.** Iliotibial band friction syndrome in runners. *Phys. Sportsmed.,* 1984; 12: 118–130.
295. **Lysholm, J. and Wikllander, J.** Injuries in runners. *Am. J. Sports Med.,* 1987; 15: 168–171.
296. **Macintyre, J.G., Taunton, J.E., Clement, D.B. et al.** Running injuries: a clinical study of 4,173 cases. *Clin. J. Sport Med.,* 1991; 1: 81–87.
297. **Martens, M., Libbrecht, P., and Burssens, A.** Surgical treatment of the iliotibial band friction syndrome. *Am. J. Sports Med.,* 1989; 17: 651–654.
298. **Marti, B., Vader, J.P., Minder, C.E., and Abelin, T.** On the epidemiology of running injuries. *Am. J. Sports Med.,* 1988; 16: 285–294.
299. **Mattalino, A.J., Deese, J.M., and Campbell, E.D.** Office evaluation and treatment of lower extremity injuries in the runner. *Clin. Sports Med.,* 1989; 8: 461–475.
300. **McKenzie, D.C., Clement, D.B., and Taunton, J.E.** Running shoes, orthotics and injuries. *Sports Med.,* 1985; 2: 334–347.
301. **McNicol, K., Taunton, J.E., and Clement, D.B.** Iliotibial tract friction syndrome in athletes. *Can. J. Appl. Sport Sci.,* 1981; 6: 76–80.

302. **Messiert, S.P., Edwards, D.G., Martin, D.F. et al.** Etiology of iliotibial band friction syndrome in distance runners. *Med. Sci. Sports Exerc.*, 1995; 27: 951–960.
303. **Micheli, L.J.** Lower extremity overuse injuries. *Acta Med. Scand. Suppl.*, 1986; 711: 171–177.
304. **Muhle, C., Ahn, J.M., Yeh, L. et al.** Iliotibial band friction syndrome: MR imaging findings in 16 patients and arthrographic study of six cadaveric knees. *Radiology*, 1999; 212: 103–110.
305. **Newell, S.G. and Bramwell, S.T.** Overuse injuries to the knee in runners. *Phys. Sportsmed.*, 1984; 12: 80–92.
306. **Nishimura, G., Yamamoto, M., Tamai, K., Takahashi, J., and Uetani, M.** MR findings in iliotibial band syndrome. *Skel. Radiol.*, 1997; 26: 533–537.
307. **Noble, C.A.** The treatment of iliotibial band friction syndrome. *Br. J. Sports Med.*, 1979; 13: 51–54.
308. **Noble, C.A.** Iliotibial band friction syndrome in runners. *Am. J. Sports Med.*, 1980; 8: 232–234.
309. **Orava, S.** Iliotibial tract friction syndrome in athletes — an uncommon exertion syndrome on the lateral side of the knee. *Br. J. Sports Med.*, 1978; 12: 69–73.
310. **Orchard, J.W., Fricker, P.A., Abud, A.T., and Mason, B.R.** Biomechanics of iliotibial band friction syndrome in runner. *Am. J. Sports Med.*, 1996; 24: 375–379.
311. **Pećina, M., Bilić, R., and Buljan, M.** Tractus iliotibialis sindrom — koljeno trkaca. *Acta Orthop. Iugosl.*, 1984; 15: 91–93.
312. **Powell, K.E., Kohl, H.W., Caspersen, C.J. et al.** An epidemiological perspective on the causes of running injuries. *Phys. Sportsmed.*, 1986; 14: 100–114.
313. **Reid, D.C.** Prevention of hip and knee injuries in ballet dancers. *Sports Med.*, 1988; 6: 295–307.
314. **Renne, J.W.** The iliotibial band friction syndrome. *J. Bone Joint Surg.*, 1975; 57A: 1110–1111.
315. **Rovere, G.D., Webb, L.X., Cristina, A.G. et al.** Musculoskeletal injuries in theatrical dance students. *Am. J. Sports Med.*, 1983; 11: 195–198.
316. **Schwellnus, M.P., Theunissen, L., Noakes, T.D., and Reinach, S.G.** Anti-inflammatory and com-bined anti-inflammatory/analgesic medication in the early management of iliotibial band friction syndrome. A clinical trial. *S. Afr. Med. J.*, 1991; 79: 602–606.
317. **Staff, P.H. and Nilsson, S.** Tendoperiostitis in the lateral femoral condyle in long-distance runners. *Br. J. Sports Med.*, 1980; 14: 38–40.
318. **Sutker, A.N., Barber, F.A., Jackson, D.W. et al.** Iliotibial band syndrome in distance runners. *Sports Med.*, 1985; 2: 447–451.
319. **Taunton, J.E., McKenzie, D.C., and Clement, D.B.** The role of biomechanics in the epidemiology of injuries. *Sports Med.*, 1988; 6: 107–120.
320. **Taunton, J.E., Ryan, M.B., Clement, D.B. et al.** A retrospective case-control analysis of 2002 running injuries. *Br. J. Sports Med.*, 2002; 36: 95–101.
321. **Terry, G.C., Hughston, J.C., and Norwood, L.A.** The anatomy of the iliopatellar band and iliotibial tract. *Am. J. Sports Med.*, 1986; 14: 39–45.
322. **Weiss, B.D.** Nontraumatic injuries in amateur long distance bicyclists. *Am. J. Sports Med.*, 1985; 13: 187–192.

Breaststroker's Knee

323. **Costill, D.L., Maglischo, W.E., and Richardson, B.A.** *Handbook of Sports Medicine and Science Swimming.* Oxford: Blackwell Scientific Publications, 1992.
324. **Johnson, J.E., Sim, F.H., and Scott, S.G.** Musculoskeletal injuries in competitive swimmers. *Mayo Clin. Proc.*, 1987; 62: 289–304.
325. **Jones, J.H.** Swimming overuse injuries. *Phys. Med. Rehabil. Clin. North Am.*, 1999; 10: 77–94.
326. **Kenal, K.A. and Knapp, L.D.** Rehabilitation of injuries in competitive swimmers. *Sports Med.*, 1996; 22: 337–347.
327. **Kennedy, J.C. and Hawkins, R.J.** Breaststroker's knee. *Phys. Sportsmed.*, 1974; 2: 33–38.
328. **Keskinen, K., Eriksson, E., and Komi, P.** Breaststroke swimmer's knee. *Am. J. Sports Med.*, 1980; 8: 228–231.
329. **McMaster, W.C.** Swimming injuries. An overview. *Sports Med.*, 1996; 22: 332–336.
330. **Rodeo, S.A.** Knee pain in competitive swimming. *Clin. Sports Med.*, 1999; 18: 379–387.
331. **Rovere, G.D. and Nichols, A.W.** Frequency, associated factors, and treatment of breaststroker's knee in competitive swimmers. *Am. J. Sports Med.*, 1985; 13: 99–104.

332. **Stulberg, S.D., Shulman, K., Stuart, S., and Culp, P.** Breaststroker's knee: pathology, etiology, and treatment. *Am. J. Sports Med.,* 1980; 8: 164–171.

333. **Taunton, J.E., McKenzie, D.C., and Clement, D.B.** The role of biomechanics in the epidemiology of injuries. *Sports Med.,* 1988; 6: 107–120.

334. **Vizsoly, P., Taunton, J., Robertson, G. et al.** Breaststroker's knee. An analysis of epidemiological and biomechanical factors. *Am. J. Sports Med.,* 1987; 15: 63–71.

335. **Wethelund, J.O. and de Carvalho, A.** An unusual lesion in the knee of breaststroke swimmer. *Int. J. Sports Med.,* 1985; 6: 174–175.

Subchapters VI through XIII

336. **Anticevic, D.** Juvenilni osteochondritis. *Jugosl. Pedijatr.,* 1989; 32(Suppl. 1): 43–47.

337. **Apostolaki, E., Cassar-Pullicino, V.N., Tyrrell, P.N., and McCall, I.W.** MRI appearances of the infrapatellar fat pad in occult traumatic patellar dislocation. *Clin. Radiol.,* 1999; 54: 743–747.

338. **Barbuti, D., Bergami, G., and Testa, F.** Ultrasonographic aspects of Sinding-Larsen-Johansson disease. *Pediatr. Med. Chir.,* 1995; 17: 61–63.

339. **Bencur, O. and Oslanec, D.** Our experience with the Osgood-Schlatter disease. *Acta Chir. Orthop. Trauma,* 1990; 57: 15–20.

340. **Binazzi, R., Felli, L., Vaccari, V., and Borelli, P.** Surgical treatment of unresolved Osgood-Schlatter lesion. *Clin. Orthop.,* 1993; 289: 202–204.

341. **Bloom, M.H.** Differentiating between meniscal and patellar pain. *Phys. Sportsmed.,* 1989; 17: 94–106.

342. **Bourne, M.H., Hazel, W.A., Jr., and Scott, S.G.** Anterior knee pain. *Mayo Clin. Proc.,* 1988; 63: 482–491.

343. **Brody, D.M.** Running injuries. *Clin. Symp.,* 1987; 39: 1–36.

344. **Calpur, O.U., Tan, L., Gurbuz, H. et al.** Arthroscopic mediopatellar plicacectomy and lateral retinacular release in mechanical patellofemoral disorders. *Knee Surg. Sports Traumatol. Arthrosc.,* 2002; 10: 177–183.

345. **Clain, M.R. and Hershman, E.B.** Overuse injuries in children and adolescents. *Phys. Sportsmed.,* 1989; 17: 111–123.

346. **Dashefsky, J.H.** Fracture of the fabella: a case report. *J. Bone Joint Surg. Am. Vol.,* 1977; 59: 698.

347. **Dalton, S.E.** Overuse injuries in adolescent athletes. *Sports Med.,* 1992; 13: 58–70.

348. **Dandy, D.J.** *Arthroscopic Management of the Knee.* Edinburgh: Churchill Livingstone, 1987; 182–201.

349. **Dorchak, J.D., Barrack, R.L., Kneisl, J.S., and Alexander, A.H.G.** Arthroscopic treatment of symptomatic synovial plica of the knee. Long-term follow-up. *Am. J. Sports Med.,* 1991; 19: 503–507.

350. **Dupont, J.Y.** Synovial plicae of the knee. Controversies and review. *Clin. Sports Med.,* 1997; 16: 87–120.

351. **Duri, Z.A., Aichroth, P.M., and Dowd, G.** The fat pad. Clinical observations. *Am. J. Knee Surg.,* 1996; 9: 55–66.

352. **Duri, Z.A., Patel, D.V., and Aichroth, P.M.** The immature athlete. *Clin. Sports Med.,* 2002; 21: 461–482.

353. **Faletti, C., De Stefano, N., Giudice, G., and Larciprete, M.** Knee impingement syndromes. *Eur. J. Radiol.,* 1998; 27(Suppl. 1): 60–69.

354. **Flanagan, J.P., Trakru, S., Meyer, M., Mullaji, A.B., and Krappel, F.** Arthroscopic excision of symptomatic medial plica. A study of 118 knees with 1–4 year follow-up. *Acta Orthop. Scand.,* 1994; 65: 408–411.

355. **Flowers, M.J. and Bhadreshwar, D.R.** Tibial tuberosity excision for symptomatic Osgood-Schlatter disease. *J. Pediatr. Orthop.,* 1995; 15: 292–297.

356. **Forbes, J.R., Helms, C.A., and Janzen, D.L.** Acute pes anserine bursitis: MR imaging. *Radiology,* 1995; 194: 525–527.

357. **Frey, C., Bjorkengen, A., Sartoris, D., and Resnick, D.** Knee dysfunction secondary to dislocation of the fabella. *Clin. Orthop.,* 1987; 222: 223–227.

358. **Garcia-Valtruille, R., Abascal, F., Cerezal, L. et al.** Anatomy and MR imaging appearances of synovial plicae of the knee. *Radiographics,* 2002; 22: 775–784.

359. **Gerbino, P.G., II and Micheli, L.J.** Bucket-handle tear of the medial plica. *Clin. J. Sports Med.*, 1996; 6: 265–268.
360. **Glynn, M.K. and Regan, B.F.** Surgical treatment of Osgood-Schlatter's disease. *J. Pediatr. Orthop.*, 1983; 3: 216–219.
361. **Grana, W.A. and Coniglione, T.C.** Knee disorders in runners. *Phys. Sportsmed.*, 1985; 15: 127–133.
362. **Handy, J.R.** Anserine bursitis: a brief review. *South Med. J.*, 1997; 90: 376–377.
363. **Hardaker, W.T., Whipple, T.L., and Bassett, F.H., III.** Diagnosis and treatment of the plica syndrome of the knee. *J. Bone Joint Surg.*, 1980; 62(A): 221–225.
364. **Hess, G.P., Cappiello, W.L., and Poole, R.M.** Prevention and treatment of overuse tendon injuries. *Sports Med.*, 1989; 8: 371–384.
365. **Houghton-Allen, B.W.** In the case of the fabella a comparison view of the other knee is unlikely to be helpful. *Aust. Radiol.*, 2001; 45: 318–319.
366. **Hulkko, A. and Orava, S.** Stress fractures in athletes. *Int. J. Sports Med.*, 1987; 8: 221–226.
367. **Hur, J., Damron, T.A., Vermont, A.I., and Mathur, S.C.** Fibroma of the tendon sheath of the infrapatellar fat pad. *Skel. Radiol.*, 1999; 28: 407–410.
368. **Jacobson, K.E. and Flandry, F.C.** Diagnosis of anterior knee pain. *Clin. Sports Med.*, 1989; 8: 179–195.
369. **Jacobson, J.A., Lenchik, L., Ruhoy, M.K., Schweitzer, M.E., and Resnick, D.** MR imaging of the infrapatellar fat pad of Hoffa. *Radiographics*, 1997; 17: 675–691.
370. **Jee, W.H., Choe, B.Y., Kim, J.M., Song, H.H., and Choi, K.H.** The plica syndrome: diagnostic value of MRI with arthroscopic correlation. *J. Comput. Assist. Tomogr.*, 1998; 22: 814–818.
371. **Johnson, D.P., Eastwood, D.M., and Witherow, P.J.** Symptomatic synovial plicae of the knee. *J. Bone Joint Surg. Am. Vol.*, 1993; 75: 1485–1496.
372. **Kang, I. and Han, S.W.** Anserine bursitis in patients with osteoarthritis of the knee. *South Med. J.*, 2000; 93: 207–209.
373. **Kerlan, R.K. and Glousman, R.E.** Tibial collateral ligament bursitis. *Am. J. Sports Med.*, 1988; 16: 344–346.
374. **Kim, S.J. and Choe, W.S.** Arthroscopic findings of the synovial plicae of the knee. *Arthroscopy*, 1997; 13: 33–41.
375. **Kim, S.J., Kim, J.Y., and Lee, J.W.** Pathologic infrapatellar plica. *Arthroscopy*, 2002; 18: E25.
376. **Kobayashi, Y., Murakami, R., Tajima, H. et al.** Direct MR arthrography of plica synovialis medio-patellaris. *Acta Radiol.*, 2001; 42: 286–290.
377. **Kosarek, F.J. and Helms, C.A.** The MR appearance of the infrapatellar plica. *Am. J. Roentgenol.*, 1999; 172: 481–484.
378. **Koubaa, M., Laudrin, P., Bauer, T., Rousselin, B., and Hardy, P.** Arthroscopic treatment of intra-articular ganglion cyst of the infra-patellar fat pad. *Rev. Chir. Orthop.*, 2002; 88: 721–724.
379. **Krause, B.L., Williams, J.P.R., and Catterall, A.** Natural history of Osgood-Schlatter disease. *J. Pediatr. Orthop.*, 1990; 10: 65–68.
380. **Kujala, U.M., Kvist, M., and Heinonen, O.** Osgood-Schlatter's disease in adolescent athletes. *Am. J. Sports Med.*, 1985; 13: 236–241.
381. **Kujala, U.M., Kvist, M., and Osterman, K.** Knee injuries in athletes. *Sports Med.*, 1986; 3: 447–460.
382. **Kuur, E.** Painful fabella. A case report with review of the literature. *Acta Orthop. Scand.*, 1986; 57: 453–454.
383. **Legendre, P., Fowles, J.W., and Godin, C.** Chondromalacia of the fabella: a case report. *Can. J. Surg.*, 1986; 29: 102–103.
384. **Lehman, W.L.** Overuse syndrome in runners. *AFP*, 1984; 29: 157–161.
385. **Magi, M., Branca, A., Bucca, C., and Langerame, V.** Hoffa disease. *Ital. J. Orthop. Traumatol.*, 1991; 17: 211–216.
386. **Main, W.K. and Hershman, E.B.** Chronic knee pain in active adolescents. *Phys. Sportsmed.*, 1992; 20: 139–156.
387. **Marks, P.H., Cameron, M., and Regan, W.** Fracture of the fabella: a case of posterolateral knee pain. *Orthopedics*, 1998; 21: 713–714.
388. **Mattalino, A.J., Deese, J.M., and Campbell, E.D.** Office evaluation and treatment of lower extremity injuries in the runner. *Clin. Sports Med.*, 1989; 8: 461–475.

389. **McKeag, D.B. and Dolan, C.** Overuse syndrome of the lower extremity. *Phys. Sportsmed.,* 1989; 17: 108–123.

390. **Medlar, R.C. and Lyne, D.E.** Sinding-Larson-Johansson disease. *J. Bone Joint Surg.,* 1978; 60(A): 1113–1116.

391. **Meier, J.L.** Popliteal tenosynovitis in athletes apropos of 12 cases. *Schweiz. Z. Sportmed.,* 1986; 34: 109–112.

392. **Micheli, L.J.** The traction apophysities. *Clin. Sports Med.,* 1987; 6: 389–404.

393. **Mital, M.A., Matza, R.A., and Cohen, J.** The so-called unresolved Osgood-Schlatter lesion: a concept based on fifteen surgically treated lesions. *J. Bone Joint Surg. Am. Vol.,* 62: 732–739.

394. **Morini, G., Chiodi, E., Centanni, F., and Gattazzo, D.** Hoffa's disease of the adipose pad: magnetic resonance versus surgical findings. *Radiol. Med.* (Torino), 1998; 95: 278–285.

395. **Moyen, B., Comtet, J.J., Genety, J., and De Mourgues, G.** Le syndrome de la fabela douloureuse. *Rev. Chir. Orthop.,* 1982; 68(Suppl.): 148–152.

396. **Nakanishi, K., Inoue, M., Ishida, T. et al.** MR evaluation of mediopatellar plica. *Acta Radiol.,* 1996; 37: 567–571.

397. **Newell, S.G. and Bramwell, S.T.** Overuse injuries to the knee in runners. *Phys. Sportsmed.,* 1984; 12: 80–92.

398. **Nowinski, R.J. and Mehlman, C.T.** Hyphenated history: Osgood-Schlatter disease. *Am. J. Orthop.,* 1998; 27: 584–585.

399. **O'Neill, D.B. and Micheli, L.J.** Overuse injuries in the young athlete. *Clin. Sports Med.,* 1988; 7: 591–610.

400. **Ogilvie-Harris, D.J. and Giddens, J.** Hoffa's disease: arthroscopic resection of the infrapatellar fat pad. *Arthroscopy,* 1994; 10: 184–187.

401. **Orava, S., Malinen, L., Karpakka, J. et al.** Results of surgical treatment of unresolved Osgood-Schlatter lesion. *Ann. Chir. Gynaecol.,* 2000; 89: 298–302.

402. **Osgood, R.B.** Lesions of the tibial tubercle occurring during adolescence. *Boston Med. Surg. J.,* 1903; 148: 114–117.

403. **Patel, D.** Plica as a cause of anterior knee pain. *Orthop. Clin. North Am.,* 1986; 17: 273–277.

404. **Patel, S.J., Kaplan, P.A., Dussault, R.G., and Kahler, D.M.** Anatomy and clinical significance of the horizontal cleft in the infrapatellar fat pad of the knee: MR imaging. *Am. J. Roentgenol.,* 1998; 170: 1551–1555.

405. **Pećina, M., Bojanić, I., Smerdelj, M., and Chudy, D.** Overuse injuries of the knee in basketball players. *Basketball Med. Per.,* 1990; 5: 13–25.

406. **Ray, J. M., Clancy, W.G., Jr., and Lemon, R.A.** Semimebranosus tendinitis: an overlooked cause of medial knee pain. *Am. J. Sports Med.,* 1988; 16: 347–351.

407. **Rettori, R. and Boespflug, O.** Popliteal vein entrapment, popliteal cyst, desmoid tumor and fabella syndrome. *J. Mal. Vasc.,* 1990; 15: 182–187.

408. **Rothstein, C.P., Lasorr, A., Helms, C.A., and Tirman, P.F.** Semimembranosus-tibial collateral ligament bursitis: MR imaging findings. *Am. J. Roentgenol.,* 1996; 166: 875–877.

409. **Schlatter, C.** Verletzungen des schnabelformingen Fortsatzes der oberen Tibiaepiphyse. *Beitr. Z. Klin. Chir. Tubing.,* 1903; 38: 874–878.

410. **Schmidt, D.R. and Henry, J.H.** Stress injuries of the adolescent extensor mechanism. *Clin. Sports Med.,* 1989; 8: 343–355.

411. **Segal, P. and Jacob, M.** *The Knee.* London: Wolfe Medical Publications, 1989; 63–144.

412. **Segawa, H., Omori, G., and Koga, Y.** Multiple osteochondroses of bilateral knee joints. *J. Orthop. Sci.,* 2001; 6: 286–289.

413. **Tang, G., Niitsu, M., Ikeda, K., Endo, H., and Itai, Y.** Fibrous scar in the infrapatellar fat pad after arthroscopy: MR imaging. *Radiat. Med.,* 2000; 18: 1–5.

414. **Taunton, J.E., McKenzie, D.C., and Clement, D.B.** The role of biomechanics in the epidemiology of injuries. *Sports Med.,* 1988; 6: 107–120.

415. **Tehranzadeh, J.** Avulsion and avulsion-like injuries of the musculoskeletal system, in *Avulsion and Stress Injuries of the Musculoskeletal System,* Tehranzadeh, J., Serafini, A.N., and Pais, M.J., Eds. Basel: Karger, 1989; 1–64.

416. **Trail, I.A.** Tibial sequestrectomy in the management of Osgood-Schlatter disease. *J. Pediatr. Orthop.,* 1988; 8: 554–557.

417. **Traverso, A., Baldari, A., and Catalani, F.** The coexistence of Osgood-Schlatter's disease with Sinding-Larsen-Johansson's disease. Case report in an adolescent soccer player. *J. Sports Med. Phys. Fitness*, 1990; 30: 331–333.

418. **Tyler, W. and McCarthy, E.F.** Osteochondrosis of the superior pole of the patella: two cases with histologic correlation. *Iowa Orthop. J.*, 2002; 22: 86–89.

419. **Uson, J., Aguado, P., Bernard, M. et al.** Pes anserinus tendino-bursitis: what are we talking about? *Scand. J. Rheumatol.*, 2000; 29: 184–186.

420. **Vahlensieck, M., Linneborn, G., Schild, H., and Schmidt, H.M.** Hoffa's recess: incidence, morphology and differential diagnosis of the globular-shaped cleft in the infrapatellar fat pad of the knee on MRI and cadaver dissections. *Eur. Radiol.*, 2002; 12: 90–93.

421. **Valley, V.T. and Shermer, C.D.** Use of musculoskeletal ultrasonography in the diagnosis of pes anserine tendinitis: a case report. *J. Emerg. Med.*, 2001; 20: 43–45.

422. **Weber, D., Friederich, N.F., Nidecker, A., and Muller, W.** Deep posterior knee pain caused by a ganglion of the popliteal tendon — a case report. *Knee Surg. Sports Traumatol. Arthrosc.*, 1996; 4: 157–159.

423. **Weiner, D., Macnab, I., and Turner, M.** The fabella syndrome. *Clin. Orthop.*, 1977; 126: 213–215.

424. **Weiner, D.S. and Macnab, I.** The "fabella syndrome": an update. *J. Pediatr. Orthop.*, 1982; 2: 405–408.

425. **Werlich, T.** An interesting case — calcific tendinitis of the popliteal tendon. *Z. Orthop. Ihre Grenzgeb.*, 1999; 137: 54–56.

426. **Witvoet, J.** *Lesions Osteotendineuses des Sportifs. Cahiers d'Enseignement de la SOFCOT.* Paris: Expansion Scientifique Française, 1983; 70.

427. **Windhager, R. and Engel, A.** Zur operativen Behandlung des Morbus Osgood-Schlatter. *Z. Orthop.*, 1988; 126: 179–184.

428. **Woo, C.C.** Fracture of the fabella. *J. Manipulative Physiol. Ther.*, 1988; 11: 422–425.

429. **Yamamoto, Z., Fujita, A., Minami, G., Ishida, R., and Abe, M.** Atraumatic hemarthrosis caused by a large mediopatellar plica. *Arthroscopy*, 2001; 17: 415–417.

9 Leg

I. SHIN SPLINTS (RUNNER'S LEG)

In the sports medicine literature, the appearance of pain in the lower leg while running is referred to as shin splints. The term *shin splints* is commonly used by athletes, coaches, trainers, and physicians to describe chronic pain in the area between the knee and ankle not involving the triceps surae muscle and the Achilles tendon. Currently, the term is used widely and variably, with little consensus on its definition.[7] Obviously, the causes leading to the development of this syndrome are numerous and different in etiology,[10,35,40,56,58] but all of them share a common characteristic — they are a direct consequence of long periods of excessive strain. In other words, they are classified among the large group of overuse injuries. It is our belief that the best term for this clinical entity is *runner's leg*.

Runner's leg is most commonly seen in runners and walkers, but can also be found in all other athletes (professional and recreational) who participate in athletic activities in which running, or jumping as in classical ballet,[15,19] plays an important part.[37,49,51] Even before the massive recreational jogging movement in the U.S., Slocum[52] attempted to describe the term shin splints terminologically and etiologically. According to Slocum,[52] the term shin splints describes a complex clinical entity characterized by the appearance of pain and tenderness in the anterior part of the lower leg, which occurs as a consequence of repeated excessive strain produced while walking and/or running. With the advance of knowledge and the development of various diagnostic tools, specific diagnosis and treatment of shin splints are now possible.[4,11,34,48] Because the term is no more specific than "headache" or "chest pain," the physician must be able to distinguish the various pathological conditions that cause lower leg pain in the athlete.[22] Thus, shin splints is not a specific diagnosis.[6] It is merely a descriptive term that describes chronic exertional shin pain in an athlete. The evidence seems clear that shin splint pain has many different causes and reflects the variation in anatomy. It would be preferable to describe shin splint pain by location and etiology, for example, lower medial tibial pain due to periostitis or upper lateral tibial pain due to elevated compartment pressure. This would aid communication between physicians and also direct therapy more accurately. Pearl[42] thinks that the term shin splints should be utilized only for pain localized to the posteromedial border of the tibia at the origin of the posterior tibial muscle.

Benas and Jolk[9] cite three possible causes of runner's leg: (1) stress fracture of the tibia (osseous origin), (2) myositis, fascitis, and tendinitis of the posterior tibial muscle (soft-tissue origin), and (3) periositis of the tibia. This belief is shared by a majority of other authors,[12,25] so that today the most common causes of runner's leg are thought to be the following:

1. Tibialis posterior syndrome
2. Periostitis of the tibia
3. Chronic (exertional) compartment syndrome
4. Stress fracture of the tibia

In addition to these causative factors, other predisposing factors such as popliteal artery entrapment syndrome and soleus syndrome are mentioned in the medical literature,[29,33,46] although it is our opinion that the latter represents a different clinical entity. Further, Garrick and Webb[16] report that today there exist athletes suffering from symptoms characteristic of runner's leg in whom not even the most sophisticated current diagnostic tools have been able to positively identify the causes leading to the development of this syndrome. Depending on the localization of the pain in the lower leg, Kulund[27] speaks of anterior shin splints and posteromedial shin splints. We feel, however, that for didactic and practical reasons (i.e., for purposes of prevention and therapy), it is more useful to describe the various causative factors leading to the development of runner's leg individually, as specific clinical entities of osseous, vascular, and soft-tissue origin. Batt[7] proposed that the term shin splints be recognized as generic, rather than diagnostic, and that specific conditions that currently exist under this term be differentiated. According to Ashford[5] a shin splint is a symptom, not a diagnosis. This partially contradicts the standard nomenclature of the American Medical Association, which encourages a more precise definition of the term. It uses the term to describe the appearance of pain and tenderness in the lower leg resulting from repeated running on hard surfaces or from strong and excessive use of the dorsal flexors of the foot. The diagnosis in this case should be limited to musculotendinous inflammation and would not include stress fractures or ischemic changes. The term *medial tibial stress syndrome* is also encountered in medical literature (in the terminology selected by Drez[36]). Medial tibial stress syndrome has been reported to be either tibial stress fracture or microfracture, tibial periostitis, or distal deep posterior chronic compartment syndrome.[12] According to Mubarak et al.[36] the medial tibial stress syndrome is a symptom complex seen in athletes who complain of exercise-induced pain along the distal posteromedial aspect of the tibia. Three chronic types exist and may coexist:

Type 1: Tibial microfracture, bone stress reaction, or cortical fracture
Type 2: Periostalgia from chronic avulsion of the periosteum at the periosteal-fascial junction
Type 3: Chronic compartment syndrome

Detmer[12] recommends operative treatment for resistant types 2 and 3 with a reasonable chance for athletes of return to full activity. Abramowitz et al.[1] describe five patients whose seven affected limbs required surgery.

However, in everyday clinical practice and in sports medicine literature, the term shin splints is deeply rooted and linked with the four most common causes of its development. From an etiological point of view, it is also correct to include all possible causative factors because, according to *Webster's* dictionary, the noun "shin" describes the anterior part of the leg (beneath the knee), the frontal edge of the tibia, and the lower part of the leg.

Whatever the causes leading to runner's leg, prevention of this syndrome is based on avoiding problems in training, in the surface on which the runner habitually runs, in muscle dysfunction and inflexibility, in athletic footwear, and in the biomechanics of running. According to James et al.,[23] problems and pain can appear in runners as a consequence of training errors because of anatomical factors and inadequate athletic footwear and surfaces. Orthotic shoe inserts were most effective in the treatment of symptoms arising from biomechanical abnormalities, such as excessive pronation or leg length discrepancy, in a study by Gross et al.[20] of 500 long-distance runners. According to Thacker et al.[57] the most encouraging evidence for effective prevention of shin splints involves the use of shock-absorbing insoles.

The principal symptom of runner's leg is pain, whatever the etiology. In the early stages, the pain appears exclusively after running; in later stages, tenderness and pain are present at the beginning, middle, and end of running and during normal everyday activities, including walking. Location of the pain is important and helps differentiate the various syndromes. Pain in the medial area of the distal third of the leg suggests tibialis posterior syndrome, pain along the anterolateral side of the leg indicates a chronic anterior compartment syndrome, and pain over the anterior surface of the tibia in the central (middle) leg is characteristic for tibial stress fracture. Pain that always occurs during a workout suggests a chronic (exertional) compartment syndrome, whereas pain that appears at the start of a workout and later disappears, only to reappear afterward, indicates tibialis posterior syndrome. Tenderness, swelling, and other clinical indicators are characteristic of specific causes leading to runner's leg; the specific causes are described in the following subsections.

A. TIBIALIS POSTERIOR SYNDROME

The tibialis posterior muscle originates at one end of the posterior plane of the tibia below the linea m. solei. Its muscle fibers converge distally and attach themselves to the aponeurosis, which is located in the middle of the muscle, and passes into the tendon in the distal part of the leg. The tendon passes behind the medial malleolus, below the calcaneonavicular ligament, and below the caput tali. It, to a large degree, holds up the caput tali and inserts into the navicular tuberosity, the cuneiform bones, the cuboid bone, and to the bases of the first three metatarsal bones (Figure 9.1). The anatomical description of the muscle indicates the importance of this muscle in maintaining the arch of the foot. With a pronated foot and a lowered arch, overuse of the muscle, e.g., during running, appears. This excessive pressure leads gradually to a "separation" of the muscle fibers at the insertion site of the muscle to the posterior side of the tibia. In other words, partial ruptures appear. As this is a gradual process, the symptomatology of the syndrome develops gradually.[39] Tenderness felt along the medial side of the leg, behind the medial edge of the tibia in the middle and distal thirds of the leg, is characteristic for this syndrome (Figure 9.2).

The diagnosis can be confirmed by palpation. Tenderness is limited to the localization of the pain, but a noteworthy characteristic of this syndrome is that pressure solely with the finger above the medial plane of the tibia does not produce pain. To demonstrate tenderness by palpation, the physician "slips" a finger behind the medial edge of the tibia and continues moving the finger from the proximal to the distal end of the tibia. Only by this method is tenderness produced — generally in the middle and distal thirds of the tibia and in length from 8 to 12 cm. Pain is also present during plantar flexion and inversion of the foot against resistance. Radiographic and scintigraphic examination rules out the possibility of stress fracture of the tibia, and bone scanning eliminates the possibility of tibial periostitis.

The initial treatment of runner's leg, of any etiology, is cessation of painful activities. The treatment, among other things, depends on the stage of development of the syndrome. If, for

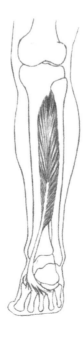

FIGURE 9.1 Tibialis posterior muscle.

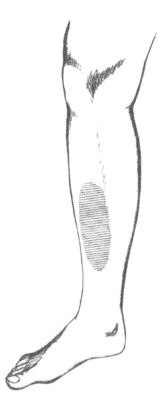

FIGURE 9.2 Characteristic area of pain/tenderness in cases of tibialis posterior muscle syndrome.

example, pain is present during everyday activities, the physician should recommend complete rest; in other words, non-weight-bearing crutch ambulation is indicated. Treatment of tibialis posterior syndrome in the beginning stages corresponds to the standard treatment for all overuse injuries: nonsteroidal anti-inflammatory drugs and other procedures such as ultrasound and high-intensity galvanic stimulation performed with the aim of reducing pain. The most important aspect of the treatment is, however, performance of stretching and strengthening exercises for the muscles and correction of static deformation of the foot with adequate arch supports and running shoes. Depending on the stage of the syndrome, cessation of athletic activities should last for a period of 1 to 2 weeks, after which the athlete is allowed to resume training, slowly increasing the speed of running and the daily mileage. With adequate stretching exercises and modification of footwear, tibialis posterior syndrome will not recur. Of course, the patient should continue to avoid the errors that lead to runner's leg. As a note of interest, there has been an attempt, in analogy with the treatment for tennis elbow, to treat runner's leg with the application of an adhesive tape or bandage that is wrapped firmly around the leg, 5 to 10 cm proximally from the malleolus.

B. Periostitis of the Tibia (Tibial Periostitis)

This term is often used by athletes and coaches when symptoms of runner's leg appear, regardless of the real cause of the syndrome. However, this term should be used only to describe periosteal changes on the anteromedial plane of the tibia, in the area approximately 10 cm above the ankle, and 5 to 10 cm in length. The appearance of pain and the development of the syndrome are similar to tibialis posterior muscle syndrome; it is most often encountered in long-distance runners and in runners who habitually run on hard, unyielding surfaces such as asphalt.[43]

During physical examination, tenderness immediately below the skin on the anterior side of the tibia is evident, and in some cases a slight swelling and thickening above the bone can also be

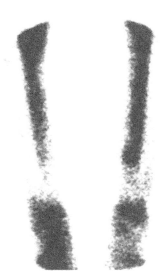

FIGURE 9.3 Bone scan demonstrating tibial periostitis.

noticed. Tibial periostitis is approximately ten times less frequently encountered than tibialis posterior syndrome. The correct etiopathogenetic explanation for its development is not yet known, although there are some indications that areas of microbleeding immediately below the periosteum are connected with the development of this injury. Bone scan can help in differential diagnosis between periostitis and stress fracture (Figure 9.3). The typical image of periostitis shows linear, vertically oriented increased uptake seen only on the delayed images.[2,16] Nielsen et al.[38] present a scintigraphic study of 29 cases of tibial periosteal reactions in soldiers and concluded that radiographs were not as sensitive as scintigraphs for differentiating the periosteal injuries seen in this study. According to Anderson et al.[3] patients with acute shin splints have a spectrum of magnetic resonance (MR) findings, which suggests this clinical entity is part of a continuum of stress response in bone. The strong association between chronic symptoms and a normal-appearing MR image implies that this modality has less utility in these patients.[32] A prospective controlled study performed by Batt et al.[8] of diagnostic imaging for acute shin splints showed that MR imagining may be used rather than triple-phase bone scan and radiographs for evaluating acute tibial pain in athletes. The type of tibial periostitis that is one of the four most frequent causes of runner's leg is periostitis on the anterior plane of the tibia. Pathological changes on the periosteum, caused by excessive pulling of the muscle fibers of the tibialis posterior muscle, are part of the clinical picture of tibialis posterior syndrome. Periostitis at the insertion site of the medial half of the soleus muscle, on the posterior side of the tibia (soleus syndrome), is part of the clinical picture and one of the causative factors of medial tibial stress syndrome.[33]

Treatment of tibial periostitis consists primarily of discontinuing activities that provoke the symptoms. Icing and nonsteroidal anti-inflammatory drugs usually produce good results. As soon as the symptoms disappear, the patient is encouraged to continue running on softer, more yielding surfaces — grass or athletic track made of synthetic materials. Strain (speed of running and daily mileage) should be increased gradually. Special consideration should be given to everyday and athletic footwear, particularly to the heel, which must absorb impact from the surface.

C. CHRONIC (EXERTIONAL) COMPARTMENT SYNDROME

The muscles of the lower leg are enveloped in the lower leg fascia (fascia cruris), from which extensions in the form of dividing walls (septa) extend deep into the leg and attach to the anterior edge of the fibula — septum intermusculare cruris anterius — and to the posterior edge of the fibula — septum intermusculare cruris posterius. This has the effect of dividing the muscle of the

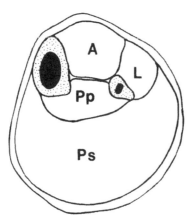

FIGURE 9.4 Schematic presentation of compartments. A = anterior; L = lateral; Ps = posterior superficial; Pp = posterior profundus.

lower leg into three compartments: anterior, lateral, and posterior. Another fascia, situated between the posterior edge of the fibula and the medial edge of the tibia, divides the muscles of the posterior compartment into two layers, a deeper layer and a shallower layer (Figure 9.4).

The etiology for chronic compartment syndrome relates in most instances to a limiting non-compliant fascia surrounding the affected muscle compartment. Sports activity leads to increased muscle volume, and if there is a noncompliant fascia, this will result in an excessive intracompartmental pressure, which interferes with muscle blood flow. If local blood is reduced to the level where it no longer meets the metabolic demands of the tissue, functional abnormalities ensue, and an exercise ischemia or exertional compartment syndrome results.

Chronic (exertional) compartment syndrome causes lower leg pain and tightness, with muscle weakness and changes in nerve sensation amplified by physical exertion. Overuse injuries trigger muscular tissue damage, fluid leakage, and increased compartment pressure, as well as ischemic muscle and nerve dysfunction under exercise stress.[45] Rest and cessation of activities typically relieve the symptoms. However, exercise triggers the process at the next exposure and a chronic pattern is established. Some athletes experience the so-called second-day phenomenon in which the amount of exercise that can be performed without pain on one day is less than the amount of exercise that could be painlessly performed on the previous day. The specific compartment involved determines the specific site of muscle weakness or paresthesia.

Lateral compartment syndrome is relatively infrequent. Analysis and measurement of intracompartmental pressure has failed to prove a significant increase in this pressure. Different opinions exist regarding the importance of posterior compartment syndrome in the development of medial tibial stress syndrome. Eriksson and Wallensten[59] have shown, for example, that normal values for pressure in the posterior compartment are found in athletes with typical medial tibial stress syndrome symptomatology. There is, however, no doubt that anterior compartment syndrome is a causative factor of runner's leg. However, it is important to differentiate between the acute type, characterized by a sudden development of ischemic changes, particularly in the tibialis anterior muscle (which is the reason it is called *tibialis anterior syndrome*), and the chronic type (chronic anterior exertional compartment syndrome), which develops gradually and belongs to the large group of overuse injuries.[43]

1. Chronic Anterior Exertional Compartment Syndrome

The etiopathogenesis and pathophysiological changes leading to the development of chronic anterior exertional compartment syndrome can best be described using the scheme compiled by Styf[54,55] (Table 9.1).

TABLE 9.1
Development of the Chronic (Exertional) Compartment Syndrome (Styf[54,55])

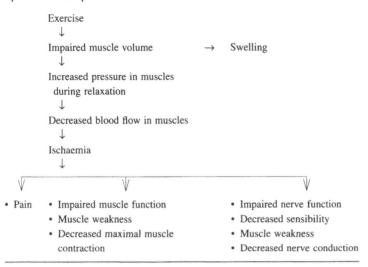

Exercise
↓
Impaired muscle volume → Swelling
↓
Increased pressure in muscles
during relaxation
↓
Decreased blood flow in muscles
↓
Ischaemia
↓

• Pain	• Impaired muscle function	• Impaired nerve function
	• Muscle weakness	• Decreased sensibility
	• Decreased maximal muscle contraction	• Muscle weakness
		• Decreased nerve conduction

The main symptom indicating the presence of this syndrome is the appearance of pain felt during athletic activities, pain that is localized along the anterior side of the lower leg (Figure 9.5), along the lateral side of the tibia, and usually in the middle third or along the whole leg. The intensity of the pain increases with time. Another characteristic of this syndrome is that the pain appears after a certain duration of activity, i.e., after a certain distance has been run. In the beginning stages of the syndrome, the athlete sometimes continues to run, disregarding the pain, which quickly worsens the symptoms. The appearance of a swelling, paresthesias in the area between the great

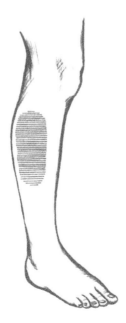

FIGURE 9.5 Characteristic area of pain/tenderness in cases of chronic (exertional) anterior compartment syndrome.

toe and the second toe, loss of active muscle strength in the anterior compartment of the lower leg, and appearance of pain during passive stretching confirm the diagnosis of this syndrome. Another characteristic of this syndrome is that during rest the symptoms can completely disappear. An objective criterion for diagnosing this syndrome is measuring the intramuscular pressure, which can be accomplished using various methods. The measurement can be taken during physical activity, but is most commonly taken during rest after physical exertion. Increased pressure after physical activity and a prolonged time for its return to normal values are considered positive indicators of the presence of chronic anterior compartment syndrome. Today, most authors agree that intramuscular pressure above 35 mmHg after physical activity and a return to normal time longer than 6 to 15 min positively confirm the diagnosis of this syndrome. However, a handheld miniature fluid pressure monitor has been developed that produces reproducible measurements of interstitial fluid, making testing potentially practical for the clinician.[17]

Non-operative treatment for this syndrome includes icing after athletic activities and reducing the level of strain. As the latter is difficult to accomplish in active athletes, most authors agree that surgical treatment (fasciotomy) is, in this case, the best solution.[4,16,27,31,41] Their reasoning is that 2 to 3 weeks after surgery, the athlete is able to continue training.[24] The fasciotomy is performed through two to three small skin incisions, through which the fascia is longitudinally cut. The whole procedure can be carried out under local anesthesia. According to Schissel and Godwin[50] the only appropriate conservative treatment is cessation of the offending activity. Early suspicion of the condition is paramount, because the definitive treatment is fasciotomy.

D. STRESS FRACTURES OF THE TIBIA

The most common localization of stress fractures of the tibia is in the area between the proximal and middle thirds of the bone. The symptoms include dull pain, localized in the same place and in a relatively small area (2 to 3 cm in circumference), and sometimes concomitant swelling. Palpation confirms the localization of the pain, which is important in differential diagnosis. In stress fractures of the tibia, the pain, whether spontaneous or caused by palpation, is always strictly localized and never diffused, which serves to differentiate this syndrome from other possible causes leading to the development of runner's leg.

In the diagnostics of stress fractures of the tibia, important auxiliary methods include radiographic examination and radionuclide scanning (Figure 9.6), with the provision that the latter can confirm the diagnosis of a stress fracture considerably before the fracture becomes radiologically visible.[8,13,14,18,30,38,53] Special emphasis must be placed on a specific type of tibial stress fracture — stress fractures of the anterior cortex of the mid-third of the tibia (Figure 9.7) — also known as

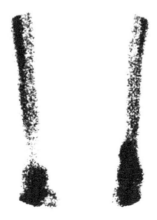

FIGURE 9.6 Bone scan demonstrating distal tibial stress fracture.

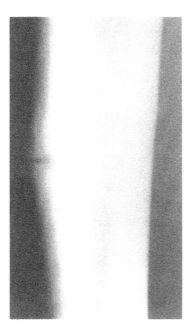

FIGURE 9.7 Roentgenogram demonstrating anterior tibial midshaft stress fracture.

anterior midshaft tibial stress fracture.[44] This fracture commonly progresses to delayed union or nonunion and frequently fractures completely. Pozderac[47] reports three cases of longitudinal tibial fatigue fractures in three runners who had exercise-related leg pain and whose clinical symptoms suggested either stress fractures or shin splints. In contrast to the focal, elliptical, cortex-based abnormal scintigraphic findings usually seen in the upper or middle tibia in patients with tibial stress fractures, all the patients had a long area of abnormal diffusely increased tibial activity that extended from tibiotalar region proximally.

Stress fracture of the fibula, which usually appears in the distal third of the fibula, is also considered by some authors to be a cause of runner's leg.

E. CONCLUSION

In conclusion, although runner's leg, or shin splints, in the past has been both a terminological and a diagnostic problem, at present this is no longer the case. Still, patients presenting with complaints of chronic exercise-induced lower leg pain can be a diagnostic challenge.[21] However, myriad specialized diagnostic studies and modalities are at one's disposal, and an emphasis on a local history and physical usually can identify the underlying cause without exposing the patient to unnecessary testing. A well-directed history and physical, coupled with an understanding of the current state of knowledge regarding the pathophysiology and pathomechanics of shin splints, help meet this challenge effectively.

II. OVERUSE INJURIES OF THE ACHILLES TENDON

A. ACHILLES TENDINITIS OR TENDINOSIS

The Achilles tendon is a common site for the development of overuse injuries. Depending on the localization of the inflammatory changes, miotendinitis, tendinitis, peritendinitis, or enthesitis can be present, according to old terminology. The new terminology recommends the following terms and definitions: *paratenonitis* — an inflammation of the paratenon; *paratenonitis with tendinosis* — paratenon inflammation associated with intratendinous degeneration; *tendinosis* —

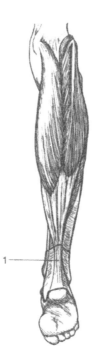

FIGURE 9.8 Muscles of the leg: triceps surae with Achilles tendon (1).

intratendinous degeneration due to atrophy (aging, microtrauma, vascular compromise, etc.); *tendinitis* — symptomatic degeneration of the tendon with vasular disruption and inflammatory repair response. Jozsa and Kannus[26] prefer to maintain the distinction between "tendinosis" and "tendinitis" so that both are considered different entities that may occur independently or together, as is the case with tendinosis and peritendinitis. Thus, they do not deny the possibility of pure tendinitis. Achilles tendinitis is the most frequently encountered entity, affecting 11% of runners and having a high frequency of recurrence.[66,89,97,101,105,111,114,117,121,136,140] Apart from runners, Achilles tendinitis is also found in other athletes, primarily those who participate in sports activities where running and jumping represent the basic components of the sport. Typical examples include basketball, handball, soccer, and tennis, as well as ballet.[79]

The Achilles tendon is the common tendon of the gastrocnemius and soleus muscles (Figure 9.8). It is the strongest tendon in the human body. It inserts on the lower half of the posterior side of the calcaneus. The insertion of the Achilles tendon is protected by two synovial bursae: (1) the subcutaneus bursa, located between the skin and the tendon, and (2) the retrocalcaneal bursa, lying between the tendon and the calcaneus. The tendon does not have a true synovial sheath (vagina synovialis), but is surrounded by a fine connective tissue sheath, the peritenon externum or the epitenon, which is continuous on its inner surface with the endotenon. In the Achilles tendon, the epitenon is surrounded by a thin, filmy layer of transparent areolar tissue, the paratenon. The paratenon functions as an elastic sleeve, permitting force movement against the surrounding tissue while maintaining continuity with adjacent structures. The epitenon and paratenon are collectively referred to as the *peritenon.*

1. Etiopathogenesis

The development of Achilles tendinitis is correlated, according to most authors, with placement of excessive force on the Achilles tendon during walking or running. The force placed on the tendon can be of different types, including stretching force (contraction of the triceps surae muscle);

compression force (the reactive force of the surface), and torsion force (walking on uneven terrain).[84,89,97,101,105,111,121,129,136,140] As the result of predisposing factors (flat or pronated foot, highly arched foot, "tight" Achilles tendon, etc.), the effects of these forces can, either individually or collectively, be increased.

The etiology of Achilles tendinitis is multifactorial. Numerous internal and external predisposing factors, acting synchronistically, lead to the development of this syndrome.[28,64,71,72,75,78,80,102,105,119,121,130,134,136,138,144] Among the many internal predisposing factors, the most frequently cited are anatomical deviations of the lower extremity, which lead to excessive and/or prolonged pronation of the foot. These include a forefoot varus, flat foot, and highly arched foot (pes cavus). Another frequently cited predisposing factor is excessive tightness of the Achilles tendon, i.e., imbalance between the strength and flexibility of the muscles that form the Achilles tendon. Vascularization of the tendon is another predisposing factor that can lead to the development of Achilles tendinitis,[69,103] because the tendon is supplied with blood at the musculotendinous junction, the bone–tendon junction, and along its length through the paratenon (small vessels from branches of the posterior tibial and peroneal arteries). Microangiographic investigations have shown that blood supply is decreased in the middle third of the tendon (2 to 6 cm above its insertion on the calcaneus). Recently, this finding has been confirmed by quantitative analysis of the number of blood vessels in the tendon.[100,103] According to many authors, this explains why the tendon is particularly prone to injury (development of tendinitis), and, accordingly, why the tendon ruptures (the final stage of Achilles tendinitis) in this area. Degeneration of the fat pad below the calcaneus is another frequently cited predisposing factor.[72,94] In this case, because of lessened impact absorption when the heel hits the surface during running, excessive force is placed on the Achilles tendon. Increased Achilles tendon strain has also been proved in individuals with unstable ankle joints. Age is another factor that plays a role in the development of overuse injury of the Achilles tendon, because, with aging, the elasticity of the tendon decreases, which increases the potential for injury.

In general, the most common cause leading to the development of overuse injuries in runners, including the development of Achilles tendinitis, is training errors. These include sudden increases in training intensity, sudden changes in the duration and/or frequency of training, and an excessively quick return to full athletic activities after a prolonged interruption in training. Running on steeply inclined or uneven terrain or hard surface also has implications in Achilles tendinitis. According to Clement et al.,[72] these causes lead to the development of Achilles tendinitis in 75% of the cases they have investigated, and Nelen et al.[121] have reported an incidence of 63% for their patients suffering from Achilles tendinitis. Inadequate running surfaces, such as hard (e.g., asphalt) or uneven surfaces, and frequent changes of running surfaces, as well as old or inadequate running shoes, also significantly increase the risk of injury.

2. Clinical Picture and Diagnostics

Achilles tendinitis can develop either suddenly, the acute form, or gradually, the chronic form (which occurs more frequently). Inflammatory changes in the tendon and/or paratenon are situated 2 to 6 cm above its insertion on the calcaneus. The main symptom is the appearance of localized pain in this area, which is typically felt during athletic activities appearing at the beginning, decreasing or disappearing during, and increasing after athletic activities. Another characteristic symptom is the appearance of pain and stiffness in the ankle joint when the patient rises from bed in the morning; this pain subsides after the first few steps. In later stages, pain impedes normal walking. Patients frequently complain that they cannot walk barefoot and feel most comfortable in shoes with higher heels. In some cases, particularly in those that develop suddenly, patients complain of "creaking" along the length of the tendon, an auditory phenomenon that they describe as similar to the sound produced when walking on freshly fallen snow.

Physical examination reveals local tenderness directly on the Achilles tendon and a local or diffuse swelling around the tendon. In some acute cases, crepitus may be felt. Detailed palpation

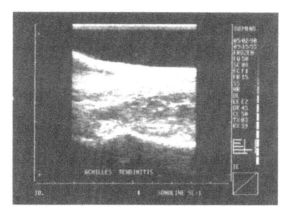

FIGURE 9.9 Sonogram of the Achilles tendon demonstrating Achilles tendinosis.

along the tendon, performed by squeezing the tendon between thumb and index finger, usually reveals one small segment that is considerably more tender than the surrounding area. Pain can also be produced by passive dorsiflexion of the ankle with the knee extended. Pain appears even more frequently during active plantar flexion against resistance. This is tested by having the patient stand on tiptoe. Pain typically appears when the patient tries to stand on tiptoe on the injured leg. Less frequently, pain appears when the physician applies resistance (by pressing down on the patient's shoulders) while the patient attempts to stand on tiptoe. In acute cases of Achilles tendinitis, a localized swelling around the tendon is frequently found, whereas chronic cases are characterized by the presence of diffuse swelling, which is felt during palpation as a thickening around the tendon. The latter are, in fact, fibrous extensions, which Pećina[83] calls *tendon scarf*. Palpable and visible masses within the tendon (nodular swelling), representing swollen, poorly healed partial ruptures, can occasionally be observed.

Physical examination should also be directed toward identifying anatomical deviations of the foot and/or ankle. These include a forefoot varus, a varus position of the heel, a valgus position of the heel, flat foot (pes planovalgus), and highly arched foot (pes cavus). For these reasons, adequate footwear is of the utmost importance — old and worn-out running shoes, especially those with worn-out soles, negatively affect the biomechanics of walking and/or running.[66,68,73] An excessively worn-out outer heel edge, for example, indicates a varus position of the heel.

Radiographic analysis of the foot and distal part of the lower leg can reveal an abnormally shaped calcaneus, bony spurs on the calcaneus, and ossification of the Achilles tendon. Today, however, a complete physical examination of the Achilles tendon must also include ultrasound examination.[65,80,83,108,109,118,125] A detailed ultrasound examination of the Achilles tendon, in both the longitudinal and perpendicular direction, can reveal details in the tendon structure (Figure 9.9) and the shape of the tendon sheath, and a dynamic examination (one carried out during passive and active movements of the ankle) enables the physician to precisely diagnose possible tendon damage. Besides its use in diagnostics, thermography is also useful in monitoring the success of the prescribed treatment. Recently, MR imaging has also been used to evaluate damage and/or changes to the Achilles tendon (see Chapter 2).[126]

3. Treatment

Treatment of Achilles tendinitis is directed toward lessening or eliminating pain, controlling the inflammatory reaction, facilitating the healing process, controlling the biomechanical parameters, and completely rehabilitating the tendon as well as protecting it from further injury. Treatment is non-operative in the vast majority of cases; surgical treatment is indicated only in exceptional cases.[61,72,81,98–101,105,106,121,131,132,136] It is crucial that treatment begin as soon as possible — ideally as soon as the first symptoms appear.

a.   Non-Operative Treatment

The program for non-operative treatment includes the following:

- Short-term cessation or modification of athletic activities
- Lifting of the heel 1 to 2 cm by inserting a heel wedge
- Ice massage of the tender area
- Application of nonsteroidal anti-inflammatory drugs
- Stretching exercises and strengthening the triceps surae muscle and Achilles tendon
- Correction of predisposing factors

In the beginning stages of Achilles tendinitis, a complete cessation of athletic activities is not mandatory. Reducing the intensity of training, principally running, along with the application of other non-operative procedures is sufficient. In later stages of the syndrome, a complete rest from athletic activities, lasting at least 1 month, is mandatory. During this interval, the functional capabilities of the athlete can be maintained with alternative training — swimming freestyle and backstroke and running in deep water without touching the bottom.

Relaxing the Achilles tendon is accomplished by inserting a heel wedge and lifting the heel for a height of 1 to 2 cm. The patient must be made aware that heel wedges should be worn in all footwear; in other words, the heel must be lifted in "everyday" activities as well as in athletic ones. After treatment is completed, the height of the heel wedge is gradually decreased.

Cryotherapy is recommended in the beginning stages of Achilles tendinitis. Tender areas should be massaged with ice after athletic activities. In later stages of the injury, cryotherapy is performed two to three times daily during the first week of therapy; following this interval, various physical procedures are used (laser or ultrasound) to increase the temperature of the injured tendon. Nonsteroidal anti-inflammatory drugs, taken in maximal daily dosages, are recommended during the first 10 days of therapy.

The principal component of non-operative Achilles tendinitis therapy consists of stretching exercises. Passive stretching exercises should begin at once and (equally important) the patient must be taught how to perform them correctly (Figure 9.10). Starting with the seventh day of therapy, the patient should begin strengthening exercises for the lower leg muscles, particularly the gastrocnemius-soleus complex.

Recognizing and correcting predisposing factors plays an important part in the treatment, as well as in prevention of Achilles tendinitis. Achilles tendinitis is an excellent example of how correctly carried out prevention, targeting predisposing factors, can significantly decrease the frequency of an overuse injury in athletes. Prevention carried out with the aim of avoiding mistakes in training (i.e., avoiding sudden increases in the intensity of training), in the choice of running surface (i.e., avoiding running on uneven and hard terrain), and in the choice of athletic footwear (i.e., wearing adequate running shoes), as well as orthotic correction of biomechanical irregularities that lead to excessive and/or prolonged pronation of the foot during running, has during the time decreased the frequency of Achilles tendinitis by more than 50%. To illustrate this, we cite the results of investigations performed by James et al.[89] and Krissoff and Ferris[97] who reported an overall frequency of Achilles tendinitis in athletes suffering from sports-related injuries of, in the former investigation, 11%, and in the later investigation, 18%. The frequencies, as reported by Taunton et al.[138] and Nelen et al.,[121] constitute significantly less, around 6% of all sports-related injuries.

Corticosteroid injections into and around the Achilles tendon are contraindicated because of the risk of tendon rupture. Only in some cases of peritenonitis are these injections allowed, but

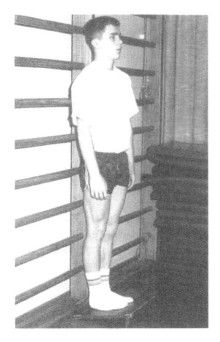
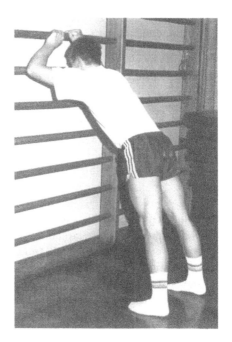
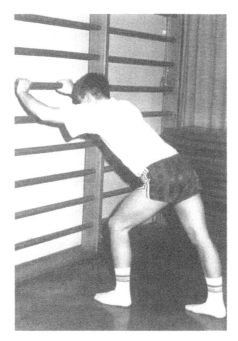

FIGURE 9.10 Various stretching exercises for the gastrocnemius-soleus complex.

only in the area around the Achilles tendon or in its sheath and never in the tendon itself (see Chapter 1, References 51 and 52).

An important point to stress is that non-operative treatment should be carried out persistently, over the course of at least a couple of months, and that surgical treatment is recommended only in resistant cases in which the symptoms fail to disappear after a long-term application of correctly applied nonsurgical therapy.

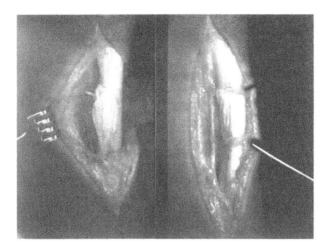

FIGURE 9.11 Intraoperative finding of inflamed peritendon sheath.

b. Surgical Treatment

Surgical treatment of Achilles tendinitis is based on the location of the pathological changes and on intraoperatively found changes in and on the tendon and tendon sheath.[61,72,81,98–101,105–107,112,121,131–133,136] If only the tendon sheath (peritendon) exhibits pathological changes, which is often the case, an adhesiolysis of the tendon is performed; the peritendon, in its entire length and circumference, is completely removed (Figure 9.11). This has the effect both of removing the injured tendon sheath and of creating a new tendon sheath, which is not pathologically changed. With regard to the latter, postoperative rehabilitation plays an important role and must strive, by means of functional adaptation, to form a new tendon sheath, while taking care not to cause irritation of the newly formed peritendon. Postoperative rehabilitation should immediately begin with the functional animation necessary for the formation of the new tendon sheath, the so-called neoperitenon of the Achilles tendon.

If the physician, during surgery, palpates degeneratively changed areas in the Achilles tendon (which could also have been discovered preoperatively, e.g., by ultrasound examination), these parts of the tendon are excised. Some authors recommend an "untangling" of that area of the tendon into fascicles, which, besides performing excision of the degeneratively changed part of the tendon, has the side effect of producing an intratendon decompression. The same procedure applies to calcificates in the tendon (Figure 9.12). However, if the calcificates are large, or if they infiltrate the tendon to such a degree that their excision will result in a significant loss of strength in the tendon, the tendon should be reinforced with tendon flaps.

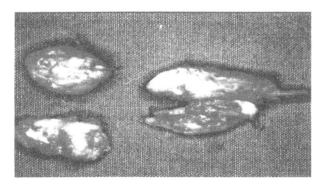

FIGURE 9.12 Calcificates removed from the Achilles tendon.

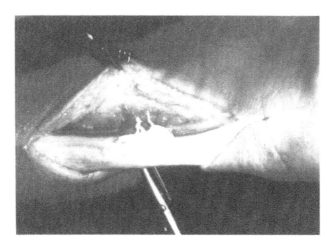

FIGURE 9.13 Intraoperative finding of iatrogenic partial rupture of Achilles tendon.

In cases with partial tendon ruptures (which can also develop as an iatrogenous consequence of corticosteroid injections into the tendon) (Figure 9.13), the injured area of the tendon is excised; in addition, depending on the size of the newly developed defect, the part is reinforced with tendon flaps. Total ruptures of the Achilles tendon, which are the result of the final stage of Achilles tendinitis, are treated surgically[96] using different operative techniques (open, percutaneous, percutaneous with mini-open, or endoscopy-assisted percutaneous repair of the tendon.[67,82,116,127,141,143]

B. Enthesitis of the Achilles Tendon

Unlike Achilles tendinitis, enthesitis of the Achilles tendon is characterized by pathological changes in the tendon–bone junction. For this reason, Achilles enthesitis is regarded as belonging to the group of insertion tendinopathies.[68,81,105,136] As with other insertion tendinopathies, a change in the tendon–bone junction zones is evident; i.e., the border between the mineralized and nonmineralized adhesive cartilage is missing (Figure 9.14) and cystic formations frequently develop. Clinically, enthesitis is differentiated from Achilles tendinitis solely by the localization of the pain; i.e., the tenderness is localized in the tendon–bone junction area. Treatment follows the same principles as in Achilles tendinitis; the only difference is that enthesitis is generally more resistant and necessitates surgical treatment more frequently. Depending on the stage of the enthesitis, various types of surgical procedures are recommended. In long-term cases with radiologically visible changes on the bone insertion site (demineralization), drilling of the bone insertion site and longitudinal cutting into the tendon at the tendon––bone junction is recommended. The aim of this procedure is to decompress the tendon and to initiate the healing process. In cases where, as a consequence of long-term enthesitis, complete tendon rupture has occurred in the tendon–bone junction area, reinsertion of the tendon through a drilled canal in the calcaneus is indicated.

C. Retrocalcaneal Bursitis and Haglund Syndrome

Retrocalcaneal bursitis is a term used to describe an inflammation of the bursa between the Achilles tendon and the calcaneus. Two bursae lie near the insertion of the Achilles tendon on the calcaneus (Figure 9.15A). The retrocalcaneal (subachilleal) bursa is located between the Achilles tendon insertion and the posterior angle of the calcaneus. The retroachilleal (subcutaneous) bursa is situated between the skin and the Achilles tendon. Retrocalcaneal bursitis may manifest as an inflammatory arthropathy (rheumatoid arthritis, seronegative spondyloarthropathies), accompany Achilles tendinitis, or occur as an isolated disorder, usually as a result of repetitive trauma due to athletic overactivity, particularly in runners. It can develop as a consequence either of irritation caused by

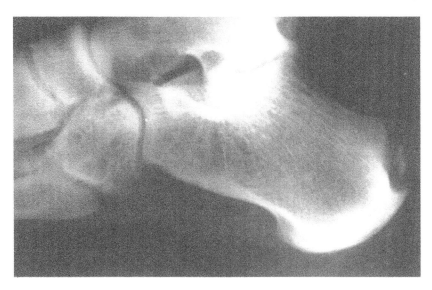

FIGURE 9.14 Ossification of the insertion of the Achilles tendon.

inadequate footwear or of a calcaneus with prominent superior and inferior ends (Figure 9.15B). Calcaneus shaped in this manner are called *Haglund's heel* and are easily visible on lateral roentgenograms.[84,85,87,88,123,128,140] If retrocalcaneal bursitis is accompanied by enthesitis of the Achilles tendon (this combination is known as Haglund syndrome or Haglund disease), tenderness is localized somewhat proximally from the insertion site of the tendon to bone and, unlike tendinitis, increases when pressure is applied. Retrocalcaneal bursitis is associated with posterior heel pain, worsened by passive dorsiflexion of the ankle. Bursal distention produces tender swelling behind the ankle with bulging on both sides of the tendon. Initial evaluation of the retrocalcaneal bursa and Haglund's heel includes radiography and ultrasonography. The retrocalcaneal and subcutaneous calcaneal bursa is not demonstrable by ultrasonography in healthy people. Exudation and proliferation of the bursa, however, facilitate detection by ultrasonography.[115] MR imaging can help establish the diagnosis by showing a bursal collection with low signal intensity on T1-weighted images and with high signal intensity on T2-weighted and STIR images.[120] Retroachilleal (subcutaneous) bursitis produces a painful, tender subcutaneous swelling, usually at the level of the shoe counter. This condition occurs predominantly in women and is generally due to local irritation from the upper edge of a rigid shoe counter. Diagnosis is essentially clinical.

Along with all the other methods of non-operative treatment that are applied in cases of tendinitis, corticosteroid injections directly into the bursa are also recommended. Occasionally, surgical treatment of retrocalcaneal bursitis and Haglund disease is indicated, in which case it consists of removing the bursa and performing an osteotomy (Figure 9.15C,D) of the prominent superior pole of the calcaneus.[62,84,87,90,91,93,110,122,135,137,140]

From 1986 to 2001, 16 active athletes, 2 of them with a bilateral condition yielding a total of 18 resected calcaneal bones, were operated on in our department in Zagreb.[124] During preoperative treatment, attention was paid to radiological measurements of the superior calcaneal angle, which is considered pathological if exceeding 75° (Figure 9.15E). Parallel pitch lines were also used to assess abnormal development of the calcaneal tuberosity (Figure 9.15F). The age of the treated athletes was from 16 to 36 years with one ultramarathon athlete aged 46 years. Two of the athletes were female. Tenderness and/or pain was present from 1 to 10 years before surgery. The athletes participated in the following sports: soccer in 5 (two bilateral) cases, basketball in 3, field hockey in 2, alpinism in 2 cases, and skiing, handball, hockey, and ultramarathon in 1 case each. All patients were operated with the same method; resection of the calcaneal tuberosity, in other words, osteotomy of the posterior calcaneus was performed from the anteroproximal to posterodistal direction, with

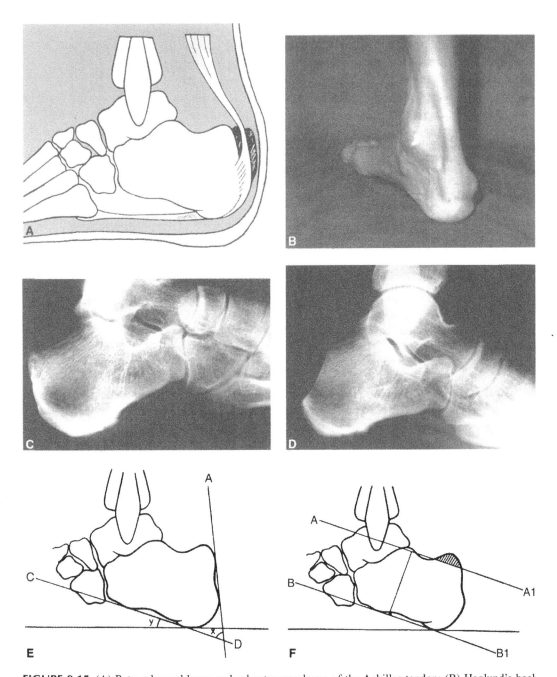

FIGURE 9.15 (A) Retrocalcaneal bursa and subcutaneous bursa of the Achilles tendon; (B) Haglund's heel in top-level basketball player; (C) preoperative roentgenogram in patient with Haglund disease; (D) postoperative roentgenogram after osteotomy of the prominent superior of the calcaneal tuberosity; (E) angles to describe Haglund's deformity, x = superior calcaneal angle, y = calcaneal inclination; (F) parallel pitch lines.

the angle of resection of about 50°. Most commonly we used the lateral paratendinous approach. The medial approach was used in cases with more prominent superolateral parts of the calcaneus. In most cases a bursectomy was also performed. The wound was closed over a suction drain that remained for 24 h. A below-knee cast was left 8 to 10 days until the cutaneous stitches were removed, after which a below-knee cast with a walking heel was put on and left for 2 weeks. This was followed by a period of physical therapy consisting primarily of stretching and strengthening. A return to full athletic activities was permitted after 2 to 6 months based on individual progress. All athletes returned to full training programs and continued competing, with some achieving their best results after surgery. Only one complication arose — in one athlete resection of the tuber was performed too deep and distal, weakening the attachment of the Achilles tendon and requiring immobilization for an additional 2 months. In two patients, in which the lateral paratendinous approach was used, some transitory damage of the cutaneous branches of the sural nerve was present. Based on our experience, we believe there is no benefit to deferring surgical treatment for longer than 1 year after the first symptoms of Haglund disease (syndrome) are noted. Adequate resection of the calcaneus is of primary importance, as is good postoperative rehabilitation. A return to full athletic activities should be based on each individual's program and rehabilitation.

Watson et al.[142] recommend a retrocalcaneal decompression for retrocalcaneal bursitis and insertional Achilles tendinitis with calcific spur. Yodlowski et al.[145] reported that 90% of patients had complete or significant relief of symptoms after surgical treatment of Achilles tendinitis by decompression of the retrocalcaneal bursa and the superior calcaneal tuberosity. Endoscopic calcaneoplasty offers access to the retrocalcaneal space, thereby making it possible to remove inflamed retrocalcaneal bursa as well as the posterosuperior part of the calcaneus in applicable cases of painful hindfoot.[76] In a study by van Dijk et al.,[76] endoscopic calcaneoplasty was performed in 21 procedures in 20 patients. One patient had a fair result, 4 patients had good results, and the remaining 15 patients had excellent results. Endoscopic calcaneoplasty is a minimally invasive technique performed in an outpatient setting and combined with a functional rehabilitation program. The procedure has low morbidity. Patients have a short recovery time and quickly resume work and sports. We agree with van Dijk et al.:[76] "Whether this operation is performed by endoscopic or open technique, enough bone must be removed to prevent impingement of the bursa between the calcaneus and Achilles tendon."

D. RUPTURE OF THE ACHILLES TENDON

The Achilles tendon is subject to the last stage of overuse injuries — total rupture of the tendon.[60,65,77,95,139] Most often, this occurs in middle-aged (30 to 50 years) males during recreational sports activities such as soccer, basketball, or jogging. In about 80% of the patients, the Achilles ruptures occur 3 to 6 cm above the calcaneal insertion where the poor blood supply may contribute to rupture. The high incidence of ruptures occurring in this midportion of the tendon could also be explained by a local variation in strain topography that causes a stress concentration at this level.[121,132] A positive diagnosis is made on the basis of history, physical examination, and ultrasound examination[80,83,118,125] (Figure 9.16 and Figure 9.17). During rupture, the patient, in addition to

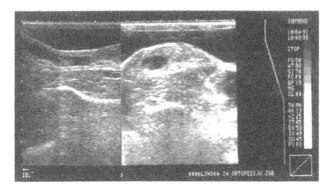

FIGURE 9.16 Sonogram of the Achilles tendon demonstrating an acute rupture.

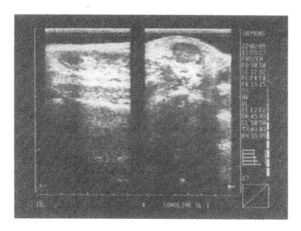

FIGURE 9.17 Sonogram of the Achilles tendon demonstrating an old rupture of the tendon.

feeling intense pain, feels "as if a stone has hit him" in the heel area. In some cases, an audible snapping sound is also heard.

Clinical signs include a painful, palpable "depression" in the Achilles tendon (Figure 9.18) and a partial or complete loss of plantar flexion. In some cases, active plantar flexion of the foot is possible, but the patient is always incapable of walking and standing on tiptoe on the injured leg. A positive Thompson "squeeze" test (loss of plantar flexion of the foot during manual compression of the lower leg muscles) is a certain indicator of tendon rupture.

The treatment of all types of acute Achilles tendon injuries (tendon strains or partial tendon ruptures, complete tendon ruptures) consists of two distinct phases, initial management and further treatment. Initial management, i.e., basic first aid, follows the mnemonic PRICES:[74] protection, rest, ice, compression, elevation, and support. Further treatment depends on injury and opinion of the surgeon and can be either non-operative or operative. In our opinion, which is shared by the other authors,[70] the best results in treating Achilles tendon rupture in young people and athletes are achieved by surgical treatment. Overall, studies support the conclusion that a complete rupture of the Achilles tendon in young active people should be treated with early surgery, whereas people involved in less strenuous recreational activities or nonathletes, especially those older than 50 years of age, can be treated primarily without surgery. Zwipp et al.[158] present long-term results that may support the use of functional treatment alone (the use of brace or splint for immobilization for 1 week, followed by a gradual increase in remobilization and rehabilitation) in complete Achilles tendon ruptures of young people as well.

The rate of Achilles reruptures varies among studies, and seems to depend on the treatment method used. In the literature, the rerupture rates following surgery have ranged from 0 to 11%, and with nonsurgical treatment from 0 to 50%.[70,104,113] A true comparison can only be made from a prospective randomized trial using a long-term follow-up study design. The prospective random-ized studies have been conducted, but with different results and conclusion.[70,86] According to Cetti et al.[70] extensive literature analysis of complete Achilles tendon ruptures, 62% of patients treated surgically and 52% of the patients treated nonsurgically were able to resume sports activities at the same level as before the injury, i.e., the difference in actual results between treatments was not very dramatic. McClelland and Maffulli[116] recommend percutaneous repair of a ruptured Achilles tendon as a safe and reliable method of treating such injuries in patients with low sporting requirements. It has a lower incidence of wound complications compared with open techniques but a slightly higher incidence of rerupture. On the basis of their results, Rebeccato et al.[127] prefer to perform the combined percutaneous and mini-open repair of Kakiuchi for the repair of acute Achilles tendon ruptures. According to Webb and Bannister[143] percutaneous repair of the ruptured tendo Achillis is simple to undertake and has a low rate of complications. A comparative study

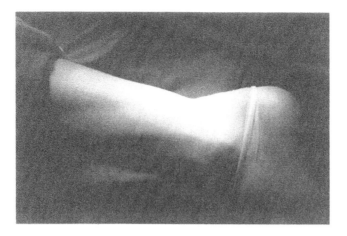

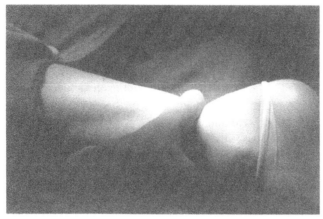

FIGURE 9.18 Characteristic clinical sign of the complete rupture of the Achilles tendon.

between percutaneous repair and open surgical repair of acute spontaneous Achilles tendon ruptures in young athletic patients is presented by Bradley and Tibone.[67] After evaluation of both subjective and objective data they recommend percutaneous repair in the recreational athlete and in patients concerned with cosmetics. Open repair is recommended for all high-caliber athletes who cannot afford any chance of rerupture. Endoscopy-assisted percutaneous repair of Achilles tendon ruptures seems to overcome certain problems of conservative, surgical, or percutaneous repair of the Achilles tendon ruptures.[141]

E. SEVER DISEASE (CALCANEAL APOPHYSITIS)

Calcaneal apophysitis (Sever disease) is a common cause of heel pain, particularly in the athletically active child. Sever disease often occurs in running and jumping sports, particularly soccer.[151] Wirtz et al.[157] described calcaneal apophysitis associated with Tae Kwon Do injuries. Patients present with intermittent or continuous heel pain occurring with weight bearing. Findings include a positive squeeze test and tight heel cords. Micheli and Ireland[153] reviewed 85 children with calcaneal apophysitis. Both heels were affected in 61% patients. The most common associated foot condition was pronation, occurring in 16 patients. In the study, 68 patients complained that pain was made worse by a specific sport, with soccer leading the list. Symptoms of pain in the region of the heel, local tenderness at the posteroinferior or inferior surface of the heel, and roentgenographic evidence of disordered ossification of the calcaneal apophysis are the classical criteria for the diagnosis of Sever disease.[152-154] Tenderness over the os calcis apophysis at the insertion of the Achilles tendon

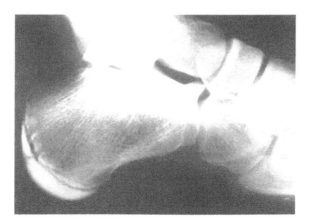

FIGURE 9.19 Typical roentgenologic findings of Sever disease.

along with a tight gastrosoleus mechanism is usually sufficient to diagnose os calcis apophysitis. This condition can frequently be bilateral. The syndrome of heel pain and tenderness localized to the os calcis apophysis in children and adolescents was first described in 1912 by Sever.[154] Sever, in his original paper, hypothesized that this heel pain was due to an inflammatory apophysitis associated with increased muscular activity in the growing child and he believed it was traumatic in origin. Roentgenograms of the feet usually show some type of disorderly ossification of the calcaneal apophysis: fragmentation, incomplete appearance, or complete formation but with increased sclerosis (Figure 9.19). There is still controversy about the significance of the radiographic changes in children with heel pain. One of the reasons is that normal children display a considerable variation in the radiographic aspects of the secondary ossification center of the calcaneus at different ages.[156] Hubbard et al.[147] present an MR imaging study of the relationship between the ossification center and cartilaginous anlage in the normal hindfoot in children. Radiography and computer-aided analysis of tomography of the os calcis in 35 children with Sever disease and of 52 control children were concurrently evaluated with histologic appearance of six calcanei of victims of road accidents, which were radiographically compatible with the same syndrome.[149] Computer-aided analysis of orientation of the "fragmentation" lines and histologic data both support the hypothesis of stress remodeling process owing to excessive bending forces acting on the calcaneal apophysis. The natural history of calcaneal apophysitis is spontaneous recovery and remodeling of an irregular apophysis and its normal fusion with the main mass of os calcis. Lokiec and Wientroub[150] reported a case of osteochondritis of the medial plantar apophysis of the calcaneus presenting as medial plantar heel pain in a 15-year-old basketball player. The lesion was detected radiographically and by increased focal uptake on bone scan. Conservative treatment resulted in complete pain relief and normal calcaneal appearance with union of the osteochondral fragment. Treatment is based on the hypothesis that the etiology of this condition is related to overgrowth. The relative increased tightness of the gastrosoleus mechanism and weakness of the dorsiflexors, when associated with repetitive microtraumas, initiate the occurrence of tiny microfractures at the junction of the apophysis with the bone.[155]

Treatment serves exclusively to modify discomfort and restore function and does not influence the natural history of spontaneous full recovery.[146,148] All children are managed with supervised therapeutic exercises, which include lower extremity flexibility and dorsiflexion strengthening, as well as the prescription of heel cups or total foot orthotics. Total foot orthotics are prescribed in children with associated biomechanical abnormalities of the foot or lower extremities, such as pronation or forefoot supination; heel cups or lifts are used in children with normal alignment and discontinued when the child becomes asymptomatic.

REFERENCES

Shin Splints (Runner's Leg)

1. **Abramowitz, A.J., Schepsis, A., and McArthur, C.** The medial tibial syndrome. The role of surgery. *Orthop. Rev.*, 1994; 23: 875–881.
2. **Allen, M.J., O'Dwyer, F.G., Barnes, M.R., Belton, I.P., and Finlay, D.B.** The value of 99Tcm-MDP bone scans in young patients with exercise-induced lower leg pain. *Nucl. Med. Commun.*, 1995; 16: 89–91.
3. **Anderson, M.V., Ugalde, V., Batt, M., Gacayan, J.** Shin splints: MR appearance in a preliminary study. *Radiology*, 1997; 204: 177–180.
4. **Andrish, J.T., Bergfeld, J.A., and Walheim, J.** A prospective study on the management of shin splints. *J. Bone Joint Surg.*, 1974; 56(A): 1697–1700.
5. **Ashford, R.** Trauma related shin splints. Shin splints are symptoms, not diagnosis. *Br. Med. J.*, 1999; 318: 1560.
6. **Bates, P.** Shin splints — a literature review. *Br. J. Sports Med.*, 1985; 19: 132–137.
7. **Batt, M.E.** Shin splints — a review of terminology. *Clin. J. Sports Med.*, 1995; 5: 53–57.
8. **Batt, M.E., Ugalde, V., Anderson, M.W., and Shelton, D.K.** A prospective controlled study of diagnostic imaging for acute shin splints. *Med. Sci. Sports Exerc.*, 1998; 30: 1564–1571.
9. **Benas, D. and Jolk, P.** Shin splints. *Am. Correct. Ther. J.*, 1978; 32: 53–57.
10. **Cibulka, M.T., Sinacore, D.R., and Mueller, M.J.** Shin splints and forefoot contact running: a case report. *J. Orthop. Sports Phys. Ther.*, 1994; 20: 98–102.
11. **Clement, D.B.** Tibial stress syndrome in athletes. *J. Sports Med.*, 1974; 2: 81–85.
12. **Detmer, D.E.** Chronic shin splints. Classification and management of medial tibial stress syndrome. *Sports Med.*, 1986; 3: 436–446.
13. **Di Leo, C., Tarolo, G.L., Aliberti, G. et al.** Stress fracture and coexistent periosteal reaction (shin splints) in a young athlete revealed by bone scintigraphy. *Nuklearmedizin*, 2000; 39: 50–51.
14. **Etchebehere, E.C., Etchebehere, M., Gamba, R., Belangero, W., and Camarga, E.E.** Orthopedic pathology of the lower extremities: scintigraphic evaluation in the thigh, knee, and leg. *Semin. Nucl. Med.*, 1998; 28: 41–61.
15. **Gans, A.** The relationship of heel contact in ascent and descent from jumps to the incidence of shin splints in ballet dancers. *Phys. Ther.*, 1985; 65: 1192–1196.
16. **Garrick, J.G. and Webb, D.R.** *Sports Injuries: Diagnosis and Management.* Philadelphia: W.B. Saunders, 1990.
17. **Gerow, G., Matthews, B., Jahn, W., and Gerow, R.** Compartment syndrome and shin splints of the lower leg. *J. Manipulative Physiol. Ther.*, 1993; 16: 245–252.
18. **Gibbon, W.** Shin splints. *Radiology*, 1998; 207: 826–827.
19. **Goertzen, M., Ringelband, R., and Schulitz, K.P.** Injuries and damage caused by excessive stress in classical ballet. *Z. Orthop. Ihre Grenzgeb.*, 1989; 127: 98–107.
20. **Gross, M.L., Davlin, L.B., and Evanski, P.M.** Effectiveness of orthotic shoe inserts in the long-distance runner. *Am. J. Sports Med.*, 1991; 19: 409–412.
21. **Hester, J.T.** Diagnostic approach to chronic exercise-induced leg pain. A review. *Clin. Podiatr. Med. Surg.*, 2001; 18: 285–306.
22. **Jackson, R., Fitch, K., and O'Brien, M., Eds.** *Sport Medicine Manual.* Lausanne, Switzerland: International Olympic Committee, 1990.
23. **James, S.L., Bates, B.T., and Ostering, L.R.** Injuries to runners. *Am. J. Sports Med.*, 1978; 6: 40–49.
24. **Jarviennen, M., Aho, H., and Nuttymaki, S.** Results of the surgical treatment of the medial tibial syndrome in athletes. *Int. J. Sports Med.*, 1989; 10: 55–57.
25. **Jones, D.C. and James, S.L.** Overuse injuries of the lower extremity. *Clin. Sports Med.*, 1987; 6: 273–290.
26. **Jozsa, L. and Kannus, P.** Human tendons. *Anatomy, Physiology and Pathology.* Champaign, IL: Human Kinetics, 1997.
27. **Kulund, N.D.** *The Injured Athlete,* 2nd ed. Philadelphia: J.B. Lippincott, 1988.
28. **Leadbetter, W.B.C.** Cell-matrix response in tendon injury. *Clin. Sports Med.*, 1992; 11: 533–578.

29. **Lysens, R.J.** Intermittent claudication in young athletes: popliteal artery entrapment syndrome. *Am. J. Sports Med.,* 1983; 11: 177–179.

30. **Macleod, M.A., Houston, A.S., Sanders, L., and Anagnostopoulos, C.** Incidence of trauma related stress fractures and shin splints in male and female army recruits: retrospective case study. *Br. Med. J.,* 1999; 318: 29.

31. **Martens, M.A. and Moeyersoons, J.P.** Acute and recurrent effort-related compartment syndrome in sports. *Sports Med.,* 1990; 9: 62–68.

32. **Meyer, X., Boscagli, G., Tavernier, T. et al.** Magnetic resonance imaging of tibial periostitis. *J. Radiol.,* 1998; 79: 45–48.

33. **Michael, R.H. and Holder, L.E.** The soleus syndrome. A cause of medial tibial stress (shin splints). *Am. J. Sports Med.,* 1985; 13: 87–94.

34. **Milgrom, C., Giladi, M., Stein, M. et al.** Medial tibial pain. *Clin. Orthop.,* 1986; 213: 167–171.

35. **Moore, M.P.** Shin splints. Diagnosis, management, prevention. *Postgrad. Med.,* 1988; 199–200, 203–205, 208–210.

36. **Mubarak, S.J., Gould, R.N., Lee, Y.F. et al.** The medial tibial stress syndrome. A cause of shin splints. *Am. J. Sports Med.,* 1982; 10: 201–205.

37. **Murtagh, J.** Pain in the leg. *Aust. Fam. Physician,* 1991; 20: 670–673.

38. **Nielsen, M.B., Hansen, K., Holmer, P., and Dyrbye, M.** Tibial periosteal reactions in soldiers. A scintigraphic study 29 cases of lower leg pain. *Acta Orthop. Scand.,* 1991; 62: 531–534.

39. **Oloff, L.M. and Schulhofer, S.D.** The tibialis posterior tendinitis/dysfunction in either early or more advanced stages. *J. Foot Ankle Surg.,* 1998; 37: 362–366.

40. **Onieal M.E.** Shin splints. *J. Am. Acad. Nurse Pract.,* 1994; 6: 214–215.

41. **Orava, S. and Puranen, J.** Athletes' leg pain. *Br. J. Sports Med.,* 1979; 13: 92–97.

42. **Pearl, A.J.** Anterior compartment syndrome: a case report. *Am. J. Sports Med.,* 1981; 9: 119–120.

43. **Pećina, M. and Bojanić, I.** Overuse injuries in track and field athletes. *Croat. Sports Med. J.,* 1991; 6: 24–37.

44. **Pećina, M. and Bojanić, I.** Compressive osteosynthesis in the treatment of tibial midshaft stress fracture. *Croat. Sportsmed. J.,* 1994; 9: 24–27.

45. **Pećina, M., Bojanić, I., and Markiewitz, A.D.** Nerve entrapment syndromes in athletes. *Clin. J. Sports Med.,* 1993; 3: 36–43.

46. **Pećina, M., Krmpotic-Nemanic, J., and Markiewitz, A.D.** *Tunnel Syndromes. Peripheral Nerve Compression Syndromes,* 3rd ed. Boca Raton, FL: CRC Press, 2001.

47. **Pozderac, R.V.** Longitudinal tibial fatigue fracture: an uncommon stress fracture with characteristic features. *Clin. Nucl. Med.,* 2002; 27: 475–478.

48. **Puranen, J.** The medial tibial syndrome. *Ann. Chir. Gynaecol.,* 1991; 80: 215–218.

49. **Rudt, R.** What is your diagnosis? Shin splints. *Schweiz. Rundsch. Med. Prax.,* 1991; 80: 281–282.

50. **Schissel, D.J. and Godwin, J.** Effort-related chronic compartment syndrome of the lower extremity. *Mil. Med.,* 1999; 164: 830–832.

51. **Sepulchre, P., Blaimont, P., and Pasteels, J.L.** Douleurs tibiales interenes chez les coureurs a pied. *Int. Orthop. (SICOT),* 1988; 12: 217–221.

52. **Slocum, D.B.** The shin splint syndrome. Medical aspects and differential diagnosis. *Am. J. Surg.,* 1967; 114: 875–881.

53. **Spencer, R.P., Levinson, E.D., Baldwin, R.D. et al.** Diverse bone scan abnormalities in "shin splints." *J. Nucl. Med.,* 1979; 20: 1271–1272.

54. **Styf, J.** Diagnosis of exercise — induced pain in the anterior aspect of the lower leg. *Am. J. Sports Med.,* 1988; 16: 165–169.

55. **Styf, J.** Chronic exercise-induced pain in the anterior aspect of the lower leg. An overview of diagnosis. *Sports Med.,* 1989; 7: 331–339.

56. **Taunton, J.E., McKenzie, D.C., and Clement, D.B.** The role of biomechanics in the epidemiology of injuries. *Sports Med.,* 1988; 6: 107–120.

57. **Thacker, S.B., Gilchrist, J., Stroup, D.F., and Kimsey, C.D.** The prevention of shin splints in sports: a systematic review literature. *Med. Sci Sports Exerc.,* 2002; 34: 32–40.

58. **Viitasalo, J.T. and Kvist, M.** Some biomechanical aspects of the foot and ankle in athletes with and without shin splints. *Am. J. Sports Med.,* 1983; 11: 125–130.

59. **Wallensten, R.** Results of fasciotomy in patients with medial tibial syndrome or chronic anterior-compartment syndrome. *J. Bone Joint Surg.,* 1983; 65(A): 1252–1255.

Overuse Injuries of the Achilles Tendon

60. **Aldam, C.H.** Repair of calcaneal tendon ruptures. A safe technique. *J. Bone Joint Surg.,* 1989; 71(B): 486–488.
61. **Anderson, D.L., Taunton, J.E., and Davidson, R.G.** Surgical management of chronic Achilles tendinitis. *Clin. J. Sport Med.,* 1992; 2: 38–42.
62. **Angermann, P.** Chronic retrocalcaneal bursitis treated by resection of the calcaneus. *Foot Ankle,* 1990; 10: 285–287.
63. **Astrom, M. and Westlin, N.** Blood flow in chronic Achilles tendinopathy. *Clin. Orthop.,* 1994; 308: 166–172.
64. **Astrom, M. and Rausing, A.** Chronic Achilles tendinopathy: a survey of surgical and histopathologic findings. *Clin. Orthop.,* 1995; 316: 151–164.
65. **Beskin, J.L., Sanders, R.A., Hunter, S.C., and Hughston, J.C.** Surgical repair of Achilles tendon ruptures. *Am. J. Sports Med.,* 1987; 15: 1–8.
66. **Bordelon, R.L.** Orthotic, shoes and braces. *Orthop. Clin. North Am.,* 1989; 20: 751–757.
67. **Bradley, J.P. and Tibone, J.E.** Percutaneous and open surgical repairs of Achilles tendon ruptures. *Am. J. Sports Med.,* 1990; 18: 188–195.
68. **Brody, D.M.** Running injuries. *Clin. Symp.,* 1980; 39: 1–36.
69. **Carr, A.J. and Norris, S.H.** The blood supply of the calcaneal tendon. *J. Bone Joint Surg.,* 1989; 71(B): 100–101.
70. **Cetti, R., Christensen, S.E., Ejsted, R., Jensen, N.M., and Jorgensen, U.** Operative versus nonoperative treatment of Achilles tendon rupture. A prospective randomized study and review of the literature. *Am. J. Sports Med.,* 1993; 21: 791–799.
71. **Clain, M.R. and Baxter, D.E.** Achilles tendinitis. *Foot Ankle,* 1992; 13: 482–487.
72. **Clement, D.B., Taunton, J.E., and Smart, G.W.** Achilles tendinitis and peritendinitis: etiology and treatment. *Am. J. Sports Med.,* 1984; 12: 179–184.
73. **Cook, S.D., Brinker, M.R., and Poche, M.** *Sports Med.,* 1990; 10: 1–8.
74. **Curl, W.W. and Martin, D.F.** Initial management of acute injuries, in *Sports Injuries: Basic Principles of Prevention and Care,* Renstrom, P.A.F.H., Ed. Oxford: Blackwell, 1993.
75. **Davidson, R.G. and Taunton, J.E.** Achilles tendinitis. *Med. Sport Sci.,* 1987; 23: 71–79.
76. **van Dijk, C.N., van Dyk, G.E., Scholten, P.E., and Kort, N.P.** Endoscopic calcaneoplasty. *Am. J. Sports Med.,* 2001; 29: 185–189.
77. **De Tullio, B., Guaganini, M., Orsi, R., and Sarda, G.** Rottura sottocutanea del tendine di Achille: trattamento chirurgico e recupero funzionale. *Riv. Patol. Appar. Locom.,* 1988; 8: 203–206.
78. **Fallon, K.E.** Musculoskeletal injuries in the ultramarathon: the 1990 Westfield Sydney to Melbourne run. *Br. J. Sports Med.,* 1996; 30: 319–323.
79. **Fernandez-Palazzi, F., Rivas, S., and Mujica, P.** Achilles tendinitis in ballet dancers. *Clin. Orthop.,* 1999; 257: 257–261.
80. **Fornage, B.D.** Achilles tendon: U.S. examination. *Radiology,* 1986; 159: 759–764.
81. **Frey, C.C. and Shereff, M.J.** Tendon injuries about ankle in athletes. *Clin. Sports Med.,* 1988; 7: 103–118.
82. **Gorschewski, O., Vogel, U., Schweizer, A., and van Laar, B.** Percutaneous tenodesis of the Achilles tendon. A new surgical method for the treatment of acute Achilles tendon rupture through percutaneous tenodesis. *Injury,* 1999; 30: 315–321.
83. **Hašpl, M. and Pećina, M.** Ultrazvucna dijagnostika koljena i potkoljenice, in *Ultrazvucna Dijagnostika Sustava za Kretanje,* Matasovic, T., Ed. Zagreb: Skolska Knjiga, 1988; 71–98.
84. **Heneghan, M.A. and Pavlov, H.** The Haglund painful heel syndrome. *Clin. Orthop.,* 1984; 187: 228–234.
85. **Hintermann, B. and Holzach, P.** Die Bursitis subachilla — eine biomechanische Analyse und klinische Studie. *Z. Orthop.,* 1992; 130: 114–119.
86. **Holch, M., Biewener, A., Thermann, H., and Zwipp, H.** Non-operative treatment of acute Achilles tendon ruptures. A clinical concept and experimental results. *Sports Exerc. Injury,* 1994; 1: 18–22.

87. **Huber, H. and Waldis, M.** Die Haglund Exostose — eine Operationsindikation und ein kleiner Eingriff? *Z. Orthop.*, 1989; 127: 286–290.

88. **Ippolito, E. and Ricciardi-Pollini, P.T.** Invasive retrocalcaneal bursitis: a report of three cases. *Foot Ankle*, 1984; 4: 204–208.

89. **James, S.L., Bates, B.T., and Ostering, L.R.** Injuries to runners. *Am. J. Sports Med.*, 1978; 6: 40–50.

90. **Jarde, O., Quenot, P., Trinquier-Lautard, J.L., Tran-Van, F., and Vives, P.** Haglund disease treated by simple resection of calcaneal tuberosity. An angular and therapeutic study. A propos of 74 cases with 2 years follow-up. *Rev. Chir.*, 1997; 83: 566–573.

91. **Jarvinen, M.** Sports traumatology expands the art of surgery. *Ann. Chir. Gynaecol.*, 1991; 80: 79–80.

92. **Jarvinen, M., Kvist, H., and Jozsa, L.** The intratendineal ossification with fracture in the Achilles tendon of the top-level athlete. *Clin. Sports Med.*, 1990; 2: 47–51.

93. **Jones, D.C. and James, S.L.** Partial calcaneal osteotomy for retrocalcaneal bursitis. *Am. J. Sports Med.*, 1984; 12: 72–73.

94. **Jorgensen, U.** Achillodinya and loss of heel pad shock absorbency. *Am. J. Sports Med.*, 1984; 13: 128–132.

95. **Jozsa, L., Kvist, M., Balint, B.J. et al.** The role of recreational sport activity in Achilles tendon rupture. *Am. J. Sports Med.*, 1989; 17: 338–343.

96. **Kahn, M.E.** Achilles tendinitis and ruptures. *Br. J. Sports Med.*, 1998; 32: 266.

97. **Krissoff, W.B. and Ferris, W.D.** Runners injuries. *Phys. Sportsmed.*, 1979; 7: 55–64.

98. **Kvist, H. and Kvist, M.** The operative treatment of chronic calcaneal paratenonitis. *J. Bone Joint Surg.*, 1980; 62(B): 353–357.

99. **Kvist, M., Lehto, M.K., Jozsa, L., Jarvinen, M., and Kvist, H.T.** Chronic Achilles paratenonitis — an immunohistologic study of fibronectin and fibrinogen. *Am. J. Sports Med.*, 1988; 16: 616–623.

100. **Kvist, M., Jozsa, L., Jarvinen, M. et al.** Chronic Achilles paratenonitis in athletes — histological and histochemical study. *J. Pathol.*, 1987; 19: 1–11.

101. **Kvist, M.** Achilles tendon injuries in athletes. *Ann. Chir. Gynecol.*, 1991; 80: 188–201.

102. **Kvist, M.** Achilles tendon injuries in athletes. *Sports Med.*, 1994; 18: 173–201.

103. **Lagergen, C. and Lindholm, A.** Vascular distribution in the Achilles tendon — an angiographic and microangiographic study. *Acta Chir. Scand.*, 1958/59; 116: 491–495.

104. **Landvater, S.J. and Renstrom, P.A.F.H.** Complete Achilles tendon ruptures. *Clin. Sports Med.*, 1992; 11: 741–758.

105. **Leach, R.E., James, S., and Wasilewski, S.** Achilles tendinitis. *Am. J. Sports Med.*, 1981; 9: 93–98.

106. **Leach, R.E.** Leg and foot injuries in racquet sports. *Clin. Sports Med.*, 1988; 7: 359–370.

107. **Leach, R.E., Schepsis, A.A., and Takai, H.** Long term results of surgical management of Achilles tendinitis in runners. *Clin. Orthop.*, 1992; 282: 208–212.

108. **Lehtinen, A., Peltokallio, P., and Taavitsainen, M.** Sonography of Achilles tendon correlated to operative findings. *Ann. Chir. Gynaecol.*, 1994; 83: 322–327.

109. **Lehtinen, A., Bondestam, S., and Taavitsainen, M.** Use of angulation in the detection of tendinitis with US. *Eur. J. Radiol.*, 1994; 18: 175–179.

110. **Lehto, M.U., Jarvinen, M., and Suominen, P.** Chronic Achilles peritendinitis and retrocalcanear bursitis. Long-term follow-up of surgically treated cases. *Knee Surg. Sports Traumatol. Arthrosc.*, 1994; 2: 182–185.

111. **Leppilahati, J., Orava, S., Karpakla, J., and Takala, T.** Overuse injuries of the Achilles tendon. *Ann. Chir. Gynaecol.*, 1991; 80: 202–207.

112. **Leppilahati, J., Karpakka, J., Gorra, A., Puranen, J., and Orava, S.** Surgical treatment of overuse injuries to the Achilles tendon. *Clin. J. Sports Med.*, 1994; 4: 100–107.

113. **Leppilahti, J. and Orava, S.** Results of surgical treatment of ruptured Achilles tendon. *Fin. J. Orthop. Trauma*, 1994; 17: 253–256.

114. **Lysholm, J. and Wiklander, J.** Injuries in runners. *Am. J. Sports Med.*, 1987; 15: 168–171.

115. **Mahlfeld, K., Kayser, R., Mahlfeld, A., Grasshoff, H., and Franke, J.** Value of ultrasound in diagnosis of bursopathies in the area of the Achilles tendon. *Ultraschall Med.*, 2001; 22: 87–90.

116. **McClelland, D. and Maffulli, N.** Percutaneous repair of ruptured Achilles tendon. *J. R. Coll. Surg. Edinburgh*, 2002; 47: 613–618.

117. **McCrory, J.L., Martin, D.F., Lowery, R.B. et al.** Etiologic factors associated with Achilles tendinitis in runners. *Med. Sci. Sports Exerc.*, 1999; 31: 1374–1381.

118. **Milbradt, H., Reiner, P., and Thermann, H.** Die Sonomorphologie der normalen Achillessehne und Muster pathologischer Veränderungen. *Radiology,* 1988; 28: 330–333.

119. **Myerson, M.S. and McGarvey, W.** Disorders of the Achilles tendon insertion and Achilles tendinitis. *Instr. Course Lect.,* 1999; 48: 211–218.

120. **Narvaez, J.A., Narvaez, J., Ortega R. et al.** Painful heel: MR imaging findings. *Radiographics,* 2000; 20: 333–352.

121. **Nelen, G., Martens, M., and Burssens, A.** Surgical treatment of chronic Achilles tendinitis. *Am. J. Sports Med.,* 1989; 17: 754–759.

122. **Nesse, E. and Finsen, V.** Poor results after resection for Haglund's heel. Analysis of 35 heels in 23 patients after 3 years. *Acta Orthop. Scand.,* 1994; 84: 734–738.

123. **Pavlov, H., Heneghan, M., Hersh, A., Goldmann, A., and Vigorita, V.** The Haglund syndrome: initial and differential diagnosis. *Radiology,* 1982; 144: 83–88.

124. **Pećina, M., Madarević, M., Pećina, H.I., and Burić, M.** Resection of calcaneus tuberosity in the treatment of Haglund's syndrome in athletes. *Croat. Sportsmed. J.,* 2000; 15: 85–91.

125. **Pfister, A.** Experimentelle und klinische Ergebnisse der Ultraschallsonographie bei sportorthopädischen Weichteilerkrankungen. *Sportverletz. Sportschaden,* 1987; 3: 130–141.

126. **Quinn, S.F., Murray, W.T., Clark, R.A. et al.** Achilles tendon: MR imaging at 1.5 T. *Radiology,* 1987; 164: 767–770.

127. **Rebeccato, A., Santini, S., Salmaso, G., and Nogarin, L.** Repair of the Achilles tendon rupture: a functional comparison of three surgical techniques. *J. Foot Ankle Surg.,* 2001; 40: 188–194.

128. **Rossi, F., La Cava, F., Amato, F., and Pincelli, G.** The Haglund Syndrome: clinical and radiological features and sports medicine aspects. *J. Sports Med.,* 1987; 27: 258–265.

129. **Saillant, G., Radinean, J., Thoraeux, P., and Roy-Camille, R.** La tendinite d'Achille. *Rev. Prat.,* 1991; 41: 1644–1649.

130. **Saltzman, C.L. and Tearse, D.S.** Achilles tendon injuries. *J. Am. Acad. Orthop. Surg.,* 1998; 6: 316–325.

131. **Santilli, G.** Achilles tendinopathies and paratendinopathies. *J. Sports Med.,* 1979; 19: 245–259.

132. **Schepsis, A.A. and Leach, R.E.** Surgical management of Achilles tendinitis. *Am. J. Sports Med.,* 1987; 15: 308–315.

133. **Schepsis, A.A., Wagner, C., and Leach, R.E.** Surgical management of Achilles tendon overuse injuries. A long-term follow-up study. *Am. J. Sports Med.,* 1994; 22: 611–619.

134. **Scioli, M.W.** Achilles tendinitis. *Orthop. Clin. North Am.,* 1994; 25: 177–182.

135. **Sella, E.J., Caminear, D.S., and McLarney, E.A.** Haglund's syndrome. *J. Foot Ankle Surg.,* 1998; 37: 110–114.

136. **Smart, G.W., Taunton, J.E., and Clement, D.B.** Achilles tendon disorders in runners — a review. *Med. Sci. Sports Exerc.,* 1980; 12: 231–243.

137. **Stephens, M.M.** Haglund's deformity and retrocalcaneal bursitis. *Orthop. Clin. North Am.,* 1994; 25: 41–46.

138. **Taunton, J.E., McKenzie, D.C., and Clement, D.B.** The role of biomechanics in the epidemiology of injuries. *Sports Med.,* 1988; 6: 107–120.

139. **Thermann, H. and Zwipp, H.** Achillessehnenruptur. *Orthopade,* 1989; 18: 321–335.

140. **Torg, J.S., Pavlov, H., and Torg, E.** Overuse injuries in sport: the foot. *Clin. Sports Med.,* 1987; 6: 291–320.

141. **Turgut, A., Gunal, I., Marlcan, G., Kose, N., and Gokturk, E.** Endoscopy, assisted percutaneous repair of Achilles tendon ruptures. *Knee Surg. Sports Traum. Arthrosc.,* 2002; 10: 130–133.

142. **Watson, A.D., Anderson, R.B., and Davis, W.H.** Comparison of results of retrocalcaneal decompression for retrocalcaneal bursitis and insertional Achilles tendinosis with calcific spur. *Foot Ankle Int.,* 2000; 21: 638–642.

143. **Webb, J.M. and Bannister, G.C.** Percutaneous repair of the ruptured tendo Achillis. *J. Bone Joint Surg. (Br.),* 1999; 81: 877–880.

144. **Williams, J.G.P.** Achilles tendon lesion in sport. *Sports Med.,* 1986; 3: 114–135.

145. **Yodlowski, M.L., Scheller, A.D., Jr., and Minos, L.** Surgical treatment of Achilles tendinitis by decompression of the retrocalcaneal bursa and the superior calcaneal tuberosity. *Am. J. Sports Med.,* 2002; 30: 318–321.

Sever Disease (Calcaneal Apophysitis)

146. **Clain, R.M. and Hershman, E.B.** Overuse injuries in children and adolescents. *Phys. Sportsmed.*, 1989; 17: 111–123.

147. **Hubbard, A.M., Meyer, J.S., Davidson, R.S., Mahboubi, S., and Harty, M.P.** Relationship between the ossification center and cartilaginous anlage in the normal hindfoot in children: study with MR imaging. *Am. J. Roentgenol.*, 1993; 161: 849–853.

148. **Katz, J.F.** Nonarticular osteochondroses. *Clin. Orthop.*, 1981; 158: 70–76.

149. **Liberson, A., Liberson, S., Mendes, D.G. et al.** Remodeling of the calcaneus apophysitis in the growing child. *J. Pediatr. Orthop. B.*, 1995; 4: 74–79.

150. **Lokiec, F. and Wientroub, S.** Calcaneal osteochondritis: a new overuse injury. *J. Pediatr. Orthop. B.*, 1998; 7: 243–245.

151. **Madden, C.C. and Mellion, M.B.** Sever's disease and other causes of heel pain in adolescents. *Am. Fam. Physician*, 1996; 54: 1995–2000.

152. **Micheli, L.J.** The traction apophysities. *Clin. Sports Med.*, 1987; 6: 389–404.

153. **Micheli, L.J. and Ireland, M.L.** Prevention and management of calcaneal apophysitis in children: an overuse syndrome. *J. Pediatr. Orthop.*, 1987; 7: 34–38.

154. **Sever, J.W.** Apophysitis of the os calcis. *N.Y. Med. J.*, 1912; 95: 1025–1029.

155. **Stanitski, C.L.** Management of sports injuries in children and adolescents. *Orthop. Clin. North Am.*, 1988; 19: 689–697.

156. **Volpon, J.B. and de Carvalho Filho, G.** Calcaneal apophysitis: a quantitative radiographic evaluation of the secondary ossification center. *Arch. Orthop. Trauma Surg.*, 2002; 122: 338–341.

157. **Wirtz, P.D., Vito, G.R., and Long, D.H.** Calcaneal apophysitis (Sever's disease) associated with Tae Kwon Do injuries. *J. Am. Podiatr. Med. Assoc.*, 1988; 78: 474–475.

158. **Zwipp, H., Therman, H. et al.** An innovative concept for primary functional treatment of Achilles tendon rupture. *Sportverletz. Sportschaden*, 1990; 4: 29–35.

10 Foot and Ankle

I. PLANTAR FASCIITIS

Plantar fasciitis is an overuse injury manifested by pain at the medial tubercle of the calcaneus and/or along the medial longitudinal arch. It usually develops when repetitive and prolonged stress is placed on the plantar fascia, which may cause microtears and inflammation in the fascia at or near its insertion on the calcaneus, i.e., when the activity of mechanical force overbalances the healing capacity of the tissue. Plantar fasciitis was first described by Wood in 1812, and its development was erroneously attributed to complications of tuberculosis.[20]

Plantar fasciitis occurs most commonly in runners, especially in long-distance runners, but may also be seen in basketball players, tennis players, and dancers. In various studies, the incidence of plantar fasciitis is about 5% of running injuries seen.[26,27,45,54,55]

A. ETIOPATHOGENESIS

Originating as a thick, fibrous band of connective tissue attached to the medial tubercle of the calcaneus, the plantar fascia (Figure 10.1) spreads distally in a fanlike manner.[5,18,21,35,40] It forms three slips (medial, central, and lateral), which proceed toward the toes where they insert on the base of each of the proximal phalanx of the toes. In histology, fascia and fibroblasts are arranged in layers and usually classified in the group of differentiated connective tissue.[28,55]

The analysis of biomechanical events taking place in the foot during walking has made it clear that the role of the plantar fascia is twofold.[16,18,27,33] When the foot touches the ground, the plantar fascia extends because of plantar dorsiflexion at the ankle joint and simultaneous dorsiflexion of proximal phalanxes of the toes.[18,27] By its extension, the plantar fascia stabilizes metatarsal joints, thus enabling the foot to be prepared for accommodation of the reactive force of the ground (Figure 10.2). The cushioning role of the plantar fascia is called a *mechanical shock absorbing effect.*[18,27,33] At the same time, it is an active load placed on the plantar fascia, as it is caused by contraction of extensor muscles of the foot (dorsiflexion of the toes). The second role of the plantar fascia is displayed during the take-off phase. Because of inertia, the body weight is transferred to the anterior region of the foot, causing the take-off of the heel and extension of the toes. The movement leads to passive stretching of the fascia, resulting in its lifting the longitudinal foot arch to prepare it for take-off (Figure 10.3). This function of the fascia is called the *windlass effect.*[18,23,27,28] The static qualities of plantar fascia were identified by mechanical analysis.[33] A longitudinal 90-kp extension force load on the plantar fascia in postmortem specimens yielded the value of 4% of the normal fascial length as the maximum ability of adjustment to stretching without tearing the fascial tissue.[33] However, *in vivo* studies have shown that the ability of fascia to adjust to stretching is smaller than in postmortem specimens, i.e., only 1.7% of its normal length.[33] Along the lines of these findings, it has also been observed that the fascia is relatively nonresistant to strong stretching force, which is probably why during activity of greater mechanical force overuse injury develops in the plantar fascia.[2,14,22]

The actions of supination and pronation are essential for the normal functioning of the foot. Different anatomical and functional alterations in the foot may result in excessive pronation. This causes the normal force of mechanical load acting on the foot to be supported not by basic structures, i.e., bones and ligaments, but rather by joint capsules and plantar fascia, thus enabling easy damage of these structures.[23,28,35,37,41,54,55]

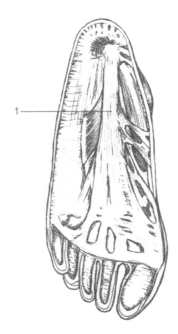

FIGURE 10.1 Plantar aponeurosis.

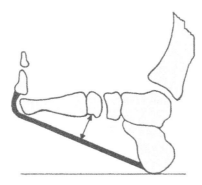

FIGURE 10.2 Action of the plantar fascia: active loading of the foot in the pre-stance phase as a shock-absorbing mechanism.

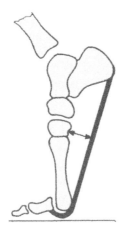

FIGURE 10.3 Action of plantar fascia: passive action in late stance phase producing so-called windlass effect.

Other commonly stated predisposing conditions of plantar fasciitis are a rigid cavus foot, flat feet, and a tight Achilles tendon.[5,13,18,28,35,40,41] The majority of cases of plantar fasciitis are associated with training errors.[26,45] Occasionally, plantar fasciitis signifies an underlying systemic disorder, e.g., rheumatoid arthritis, systemic lupus erythematosus, gout, psoriatic arthritis, ankylosing spondylitis, or Reiter's syndrome.[5,13,18,28,32,35,40,50]

B. CLINICAL PICTURE AND DIAGNOSTICS

The clinical manifestation of plantar fasciitis is painful heel or, more specifically, painful sensation in the bottom of the heel bone. Various terms and expressions have been used to describe painful heel syndrome, such as subcalcaneal pain, subcalcaneal heel pain, stone bruise, bone bruise, runner's heel, policeman's heel, heel pain syndrome, medial arch sprain, medial calcaneal neuritis, fat pad syndrome, heel spurs, calcaneal periostitis, and calcaneodynia.[3,8,19,21,33] Different causes of this clinical syndrome have also been identified, such as entrapment of the medial calcaneal branch of the posterior tibial nerve or entrapment of the nerve to abductor digiti quinti.[18,35] Painful heel syndrome is also often described as an inflammation of common origin of plantar fascia and smaller foot muscles or as a consequence of certain systemic diseases. It has been reported that the calcaneal stress fracture and calcaneal periostitis may easily be mistaken for plantar fasciitis.[5,47,56] For these reasons, it is very important to determine the exact cause of painful heel syndrome (Table 10.1). The site and quality of pain are essential to differentiate plantar fasciitis from other possible causes of painful heel syndrome.

The pinpoint, knifelike pain of plantar fasciitis is localized specifically at the medial tubercle of the calcaneus, i.e., at the site of the medial plantar fascia origin. There are cases when pain radiates along the medial longitudinal arch of the foot, but swelling occurs quite rarely. Swelling is usually localized to the area just anterior to the calcaneus (Figure 10.4).

Similar to other overuse injuries, pain is usually of gradual onset. The pain is usually insidious, with no history of acute trauma. Initially, the symptoms are noticed only with athletic activity. Pain is present at the beginning of an activity, becomes bearable after a few minutes, and will recur with increased severity toward the end of the activity. As the condition progresses, pain may be present with all activities of daily living. Most patients have severe pain in the morning upon getting up, which disappears after a few dozen steps. The early morning pain is believed to be related to the plantary flexed position patients assume while in bed. While the Achilles tendon and plantar fascia are relaxed, a contracture can develop during the night. On awaking, the first steps will then stretch these tissues.

Even in this age of modern technology, the diagnosis of plantar fasciitis is based mainly on the medical history and clinical presentation. Physical examination should include musculoskeletal examination of the lower leg, pulses, neurological examination, and observation of gait and stance. Examination of the patient's footwear is essential. On physical examination, the patient feels tenderness on firm palpation at the medial tubercle of the calcaneus, as well as diffuse tenderness along the medial longitudinal arch. Passive dorsiflexion of the great toe (with or without simultaneous dorsiflexion of the foot) increases the pain because of the stretching of the plantar fascia.

The usual radiographic findings in plantar fasciitis are more or less limited to imaging a bone spur on the calcaneus, which is more common in patients with plantar fasciitis, although it was observed in about 15% of patients without symptoms of the disease.[3,5,13,39,40] The spur is thought to be the result, not the cause, of chronic fascial inflammation. The most recent research has shown that, on 45° medial oblique radiographic examination, changes in the cortex and/or trabecular pattern in 85% of the patients with painful heel syndrome may be seen, whereas, on lateral roentgenograms, the majority of the images demonstrated thickening of heel fat pad and subfascial area.[3,39]

Bone scan is used to differentiate calcaneal stress fractures from calcaneal periostitis and plantar fasciitis. In patients with plantar fasciitis, there is an early increase in the flow of blood through the damaged area of the fascia, but there is no late accumulation of radionuclides in the calcaneus,

TABLE 10.1
Possible Causes of Calcaneodynia[18]

Inflammatory
    Juvenile rheumatoid arthritis
    Rheumatoid arthritis
    Ankylosing spondylitis
    Reiter's syndrome
    Gout
Metabolic
    Migratory osteoporosis
    Osteomalacia
Degenerative
    Osteoarthritis
    Atrophy of the heel fat pad
Nerve entrapment
    Tarsal tunnel syndrome
    Entrapment of the medial calcaneal branch of the posterior tibial nerve
    Entrapment of the nerve to abductor digiti quinti
Traumatic
    Calcaneal fractures
    Calcaneal malunions
    Traumatic arthritis
    Rupture of the fibrous septae of the fat pad
    Puncture of the fat pad
Overuse injuries
    Plantar fasciitis
    Stenosing tenosynovitis of the flexor digitorum longus and flexor hallucis longus
    Calcaneal apophysitis (Sever's disease)
    Subcalcaneal bursitis
    Periostitis
    Calcaneal stress fractures
    Achilles tendinitis and peritendinitis
    Haglund's deformity

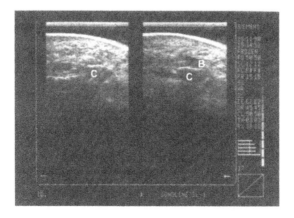

FIGURE 10.4 Sonogram of the sole of the foot showing bursa at the origin of the plantar fascia. C = calcaneus; B = bursa.

otherwise a characteristic feature in stress fracture or calcaneal periostitis.[5,13,39] Magnetic resonance (MR) imaging is rarely indicated but may show thickening of the plantar fascial medial column in chronic cases and can also be used to evaluate other soft-tissue and bony pathology.[17,57]

Plantar fasciitis is usually unilateral, but it is bilateral in up to 15% of patients. The majority of patients with plantar fasciitis are between 40 and 60 years of age. Distribution among men and women is equal.[14] The history should include the patient's general medical condition. Obesity in patients with plantar fasciitis occurs in 40% of men and 90% of women. A higher tendency toward plantar fasciitis has been observed in those patients who have engaged in activities requiring maximum plantar flexion with simultaneous metatarsophalangeal dorsiflexion. Thus, plantar fasciitis occurs much more frequently in runners and ballet dancers.

C. TREATMENT

1. Non-Operative Treatment

The first line of treatment is always prevention. In the case of plantar fasciitis patient education is imperative. Patients must understand the etiology of their pain, including the biomechanical factors that cause their symptoms. They should learn about therapy (stretching exercises) that may relieve some discomfort and about recommended changes in daily activities, such as wearing appropriate athletic shoes with a significant medial arch while walking.

Treatment of plantar fasciitis is directed at relieving the inflammatory process of the fascia and correcting predisposing factors. Initial management should include local application of ice, administration of nonsteroidal anti-inflammatory drugs, plantar fascia and Achilles stretching exercises, use of a plantar fascia night splint, othoses, and cessation of athletic activities. A 15- to 20-min ice massage applied several times daily is recommended for quickly relieving pain. However, it has been noted that when cryotherapy is applied for a longer period of time, the results are less satisfactory.[27,47]

It is often advantageous for patients with no contraindication to take nonsteroidal anti-inflammatory drugs, which provide pain relief and are useful in decreasing the inflammation. We believe that steroid injections should be avoided in the initial treatment of plantar fasciitis. We use them only as supplemental treatment in patients with refractory symptoms after achieving adequate biomechanical control. During the application of steroid injections, caution is necessary to avoid possible adverse reactions such that no more than three injections should be given in any one series. Atrophy of calcaneal fat tissue, affected nerves, or resistance to applied treatment may accompany repeated application of steroid injection.[1,49] Although there have been reports of dramatic improvements in plantar fasciitis by athletes given steroid injections, these are temporary improvements, which must be accompanied by correction of training errors, running on appropriate surfaces, orthotic treatment, and flexibility and strength exercises. To provide immediate relief from plantar fasciitis symptoms, reduced physical activity or even complete rest is often very useful.

Most patients with plantar fasciitis also have tightness of the Achilles tendon; stretching interrupts a cycle in which two disorders aggravate each other. Patients should be instructed to stretch plantar fascia, Achilles tendon, gastrocnemius–soleus complex, and foot muscles.[6,43] Patients should be encouraged to repeat the gentle, sustained stretches at least ten times, five or six times daily.

The use of the plantar fascia night splint has been effective in decreasing discomfort. It holds the ankle fixed in 5% of dorsiflexion and the toes slightly dorsiflexed.[29,34,52] When the foot is held in constant neutral position, the inflamed plantar fascia does not shorten during sleep. As a result, the vicious cycle of nocturnal contracture and early morning stretching of the plantar fascia with weight bearing is broken. For most patients this orthosis reduces morning pain considerably; Wapner and Sharkey[52] had a 79% cure rate after patients used the splint for an average of 4 months.

Ultrasound, high-voltage galvanic stimulation, and deep transverse friction massage are also used with treatment of plantar fasciitis.[5,13,39,44] In addition, alternating use of ultrasound and ice or contrast bath has shown beneficial effects on the course of plantar fasciitis.

Despite its usefulness, quick alleviation of symptoms has only temporary effects in the treatment of plantar fasciitis unless it is used in combination with orthotic therapy.[5,13,39,44] The purpose of orthotic therapy is to decrease the stretching of plantar fascia caused by excessive and/or prolonged foot pronation. Because the plantar fascia is stretched during flattening of the foot, we prefer orthoses designed to maintain the medial longitudinal arch during ambulation. Correction of biomechanical foot abnormalities may also be achieved by special technique of fixation of the foot with an adhesive strapping, the so-called low Dye strapping technique.[47] In the treatment of plantar fasciitis, a variety of orthotic devices may be used, such as heel lifts or ready-made arch supports (rigid, semirigid, and flexible).[11]

2. Surgical Treatment

Although there are numerous non-operative therapeutic measures used for the treatment of plantar fasciitis, a minority of patients do not exhibit satisfactory improvement. Surgical intervention is recommended when symptoms last longer than 1 year and do not recede in spite of non-operative treatment measures and complete rest.

It is well documented that open plantar fasciotomy alone, without inferior calcaneal exostectomy, is an effective surgical approach to this condition.[12,20,24,38,42,48,53] The procedure involves division of the plantar fascia approximately 1 cm distal from its attachment at the medial tuberosity of the calcaneus. This release has a beneficial effect on the inflammation of plantar fascia, probably because afterward the fascia assumes the position at which it possesses weaker internal tension and at the same time the natural healing process of the fascia is stimulated. During an open plantar fasciotomy, the patient is placed in a fixed ankle cast and is non-weight-bearing for 2 to 3 weeks. Stretching and exercises are resumed at this point, and sports are resumed 6 to 8 weeks postoperatively.

Recently, techniques have been described whereby the plantar fasciotomy can be performed endoscopically.[4,5,7,15,25,31,46] The endoscopic procedure has been reported to be less traumatic than traditional open surgery, to allow patients to return to their daily lifestyles earlier and often with better functional results. Some authorities consider the technique controversial, but a study of 652 endoscopic plantar fasciotomy procedures, performed by 25 different surgeons, reported a success rate (resolution of chronic plantar fasciitis) as high as 97%.[4]

Alternatives to surgery such as extracorporeal shock wave therapy are still in their infancy, but show promise.[9,10,30,36,51]

II. ANTERIOR IMPINGEMENT SYNDROME OF THE ANKLE

Repeated maximal dorsiflexion of the foot leads to the development of bony growths (osteophytes, spurs) on the anterior edge of the tibia, the neck of the talus, and occasionally the navicular bone. This is caused by the repetitive collisions of the anterior edge of the tibia against the neck of the talus. The newly developed osteophytes incapacitate maximal dorsiflexion of the ankle, and repeated efforts to perform this movement lead to pain and swelling limited to the anterior side of the ankle, i.e., anterior impingement syndrome of the ankle.[61,85,99,103,109,118,119,120]

This syndrome is most often encountered in soccer players, especially older soccer players. For this reason, some authors refer to this syndrome as soccer players' exostosis on the neck of the talus (Figure 10.5). In soccer players, the development of this syndrome is linked with, in addition to the previously mentioned causes, repeated maximal plantar flexion movements of the foot performed while kicking the ball. The explanation is that during these movements the joint capsule is subjected to stress localized at its insertion points. The development of osteophytes in the anterior ankle area is also described in other athletes and, most frequently, in ballet dancers.

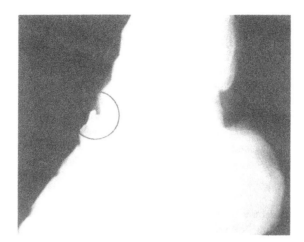

FIGURE 10.5 Soccer player's exostosis on the neck of the talus.

For ballet dancers, limited dorsiflexion reduces the depth obtained while performing the *plié*, and the patient complains of pain, swelling, and localized tenderness during palpation of the area between the medial malleolus and the tibialis anterior muscle tendon, and between the lateral malleolus and the extensor digitorum longus muscle tendon.

Symptoms of anterior impingement syndrome of the ankle are anterior ankle pain and limitation of dorsiflexion. On examination of the ankle, there is localizing tenderness along the anterior ridge of the tibia. Tenderness is accentuated with dorsiflexion and relieved with plantar flexion. Forced dorsiflexion is often painful as a result of the catching of synovium or capsular tissue between a tibial osteophyte and the talus or between tibiotalar osteophytes. The limited dorsiflexion characteristic of this syndrome is often incorrectly attributed to an excessively "tight" Achilles tendon; this results in the unsuccessful application of stretching exercises, which are generally extremely painful to the patient.

The size of osteophytes on the anterior tibia and talus can be estimated on lateral radiographs of the ankle.[70,109] But in early stages of the anterior impingement syndrome of the ankle radiographs are negative. However, bone scan will show increased uptake along the anterior tibial crest. A computerized tomography (CT) scan may demonstrate osteophyte formation, which is better seen with the MR imaging technique.

Scranton and McDermott[119] developed the following classification system for tibiotalar osteophytes:

Grade I: Synovial impingement. Radiographs show inflammatory reaction with spurs as large as 3 mm.
Grade II: Osteochondral reaction exostosis. Anterior tibial spur formation greater than 3 mm in size, with no talar spur.
Grade III: Severe exostosis with or without fragmentation. Large anterior tibial spur with or without fragmentation, accompanied by spur formation on the talar neck, often with fragmentation.
Grade IV: Plantarocrural osteoarthrotic destruction. Radiographs suggest degenerative osteoarthritic changes medially, laterally, or posteriorly.

The Scranton and McDermott[119] classifications can assist in the treatment plan, as well. At grade I, modification of activities, the use of a heel lift (1 to 2 cm), and the use of nonsteroidal anti-inflammatory medication may suffice. If symptoms persist, arthroscopic resection of hyperplastic reaction would be the treatment option. At grade II, III, or IV patients are unlikely to improve with non-operative measures, and thus are candidates for arthroscopic resection of the anterior tibial and talar spurs. The use of arthroscopic technique vs. open technique for anterior impingement syndrome of the ankle has been shown to reduce the morbidity following surgery and eliminate the need for hospitalization.[72,73,85,103,110,120] Branca et al.[61] noted improvement in all four stages of disease with arthroscopic management, and reported significant improvement in pain, reduced limitation in day-to-day activities and joint stiffness, and improvement in ankle function as manifested by limping in all four stages. Van Dijk and colleagues[66] demonstrated that the degree of osteoarthritic changes is a better prognostic factor for the outcome of arthroscopic surgery for anterior ankle impingement than size and location of the spurs.

III. POSTERIOR IMPINGEMENT SYNDROME OF THE ANKLE

Repeated maximal plantar flexion may lead to posterior impingement syndrome of the ankle by virtue of the presence of os trigonum or Stieda's process on the talus.[77,89,105] This syndrome can also be caused by an exceptionally developed posterior process of the calcaneus, by the presence of an ankle meniscus, or by the thickening of soft tissues resulting from repeated injuries sustained during maximal plantar flexion of the foot. The posterior aspect of the talus is grooved by the tendon of flexor hallucis longus, producing the medial and lateral tubercles. The lateral tubercle is either short or long. If it is long, it is called *Stieda's process*. Instead of this process, there may be an ossicle attached to the body of the talus by a fibrous tissue. This accessory ossicle is known as the os trigonum and is present in 5 to 20% of individuals, appearing unilaterally in two thirds.[99,104]

Because most individuals who have an os trigonum are not aware of its presence, it is accidentally spotted while radiographing the ankle. Nevertheless, os trigonum or Stieda's process may cause trouble. During extreme plantar flexion, Stieda's process is trapped between the calcaneus and tibia like "a nut in a nutcracker," limiting extreme plantar flexion (Figure 10.6). Its entrapment causes compression and irritation of the adjacent synovial and capsular tissue. With repeated entrapment and irritation, the soft tissue undergoes inflammatory changes and eventually thickens, preventing already reduced plantar flexion from flexing any further (Figure 10.7). The pain located on the posterior side of the ankle is caused by trying to force the foot farther down than it can go. This syndrome, commonly seen in ballet dancers and therefore called *dancer's heel,* is also encountered in soccer players, high jumpers, and pole vaulters.[82–84,87,90,91,107,108,112,113,117]

In differential diagnosis, posterior impingement syndrome must be distinguished from other conditions that can produce similar posterior ankle pain, especially Achilles tendinitis and peroneal and flexor hallucis longus tendinitis. These conditions are also common in ballet

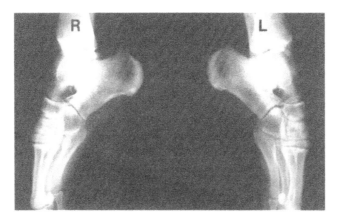

FIGURE 10.6 Lateral roentgenogram of the both ankles taken in a plantar flexed position. Note the limitation in plantar flexion of the right ankle.

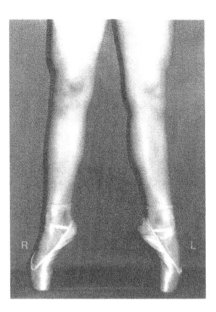

FIGURE 10.7 Lack of maximal plantar flexion in the right ankle (R) in *pointe* position.

dancers.[74,79,82–84,87,91,108,112,113] The symptoms of Achilles tendinitis occur 2 to 6 cm above the insertion of the tendon into the calcaneus, or in the tendon–bone junction in the case of insertional Achilles tendinitis or enthesitis. Symptoms and signs of peroneal tendinitis include pain, swelling, and tenderness in the posterior lateral malleolar area. The most difficult differential diagnosis is to distinguish the syndrome from flexor hallucis longus tendinitis whose symptoms include pain, swelling, and tenderness localized in the posterior medial malleolar region; the most significant finding on physical examination is functional (pseudo) hallux valgus. In some patients, flexor hallucis longus tendinitis may coexist with posterior impingement syndrome.

Initial treatment of posterior impingement syndrome of the ankle involves cessation or moderation of activities that provoke entrapment and irritation of the tissue, physical therapy to increase flexibility of the ankle, and application of nonsteroidal anti-inflammatory drugs. In cases in which this therapy does not produce the expected results, infiltration of the tender area with corticosteroids and anesthetics may be performed. In resistant cases, surgical treatment — excision of the os trigonum along with the surrounding thickened fibrous tissue — is considered.[69,77,95,105] If symptoms of tendinitis of the flexor hallucis longus muscle are also present, tenolysis, which requires opening of the ankle, is indicated. The results of surgical treatment confirm the opinion held by many authors that too much time should not be expended on non-operative treatment especially when dealing with professional dancers and athletes.

IV. FLEXOR HALLUCIS LONGUS TENDINITIS

Tendinitis of the flexor hallucis longus muscle is a common entity in ballet dancers; therefore, it is known as dancer's tendinitis.[74,79,80,82–84,87,91,92,96,112–114,121] Dancers, especially ballerinas, are constantly stressing the flexor hallucis longus tendon in *pointe* work, dancing on the tips of their toes in hyperplantar flexion of the ankle. The main dynamic stabilizing factor of the medial region of the foot in this position is the flexor hallucis longus muscle. Because of its functional importance, the flexor hallucis longus muscle has been referred to as the "Achilles tendon of the foot."

The flexor hallucis longus tendon is formed above the ankle, crosses behind the medial malleolus traveling through a groove in the talus, and travels under the sustentaculum tali as it passes into the foot (Figure 10.8). The tendon, encased in the synovial sheath (vagina synovialis), courses

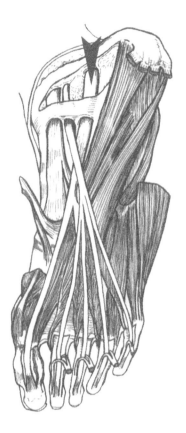

FIGURE 10.8 The flexor hallucis longus muscle (arrowhead).

through the tarsal tunnel as it passes into the foot and then goes along the lower medial side of the foot to its origin on the base of the distal phalanx of the great toe. Repeated overuse of the foot may lead to degenerative changes within the tendon, ranging from characteristic inflammatory changes to formation of a knot, thickening of the tendon, development of cysts in the tendon, and even partial rupture of the collagen fibers in the tendon (Figure 10.9).[86] Thickening of the tendon usually develops in the lacuna tendinum, below and behind the medial malleolus and, in rare cases,

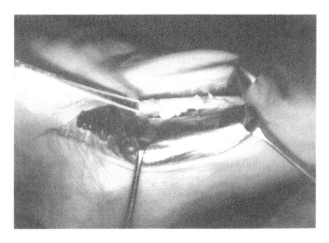

FIGURE 10.9 Intraoperative finding of partial rupture of the flexor hallucis longus muscle in a long-distance runner.

at the exit of the lacuna tendinum. Development of this thickening can lead to stenosing tenosynovitis of the flexor hallucis longus muscle with a clinical picture resembling trigger finger.[96,121]
Functional hallux rigidus also develops because of the barrier effect of the thickened tendon. This
disables flexion of the great toe during dorsiflexion of the foot until the resistance of the thickened
tendon passing through the lacuna tendinum is overcome, either passively or actively.

Clinical findings include pain and swelling in the medial aspect of the ankle, behind the medial
malleolar region. If the tendon is inflamed, pain and swelling behind the medial malleolus of the
ankle occur. Physical findings include localized tenderness over the course of the flexor hallucis
longus. Palpation of the sheath with active and passive motion of the hallux will painfully reproduce
the patient's symptoms. If stenosing tenosynovitis develops, the signs and symptoms are more
dramatic. In these cases, during passive movements of the great toe, crepitations are felt in the
same region, and sometimes the trigger finger phenomenon is also felt. Flexion of the great toe
against resistance will produce pain in the area posterior to the medial malleolus. The pain is blunt
and increases in severity during physical activity while disappearing after rest, depending, of course,
on the stage and severity of the tendinitis. In diagnosing this symptom, tenography was frequently
employed in the past, but today ultrasound examination is generally used. Differential diagnostics
include ruling out Achilles tendon overuse syndrome. Posterior impingement syndrome of the ankle,
however, is the most difficult clinical entity to differentiate, especially because both syndromes
may be present.[74,91,95,108]

The basic non-operative treatment for tendinitis of the flexor hallucis longus muscle consists
of cessation or reduction of athletic activities (especially those involving standing on the toes),
physical therapy (stretching exercises), and use of nonsteroidal anti-inflammatory drugs. Dancers
are encouraged to exercise in a pool because this enables them to imitate exercises done on dry
land but with considerably less pressure. Local applications of corticosteroids with anesthetics are
also indicated in some cases. Surgical treatment should remain as the last option and consists of
tenolysis, whereas in cases of stenosing tenosynovitis freeing of the tendon in the tarsal canal is
indicated.[74,91,95,108]

A rarer, more distal form of flexor hallucis longus tenosynovitis occurs at the point where the
flexor hallucis longus tendon passes through its sheath between sesamoids.[115] As a second pulley
system, it is prone to trauma, particularly in runners. The sheath becomes chronically or intermittently inflamed and eventually heals with a constricted area, which impairs passage of the tendon.
It often expresses itself as tenderness and swelling in the region of the sesamoids. Frequently, the
patient has difficulty flexing the interphalangeal joint of the great toe while the metatarsophalangeal
joint is stabilized. Non-operative treatment includes rest, nonsteroidal anti-inflammatory drugs, ice,
stretching exercises, and shoe modification including an inflexible shoe to improve push-off. If the
patient fails to respond to this treatment, tenolysis may be required.

V. TENDINITIS OF THE COMMON EXTENSOR MUSCLE

The tendons of the long and short extensors of the toes and the long extensor of the great toe stretch
along the dorsal side of the foot (Figure 10.10). Excessive pressure from footwear or too tightly
laced shoestrings can lead to overstimulation of these tendons and/or their enveloping synovial
sheaths, resulting in tendinitis or tendovaginitis.[63,65,71,76,94,107] In most cases, the symptoms of tendinitis gradually increase; cases of tendinitis resulting from one episode of excessive irritation are
rare. Pain located on the dorsal side of the foot that increases during running is the most common
and indicative sign of tendinitis. Another very characteristic symptom is the appearance of a
localized swelling on the dorsal side of the foot, which can best be noticed by comparing the
affected foot with the other unaffected foot (bilateral tendinitis of the toe extensors of the foot is
rare). Tendinitis of the extensors of the toes is characterized by pain and tenderness felt when
moving the toes. Later stages of the syndrome are characterized by painful limping during running
and, in long-standing cases, by the inability to walk without a limp. Differential diagnosis should

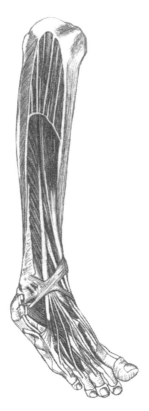

FIGURE 10.10 Anterior muscles of the leg.

take into account the possibility of stress fractures of the metatarsal bones of the foot (marching fracture), which manifest with similar symptoms.

Tendinitis of the toe extensors is treated according to the principles that apply to all overuse syndromes of the musculoskeletal system. Athletic activities should be stopped for a period of at least 7 days, nonsteroidal anti-inflammatory drugs and local cryotherapy should be applied (twice a day for a period of 20 min), and the way that the shoelaces are laced should be corrected. The shoelaces should be laced in a steplike manner (not criss-crossed), and in some cases, the tongue of the shoe should be thickened with a sponge or similar substance. In cases where this therapy does not produce results, local infiltration of corticosteroids and anesthetics is recommended.

VI. TENDINITIS OF THE POSTERIOR TIBIAL MUSCLE AND POSTERIOR TIBIAL TENOSYNOVITIS

The contribution of the posterior tibial muscle to forming the arch of the foot is of paramount importance. For this reason, the exertion of that muscle during athletic activities in individuals with flat-foot deformity is considerable. Excessive exertion of this muscle can manifest either by the appearance of pain in the region of its origin on the posterior side of the tibia (runner's leg or shin splints), or by the development of an overuse syndrome that can appear at two locations. If the pain is in the region of the muscle tendon unit and its insertion on tarsal bones, then it is called tendinitis of the posterior tibial muscle, whereas if the pain is in the area behind the posterior part of the medial malleolus, then it is called posterior tibial tenosynovitis.

Tendinitis of the posterior tibial muscle is rare and usually develops in older athletes who habitually run for long periods of time. The usual symptoms are a gradually increasing pain localized in the mid-arch region, i.e., in the area of insertion of tendon; difficulty while pushing off with

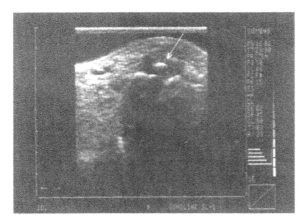

FIGURE 10.11 Sonogram of the leg showing posterior tibial tenosynovitis (arrow).

running; and a flattened arch. Differential diagnostics includes ruling out stress fractures. Treatment is conducted according to the principles that apply to treatment of all tendinitis syndromes (rest, ice, stretching exercises, nonsteroidal anti-inflammatory drugs), with special emphasis on the static correction of the foot by using semirigid orthosis. In resistant cases, local infiltration of corticosteroids and anesthetics often produces good results. Surgical treatment (tenolysis and decompression) is rarely needed.[76,117]

Posterior tibial tenosynovitis is most commonly seen during athletic activities requiring quick changes in direction, such as basketball, soccer, tennis, and ice hockey. It is characterized by diffuse swelling, pain at the medial aspect of the ankle, tenderness over the tendon course, and frequently there is associated crepitance (Figure 10.11). On physical examination, pain can be elicited over the medial aspect of the ankle by active inversion of the foot against resistance. Non-operative treatment consists of rest, ice, nonsteroidal anti-inflammatory drugs, and a medially posted orthosis to decrease pronation during the weight-bearing phase. In the young athlete with acute inflammation, immobilization in a non-weight-bearing short leg cast with the foot in slight inversion for several weeks often relieves symptoms dramatically. In the event of failure of non-operative treatment, posterior tibial tenosynovitis can be treated by open surgery or by endoscopic procedure — tendon sheath endoscopy.[67]

VII. DISLOCATION OF THE PERONEAL TENDONS AND PERONEAL TENOSYNOVITIS

Monteggia first described dislocation of the peroneal tendons in 1803.[124] This entity occurs more frequently than is usually diagnosed. It is more common in younger athletes, particularly those participating in such sports as skiing, soccer, ice skating, and basketball. The tendons of the long and short peroneal muscle pass behind the lateral malleolus in a variably deep groove, which, together with the retinaculum mm. peroneorum proximale et distale, forms a channel (Figure 10.12). The most common mechanism of injury includes forceful passive dorsiflexion with a violent reflex contracture of the peroneal tendons; for example, when a skier catches a tip of his or her skis and falls forward over the ski, these retinaculs can snap (sometimes audibly) and the muscle tendons can dislocate.[62,102] Another common mechanism is inversion of the slightly plantar-flexed foot, as would occur with a lateral ankle sprain.[62] The patient may report a cracking sensation, accompanied by an intense flash of pain. The patient will usually have been unable to continue the activity and often be unable to ambulate.

Physical examination reveals swelling and tenderness to palpation localized in the area behind the lateral malleolus. After several hours, subcutaneous bleeding appears while the pain diffusely

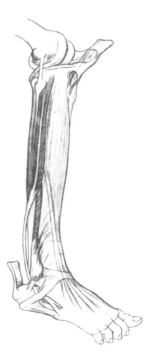

FIGURE 10.12 Peroneal group of muscles of the leg.

spreads, which often leads to incorrect diagnosis of dislocation of the ankle. In some cases, the dislocated peroneal tendons can be palpated. In clinical diagnostics, the eversion and dorsiflexion test for the sole of the foot is helpful (Figure 10.13). In this test, eversion and dorsiflexion of the sole of the foot against resistance produces pain in the retromalleolar region if dislocation of the peroneal tendons is present. These symptoms can be mistaken for anterior impingement syndrome of the ankle.

In cases of acute dislocation of the peroneal tendons, surgical treatment is indicated, although some authors recommend immobilization and refrain from surgery except in cases where repeated dislocations of the peroneal tendons develop. In those cases of repeated dislocations, the peroneal tendons are placed retromalleolarly during plantar flexion, while during dorsiflexion, they dislocate. These repeated dislocations are extremely unpleasant and lead to instability of the ankle. Numerous procedures have been described in attempts to hold the peroneal tendons within the retrofibular sulcus.[58,64,97,100,101,116,123]

The mechanical stress on the peroneal tendons as they ride in the retrofibular sulcus may result in decreased vascularity, inflammation, and degenerative changes. Symptoms and signs of peroneal tenosynovitis include pain, swelling, and tenderness in the retromalleolar region over the peroneal tendons. On physical examination pain may be elicited over the lateral aspect of the ankle with active eversion against resistance. Most authors report good results with non-operative treatment: decrease in activity, rest, and orthosis. In milder cases, a lateral heel wedge decreases stress on the peroneal tendons by limiting their excursion. Casting may be necessary in severe acute cases. When non-operative treatment fails, tenosynovectomy (release and debridement) can be performed, today even endoscopically — tendon sheath endoscopy.[68]

VIII. SESAMOIDITIS

Two small sesamoid bones of the great toe, medial (tibial) and lateral (fibular), are located within the tendon of the flexor hallucis brevis on the plantar aspect of the foot. The primary functions of the sesamoids include absorbing the weight-bearing stress on the medial forefoot, increasing the

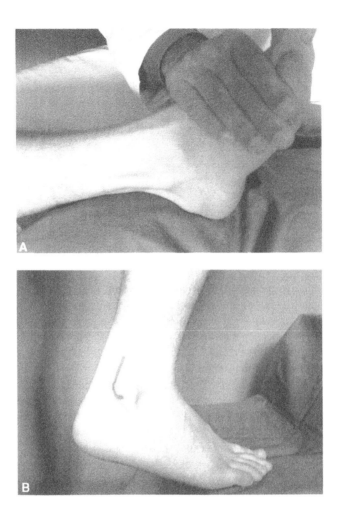

FIGURE 10.13 (A) Peroneal dislocation testing (maximal dorsal flexion and eversion of the foot). (B) Spontaneous peroneal tendon dislocation during walking.

mechanical advantage of the flexor hallucis brevis or increasing its lever arm, and protecting the flexor hallucis longus tendon. Unfortunately, these small but important bones and support structures are subject to a variety of acute and chronic injuries in the athlete.

The sesamoid bones are formed from multiple ossification centers and nonunion of the centers, which appear radiographically as bipartite, tripartite, and quadripartite sesamoid bones. Multipartite sesamoids occur more frequently in females and are often bilateral. Bipartite and multipartite medial sesamoid occur in 10 to 33% of all feet.[93,98] Differentiating between bipartite sesamoid and sesamoid fracture is a common clinical problem. Fracture is associated with pain localized at the sesamoid, sharp radiographic margins, and unilateral involvement. A bipartite sesamoid has smooth radiographic margins and is not painful in the absence of injury. Occasionally, because of repetitive overloading, stress fractures of the sesamoids occur (described in Chapter 12).[122]

The most common sesamoid problem, termed *sesamoiditis,* in athletes is caused by repetitive stress on the sesamoids. The problem occurs most frequently in those athletes who require maximum dorsiflexion of the great toe, but may also be associated with trauma from direct pressure of the athletic shoe. Athletes at risk include joggers, sprinters, figure skaters, and basketball and football players.[59,75,78,81,88] In ballet dancers, sesamoiditis results when the sole of the foot is in the *releve* position, which creates maximal loading of the head of the first metatarsal bone. There is some suggestion that the development of sesamoiditis is facilitated by a highly arched (cavus), rigid foot.

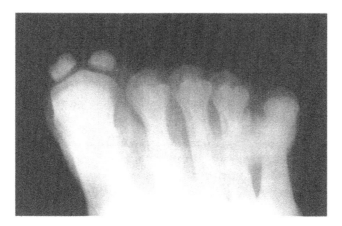

FIGURE 10.14 Axial roentgenogram of the foot demonstrating great toe sesamoids.

The most characteristic symptoms are pain and swelling in the ball of the foot. Rolling through the foot to stand on the toes is painful, as are running and, eventually, walking. In later stages of the disease, pain appears on the lateral aspect of the foot because the patient walks in inversion in an attempt to protect the painful first metatarsophalangeal joint. Physical examination reveals tenderness to palpation over the involved sesamoid. With dorsiflexion of the great toe, the sesamoids move distally, as does the area of maximal tenderness. Passive dorsiflexion and resisted plantar flexion of the great toe often increase the pain. Swelling may be present but is often difficult to note because of the presence of the subcutaneous fat. Ultrasound examination is generally helpful in determining the potential presence of swelling. Radiological diagnostics and scintigraphy are also useful (Figure 10.14).

Sesamoiditis is difficult to treat, primarily because it is hard to avoid placing pressure on the sesamoid bones when walking. To decrease the pressure, we recommend placing a small sponge, or other soft material (felt, for example, is particularly good), cut out in the shape of a crescent below the head of the first metatarsal bone. Taping the great toe in neutral or slight plantar flexion also may relieve pressure on the sesamoids. Occasionally, a stiff-soled shoe will alleviate the pain with weight bearing. Nonsteroidal anti-inflammatory drugs and physical therapy can also be applied. Orthopedic implants can correct the biomechanics of the sole of the foot, thus eliminating the cause of the sesamoiditis.[60] In long-standing cases surgical excision can be performed.[106,111] However, because of the concomitant degenerative changes in the cartilage of the head of the first metatarsal bone, this procedure can be unsuccessful.

REFERENCES

Plantar Fasciitis

1. **Acevedo, J.I. and Beskin, J.L.** Complications of plantar fascia rupture associated with corticosteroid injection. *Foot Ankle*, 1998; 19: 91–97.
2. **Ahstrom, J.P.** Spontaneous rupture of the plantar fascia. *Am. J. Sports Med.,* 1988; 16: 306–307.
3. **Amis, J., Jennings, L., Graham, D., and Graham, C.E.** Painful heel syndrome: radiographic and treatment assessment. *Foot Ankle,* 1988; 9: 91–95.
4. **Barrett, S.L. and Day, S.V.** Endoscopic plantar fasciotomy: a multi-surgeon prospective analysis of 652 cases. *J. Foot Ankle Surg.,* 1995; 34: 400–406.
5. **Barrett, S.L. and O'Malley, R.** Plantar fasciitis and other causes of heel pain. *Am. Fam. Physician,* 1999; 59: 2200–2206.

6. **Barry, L.D., Barry, A.N., and Chen, Y.** A retrospective study of standing gastrocnemius-soleus stretching versus night splinting in the treatment of plantar fasciitis. *J. Foot Ankle Surg.*, 2002; 41: 221–227.
7. **Blanco, C.E., Leon, H.O., and Guthrie, T.B.** Endoscopic treatment of calcaneal spur syndrome: a comprehensive technique. *Arthroscopy,* 2001; 17: 517–522.
8. **Bordelon, R.L.** Subcalcaneal pain. A method of evaluation and plan for treatment. *Clin. Orthop.,* 1983; 177: 49–53.
9. **Buch, M., Knorr, U., Fleming, L. et al.** Extrakorporale Stosswellentherapie beim symptomatischen Ferensporneine Übersicht. *Orthopade,* 2002; 31: 637–644.
10. **Buchbinder, R., Ptasznik, R., Gordon, J. et al.** Ultrasound-guided extracorporeal shock wave therapy for plantar fasciitis: a randomized controlled trial. *J. Am. Med. Assoc.,* 2002; 288: 1364–1372.
11. **Campbell, J.W. and Inmann, V.T.** Treatment of plantar fasciitis and calcaneal spurs with the UCBL shoe insert. *Clin. Orthop.,* 1974; 103: 57–62.
12. **Davies, M.S., Weiss, G.A., and Saxby, T.S.** Plantar fasciitis: How successful is surgical intervention? *Foot Ankle,* 1999; 20: 803–807.
13. **Gill, L.H.** Plantar fasciitis: diagnosis and conservative management. *J. Am. Acad. Orthop. Surg.,* 1997; 5: 109–117.
14. **Herrick, R.T., and Herrick, S.** Rupture of the plantar fascia in a middle-aged tennis player. *Am. J. Sports Med.,* 1983; 11: 95.
15. **Jerosch, J.** Endoscopic release of plantar fasciitis: A benign procedure? *Foot Ankle,* 2000; 21: 511–513.
16. **Kibler, W.B., Goldberg, C., and Chandler, T.J.** Functional biomechanical deficits in running athletes with plantar fasciitis. *Am. J. Sports Med.,* 1991; 19: 66–71.
17. **Kier, R.** Magnetic resonance imaging of plantar fasciitis and other causes of heel pain. *MRI Clin. North Am.,* 1994; 2: 97–107.
18. **Kwong, P.K., Kay, D., Voner, R.T. et al.** Plantar fasciitis: mechanics and pathomechanics of treatment. *Clin. Sports Med.,* 1988; 7: 119–127.
19. **Lapidus, P.W. and Guidotti, F.P.** Painful heel: reports of 323 patients with 364 painful heels. *Clin. Orthop.,* 1965; 39: 178–186.
20. **Leach, R.E., Seavey, M.S., and Salter, D.K.** Results of surgery in athletes with plantar fasciitis. *Foot Ankle,* 1986; 7: 156–161.
21. **Leach, R.E., Dilorio, E., and Harney, R.A.** Pathologic hindfoot condition in the athlete. *Clin. Orthop.,* 1982; 177: 116–119.
22. **Leach, R.E., Jones, R., and Silva, T.** Rupture of the plantar fascia in athletes. *J. Bone Joint Surg.,* 1978; 60(A): 537–539.
23. **Leach, R.E.** Leg and foot injuries in racquet sports. *Clin. Sports Med.,* 1988; 7: 359–370.
24. **Lester, K.D. and Buchanan, J.R.** Surgical treatment of plantar fasciitis. *Clin. Orthop.,* 1984; 186: 202–204.
25. **Lundeen, R.O., Aziz, S., Burks, J.B., and Rose, J.M.** Endoscopic plantar fasciotomy: a retrospective analysis of results in 53 patients. *J. Foot Ankle Surg.,* 2000; 39: 208–217.
26. **Macintyre, J.G., Taunton, J.E., Clement, D.B. et al.** Running injuries. A clinical study of 4173 cases. *Clin. J. Sports Med.,* 1991; 1: 81–87.
27. **Marshall, P.** Overuse foot injuries in athletes and dancers. *Clin. Sports Med.,* 1988; 7: 175–191.
28. **McBryde, A.M.** Plantar fasciitis. *AAOS Instr. Course Lect.,* 1984; 33: 278–282.
29. **Mizel, M.D., Marymont, J.V., and Trapman, E.** Treatment of plantar fasciitis with a night splint and shoe modification consisting of a steel shank and anterior rocker bottom. *Foot Ankle,* 1997; 17: 732–735.
30. **Ogden, J.A., Alvarez, R., Levitt, R., Cross, G.L., and Marlow, M.** Shock wave therapy for chronic proximal plantar fasciitis. *Clin. Orthop.,* 2001; 387: 47–59.
31. **Oglivie-Harris, D.J. and Lobo, J.** Endoscopic plantar fascia release. *Arthroscopy,* 2000; 16: 290–298.
32. **Paice, E.W. and Hoffbrand, B.I.** Nutritional osteomalacia presenting with plantar fasciitis. *J. Bone Joint Surg.,* 1987; 69(B): 38–40.
33. **Perry, J.** Anatomy and biomechanics of the hindfoot. *Clin. Orthop.,* 1983; 177: 9–15.
34. **Probe, R.A., Baca, M., Adams, R., and Preece, C.** Night splint treatment for plantar fasciitis. *Clin. Orthop.,* 1999; 368: 190–195.

35. **Ribarić, G., Pećina, M., and Bojanić, I.** Plantarni fascitis. *Acta Orthop. Iugosl.,* 1989; 20: 18–22.

36. **Rompe, J.D., Schoellner, C., and Nafe, B.** Evaluation of low-energy extracorporeal shock-wave application for treatment of chronic plantar fasciitis. *J. Bone Joint Surg.,* 2002; 84(A): 335–341.

37. **Roy, S.** How I manage plantar fasciitis. *Phys. Sportsmed.,* 1983; 11: 27–31.

38. **Sammarco, G.J. and Helfrey, R.B.** Surgical treatment of recalcitrant plantar fasciitis. *Foot Ankle,* 1996; 17: 520–526.

39. **Shereff, M.J. and Johnson, K.A.** Radiographic anatomy of the hindfoot. *Clin. Orthop.,* 1983; 177: 16–22.

40. **Singh, D., Angel, J., Bentley, G., and Trevino, S.G.** Plantar fasciitis. *Br. Med. J.,* 1997; 315: 172–175.

41. **Smerdelj, M., Maďarević, M., and Oremuž, K.** Overuse injuries of the calf and foot. *Arh. Hig. Rada Toksikol.,* 2001; 52: 451–464.

42. **Snider, M.P., Clancy, W.G., and McBeath, A.A.** Plantar fascia release for chronic plantar fasciitis in runners. *Am. J. Sports Med.,* 1983; 11: 215–219.

43. **Stanish, W.D., Rubinovich, R.M., and Curwin, S.** Eccentric exercise in chronic tendinitis. *Clin. Orthop.,* 1986; 208: 65–68.

44. **Tanner, S.M. and Harvey, J.S.** How we manage plantar fasciitis. *Phys. Sportsmed.,* 1988; 16: 39–47.

45. **Taunton, J.E., Ryan, M.B., Clement, D.B., McKenzie, D.C., Lloyd-Smith, D.R., and Zumbo, B.D.** A retrospective case-control analysis of 2002 running injuries. *Br. J. Sports Med.,* 2002; 36(2): 95–101.

46. **Tomczak, R.L. and Haverstock, B.D.** A retrospective comparison of endoscopic plantar fasciotomy to open plantar fasciotomy with heel spur resection for chronic plantar fasciitis/heel spur syndrome. *J. Foot Ankle Surg.,* 1995; 34: 305–311.

47. **Torg, J.S., Pavlov, H., and Torg, E.** Overuse injuries in sport: the foot. *Clin. Sports Med.,* 1987; 6: 291–320.

48. **Tountas, A.A. and Fornasier, V.L.** Operative treatment of subcalcaneal pain. *Clin. Orthop.,* 1996; 332: 170–178.

49. **Tsai, W.C., Wang, C.L., Tang, F.T., Hsu, T.C., Hsu, K.H., and Wong, M.K.** Treatment of proximal plantar fasciitis with ultrasound-guided steroid injection. *Arch. Phys. Med. Rehabil.,* 2000; 81: 1416–1421.

50. **Vasavada, P.J., DeVries, D.F., and Nishiyama, H.** Plantar fasciitis — early blood pool images in the diagnosis of inflammatory process. *Foot Ankle,* 1984; 5: 74–76.

51. **Wang, C.J., Chen, H.S., and Huang, T.W.** Shockwave therapy for patients with plantar fasciitis: a one-year follow-up study. *Foot Ankle,* 2002; 23: 204–207.

52. **Wapner, K.L. and Sharkey, P.F.** The use of night splints for treatment of recalcitrant plantar fasciitis. *Foot Ankle,* 1991; 12: 135–137.

53. **Ward, W.G. and Clippinger, F.W.** Proximal medial longitudinal arch incision for plantar fascia release. *Foot Ankle,* 1987; 8: 152–155.

54. **Warren, B.L. and Jones, C.J.** Predicting plantar fasciitis in runners. *Med. Sci. Sports Exerc.,* 1987; 19: 71–73.

55. **Warren, B.L.** Plantar fasciitis in runners. *Sports Med.,* 1990; 10: 338–345.

56. **Williams, P.L., Smibert, J.G., Cox, R. et al.** Imaging study of the painful heel syndrome. *Foot Ankle,* 1987; 7: 345–349.

57. **Yu, J.S.** Pathological and postoperative conditions of the plantar fascia: review of MRI imaging appearances. *Skel. Radiol.,* 2000; 29: 491–501.

Anterior Impingement Syndrome and Other Subchapters
(III, IV, V, VI, VII, and VIII)

58. **Alanen, J., Orava, S., Heinonen, O.J., Ikonen, J., and Kvist, M.** Peroneal tendon injuries. Report of thirty-eight operated cases. *Ann. Chir. Gynaecol.,* 2001; 90: 43–46.

59. **Allen, M.A. and Casillas, M.M.** The passive axial compression (PAC) test: a new adjunctive provocative maneuver for the clinical diagnosis of hallucal sesamoiditis. *Foot Ankle,* 2001; 22: 345–346.

60. **Axe, M.J. and Ray, R.L.** Orthotic treatment of sesamoid pain. *Am. J. Sports Med.,* 1988; 16: 411–416.

61. **Branca, A., DiPalma, L., Bucca, C., Visconti, C.S., and DiMille, M.** Arthroscopic treatment of anterior ankle impingement. *Foot Ankle,* 1997; 18: 413–418.

62. **Brukner, P.** Calf and ankle swelling. *Aust. Fam. Physician,* 2000; 29(1): 35–40

63. **Chung, Y., Rosenberg, Z.S., Mogee, T., and Chinitz, L.** Normal anatomy and pathologic conditions of ankle tendons: current imaging techniques. *Radiographics,* 1992; 12: 429–444.

64. **Clarke, H.D., Kitaoka, H.B., and Ehman, R.L.** Peroneal tendon injuries. *Foot Ankle,* 1998; 19: 280–288.

65. **Coughlin, R.R.** Common injuries of the foot. *Postgrad. Med.,* 1989; 86: 175–85.

66. **Dijk, van, C.N., Tol, J.L., and Verheyen, C.P.P.M.** A prospective study of prognostic factors concerning the outcome of arthroscopic surgery for anterior ankle impingement. *Am. J. Sports Med.,* 1997; 25: 737–745.

67. **Dijk, van, C.N. and Scholte, D.** Arthroscopy of the ankle joint. *Arthroscopy,* 1997; 13: 90–96.

68. **Dijk, van, C.N. and Kort, N.** Tendoscopy of the peroneal tendons. *Arthroscopy,* 1998; 14: 471–478.

69. **Dijk, van, C.N., Scholten, P.E., and Krips, R.** A 2-portal endoscopic approach for diagnosis and treatment of posterior ankle pathology. *Arthroscopy,* 2000; 16: 871–876.

70. **Dijk, van, C.N., Wessel, R.N., Tol, J.L., and Maas, M.** Oblique radiograph for the detection of bone spurs in anterior ankle impingement. *Skel. Radiol.,* 2002; 31: 214–221.

71. **Duddy, R.K., Meredith, R., Visser, J., and Brooks, J.S.** Tendon sheath injuries of the foot and ankle. *J. Foot Surg.,* 1991; 30: 179–186.

72. **Ewing, J.W.** Arthroscopic management of transchondral talar-dome fractures (osteochondritis dissecans) and anterior impingement lesions of the ankle joint. *Clin. Sport Med.,* 1991; 10: 677–687.

73. **Ferkel, R.D., Karzel, R.P., Del Pizzo, W., Friedman, M.J., and Fischer, S.P.** Arthroscopic treatment of anterolateral impingement of the ankle. *Am. J. Sports Med.,* 1991; 19: 440–446.

74. **Fond, D.** Flexor hallucis longus tendinitis — a case of mistaken identity and posterior impingement syndrome in dancers: evaluation and management. *J. Orthop. Sports Phys. Ther.,* 1984; 5: 204–206.

75. **Frankel, J.P. and Harrington, J.** Symptomatic bipartite sesamoids. *J. Foot Surg.,* 1990; 29: 318–323.

76. **Frey, C.C. and Shereff, M.J.** Tendon injuries about the ankle in athletes. *Clin. Sports Med.,* 1988; 7: 103–118.

77. **Fricker, P.A. and Williams, J.G.P.** Surgical management of os trigonum and talar spur in sportsmen. *Br. J. Sports Med.,* 1979; 13: 55–57.

78. **Garrick, J.G. and Webb, D.R.** *Sports Injuries: Diagnosis and Management.* Philadelphia: W.B. Saunders, 1990.

79. **Garth, W.P.** Flexor hallucis tendinitis in a ballet dancer. A case report. *J. Bone Joint Surg.,* 1981; 63A: 1489.

80. **Gould, N.** Stenosing tenosynovitis of the flexor hallucis longus at the great toe. *Foot Ankle,* 1981; 2: 46–48.

81. **Grace, D.L.** Sesamoid problems. *Foot Ankle Clin.,* 2000; 5: 609–627.

82. **Hamilton, W.G.** Foot and ankle injuries in dancers. *Clin. Sports Med.,* 1988; 7: 143–173.

83. **Hardaker, W.T., Jr., Margello, S., and Goldner, J.L.** Foot and ankle injuries in theatrical dancers. *Foot Ankle,* 1985; 6: 59–69.

84. **Hardaker, W.T., Jr.** Foot and ankle injuries in classical ballet dancers. *Orthop. Clin. North Am.,* 1989; 20: 621–627.

85. **Hawkins, R.B.** Arthroscopic treatment of sports — related anterior osteophytes in the ankle. *Foot Ankle,* 1988; 9: 87–90.

86. **Holt, K.W.G. and Cross, M.J.** Isolated rupture of the flexor hallucis longus tendon. A case report. *Am. J. Sports Med.,* 1990; 18: 645–646.

87. **Howse, A.J.G.** Orthopedists aid ballet. *Clin. Orthop.,* 1972; 89: 52–63.

88. **Jahss, M.H.** The sesamoids of the hallux. *Clin. Orthop.,* 1981; 157: 88–97.

89. **Johnson, R.P., Collier, D.B., and Carrera, G.F.** The os trigonum syndrome: use of bone scan in the diagnosis. *J. Trauma,* 1984; 24: 761–764.

90. **Keene, J.S. and Lange, R.H.** Diagnostic dilemmas in foot and ankle injuries. *J. Am. Med. Assoc.,* 1986; 256: 247–251.

91. **Khan, K., Brown, J., Way, S., Vass, N., Crichton, K., Alexander, R., Baxter, A., Butler, M., and Wark, J.** Overuse injuries in classical ballet. *Sports Med.,* 1995; 19: 341–357.

92. **Kolettis, G.J., Micheli, L.J., and Klein, J.D.** Release of the flexor hallucis longus tendon in ballet dancers. *J. Bone Joint Surg.,* 1996; 78: 1386–1390.

93. **Leventen, E.O.** Sesamoid disorders and treatment — an update. *Clin. Orthop.,* 1991; 269: 236–240.

94. **Lillich, J.S. and Baxter, D.E.** Common forefoot problems in runners. *Foot Ankle,* 1986; 7: 145–151.

95. **Lombardi, C.M., Silhanek, A.D., and Connolly, F.G.** Modified arthroscopic excision of the symptomatic os trigonum and release of the flexor hallucis longus tendon: operative technique and case study. *J. Foot Ankle Surg.*, 1999; 38: 347–351.

96. **Lynch, T. and Pupp, G.R.** Stenosing tenosynovitis of the flexor hallucis longus at the ankle joint. *J. Foot Surg.*, 1990; 29: 345–352.

97. **Mason, R.B. and Henderson, J.P.** Traumatic peroneal tendon instability. *Am. J. Sports Med.*, 1996; 24: 652–658.

98. **McBryde, A.M. and Anderson, R.B.** Sesamoid foot problems in the athlete. *Clin. Sports Med.*, 1988; 7: 51–60.

99. **McCarroll, J.R., Schrader, J.W., Shelbourne, K.D. et al.** Meniscoid lesions of the ankle in soccer players. *Am. J. Sports Med.*, 1987; 15: 255–257.

100. **McDougall, A.** The os trigonum. *J. Bone Joint Surg.*, 1955; 37(B): 257–265.

101. **McLennan, J.G.** Treatment of acute and chronic luxations of the peroneal tendons. *Am. J. Sports Med.*, 1980; 8: 432–436.

102. **Micheli, L.J., Waters, M.P., and Sanders, D.P.** Sliding fibular graft repair for chronic dislocation of the peroneal tendons. *Am. J. Sports Med.*, 1989; 17: 68–71.

103. **Oden, R.R.** Tendon injuries about the ankle resulting from skiing. *Clin. Orthop.*, 1987; 216: 63–69.

104. **Ogilvie-Harris, D.J., Mahomed, N., and Demaziere, A.** Anterior impingement of the ankle treated by arthroscopic removal of bony-spurs. *J. Bone Joint Surg.*, 1993; 75(B): 437–440.

105. **Paulos, L.E., Johnson, C.L., and Noyes, F.R.** Posterior compartment fractures of the ankle. *Am. J. Sports Med.*, 1983; 11: 439–443.

106. **Pećina, M. and Bojanić, I.** Posterior impingement syndrome of the ankle. *Acta Orthop. Iugosl.*, 1989; 20: 120–123.

107. **Perez Carro, L., Echevarria Llata, J.I., and Martinez Agueros, J.A.** Arthroscopic medial bipartite sesamoidectomy of the great toe. *Arthroscopy*, 1999; 15: 321–323.

108. **Plattner, P.F.** Tendon problems of the foot and ankle. *Postgrad. Med.*, 1989; 86: 155–170.

109. **Quirk, R.** Common foot and ankle injuries in dance. *Orthop. Clin. North Am.*, 1994; 25: 123–133.

110. **Raikin, S.M. and Cooke, P.H.** Divot sign: a new observation in anterior impingement of the ankle. *Foot Ankle*, 1999; 20: 532–533.

111. **Rasmussen, S. and Hjorth Jensen, C.** Arthroscopic treatment of impingement of the ankle reduces pain and enhances function. *Scand. J. Med. Sci. Sports*, 2002; 12: 69–72.

112. **Richardson, E.G.,** Hallucal sesamoid pain: causes and surgical treatment. *J. Am. Acad. Orthop. Surg.*, 1999; 7: 270–278.

113. **Sammarco, G.J.** The foot and ankle in classical ballet and modern dance, in *Disorders of the Foot,* Jahss, M.H., Ed. Philadelphia: W.B. Saunders, 1982; 1626–1659.

114. **Sammarco, G.J.** Diagnosis and treatment in dancers. *Clin. Orthop.*, 1984; 187: 176–187.

115. **Sammarco, G.J. and Cooper, P.S.** Flexor hallucis longus tendon injury in dancers and nondancers. *Foot Ankle*, 1998; 19: 356–362.

116. **Sanhudo, J.A.** Stenosing tenosynovitis of the flexor hallucis longus tendon at the sesamoid rea. *Foot Ankle*, 2002; 23: 801–803.

117. **Sarmiento, A. and Wolf, M.** Subluxation of the peroneal tendons. *J. Bone Joint Surg.*, 1975; 57(A): 115–116.

118. **Scheller, A.D., Kasser, J.R., and Quigley, T.B.** Tendon injuries about the ankle. *Orthop. Clin. North Am.*, 1980; 11: 801–811.

119. **Scranton, P.E., Jr., and McDermott, J.E.** Anterior tibiotalar spurs: a comparison of open versus arthroscopic debridement. *Foot Ankle*, 1992; 13: 125–129.

120. **Stoller, S.M., Hekmat, F., and Kleiger, B.** A comparative study of the frequency of anterior impingement exostoses of the ankle in dancers and nondancers. *Foot Ankle*, 1984; 4: 201–203.

121. **Tol, J.L., Verheyen, C.P.P.M., and van Dijk, C.N.** Arthroscopic treatment of anterior impingement in the ankle. *J. Bone Joint Surg.*, 2001; 83(B): 9–13.

122. **Tudisco, C. and Puddu, G.** Stenosing tenosynovitis of the flexor hallucis longus tendon in a classical ballet dancer. A case report. *Am. J. Sports Med.*, 1984; 12: 403–404.

123. **Van Hal, M.E., Keene, J.S., and Lange, T.A.** Stress fractures of the great toe sesamoids. *Am. J. Sports Med.*, 1982; 10: 122–128.

124. **Zoelner, G. and Clancy, W., Jr.** Recurrent dislocation of the peroneal tendon. *J. Bone Joint Surg.*, 1979; 61(A): 292–294.

Part V

Other Overuse Injuries

11 Bursitis

Synovial bursae constitute an integral part of the bone–tendon–joint complex. They are particularly susceptible to injuries and damage in athletes. Direct acute trauma leads to bleeding into the bursal space, causing acute swelling and pain with limited motion; this is usually called *acute hemorrhagic bursitis*. Repetitive microtraumas, such as permanently increased friction of tendon over the bursa or constant outer pressure on bursa (ill-fitting shoes or athletic equipment), can cause chronic inflammation clinically referred to as *chronic bursitis*. Bursitis may be infected either primarily or secondarily, and these cases are referred to as *septic bursitis*.[65] Overuse injuries include chronic bursitis as well.[4,7,16,33,34,47]

I. ANATOMY

Synovial bursae are either small or large closed saclike structures that lie in continuity with, but not normally in communication with, a joint. They are found between skin and bone (prepatellar bursa), tendon and tendon (semitendinosus bursa), bone and tendon (deep infrapatellar bursa), tendon and ligament (between fibular collateral ligament and popliteus tendon), tendon and capsule (semimembranosus bursa), and also in the subfascial planes noted under the iliotibial tract.

The structure of the mucous sac membranous wall is similar to that of the joint capsule synovial membrane; it normally secretes a small amount of fluid, which acts as a lubricant, enabling the two bursal surfaces to glide easily over one another. The basic function of the mucous sacs is to improve the gliding motion of two adjoining structures by dissipating friction.

More than 150 synovial sacs are found in a human body, and each may show clinical symptoms. We emphasize only a few, specifically those most commonly affected in athletes. Although the shoulder area contains eight synovial sacs (Figure 11.1), only the subacromial bursa is of great clinical significance.[1,9] The subacromial bursa is located between the acromion, coracoacromial ligament, and deltoid muscle on one side, and joint capsule with coracohumeral ligament and rotator cuff tendons of the shoulder on the other side (Figure 11.2). Several bursae are found in the elbow region — the olecranon bursa, the radial and ulnar epicondylar bursae, the radiohumeral bursa, the supinator bursa, and the bicipital radial bursa. Only the olecranon bursa (Figure 11.3) is of practical clinical significance.[10,60] The wrist region is characterized by frequent synovial herniation or synovial cyst at the volar or dorsal side of the joint. Due to weak membrane of the joint capsule, usually resulting from long-term and chronic overuse, part of the synovial membrane herniates under the skin, forming a relatively hard node that may be either large or small in size. The lesion is known as *ganglion cyst* and is not to be confused with bursitis.[58]

The hip region is known for many synovial sacs. Specific mention should be made of the great trochanter bursa, the subgluteal, ischiogluteal, and iliopectineal bursae, and the iliopsoas tendon attachment bursa.[11,19,20,28,50,55] The trochanteric bursa is the most important from a practical and clinical viewpoint (Figure 11.4). A number of synovial sacs are found in the knee region (Figure 11.5): prepatellar bursa, infrapatellar bursa, suprapatellar bursa, semimembranosus bursa, pes anserina bursa, bursa between the fibular collateral ligament and popliteal tendon, bursa between popliteal tendon and lateral femoral condyle, bursa of the lateral head of the gastrocnemius, bursa between the fibular collateral ligament and biceps tendon, medial collateral ligament bursa, and medial head of the gastrocnemius muscle bursa.[8,15,23,24,25,48] Some of the bursae communicate with the joint space (articular cavity). For example, the bursa between the medial head of the

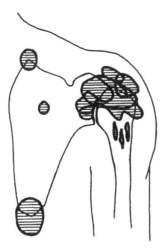

FIGURE 11.1 Bursae in the shoulder region.

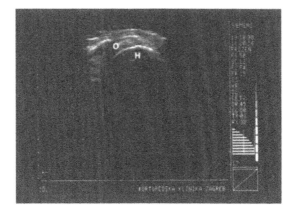

FIGURE 11.2 Sonogram showing ossification in the subacromial bursa. H = humeral head; O = ossification.

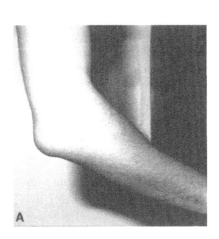

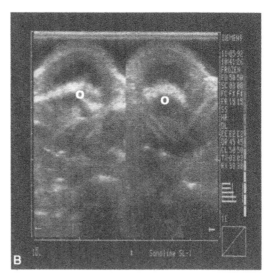

FIGURE 11.3 (A) Olecranon bursa. Native. (B) Olecranon bursa. Sonogram. O = olecranon.

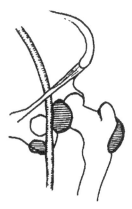

FIGURE 11.4 Bursae in the hip region.

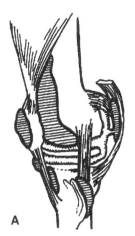

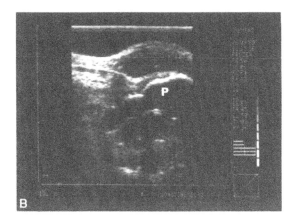

FIGURE 11.5 (A) Bursae in the knee region. (B) Sonogram demonstrating prepatellar bursitis. P = patella.

gastrocnemius and the semimembranosus muscle communicates through the posterior joint capsule with the knee joint (Figure 11.6). Frequent swelling of the bursa results in the formation of popliteal cyst (Baker's cyst).[16,51,64]

Regarding the ankle and the foot, the bursae located in the region of the heel bone and Achilles tendon attachment are of greater clinical significance, as are those in the region of the metatarsophalangeal joint of the big toe. The retrocalcaneal bursa is located between the posterior plane of the heel bone and the anterior aspect of the Achilles tendon (Figure 11.7), and the superficial Achilles tendon bursa is located between the posterior aspect of the tendon and the skin.[17,27,49] As a result of long-term pressure on the foot caused by ill-fitting shoes, bursitis may occur in different sites, while septic bursitis commonly develops in the big toe region.[47]

II. ETIOPATHOGENESIS

A direct blow as either in a collision with an athletic competitor or through contact with a hard surface may cause an acute hemorrhagic bursitis.[4,16,33,34,37,47] Direct trauma causes bleeding into the bursal space, which results in acute swelling, pain, and limited mobility. Bursae may also be injured by a less violent but constant repetitive stress, usually occurring during athletic or some other work-related activities.[4,16,33,34,47] The repetitive stress in sports may be caused by artificial surfaces, wrestling mats, and gymnastic floor exercise mats.[26,47] However, repetitive joint motion is the most common cause. The most characteristic example is the development of chronic bursitis of the shoulder joint

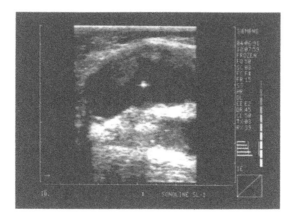

FIGURE 11.6 Sonogram of the posterior part of the knee, demonstrating a large Baker's cyst.

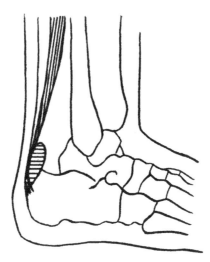

FIGURE 11.7 Retrocalcaneal bursa.

in throwers because of the repetitive swinging motions of their arm.[18,47] The initial physiologic reaction to repetitive stress is vasodilation resulting from the increased blood flow into the injured area. The bursa becomes warm and sometimes erythematous. Changes take place in the permeability of the capillary wall, and extracellular fluid and serum protein accumulate in the bursa. These processes are clinically manifested as swelling. If the condition persists, the bursal wall thickens and calcium may be deposited, causing the bursal fluid to acquire a consistency similar to toothpaste.[38] The condition is referred to as *chemical bursitis*. This type of bursitis causes degeneration and calcification of tendons, very much like calcification of the supraspinatus tendon. The direct cause of calcification in tendon and bursa has not yet been fully explained. According to Reilly and Nicholas,[47] changes in the collagen structure of the bursa and its neighboring tendons result in increased affinity for calcium salts, possibly with a local increase in hydrogen ion concentration.

Chronic subacromial bursitis is caused by repetitive motions in sports requiring a significant amount of overhead throwing-type motions, such as swimming, gymnastics, baseball, tennis, and weightlifting.[18,40,47] Bursitis may precede rotator cuff tendinitis, although in most cases it is a secondary sign.[18] Bursal reaction and swelling result from the need to decrease friction, i.e., an effort to create a soft cushion in the area of tendinous lesions.

Acute olecranon bursa injuries have often been noted in athletes participating in such sport activities as football, hockey, handball, and basketball.[10,61] Weight lifters and gymnasts often suffer from chronic inflammation of this bursa.[61] A specific feature of this lesion is the so-called student's elbow, which is marked by inflammation of the olecranon bursa caused by long-term pressure on the bursa as a result of a characteristic position when studying (leaning on the elbows on a table).[47]

According to the findings of some authors, bursitis in the hip region may develop as a result of abductor tendinitis, i.e., dancing activities or gymnastics (bursitis of the medial gluteal muscle and the piriformis muscle).[29,46] The best illustration of bursitis resulting from repetitive friction of an anatomic structure over the bursa is trochanteric bursitis. In cases when the iliotibial band is excessively tight, during flexion and extension in the hip joint, the friction of the iliotibial band against the greater trochanter of the femur and the underlying bursa leads to chronic bursitis.[42]

Bursitis in the knee region most commonly develops as a consequence of overuse. Anatomical malalignment of the lower leg is often mentioned as a predisposing factor to bursitis. For example, lower leg valgum alignment predisposes to anserine bursitis, while an increased Q-angle predisposes to the prepatellar and infrapatellar bursitis.[23,47]

Bursitis in the ankle (retrocalcaneal and superficial Achilles tendon bursitis) is common in runners and walkers.[49] Anatomical malalignment of the lower leg, such as tibia vara, equinus or cavus feet, and tight calf muscles predispose the athlete to the development of these types of bursitis. The retrocalcaneal bursitis caused by prominence of the posterior superior portion of the calcaneus ("hatchet" sign) is considered a separate entity. This type of bursitis is usually accompanied by insertional tendinitis (enthesitis) of the Achilles tendon, commonly referred to as Haglund syndrome or disease.[14,17,47,49,54,62]

Brown et al. describe malleolar bursitis in figure skaters.[5]

III. CLINICAL PICTURE AND DIAGNOSTICS

In trying to identify the cause of pain in athletes and to treat and prevent injuries occurring in sports or recreation, bursae are rarely taken into account, although their acute or chronic injury may significantly diminish the abilities of an athlete. Swelling and pain with a limited motion are signs of acute bursitis. The major symptom of chronic bursitis is dull pain in the bursal region during certain motions of the joint. Clinical examination reveals pain when pressure is applied either on the affected bursa or on the pathologically altered tendon that is the underlying cause of bursitis.

Clinical findings greatly depend on the location of bursitis. Subacromial bursitis is characterized by pain in the position of the arm above the head and in its abduction above the axillary line. The impingement sign and test are positive in subacromial bursitis.[18] Chronic olecranon bursitis causes no pain; the patient complains of swelling in the elbow region as a major clinical symptom and difficulty in elbow flexion above 90°.[47] In contrast to chronic olecranon bursitis, trochanteris bursitis is usually rather painful and often will cause the patient to limp.[42,66] Patients complain of inability to put on their shoes because of severe pain. Clinical examination shows localized tenderness on the lateral aspect of the great trochanter and antalgic gait. Straight leg raising and quadriceps stretching elicit pain, as does Ober's test. Passive range of hip motion is normal but often weakness is detected in the hip abductors and flexors.[29,42,46] In view of its pathology, iliopsoas bursitis might be better referred to as iliopsoas syndrome.[19] Prepatellar bursitis is characterized by gradual swelling and pain in the anterior aspect of the knee and slightly limited terminal knee flexion.[23,37] Beside antalgic gait, clinical examination also shows quadriceps hypotrophy and tightness of hamstrings. As opposed to prepatellar bursitis, in the case of intra-articular effusion, pain is present and range of motion is markedly decreased. Pes anserine bursitis is manifested by tenderness in the antero-medial aspect of the proximal tibia (just below the joint line).[2,12,23,47] The tenderness may also extend proximally along the pes anserine tendons to the posteromedial corner of the knee. Pes anserine bursitis has been encountered more often in athletes with tight hamstrings, lower limb valgus alignment, increased external tibial torsion, and increased femoral anteversion. Semimembranosus bursitis causes tenderness at the posteromedial corner of the knee. The pain may be elicited by passive knee extension and resisted active flexion.[23] In retrocalcaneal bursitis, the patient usually complains of pain in the morning when getting out of bed and when getting out of a chair after a shorter period of sitting. Swelling prominence is noted on both sides of the Achilles tendon, although thickened areas or nodes do not appear and cannot be palpated on the tendon itself. Clinical examination provokes pain by placing the thumb and index fingers in the space behind the tendon and in front of the talus. Crepitation may also be noticed in this region. No limping is seen during normal walking, but it may be clearly noticed during running.[47,49]

In addition to clinical findings, radiographic diagnosis is also necessary. Radiographic findings show that certain osseous alterations may cause bursitis — enlarged prominence of the posterior superior portion of the calcaneus, changes in the acromion, abnormal iliopsoas tendon motion, and intratendinous and intrabursal calcifications.[55] By introducing noninvasive ultrasonographic diagnostic procedures, bursography (the injection of contrast media into the bursal space) is no longer of prime importance. Ultrasonography has proved to be of great help in the diagnosis of acute and chronic bursitis.[13,31,35,43,56] Diagnostic ultrasound enables evaluation not only of density and amount of bursal content but also of alterations in bursal walls. Arthroscopy has recently been used more extensively both for the diagnosis and treatment of some types of bursitis, e.g., subacromial bursitis, trochanteric bursitis, prepatellar bursitis, olecranon bursitis, and deep infrapatellar bursitis.[3,22,39–41,53] Computerized tomography (CT) and scintigraphy are also used, although magnetic resonance imaging (MRI) is the diagnostic method of choice, and on MRI the inflamed bursa is seen as fluid-filled distended sac with low signal intensity on T1-weighted images and high signal intensity on T2-weighted images.[6,12,30,32,36,44,51,57,59,60] Laboratory analysis of bursal aspirate is performed whenever nontraumatic etiology of bursitis is suspected, e.g., when bursitis could be of septic, tuberculous, rheumatoid, or gouty origin.[38]

When diagnosing sports injuries, one should always consider the possibility of bursitis.

IV. TREATMENT

Non-operative treatment is the method of choice in acute and chronic bursitis; it entails rest, reduction of the activity that provokes pain, administration of nonsteroidal anti-inflammatory medication, and aspiration of bursal content with compression dressing. In chronic bursitis, water-soluble steroid injections are applied directly into the bursa. It has been noted that in chronic bursitis the mere aspiration of the bursal content is not sufficient, as effusion tends to recur. Physical therapy of chronic bursitis is based on stretching exercises with the purpose of increasing muscle flexibility, thus reducing pressure on the bursa and achieving painless motion. Non-operative treatment procedures depend on the underlying cause and site of bursitis. It has been observed that in chronic trochanteric bursitis or subacromial bursitis good treatment outcome is achieved by corticosteroid injections.[52] Orthotic foot corrections are essential in the treatment of retrocalcaneal bursitis.[29,47] The introduction of an angiocatheter into the bursa followed by compressive dressing of the elbow for 3 days is the procedure proposed for the treatment of chronic olecranon bursitis.[10]

Surgical treatment is indicated when appropriate non-operative treatment fails. Operative treatment entails removing the bursa but only in terms of space decompression (resection of coracoacromial ligament or acromioplasty) or in terms of bursectomy (arthroscopic technique is possible for bursitis of various localizations).[39–41,47,53,66] The cause of bursitis should also be removed surgically — resection of the prominence of the posterior superior portion of the calcaneus or removal of the tip of the olecranon.[14,27,54,62]

Following operative treatment, progressive physical therapy is always prescribed, consisting primarily of stretching exercises to achieve and even increase the active range of painless motion. After that, and depending on the site of bursitis and type of athletic activity, the patient engages in gradual exercises to strengthen the affected muscles.

REFERENCES

1. **Bimbaum, K. and Lierse, W.** Anatomy and function of the bursa subacromialis. *Acta Anat.* (Basel), 1992; 145: 354–363.
2. **Boland, A.L., Jr. and Hulstyn, M.J.** Soft-tissue injuries of the knee, in *The Lower Extremity and Spine in Sports Medicine*, 2nd ed., Nicholas, J.A. and Hershman, E.B., Eds. St. Louis: Mosby, 1995.
3. **Bradley, D.M. and Dillingham, M.F.** Bursoscopy of the trochanteric bursa. *Arthroscopy*, 1998; 14: 884–887.
4. **Brody, D.M.** Running injuries. *Clin. Symp.*, 1987; 39: 1–36.
5. **Brown, T.D., Varney, T.E., and Micheli, J.J.** Malleolar bursitis in figure skaters. Indications for operative and nonoperative treatment. *Am. J. Sports Med.*, 2000; 28: 109–111.
6. **Bureau, N.J., Dussault, R.C., and Keats, T.E.** Imaging of bursae around shoulder joint. *Skel. Radiol.*, 1996; 21: 35–43.
7. **Chen, W.S. and Wang, C.J.** Recalcitrant bicipital radial bursitis. *Arch. Orthop. Trauma Surg.*, 1999; 119: 105–108.
8. **Damron, T. and Sim, F.H.** Soft-tissue tumors about the knee. *J. Am. Acad. Orthop. Surg.*, 1997; 5: 141–152.
9. **Duranthon, L.D. and Gagey, O.J.** Anatomy and function of the subdeltoid bursa. *Surg. Radiol. Anat.*, 2001; 23: 23–25.
10. **Fisher, R.H.** Conservative treatment of distended patellar and olecranon bursae. *Clin. Orthop.*, 1977; 123: 98–99.
11. **Flanagan, F.L. et al.** Symptomatic enlarged iliopsoas bursae in the presence of a normal plain hip radiograph. *Br. J. Rheumatol.*, 1995; 34: 365–369.
12. **Forbes, J.R., Helms, C.A., and Janzen, D.L.** Acute pes anserinus bursitis: MR imaging. *Radiology*, 1995; 194: 525–527.
13. **Fornage, B.D. and Rifkin, M.D.** Ultrasound examination of tendons. *Radiol. Clin. North Am.*, 1988; 26: 87–107.
14. **Heneghan, M.A. and Pavlov, H.** The Haglund painful heel syndrome. *Clin. Orthop.*, 1984; 187: 228–234.
15. **Henningan, S.P. et al.** The semimembranosus-tibial collateral ligament bursa. Anatomical study and magnetic resonance imaging. *J. Bone Joint Surg.*, 1994; 76(A): 1322–1327.
16. **Herring, S.A. and Nilson, K.L.** Introduction to overuse injuries. *Clin. Sports Med.*, 1987; 6: 225–239.
17. **Hintermann, B. and Holzach, P.** Die Bursitis subachillea — eine biomechanische Analyse und klinische Studie. *Z. Orthop.*, 1992; 130: 114–119.
18. **Jobe, F.W. and Bradley, J.P.** Diagnosis of shoulder injuries. *Clin. Sports Med.*, 1989; 8: 419–438.
19. **Johnston, C.A. et al.** Iliopsoas bursitis and tendinitis. *Sports Med.*, 1998; 25: 271–283.
20. **Jones, P.B. et al.** Iliopsoas bursa presenting as deep vein thrombosis in rheumatoid arthritis. *Br. J. Rheumatol.*, 1993; 32: 832–834.
21. **Kannangara, S. et al.** Scintigraphy of cubital bursitis. *Clin. Nucl. Med.*, 2002; 27: 348–350.
22. **Klein, W.** Endoscopy of the deep infrapatellar bursa. *Arthroscopy*, 1996; 12: 127–131.
23. **Kujala, U.M., Kvist, M., and Osterman, K.** Knee injuries in athletes. *Sports Med.*, 1986; 3: 447–460.
24. **La Prade, R.F.** The anatomy of the deep infrapatellar bursa of the knee. *Am. J. Sports Med.*, 1998; 26: 129–132.
25. **La Prade, R.F. and Hamilton, C.D.** The fibular collateral ligament-biceps femoris bursa. An anatomic study. *Am. J. Sports Med.*, 1997; 25: 439–443.
26. **Larson, R.L. and Ostering, L.R.** Traumatic bursitis and artificial turf. *Am. J. Sports Med.*, 1974; 2: 183–188.
27. **Lehto, M.U., Jarvinen, M., and Suominen, P.** Chronic Achilles peritendinitis and retrocalcanear bursitis. Long-term follow-up of surgically treated cases. *Knee Surg. Sports Traumatol. Arthrosc.*, 1994; 2: 182–185.
28. **Lin, Y.M., Ho, T.F., and Lee, T.S.** Iliopectineal bursitis complicating hemiarthroplasty: a case report. *Clin. Orthop.*, 2001; 392: 366–371.
29. **Lloyd-Smith, R. et al.** A survey of overuse and traumatic hip and pelvic injuries in athletes. *Phys. Sportsmed.*, 1985; 12: 131–141.

30. **Major, N.M.** MR imaging after therapeutic injection of the subacromial bursa. *Skel. Radiol.,* 1999; 28: 628–631.
31. **Major, N.M.** Imaging of the subcoracoid bursa. *Am. J. Roentgenol.,* 2001; 176: 812–813.
32. **Mahlfeld, K. et al.** Value of ultrasound in diagnosis of bursopathies in the area of the Achilles tendon. *Ultraschall Med.,* 2001; 22: 87–90.
33. **Mattalino, A.J., Deese, J.M., Jr., and Campbell, E.D., Jr.** Office evaluation and treatment of lower extremity injuries in the runner. *Clin. Sports Med.,* 1989; 8: 461–475.
34. **McCarthy, P.** Managing bursitis in the athlete: an overview. *Phys. Sportsmed.,* 1989; 17: 115–123.
35. **Mellerowicz, H., Stelling, E., and Kefenbaum, A.** Diagnostic ultrasound in the athlete's locomotor system. *Br. J. Sports Med.,* 1990; 24: 31–39.
36. **Miller, T.T., Ghelman, B., and Potter, H.G.** Imaging of the foot and ankle, in *The Lower Extremity and Spine in Sports Medicine,* 2nd ed., Nicholas, J.A. and Hershman, E.B., Eds. St. Louis: Mosby, 1995.
37. **Mysyk, M.C., Wroble, R.R., and Foster, D.T.** Prepatellar bursitis in wrestlers, *Am. J. Sport Med.,* 1986; 14: 46–54.
38. **Newman, R.J., Curtis, G.D.W., and Slack, M.P.E.** Bursal fluid lactate determination and the diag⸱ nosis of bursitis. *Br. Med. J.,* 1983; 286: 2022–2023.
39. **Nussbaumer, P., Candrian, C., and Hollinger, A.** Endoscopic bursa shaving in acute bursitis. *Swiss Surg.,* 2001; 7: 121–125.
40. **Ogilvie-Harris, D.J. and D'Angelo, G.** Arthroscopic surgery of the shoulder. *Sports Med.,* 1990; 9: 120–128.
41. **Ogilvie-Harris, D.J. and Gilbart, M.** Endoscopic bursal resection: the olecranon bursa and prepatellar bursa. *Arthroscopy,* 2000; 16: 249–253.
42. **Pećina, M. and Bojanić, I.** The snapping hip syndrome. *Croat. Sports Med. J.,* 1992; 7: 28–32.
43. **Pećina, M. Bojanić, I., and Janković, S.** Ultrasound diagnostics of bursitis of different localization. *Croat. Sports Med. J.,* 1993; 8: 25–34.
44. **Pfirrmann, C.W. et al.** Greater trochanter of the hip: attachment of the abductor mechanism and a complex of three bursae. MR imaging and MR bursography in cadavers and MR imaging in asymptomatic volunteers. *Radiology,* 2001; 221: 469–477.
45. **Rahme, H. et al.** The subacromial bursa and the impingement syndrome. A clinical and histological study of 30 cases. *Acta Orthop. Scand.,* 1993; 64: 485–488.
46. **Reid, D.C.** Prevention of hip and knee injuries in ballet dancers. *Sports Med.,* 1988; 6: 295–307.
47. **Reilly, J.P. and Nicholas, J.A.** The chronically inflamed bursa. *Clin. Sports Med.,* 1987; 6: 345–370.
48. **Roland, G.C., Beagley, M.J., and Cawley, P.W.** Conservative treatment of inflamed knee bursitis. *Phys. Sportsmed.,* 1992; 20: 67–77.
49. **Rossi, F. et al.** The Haglund syndrome: clinical and radiological features and sports medicine aspects. *J. Sports Med.,* 1987; 27: 238–265.
50. **Salmeron, I. et al.** Idiopathic iliopsoas bursitis. *Eur. Radiol.,* 1999; 9: 175.
51. **Sansone, V., de Ponti, A., and Paluello, G.M.** Popliteal cysts and associated disorders of the knee: critical review with MR imaging. *Int. Orthop.,* 1995; 19: 275–279.
52. **Scott, P.M.** Treating subacromial bursitis with an injection into the bursa. *JAAPA,* 2000; 13: 16–19.
53. **Steinacker, T. and Verdonck, A.J.** Endoscopic therapy of pre-patellar bursitis. *Sportverletz. Sportschaden,* 1998; 12: 162–164.
54. **Stephens, M.M.** Haglund's deformity and retrocalcaneal bursitis. *Orthop. Clin. North Am.,* 1994; 25: 41–46.
55. **Vaccaro, J.P., Sauser, D.D., and Beals, R.K.** Iliopsoas bursa imaging: efficacy in depicting abnormal iliopsoas tendon motion in patients with internal snapping hip syndrome. *Radiology,* 1995; 197: 853–856.
56. **van Holsbeeck, M. and Strouse, P.J.** Sonography of the shoulder: evaluation of the subacromialsubdeltoid bursa. *Am. J. Roentgenol.,* 1993; 160: 561–564.
57. **Varma, D.G., Parihar, A., and Richli, W.R.** CT appearance of the distended trochanteric bursa. *Comput. Assist. Tomogr.,* 1993; 17: 141–143.
58. **Wood, M.B. and Dobyns, J.H.** Sports-related extraarticular wrist syndromes. *Clin. Orthop.,* 1986; 202: 93–102.
59. **Wunderbaldinger, P. et al.** Imaging features of iliopsoas bursitis. *Eur. Radiol.,* 2002; 12: 409–415.

60. **Yamamoto, T. et al.** Bicipital radial bursitis: CT and MR appearance. *Comput. Med. Imaging Graph.,* 2001, 25: 531–533.
61. **Yocum, L.A.** The diagnosis and nonoperative treatment of elbow problems in the athlete. *Clin. Sports Med.,* 1989; 8: 439–451.
62. **Yodlowski, M.L., Scheller, A.D., Jr., and Minas, L.** Surgical treatment of Achilles tendinitis by decompression of the retrocalcaneal bursa and calcaneal tuberosity. *Am. J. Sports Med.,* 2002; 30: 318–321.
63. **Yu, W.D. and Shapiro, S.M.** Cysts and other masses about the knee. *Phys. Sportsmed.,* 1999; 27: 59–68.
64. **Zambacos, G.J. et al.** Massive prepatellar bursa: a case of natural tissue expansion: anatomic and histologic implications. *Plast. Reconstr. Surg.,* 2001; 108: 267–268.
65. **Zimmermann, B., III, Mikolich, D.J., and Ho, G., Jr.** Septic bursitis. *Semin. Arthritis Rheum.,* 1995; 24: 391–410.
66. **Zoltan, D.J., Clancy, W.G., and Keene, J.S.** A new operative approach to snapping hip and refractory trochanteric bursitis in athletes. *Am. J. Sports Med.,* 1986; 14: 201–204.

12 Stress Fractures

Stress fractures, which are classified among overuse injuries of bone, may be defined as partial or complete bone fracture that results from repeated application of stress of less strength than the stress required to fracture the bone in a single loading.[179]

Stress fractures usually occur when excessive, repetitive loads on the bone cause imbalance between bone resorption and bone formation. There are two theories explaining the etiology of stress fractures. The first states that muscle weakness reduces the capacity for shock absorption and allows the redistribution of forces to bone, increasing the stress at focal points in the bone.[208] The second theory states that mere muscle pull across a bone produces enough repetitive force to create a stress fracture.[269] Stress fractures have been described in nearly every bone of the human body. Most commonly, stress fractures occur in the lower extremity, weight-bearing bones, second most common are pars interarticularis stress fractures of the lumbar spine, and third most common are stress fractures of bones of the upper extremity, especially those not bearing a static load.[22,36,47,77,101,106,130,144,182,187,188,213,245,274,280] Thus, both theories of stress fracture occurrence might be correct. The origins of stress fractures are most likely site specific and depend on the bone density and geometry, the direction of the load, the vascular supply to the bone, the surrounding muscular attachments, the skeletal alignment, and the type of athletic activity. In addition to mechanical influences, systemic factors, including nutritional deficiencies, hormonal imbalances, collagen abnormalities, and metabolic bone disorders, can contribute to the development of stress fractures.

The first clinical description of stress fracture is credited to Breithaupt, a Prussian military physician. In 1855, he described the clinical picture and symptoms of metatarsal bone stress fractures in soldiers.[43] Since then, fractures at this specific site have been commonly called a *march fracture* or *Deutschlander fracture*. Only about 40 years later, in 1897, radiographic identification of these injuries was first delineated by Stechow.[270]

The first stress fracture in an athlete was reported in 1934 by Pirker; it was a transverse stress fracture of the femoral shaft in an 18-year-old athlete involved in skiing, swimming, and handball.[50] Runner's fracture, i.e., stress fracture of the distal fibula, was reported for the first time in 1940.[73] Since that time, more cases of stress fractures in athletes have been reported, and the first large series of stress fracture in athletes is the work of Devas. In 1975, he published a monograph series on stress fractures, the first of its kind in the medical literature.[78]

To some extent, stress fractures in athletes may be considered professional injuries or diseases. As sports become more popular, both as a profession and as recreation, the number of overuse injuries is increasing as is the number of medical publications discussing the issue. Running, as an activity per se, or as an essential part of such sports as football, basketball, soccer, handball, etc., or as part of preparatory training for almost all athletic activities, contributes to the development of overuse injuries more than any other physical activity.

I. AGE, SEX, RACE, AND TYPE OF ACTIVITY

Stress fractures are common problems in sports medicine, comprising between 1.1 and 10% of all athletic injuries; in the population of runners, they account for 15% of all injuries (although the data may vary from one medical institution to another).[22,24,26,47,77,91,101,106,130,144,182,187,188,198,213,245,274,280,290] The average age of patients ranges from 19 to 30 years.

As a result of the present-day tendency to include children and adolescents in top athletic activities, the number of overuse injuries in pediatric athletes are increasing. Stress fractures in pediatric athletes are less common than in adults.[67,75,214,292] Hulkko and Orava[130] surveyed 368 patients with stress fractures and found an incidence of 9% among children younger than 15 years of age and 32% among those age 16 to 19 years. In addition, the distribution of stress fractures is somewhat different in pediatric athletes. The tibia is the predominant site of stress fractures in pediatric athletes, with an incidence of 51%.[130] Other sites, in descending order, are the fibula 20%, pars interarticularis 15%, femur 3%, metatarsal 2%, and the tarsal navicular 2%.[130] Epiphyseal stress fractures have been reported on the humerus, olecranon, distal radius, distal femur, and proximal tibia, although when compared to apophyseal overuse injuries (Osgood-Schlatter disease, Sever disease, etc.) they occur much more rarely.

Various studies have found that women have a higher incidence of stress fractures compared with men. Identical military conditions and physical training have shown that women are 3 to 12 times more often affected by stress fractures than men.[46,144,145,227] This increased risk, ranging from 1.5 to 3.5 times, has also been observed in athletic populations.[51,106,205,223] The difference may be due to biomechanical differences between the sexes and the female athletic triad (disordered eating, amenorrhea, and osteoporosis).[8,48,136,205,206,291,305] Multiple studies have demonstrated that stress fractures occur more commonly in women with amenorrhea or oligomenorrhea than in eumenor-rheic women.[15,25,147,159] Significant sex differences have been noted in the site distribution of stress fractures. The tibia is the most common site for stress fractures in men and women who participate in jumping and running sports. However, studies suggest that women develop more metatarsal and pelvic stress fractures and fewer fibular fractures than men.

In a questionnaire-based study, the prevalence of stress fractures was much lower among black athletes than among white athletes.[15] Military studies have suggested this as well.[46,194] These studies surmised that the lower stress fracture risk in blacks may be related to their higher bone density or to different biomechanical features that may protect against stress fracture development.

The site and frequency of stress fractures in athletes depend to a large extent on the type of activity. Evidence shows that certain stress fracture sites are reported more often in some athletes than in others, e.g., rib stress fracture in golfers and rowers, tarsal navicular stress fracture in sprinters and high jumpers, etc. (Table 12.1).

II. PREDISPOSING FACTORS

A. BIOMECHANICAL FACTORS

Research evidence shows that certain anatomical deviations on lower extremities, e.g., genus varum, tibia vara, forefoot varus, flat foot, and cavus foot, by altering the distribution of load, contribute to the development of stress fracture.[103,132,162] Varus alignments are common in athletes with stress fractures, especially with femoral and tarsal stress fractures. Cavus foot is found more often in athletes with stress fracture of the metatarsal bones and the femur, and flat foot with excessive pronation significantly contributes to the development of stress fractures of the tibia, fibula, and tarsal bones.[182] In a prospective study, incidences of stress fractures were 10% in flat feet,[31] 3% in feet with average arches, and 39% in feet with high arches.[290] Leg-length discrepancy may also predispose to the development of stress fracture.[96] For example, stress fractures of the femur, tibia, and metatarsal bone occur more often in longer legs, whereas stress fractures of the fibula are more common in shorter legs. In addition, the mediolateral width of the tibia is a factor. Giladi et al.[102] found that 31% of military recruits who sustained femoral, tibial, or foot stress fractures possessed narrower mediolateral tibial widths than those recruits without stress fractures during identical training. Because bone size throughout the skeleton is proportional, narrow tibial width may provide an indicator of biomechan-ically weaker skeletal structures that are more likely to sustain a stress injury to bone.

TABLE 12.1
Sports and Activities Commonly Associated with Various Stress Fractures Sites[36]

Site of Stress Fracture	Sport or Activity
Coracoid process of scapula	Trapshooting
Humerus	Throwing, racket sports
Ulna — olecranon	Javelin throwing, pitching
Ulna — shaft	Racket sports
Radius	Gymnastics
Ribs (I)	Basketball, ballet
Ribs (IV–IX)	Rowing, golf
Pars interarticularis	Gymnastics, dancing, weight lifting, pole vaulting
Sacrum	Long-distance and marathon running
Pubic ramus	Long-distance and marathon running
Femur — neck	Long-distance running, gymnastics
Femur — shaft	Long- and middle-distance running, hurdling
Tibia — shaft	Running, ballet
Tibia — midshaft	Basketball, volleyball, pole vaulting, high jumping
Tibia — medial malleolus	Basketball, high and long jumping, sprinting
Fibula	Running, gymnastics, figure skating
Tarsal navicular	Sprinting, hurdling, basketball, high and long jumping
Metatarsal — general	Running, dancing, gymnastics
Metatarsal — second	Ballet
Metatarsal — fifth	Basketball, soccer, football, throwing (javelin, hammer)
Sesamoid bones of great toe	Running, dancing, gymnastics, basketball

B. Muscles

The condition and tone of skeletal muscles, i.e., their strength, are directly related to stress fracture. During a rapid increase of physical activity, muscular tone also increases, resulting in stresses stronger than those that the bone can withstand and a stress fracture may occur. In contrast, muscular weakness may predispose to the development of stress fracture by causing an increase or redistribution of stress to bone.[178] Clement et al.[65] have reported on the triceps surae muscle weakness in 40 to 56% of patients with tibial stress fractures. Fatigued muscles have decreased contractility and their ability to absorb shock is diminished, causing altered stress distribution and high compression loads and shear stresses. Increased tightness and poor flexibility of muscles and tendons have also been regarded as major causes of chronic stress conditions. This is precisely why stretching and strengthening exercises of muscles are essential.

C. Training Errors

Training errors are the most frequently encountered cause of stress fractures. There is extensive research evidence showing that training errors cause stress fractures in as many as 22 to 75% of cases.[51,106,130,182,187,188,213,274] They are characterized by "mileage mania" (excessive mileage), extremely intensive training, or too rapid changes in both the qualitative and quantitative aspects of training. Studies in military recruits and athletes have revealed that modification of the training regimen to include rest periods intermittently with periods of strenuous activity significantly decreases stress fracture risk by providing time for bone microdamage to be repaired and by decreasing the load applied to bone.[260]

D. Surface

The type of ground used for running (tartan, asphalt, grass, etc.), i.e., the surface quality of a playing area (parquet, concrete, asphalt, etc.), is an extremely important contributor to stress fracture.[51,182] Running on hard surfaces may be associated with an increased risk of stress fractures because of the mechanical shock introduced to the bone. Assessment of two groups of runners with stress fractures revealed that 50% had been running on a hard surface.[51,174,293] Further, running on an uneven surface may increase the risk of stress fracture by causing increased muscle fatigue and redistributing load to bone. Running along the margin of the road, i.e., on a sloped surface, leads to short–long leg syndrome, which may cause tibial stress fracture.[130]

E. Footwear

Athletic footwear is designed to reduce impact on ground contact and provide stability by controlling foot and ankle motion. Shoe age has been shown to be a better indicator of shock-absorbing quality than shoe cost.[95,99] Gardner et al.[99] have shown that training in shoes older than 6 months increases the risk for stress fracture. However, running in new shoes can also lead to the development of stress fractures. No association has been demonstrated between shoe cost and stress fracture risk. In fact, increased cushioning, which reduces the body's sensory-feedback mechanism (originating in the plantar surface of the foot), can lead to injury during running. Robbins and Gouw[246] describe this sensory disturbance as a pseudoneuropathic condition, a term that also relates to other changes (running on a different surface, using a different tennis racket, trying a different pitch, etc.).

III. PREVENTION

To prevent stress fractures and other overuse injuries, it is of utmost importance that the athlete, the coach, and the physician cooperate. It is essential to identify the group at higher risk of stress fracture, most commonly, athletes with biomechanical irregularities in lower extremities. These athletes should be kept under constant surveillance and provided with various orthotic devices. In extreme cases, surgery may be required to correct biomechanical disorders. Female athletes and their coaches and parents need to be alerted to the adverse effects of eating disorders and hormonal abnormalities. Identification of female athletes with "female athlete triad" is especially important so that early intervention may be initiated. Furthermore, athletic and training activities should be adapted to age and abilities of individual athletes, i.e., maximum load should be achieved gradually. As well, rest periods should be incorporated with periods of strenuous activity. Athletic requisites are also very important for the prevention of stress fractures, especially the condition of the running shoes and quality of playing surface. An important preventive measure also entails stretching and strengthening exercises, which also diminish stressful forces on the bone.

IV. DIAGNOSTICS

Similar to other overuse injuries, when attempting to diagnose a stress fracture, it is essential that the physician keep the possibility of such condition constantly in mind. Thus, clinical diagnosis is the basic procedure, followed by other diagnostic methods.

A. Clinical Diagnosis

The main symptom of stress fracture is pain.[19,32,33,36,47,50,77,106,158,176,182,187,188,213,216,239,272,274,280] Classically, the patient describes a history of insidious onset of pain in the area of the fracture that has its onset during activity but disappears with rest. If the activity is continued, the pain may begin earlier at an increasing intensity in the course of that activity and persist after the activity. Later on, the pain increases so much that the activity must be stopped. Finally, the pain may be present even at rest despite cessation of the activity.

A comprehensive history should include a review of the exercise or training program, in particular any recent changes in the type or level of activity, as well as changes in surface, equipment (especially shoes), and technique. A history of previous similar injury or any other musculoskeletal injury should be obtained. In addition, the patient's general health, medications, diet, occupation, and personal habits should be assessed. A careful menstrual history should be obtained from all female patients.

The hallmark of stress fracture is localized tenderness to palpation at the fracture site. Point tenderness may be best provoked over bones that can be easily palpated, such as the metatarsal bones or fibula. For bones that are deep, such as the pelvis or femoral neck and shaft, pain may be elicited through gentle range of motion or specific diagnostic tests. Deformity is usually absent at the fracture site. Physical examination may also show swelling and erythema. As reported in the literature, point tenderness has been observed in 66 to 88%, local swelling in 25 to 50%, and limping has been found in 45% of cases with stress fracture.[182] Percussion of the affected bone distal to the fracture site causes pain. Muscle atrophy, weakness, and limited range of motion are usually not present. If the diagnosis is still in doubt after palpation, applying stress to the area involved will help to reproduce a patient's symptoms. Activities such as walking, walking on toes, or running in place can reproduce a patient's symptoms in the physician's office. Passive stretching can also elicit pain in the affected area. In this case, muscle pull rather than weight bearing induces stress on the bone.

B. Radiography

Standard radiographic imaging may show bone lesions in only 30 to 70% of stress fracture cases.[32,33,36,47,52,77,101,182,213,216,268] It has also been found that the time, from the onset of pain to the moment when alterations become visible on a standard radiographic film, is 2 weeks to even 3 months, depending on the fracture site. For certain locations, e.g., tarsal bones, femur, or spine, it is often not possible to identify any changes whatsoever, even if followed up for a longer period of time.

The first noticeable radiographic signs of stress fracture in cortical bone are a periosteal reaction (in diaphyseal fractures) and medullar sclerosis and endosteal thickenings (in metaphyseal fractures). Such stress fractures usually affect only one cortex and only later on (2 to 4 weeks following the onset of symptoms) may be seen as an oblique or transverse fissure. These changes are not so easily recognized; i.e., they can be identified with greater certainty only on tangential radiographs or tomograms. Blickenstaff and Morris[30] and Hallel et al.[114] have classified stress fractures of cortical bone with regard to radiological findings into the following three groups:

1. Stress fractures in which endosteal or periosteal callus is visible only on one side of the bone, without an overt fracture line
2. Stress fractures with a fracture line through one cortex or across the bone and in which a circumferential periosteal reaction is present
3. Stress fractures with displacement, i.e., fractures with dislocation of the segments

The initial changes of cancellous bone stress fractures, known as trabecular fractures, are characterized by hardly noticeable flakelike patches of new bone that may be seen 10 to 21 days following the onset of symptoms.[52,182] Later, the patches transform into wider cloudlike areas of mineralized bone, and then an area of focal linear sclerosis oriented perpendicular to trabeculae appears within the bone; these are among the most characteristic signs of cancellous bone stress fracture.

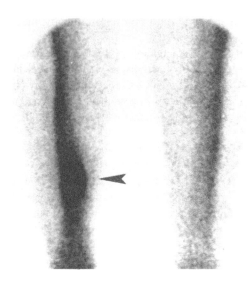

FIGURE 12.1 Bone scan demonstrating tibial stress fracture (arrowhead).

Plain radiographs are necessary in the initial assessment to rule out other causes of localized bone pain, such as complete fracture, infection, or malignancy. It is important to remember that stress fractures are dynamic in nature, and the radiographic appearance is also a continuum. However, despite a negative radiograph, the diagnosis of a stress fracture should be entertained if the prodromal signs and symptoms and clinical index of suspicion are still high. [32,33,36,47,50,52,77,101,182,213,216,268]

C. SCINTIGRAPHY

Bone scintigraphy is highly sensitive but has low specificity. On account of higher specificity of radiographic findings, a bone scan is recommended only when radiographic examination seems negative in spite of reasonable doubt that stress fracture might be present. Triple-phase technetium-99m diphosphate bone scan is today the gold standard for the diagnosis of stress fracture.[7,72,148,157,166,183,233,253,268,307] Bone scan may demonstrate bony changes within 6 to 72 h following the appearance of initial stress fracture symptoms.

A typical scintigraphic finding of a stress fracture is characterized by an oval or spindle-shaped, sharply bordered focus of increased uptake that involves one cortex or, occasionally, extension of the width of the bone (Figure 12.1). In stress fractures, all three phases (the angiogram phase, the blood-pool phase, and the delayed image phase) of the triple-phase bone scan are positive.[72,148,157,166,183,184,233,253,268,307] Some other overuse soft-tissue injuries would be positive only in the angiogram and blood-pool phase, thereby differentiating bony pathology and pathology involving soft tissue from stress fracture.[72,148,184,253,268]

Routine scintigraphy of the pelvis and lower extremities often shows multiple foci of increased activity that remain silent, i.e., are not manifested either clinically (as pain) or radiographically.[183] The asymptomatic accumulation of radionuclide, the so-called stress reaction, only indicates remodeling of bone caused by physical stress. As scintigraphic findings may remain positive for several months, clinical and radiographic findings are used as discriminative tools for follow-up of stress fracture treatment.

Quite a number of scintigraphic classifications of stress fractures have been reported in the reference literature, the most common is that of Zwas et al.[307] identifying four grades:

Grade 1: A small, ill-defined lesion with mildly increased activity in the cortical region
Grade 2: Larger than grade 1; well-defined, elongated lesion with moderately increased
    activity in the cortical region

Grade 3: A wide fusiform lesion with markedly increased activity in the corticomedullary region

Grade 4: A wide, extensive lesion with intensely increased activity in the transcorticomedullary region

D. COMPUTERIZED TOMOGRAPHY

Computerized tomography (CT) may be used in conjunction with scintigraphy to fully delineate the pathological process. CT is very useful for differentiating conditions that may mimic stress fracture: various malignancies, osteomyelitis with a Brodie's abscess, etc. CT scans can show stress fractures that are not apparent on plain radiographs and may also be used to evaluate healing when plain radiographs do not adequately demonstrate the fracture. They are particularly helpful in identifying stress fractures of the sacrum, pelvis, and spine, and in proposing treatment of tarsal navicular stress fracture.[34,36,52,153,156] A disadvantage of CT is that, in many circumstances, scanning is limited to the axial plane, which does not allow views of transversely oriented fractures. An alternative, helical or spiral CT, can be used to minimize this limitation.

E. MAGNETIC RESONANCE IMAGING

Magnetic resonance imaging (MRI) is proving useful in identifying stress fractures.[9,94,134,157,166,268] It is highly sensitive for the diagnosis of stress injury to bone, and usually allows depiction of abnormalities several weeks before the development of radiographic alterations. Its sensitivity for detection of bone abnormalities is comparable with that of bone scintigraphy. Besides having higher specificity than bone scintigraphy in distinguishing bone involvement from soft-tissue injuries, MRI is helpful in grading the stage of certain stress fractures and, therefore, predicting the time to recovery. In addition, MRI avoids exposure to ionizing radiation and requires less time to complete than triple-phase bone scan. Recent advances in MRI availability, including the increasing availability of relatively low cost, dedicated extremity scanners, likely will expand further the application of MRI for detection of bone abnormalities, and could challenge conventional radiography as the primary diagnostic tool used to detect stress injuries to bone (see Chapter 2).

F. MISCELLANEOUS TESTS

Sonography and thermography have been used to diagnose stress fracture, especially in bones located near the surface (metatarsal bones or the fibula).[107,125,200] Intentions have also been reported to use therapeutic ultrasound as a diagnostic test. Moss and Mowat[200] have found that, when applied to the fracture site, therapeutic ultrasound causes pain. Further, the test is of questionable reliability and the researchers recommend additional radiological assessment for definitive diagnosis.

V. DIFFERENTIAL DIAGNOSIS

The two major reasons for failure to diagnose a stress fracture are neglect to consider it a diagnostic possibility and acceptance of negative radiography that has been taken prematurely or examines the region inadequately. The differential diagnosis for stress fractures is extensive and includes stress reaction, periostitis, muscle strain, infection, neoplasm, bursitis, exertional compartment syndrome, and nerve entrapment. In children and adolescents, it is of utmost importance to differentiate stress fracture from osteogenic sarcoma and Ewing's tumor. A follow-up roentgenogram, repeated after 2 to 3 weeks, usually solves the problem of diagnosis. Differential diagnosis of stress fracture and overuse injuries of soft tissue cannot be based solely on clinical findings and radiological diagnosis; it also requires scintigraphy, and sometimes even MRI. The differential diagnosis between shin splints and tibial stress fracture shown by triple-phase bone scan may serve as a very good example. The fact is that the difference may be noted only at a delayed image of scintigraphic examination. The delayed image of a stress fracture is intense, solitary, and focal, whereas in shin splints, it is less intense, linear, and longitudinal. Another good example is osteoid osteoma. Osteoid osteoma is commonly mistaken for a stress fracture because it presents with pain and discrete focal area of increased uptake on bone scintigraphy. Two distinguishing features of osteoid osteoma are presence of night pain and relief of pain with use of aspirin.

VI. TREATMENT

The main treatment of stress fractures is rest from the offending athletic activity; a concept known as "relative rest."[22,32-34,36,47,50,101,106,119,130,182-188,213,216,239,245] There is a group of stress fractures, called high-risk stress fractures, that requires additional treatment to relative rest. High-risk stress fractures include those in the femoral neck (tension side), patella, anterior cortex of the tibia, medial malleolus, talus, tarsal navicular, fifth metatarsal, and great toe sesamoids.[32]

The duration of treatment may vary according to the individual patient, the bone involved, and the particular sport. Compliance is critical to the success of treatment. In some cases where the activities of daily living are painful it may be necessary to restrict the patient to non-weight-bearing activities or partially weight-bearing activities on crutches for a period of time. Exercise is very important to prevent detraining in affected athletes. General conditioning can be maintained by exercising other areas of the body, and by partaking in alternative training, such as water running, swimming, cycling, etc. The alternative activity must not produce pain or tenderness. When athletes have been free from pain for 2 to 3 weeks and full weight bearing is normal, they may gradually return to their sport. The athlete must have no bony tenderness at the time of resumption of the sport. Furthermore, the athlete must be cautioned to resume the sport at a frequency, an intensity, and a duration well below the level that previously produced symptoms. In general, increasing the volume or intensity of training no more than 10% per week will avoid recurrence of the stress fracture. Patients must be sequentially monitored during recovery. If they develop any pain during athletic participation or tenderness afterward, they should decrease or modify the activity for an additional 2-week period.[34,36]

In rare instances, surgical treatment may be indicated if there is a high-risk fracture, if the stress fracture has progressed to a complete fracture, or if the fracture has become an established nonunion.

VII. DISTRIBUTION OF STRESS FRACTURE

A. UPPER EXTREMITIES

1. Scapula

Reports of scapula stress fractures in athletes have included a coracoid stress fracture in a trap-shooter, a scapular body stress fracture in a gymnast, a stress fracture of the superomedial portion of the scapula in a jogger who had been jogging with weights in his hands, and a stress fracture of the base of the acromional process in a professional American football player.[39,204,258,289,296]

Stress fracture of the coracoid process has been described in association with trapshooting.[39] Development of this type of fracture is linked to repeated hitting of a gunstock on the coracoid process during shooting. Physical examination reveals point tenderness on the coracoid process, and tenderness along the bicipital groove. Resistance against adduction and anteflexion of the shoulder increases pain over the coracoid process. The fracture fissure occurs in the mid-third or on the base of the coracoid process and may best be seen on axillary view radiograph of the shoulder. Treatment consists of rest with elimination of trapshooting until the patient is asymptomatic (4 to 6 weeks), and then gradual resumption of activity.

2. Clavicle

Stress fractures of the clavicle have been reported in a javelin thrower, a collegiate springboard diver, a baseball player, a female gymnast, and a female lightweight rower.[1,3,87,250,295,303] Athletes presented with insidious onset of pain over the clavicle and local tenderness. The pain was maximal when the shoulder was abducted above the horizontal plane. Radiographic examination usually demonstrated periosteal reaction. Rest from the aggravating athletic activities for 8 to 10 weeks is sufficient for healing.

3. Humerus

Stress fractures of the humerus may occur in the shaft in adults or through the proximal humeral epiphysis in skeletally immature athletes.[45,49,267] Stress fractures of the humeral shaft have been reported in baseball pitchers, tennis players, shot-putters, cricket players, and in a javelin thrower, a bodybuilder, and a weight lifter.[6,16,42,124,231,238,242,271] Signs that should alert the physician to the presence of a humeral shaft stress fracture include deep aching in a region of the mid-humerus during activity and at rest. If not attended to, these symptoms may progress to an overt fracture. Physical examination reveals tenderness over the stress fracture and mild pain on manual resistance testing of shoulder movements, especially on internal rotation and abduction. Although early radiographs of the humerus are unremarkable, lately radiographs may demonstrate cortical thickening along the mid-third of the medial cortex or a fracture line, which is either transverse or spiral.

Stress fracture of the proximal humeral epiphysis is called Little League shoulder because it occurs in children and adolescents, especially in baseball throwers, i.e., the pitchers.[45,49,242] This type of fracture is caused by strong rotational forces during the cocking phase and acceleration phase of pitching. Radiographs demonstrate widening of the lateral portion of the epiphysis on external rotation anteroposterior (AP) shoulder radiographs. This widening may be associated with lateral fragmentation, sclerosis, or cystic changes.

Treatment of humeral shaft and proximal humeral epiphysis stress fractures is avoidance of the precipitating factor, usually throwing or weight lifting. Early diagnosis and proper treatment is of utmost importance because continued forces may result in a spiral fracture of the humerus or premature closure of the epiphysis. The recommended treatment involves a minimum of 8-week (in adults) and 12-week (in adolescents) absence from the aggravating activity, and then gradual resumption of activity over another 4 weeks.

4. Ulna

Ulnar stress fractures may be located on either the olecranon or the diaphysis. Olecranon stress fractures are rare injuries. There seem to be three types of stress fracture of the olecranon: stress fracture of the growth plate, stress fracture of the tip of the olecranon, and stress fracture that occurs in the middle third of the olecranon.[119,129,175,209,235,275,284,300] Stress fractures of the olecranon growth plate have been reported in gymnasts.[119,175,300] Gymnasts present with a pain and local tenderness. Radiographs reveal a radiolucency and/or a widening of the epiphyseal plate. Sclerosis of the fracture margins, persistent radiolucency, and no relief of pain are signs of delayed union or nonunion. If the diagnosis is made relatively early, there is a reasonable chance that non-operative treatment will be successful and that the athlete will resume sport in 8 to 12 weeks. In case of delayed union or nonunion of the fracture, surgical intervention is unavoidable.

Stress fractures of the tip of the olecranon and of the olecranon itself have been reported in javelin throwers and baseball pitchers.[129,209,235,275,284] Nuber and Diment[209] emphasize that these fractures are not the same entity even though they are both seen in throwers. They state that stress fractures of the tip are more likely to be seen in throwers who present with a painful elbow after a particularly strong throw, which Warris called "mal-throw." Authors think that this type of stress fracture could be the result of impingement of the olecranon in its fossa and that this was partly attributable to the hypertrophy that was present in the pitching arm. Throwers with stress fractures that occur in the middle third of the olecranon, however, are more likely to present with a longer history of pain that recurs when they resume throwing. Authors think that this type of stress fracture results from the repeated violent pull of the triceps muscle on the olecranon during the acceleration phase of the throw. The stress fracture of the tip of the olecranon can be treated non-operatively, but the treatment of choice is surgical excision of the tip fragment. Surgical intervention enables the athlete to return to sport at approximately 8 weeks. Surgical treatment is commonly recommended for olecranon mid-third stress fracture (insertion of bone graft or tension band plus two Kirschner wires), because non-operative treatment requires prolonged immobilization that might limit range of motion of the elbow.[129,209,279]

Stress fractures of the ulnar diaphysis have been described in softball pitchers, tennis players, table tennis players, weight lifters, volleyball players, a bowler, a golfer, and a polo player.[20,37,58,63,80,86,93,115,116,160,203,228,241,279,304] All reported cases of these stress fractures in tennis players concerned the nondominant forearm of tennis players using a double-handed backhand stroke.[37,93,241,304] These observations suggest that this technique is associated with such fractures. Stress fractures of the ulnar diaphysis are located at the middle third or at the junction of the middle and distal third of the ulna. Athletes often complain of pain over the ulna shaft both during and after athletic activity. Physical examination reveals tenderness over the ulna shaft and pain on resisted wrist movements. If symptoms have been noted for some time, early callus may palpable along the subcutaneous ulna shaft. Radiographs show either a crack in the cortex or subtle elevation of the periosteum at the stress fracture site. A bone scan can be used to confirm the diagnosis when radiographs are unremarkable. Rest from the aggravating athletic activities for 4 to 6 weeks is sufficient for healing.

5. Radius

Stress fractures of the radius have been described in gymnasts, a tennis player, a pool player, and a cyclist.[4,54,55,171,222,236,251,252] The most common stress fracture affecting the radius is that of its distal epiphysis found in gymnasts.[4,55,236,251,252] The main symptom is wrist pain, occurring during or after athletic activity and relieved by rest. Pain is localized mainly to the dorsal aspect of the distal radius and carpal area, and occasionally it can be localized on the volar-wrist crease and at ulnar styloid. Clinical findings include painful limitation at the extreme of forced active and passive dorsiflexion of the wrist. Tenderness is localized mainly to the distal radial epiphyseal area, particularly the dorsal surface. This stress fracture is characterized by the following radiographic changes: widening of the growth plate of the distal radial epiphysis, cystic changes, irregularity of the metaphyseal margin, or haziness of the distal radial epiphysis. Early diagnosis and non-operative management, consisting of rest from aggravating activities and immobilization, can enable a young gymnast to return to normal activity without permanent morbidity, such as chronic pain or disproportionate growth of the radius, or prolonged interruption of his or her training. It should be emphasized that this stress fracture may require many weeks or even months to heal.

6. Carpal Bones

Stress fractures of the scaphoid have been reported in gymnasts, a shot-putter, and a canoeist.[85,117,185] All the activities involve repeated wrist movements, mainly dorsiflexion. The main symptom of scaphoid stress fracture is pain within the wrist, appearing in the course of the activity and disappearing during rest, without any history of a wrist trauma. Physical examination usually shows a restriction of dorsiflexion and tenderness over the scaphoid bone. Radiographic examination usually demonstrates a transverse fracture fissure of the scaphoid waist with rather sclerotic margins.

The method of choice in the treatment of this type of stress fracture is immobilization in a thumb-spica cast that should be worn for a minimum of 10 weeks.

A stress fracture of the scaphoid combined with distal radial epiphysiolysis has been reported in a 16-year-old badminton player.[133] A stress fracture of the hook of the hamate has been described in a tennis player.[111] The patient had complained of gradual onset of pain on the ulnar aspect of the wrist after altering his grip for serving. Stress fracture of the pisiform bone has been reported in volleyball players.[135] It seems to be caused by repetitive trauma of the bone occurring during hitting and blocking the ball with the base of their palm.

7. Metacarpal Bones

Metacarpal stress fractures have been described in tennis players and in a softball player.[146,202,216,294] In cases of stress fracture of the second metacarpal bone, tennis players have described an increase in training volume and intensity as well as an alteration in technique.[202,294] The softball player who presented with a stress fracture of the fifth metacarpal had increased her training intensity and altered the grip for her curve ball.[146] Rest and avoidance of aggravating athletic activities for 4 weeks is sufficient for healing. Attention must be paid to the errors in technique (poor stroke technique, improper grip) and training overload, which first precipitate the problem.

B. TRUNK

1. Sternum

Stress fractures of the sternum have been reported in a wrestler, a golfer, and a body-builder.[12,110,152,247] All fractures were associated with a recent increase in athletic activity and gradual onset of the pain over the sternum. Physical examination revealed exquisite tenderness over the anterior sternum, about 2 cm distal to the sternal angle. Radiographic examination revealed fracture fissure and bone scan demonstrated a "hot spot" with increased uptake at the pain site. Discontinuation of aggravating athletic activities from 6 to 8 weeks is sufficient treatment for the fracture to heal.

2. Ribs

Stress fractures of the ribs occur most commonly at the first rib or ribs 4 through 9. The most plausible explanation for rib stress fractures is the repetitive contraction of muscles, which act in opposing directions on the ribs. Stress fractures of the first rib have been reported in basketball players, baseball players, weight lifters, ballet dancers, and tennis players.[13,82,113,164,193,196,254] Most stress fractures of the first rib are located in the thinnest and weakest portion of the bone, i.e., at the groove for the subclavian artery, just posterior to the scalene tubercle. The typical presentation for stress fracture of the first rib is gradual onset of pain that is aggravated by overhead activity, deep inspiration, and coughing. The pain is rarely local but more often radiates along the arm, into the anterior part of the neck, and sometimes even into the sternum and the pectoral region. Less commonly, patients are seen with acute pain when a stress fracture progresses to a complete fracture. Physical examination reveals local tenderness over the first rib. The stress fracture is often visible on an AP chest radiograph, but it can be confirmed by a bone scan. Usually, these fractures heal uneventfully with a 4-week rest from the aggravating activity. In cases when an acute fracture develops, there is a risk of delayed union with healing often requiring 6 to 12 months of activity restriction.

Stress fractures of the ribs have been reported in rowers, golfers, paddlers, tennis players, gymnasts, squash players, and a swimmer.[35,59,60,122,149,172,191,217,219,237,278,297] Often the diagnosis of stress fractures is delayed due to neglect of the symptoms by the patients, and possibly lack of

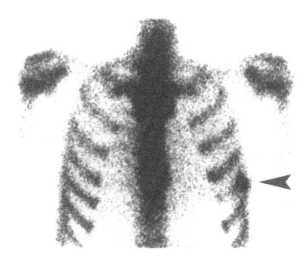

FIGURE 12.2 Bone scan (AP view) demonstrated focal uptake on the left sixth rib in rower (arrowhead).

awareness of the existence of stress fractures in the ribs by physicians, and possible confusion with intercostal muscle strains. The symptoms of rib stress fracture are mainly pain associated with activity. Physical examination often reveals point tenderness of the affected rib. Radiographs, including oblique views, should be performed and often can confirm diagnosis. If the radiograph is negative and there is a clinical suspicion, bone scan should be conducted for identifying stress fracture (Figure 12.2). Stress fractures of the ribs are treated non-operatively, and discontinuation of the aggravating activity is recommended for 4 to 6 weeks. No cases of delayed union or nonunion of lower rib stress fractures have been reported.

3. Lumbar Spine

Stress fractures of the lumbar spine occur most often in the pars interarticularis, although they may also be located in the pedicle or lamina. The most common vertebral level affected is the L5 segment followed by the L4 and L3 levels.

Stress fracture of the pars interarticularis is one of the most common stress fractures, and is especially common in sports that involve repeated hyperextension of the lower back, such as gymnastics, dancing, weight lifting, hockey, pole vaulting, football, basketball, running.[21,61,68,138,169,197,199,277,301] The basic signs of pars interarticularis stress fracture are absence of periosteal reaction and great possibility of refracturing, i.e., development of spondylolysis and sometimes even spondylolisthesis. The patients typically present with localized, unilateral low-back pain. The pain worsens with sports activities, especially extension and hyperextension, and is relieved by rest. The one-leg lumbar hyperextension test (commonly called the stork test), in which the patient is asked to hyperextend the back while standing on the ipsilateral leg of the affected side, usually reproduces the pain. They also often have diminished straight-leg raising secondary to hamstring spasm. Radiographic assessment should include AP, lateral, and oblique views of the lumbar spine. On the oblique radiograph the "Scottie dog" sign can be demonstrated with the pars interarticularis corresponding to the neck of the dog. Images that resemble a collared dog or a dog with a broken or elongated neck are diagnostic of a stress lesion or fracture through the pars. Many stress fractures may be too subtle to detect radiographically, and require nuclear imaging. Bone scanning with single-photon emission tomography (SPECT) has been particularly helpful in delineating stress injury to the pars interarticularis.[21] Advanced imaging with CT or MRI may be needed to ascertain the acuity of the lesion, assist in identifying a particular pars lesion as potentially symptomatic, and to exclude other spinal pathology that may be present. Early recognition of the fracture and rest from athletic activities together with thoracolumbar orthosis are essential to good treatment outcome. When the athlete is pain free, he or she may begin a graduated rehabilitation program emphasizing a spinal stabilization program consisting of abdominal and paraspinal muscle strengthening.

Other lumbar spine stress fractures that are reported in the literature include a pedicle fracture in a ballet dancer, and a laminar fracture in a jogger.[2,89]

4. Sacrum

Stress fractures of the sacrum have been commonly reported in competitive, long-distance, and marathon runners.[11,38,70,84,88,141,177,190,257,262] They are rare but important to recognize because the symptoms often mimic sciatica, which can lead to delay in diagnosis and treatment. Patients usually report the insidious onset of low-back and sacral pain that may radiate into the buttocks. On physical examination pain and tenderness are localized to the sacral region. Because plain radiographic findings are typically normal, the diagnosis is best made with bone scintigraphy or MRI. If treated with rest, most of these fractures heal after 6 weeks and the athlete then can gradually return to full activity.

5. Pelvis

Stress fractures of the pelvis are relatively uncommon. When discussing stress fractures of the pelvis, it has been noted that they most often occur in the ischial pubic ramus. The fracture is usually located in the inferior ischiopubic junction between the sites of origin of adductor muscles and hamstring muscles. It most frequently affects long-distance and marathon runners, as well as joggers; incidence of this type of stress fracture is also very high in women.[121,207,224,282] This fact may be due to differences in pelvic geometry and gait biomechanics, or due to the female athlete triad. The leading symptom is pain in the groin, and sometimes in the buttock or thigh. The pain appears during running and, after a while, becomes so severe that the activity must be discontinued. On physical examination, deep palpation reveals painful tenderness localized to pubic ramus and not to overlying soft tissues. Hip range of motion is usually full. Noakes and co-workers[207] report that the "positive standing sign" (frank pain or an inability to stand unsupported on the affected leg) is highly suggestive if not diagnostic of pubic rami stress fracture. Radiologically, the fracture is initially manifested as a transverse fissure or small cloudlike callus in the upper border of the obturator foramen. If, in spite of the pain, the activity is continued, a massive callus will develop and should not be confused with malignancy. When a pubic rami stress fracture is clinically suspected, but the radiographs are normal, a bone scan should be performed to confirm the diagnosis. Once the diagnosis has been made, cessation of running from 10 to 16 weeks is usually adequate treatment. The patient is free to walk, although in the case of pain and/or limping during normal walking, crutches should be used in the first few weeks of treatment. A small risk of nonunion or refracture is present if an adequate rest period is not enforced.

C. LOWER EXTREMITIES

1. Femur

A stress fracture of the femur may be located in the neck, the shaft, and supracondylar and condylar regions.

The most common stress fracture of the femur is that of its neck, which is most noteworthy not for its frequency as much as for the resulting complications: delayed union, nonunion, dislocation of fragments, and avascular femoral head necrosis.[10,30,76,83,97,98,142,248,265] Because of this the primary goal of management should be to prevent complications through early diagnosis and careful treatment. Stress fracture of the femoral neck most often occurs in military recruits during basic training and in long-distance runners. However, it has also been reported in basketball players and gymnasts. The initial and most frequent symptom is anterior groin (inguinal) pain. The pain is often exacerbated by weight bearing or activity, resulting in an antalgic gait. Night pain is occasionally present. Physical examination reveals pain at the extremes of gentle passive hip motion and slight limitation of flexion and internal rotation. Bone tenderness is often minimal owing to the depth of soft tissue overlying the femoral neck. Axial compression or percussion over the greater trochanter may also elicit pain. An additional test that has been found to be helpful is "hop test" in which the patient attempts to hop on the injured leg, inevitably reproducing the pain that these patients experience if an undisplaced stress fracture is present. If physical findings suggest a femoral neck stress fracture, it should be considered present until proved otherwise. If the diagnosis is suspected, radiographs may be obtained, keeping in mind that changes (when present) normally lag behind the onset of symptoms by 2 to 4 weeks. Bone scan or MRI should be performed to make an early, definitive diagnosis. Compared with bone scan, MRI has a similar sensitivity but an improved specificity, and is becoming the diagnostic procedure of choice.[266]

In 1988, Fullerton and Snowdy[97] presented a classification of femoral neck stress fractures based on a combination of biomechanical factors and degree of displacement, as well as position of the fracture line: (1) fracture on the inferior aspect of the neck — compression-side fracture, (2) fracture on the superior aspect of the neck — tension-side fracture, (3) displaced fracture of the femoral neck. Their classification also demonstrated the spectrum of changes: stage 1, a normal radiograph and a positive isotope bone scan; stage 2, endosteal or periosteal callus without a fracture; stage 3, a cortical crack without displacement; stage 4, a widening of the cortical crack followed by displacement. In the case of a normal radiograph and a positive bone scan (stage 1) or of sclerosis without overt fracture line (stage 2), non-operative treatment (absolute bed rest until the pain resolves) will suffice for both the "compression" and "tension" type of femoral neck stress fracture. The patient is then advanced from partial to full weight bearing on crutches as symptoms permit. Once the patient is free of pain, he or she is allowed to progress to a cane and then to unprotected weight bearing. A progressive walking, then running program is prescribed, and the patient returns over several months to full activity. If the patient presents with or develops an undisplaced cortical crack (stage 3) the type of fracture is important in planning the treatment. In the more common compression-side stress fractures a complete displacement is extremely rare and non-operative treatment as noted above is appropriate. Tension-side stress fractures have a greater propensity to become displaced with continued stress than compression-side stress fractures and, therefore, require more aggressive treatment, i.e., internal fixation. In those fractures that present with any widening or with defect in both cortices (stage 4), immediate internal fixation is recommended. Displaced femoral neck stress fracture is an orthopedic emergency. Early, accurate reduction and internal fixation are essential.

Stress fractures of the femoral shaft are uncommon in athletes and occur most commonly in the proximal third of the femur.[29,31,53,66,81,105,120,143,168,170] They have been reported in the medial subtrochanteric region (long- and middle-distance runners, hurdlers, basketball players), in the mid-shaft (long-distance runners, baseball players, football players), and in the distal femoral epiphysis in adolescents (basketball players, runners). It should be noted that diagnosis is often delayed due to scarce clinical signs. In the majority of cases, the only symptom is pain located in the groin and thigh region. There is often no localized tenderness, and a full range of motion in the hip and knee is usually present. Occasionally, an antalgic gait is present. The "fulcrum test" may aid in making the diagnosis of femoral shaft stress fractures.[143] In the test, the patient is seated on the edge of the examining table with lower legs dangling. The examiner's arm is used as a fulcrum under the thigh and is moved from distal to proximal thigh as gentle pressure is applied to the dorsum of the knee with the opposite hand. When the arm is placed under the site of the stress fracture, the patient experiences pain and apprehension. This test may also be useful in assessing the healing response. Standard radiographs may be totally within normal limits. The diagnosis of femoral shaft stress fractures can be confirmed by either bone scan or MRI (Figure 12.3). Treatment is usually

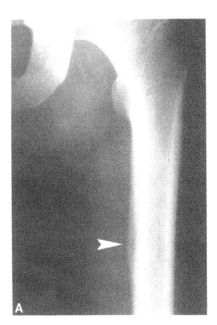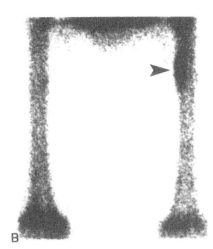

FIGURE 12.3 (A) Roentgenogram demonstrating stress fracture in the proximal third of the femoral shaft (white arrowhead); (B) bone scan of the same patient (black arrowhead).

non-operative and entails rest from athletic activity from 8 to 14 weeks. A brief non-weight-bearing period on crutches (2 to 4 weeks) is appropriate if athletes have difficulty bearing full weight. Displacement of femoral shaft stress fracture in athletes is uncommon, although it can occur.

2. Patella

The patella is an uncommon location for a stress fracture, and therefore difficulties and delays in the diagnosis and treatment may occur. The fractures have been reported in young athletes, basketball players, volleyball players, soccer players, high jumpers, and runners.[44,74,137,139,181,221,229,281] The fracture line may be either transverse or longitudinal. The transverse stress fracture is the consequence of muscular traction stresses, whereas the longitudinal stress fracture results from forces that compress the patella against the femoral condyle. Treatment of the so-called longitudinal patellar stress fracture is non-operative, i.e., rest from athletic activities for 8 to 12 weeks. For nondisplaced transverse patellar stress fracture 4 weeks of non-weight-bearing cast immobilization in knee extension is indicated. A displaced transverse patellar stress fracture requires surgical treatment for open reduction and internal fixation. Untreated or misdiagnosed patellar stress fractures may develop into complete fractures during athletic activity.

3. Tibia

The tibia is the most common stress fracture site among athletes.[22,47,91,108,119,130,182,198,216,239,290] Tibial stress fractures may be located on the posteromedial cortex of the diaphysis either at its proximal or distal (more often) end, on the proximal epiphyseal-metaphyseal area in prepubescent individuals, and on the anterior cortex of the tibial midshaft. Stress fracture of the medial malleolus also has been reported.[211,220,240,259,261,264]

Stress fractures of the tibial shaft on the posteromedial aspect (compression side of the bone) are most common in sports that include running, such as distance running, soccer, basketball, and ballet dancing[22,47,91,108,119,130,182,198,216,239,290] (Figure 12.4). The main symptom is pain appearing during activity and disappearing when resting. With time, pain may be present with activities of

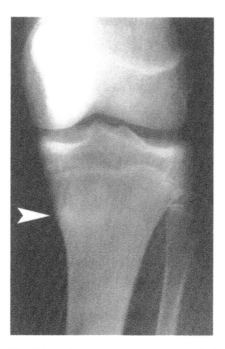

FIGURE 12.4 Stress fracture of the tibia at the proximal metaphyseal-diaphyseal junction (arrowhead).

daily living, or even at night. Physical examination reveals painful tenderness to palpation and percussion at the fracture site; at a later stage, callus may be palpated. Occasionally, swelling is present. Radiological diagnosis is possible only 2 to 5 weeks following the appearance of pain, when callus as well as the fracture line may be seen (usually oblique radiographs are also required). Bone scan is useful for early diagnosis and helps to differentiate stress fracture from the posterior tibialis muscle syndrome, tibial periostitis, and external chronic compartment syndrome. Treatment is rest, in which a non-weight-bearing period on crutches for pain relief is sometimes required, until the patient is pain free and has no bony tenderness. Most tibial stress fractures heal within 6 to 8 weeks, with an average time to return to full sports of 8 to 12 weeks. Supplemental use of a pneumatic brace can allow athletes to return to activity sooner than the above-mentioned traditional treatment.[79,276,299]

The atypical stress fracture of the anterior cortex of the midshaft of the tibia (tension side of the bone) occurs almost exclusively in athletes performing repetitive jumping and leaping activities. This type of stress fracture has been reported in basketball players, runners, pole vaulters, high jumpers, volleyball players, handball players, figure skaters, and ballet dancers.[14,17,28,41,56,109,173,215,218,230,243] These stress fractures require prolonged healing time. It is quite common for these fractures to develop delayed union or nonunion and they even fracture completely. The main symptom is diffuse, dull pain in the leg that is intensified by physical activity. Physical examination reveals point tenderness over the anterior aspect of the midshaft of the tibia. A characteristic radiograph appearance is that of V- or wedge-shaped defect in the middle third of the anterior cortex of the tibia with or without hypertrophy of this cortex with the open end of the V directed anteriorly (Figure 12.5). This defect is termed the *dreaded black line* and may be single or multiple. Callus formation is generally absent. Initial treatment consists of rest with or without immobilization for a minimum of 3 to 6 months. If after 3 to 6 months there is no evidence of healing either clinically or radiologically, surgical management is indicated. The recommended surgical intervention modalities vary from surgical excision and bone grafting, transverse drilling at the fracture site, to intramedullary tibial nailing.[14,56,109,215,218,230] Intramedullary fixation has become the favored approach for this type of stress fracture.[14,56,230]

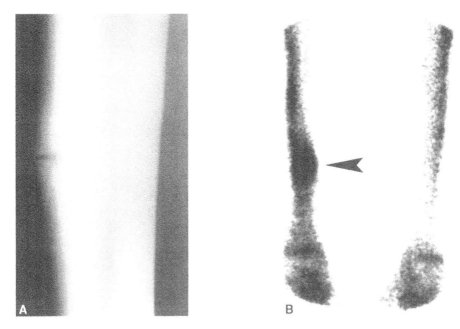

FIGURE 12.5 (A) Lateral roentgenogram demonstrating anterior midshaft stress fracture; (B) bone scan of the same patient (arrowhead).

Another variety of atypical tibial stress fracture occurs in the medial malleolus. Stress fractures of the medial malleolus have been reported in athletes participating in running and jumping activities, i.e., in basketball players, hurdlers, high and long jumpers, sprinters, and gymnasts.[211,220,240,259,261,264] Patients with medial malleolar stress fractures present with tenderness over the medial malleolus and an ankle effusion. They usually have pain during athletic activities for several weeks prior to an acute episode that results in their seeking medical attention. The fracture line extends vertically or obliquely upward at the junction of the medial malleolus and the tibial plafond (Figure 12.6). If there are clinical signs and a clinical history and if the fracture line is not detected on radiographs, a bone scan should be performed to confirm the diagnosis. CT scan and MRI are also helpful in early detection of medial malleolar stress fracture. Undisplaced stress fractures of the medial malleolus should be treated with immobilization for a period of 6 weeks; displaced fractures require open reduction and internal fixation.

Recently, longitudinal stress fractures of the tibia have been reported.[64,140,151,232,263] They occur more commonly in middle-aged to elderly adults, and are not usually associated with strenuous activity. They often have an atypical presentation and require CT or MRI for definitive diagnosis. Non-operative treatment is usually sufficient.

4. Fibula

Stress fractures of the fibula occur most commonly in the lower third of the bone, approximately 3 to 8 cm above the tip of the lateral malleolus (Figure 12.7). In sports medicine, it is commonly called runner's fracture.[73] However, basketball players, figure skaters, volleyball players, football players, soccer players, gymnasts, and squash players are also known to be affected by this type of stress fracture.[73,186,226] It has been suggested that fibular stress fractures are caused either by a combination of compression and torsion forces against the lateral malleolus or by the rhythmic contractions of flexor muscles of the foot. Pain is usually localized along the affected area, and swelling is often apparent. The pain, which may last from several days to several weeks, is aggravated by physical activity and relieved by rest. An antalgic gait is also common. Physical

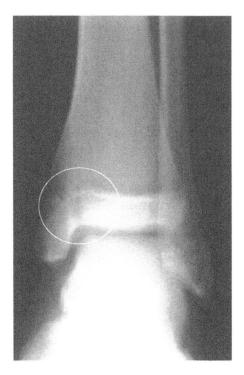

FIGURE 12.6 Roentgenogram of the medial malleolus with stress fracture in basketball player.

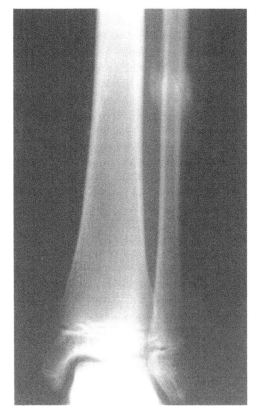

FIGURE 12.7 Stress fracture of the fibula.

examination reveals localized tenderness at the fracture site and pain by pressing the fibula toward the tibia. Callus is occasionally palpable. Radiological changes are visible only 3 or 4 weeks following the onset of symptoms. Initially, only an oblique or transverse fissure may be seen on radiographs but, later, callus appears. A bone scan can be conducted to confirm the diagnosis. Discontinuation of the athletic activity for 6 weeks is sufficient for the fracture to heal. If the inciting activity is not stopped, healing may take 3 to 6 months.

Although most stress fractures are in the lower third of the fibula, proximal fibular stress fractures have also been described.[163,167,273] The predominant symptom is diffuse proximal and lateral leg pain that is often aggravated by physical activity and/or knee range of motion. Radiographs may reveal a transverse or oblique fracture line at the neck of the fibula with periosteal new bone formation developing during the healing phase. A bone scan is useful in uncertain cases to confirm the diagnosis. This stress fracture typically heals with a 6-week period of rest.

In the literature, two unusual fibular stress fractures are reported: a stress fracture that was associated with distal tibiofibular synostosis[161] and delayed union of a fibular stress fracture secondary to rotational malunion of a lateral malleolar fracture.[112]

5. Tarsal Bones

Recent research on the incidence of stress fractures in athletes shows that the number of tarsal navicular stress fractures is increasing, as is the number of reports discussing the possibilities and results of treatment.[22,47,91,108,119,130,182,198,216,239,290] Stress fracture of the tarsal navicular bone is most common in sprinters, hurdlers, basketball players, high and long jumpers, and middle-distance runners, in other words in explosive athletic activities that involve sprinting, jumping, and hurdling.[5,34,92,100,108,128,131,153,155,156,255,256,283,285,287] They generally occur as partial or complete fractures in the sagittal plane, almost always within the central third of the bone. Because of poor vascularization of that part of the bone, the tendency to delay union or nonunion and to refracture is high. The patient usually complains of a vague pain along the dorsum of the foot, which increases during jumping (usually the take-off foot is affected) and sudden starts and which persists for a longer period of time (according to reference literature, the time span between the onset of symptoms and the diagnosis is rather long, 4.5 months on average). Physical examination reveals point tenderness over the tarsal navicular bone, especially at the proximal dorsal border, the "N-spot." Swelling in that area occurs quite rarely. Two clinical tests are helpful in the diagnosis: (1) tiptoeing on the affected leg and (2) attempting to jump from this position, which causes severe pain, thus indicating the probability of the tarsal navicular stress fracture.[34] When, after clinical examination, tarsal navicular stress fracture is suspected a bone scan is required, because radiographs in most cases do not reveal the fracture. If clinical indication of tarsal navicular stress fracture is confirmed by a positive bone scan, CT or MRI is required to distinguish stress reaction from stress fracture, and to provide information on the extent of the lesion (partial or complete fracture) (Figure 12.8). A navicular stress reaction (a positive bone scan and a negative CT or MRI scan) would be treated by rest from weight bearing and close observation. Partial tarsal navicular stress fractures should be treated by immobilization in a short-leg cast with a non-weight-bearing period of 6 to 8 weeks. Based on the results of our prospective research, we propose an algorithm of non-operative procedures in treatment of partial tarsal navicular stress fracture[34] (Figure 12.9). In the case of complete fracture, displaced fracture, delayed union, nonunion, and refracture, surgery is indicated—drilling, bone grafting, or internal fixation by compression screws — followed by immobilization and avoidance of weight bearing until union has occurred.

Calcaneal stress fractures are common in military recruits and quite rare among athletes.[33,50] Still, the fracture has been reported in joggers, long-distance runners, and ballet dancers. Patients present with a history of insidious onset of heel pain that is aggravated by running or jumping. Physical examination reveals tenderness over the medial or lateral aspects of the calcaneus, and pain with squeezing the posterosuperior calcaneus from both sides simultaneously. Radiographs

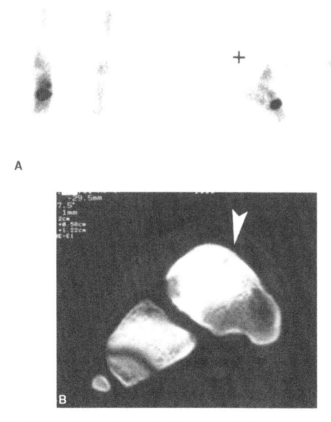

FIGURE 12.8 Navicular tarsal stress fracture. (A) Bone scan; (B) CT scan (arrowhead).

typically demonstrate a sclerotic line that on a lateral image is parallel to the posterior margin of the calcaneus. A less common location for calcaneal stress fractures is adjacent to the medial tuberosity. Treatment is rest (6 to 8 weeks), during which a non-weight-bearing period on crutches for pain relief is sometimes required, until the patient is pain free and has no bony tenderness. Then a gradual rehabilitation program is recommended, as well as the use of soft heel pads.

Stress fractures of the talus are very rare. Two types of talar stress fracture are reported. The first is a vertical lateral body fracture near the junction of the body with the lateral process of the talus, and the second, less common, is a talar neck stress fracture.[27,40,201] The fracture should be confirmed by way of either a bone scan or MRI (CT), because radiographs often fail to reveal the lesion. The recommended treatment is immobilization in a short-leg cast and avoidance of weight bearing for 6 to 8 weeks, followed by gradual rehabilitation.

The literature contains few reported cases of tarsal cuboid stress fractures.[18,57] They require a high index of suspicion to avoid misdiagnosis. A bone scan, a CT scan, or MRI is necessary to confirm the diagnosis. Treatment consists of a short-leg non-weight-bearing cast for 6 to 8 weeks, followed by gradual rehabilitation.

Very few cases of the stress fractures of the cuneiform bones are reported. A stress fracture of the lateral cuneiform bone in a basketball player, a stress fracture of the intermediate cuneiform bone in a triathlete, and a stress fracture of the medial cuneiform bone in a runner are described.[69,154,180]

6. Metatarsal Bones

Although both physicians and laypersons seem to be best acquainted with stress fractures of the metatarsal bones, either as stress fractures primarily affecting soldiers or as "march fractures,"

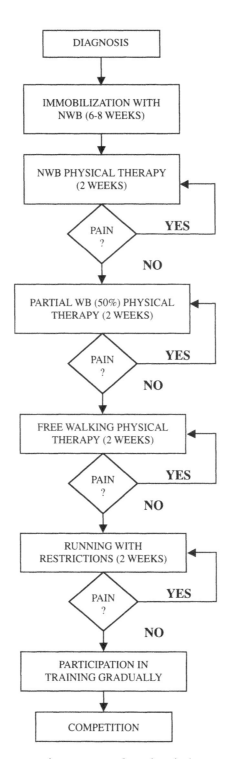

FIGURE 12.9 Algorithm of non-operative treatment of tarsal navicular stress fracture in athletes.[34]

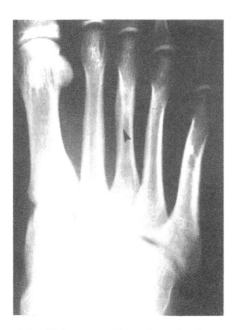

FIGURE 12.10 Stress fracture of the third metatarsal bone (arrowhead).

these fractures rank second among athletes; tibial stress fractures are first. In more than 80% of metatarsal bone stress fractures, the shaft of the second and third metatarsal bone is affected[298] (Figure 12.10). Less common locations include the base of the second metatarsal and the base of the fifth metatarsal bone.

Metatarsal shaft stress fractures are typical in runners, dancers, basketball players, soccer players, figure skaters, and gymnasts.[298] Diagnosis is very simple once the stress fracture is suspected. Patients complain of forefoot pain that is aggravated by running, jumping, or dancing activity. Although the pain is not severe at first, it gradually worsens when activity is undertaken. Physical examination reveals tenderness over the involved bone and sometimes a mass can be palpated along the shaft of the involved bone, which represents fracture callus. Radiographic changes may not be evident for at least 2 to 3 weeks following the onset of patients' symptoms, but thereafter a subtle fracture line with periosteal reaction may be present. If radiographs do not confirm that a stress fracture is present, a bone scan can be conducted. Rest from athletic activities for 4 to 6 weeks and immobilization in a boot cast with a heel for walking (2 to 4 weeks) yield good results, i.e., complete bone healing. Patients are observed clinically and allowed to commence a graduated activity program once the symptoms have resolved and there is no local tenderness at the fracture site.

a. The Base of the Second Metatarsal Bone

Stress fracture of the base of the second metatarsal is described among female ballet dancers.[118,192,212] All dancers presented with midfoot pain that was worse *en pointe* and with jumps. There was no pain when standing flat. Physical examination revealed tenderness either at the base of the first web space or on the proximal portion of the second metatarsal. Radiographs and bone scan should be used to confirm the diagnosis. Rest from dancing for 6 to 8 weeks is sufficient for healing, and then this type of stress fracture requires 4 to 6 weeks of gradual resumption of full activity.

b. The Base of the Fifth Metatarsal Bone Distal to the Tuberosity
(Jones Fracture)

Stress fractures of the proximal fifth metatarsal distal to the tuberosity, Jones fracture, should be discussed as a separate entity, especially because it tends toward delayed union, nonunion, and refracture (Figure 12.11). Jones fracture is most common in basketball players, football players, soccer players, runners, and throwers (javelin, hammer).[62,71,90,126,150,195,210,225,234,249,286,306] The main symptom is pain in the lateral foot region. Physical examination reveals pain on palpation in the proximal end of the fifth metatarsal (about 1.5 cm distally from the tuberosity). Pain is exacerbated by inversion of the foot. Based on radiography, Pećina and co-workers[225] divide Jones fracture into three types and, according to the type, suggest treatment. If the radiograph shows an evident narrow fissure of the cortex and a passable medullar cavity (type 1), immobilization in a short leg cast with a non-weight-bearing period of 6 to 8 weeks is suggested. When there is a fissure with an evident sclerosing of its edges (type 2), they suggest the same treatment with the exception of active athletes, in whose case they suggest surgery. At the time of cast removal, healing of the fracture should be assessed both clinically and radiologically. It may be sometimes necessary to immobilize the foot for another period, as long as 4 weeks. Nonunion may occur, and should be treated surgically. If radiography demonstrates that sclerosing completely obliterates the medullar cavity (type 3), they suggest that both athletes and nonathletes undergo surgery. Choices for surgical intervention include corticocancellous bone grafting and intramedullary screw fixation. Currently, the most popular choice in athletes is intramedullary screw fixation. Review of the literature shows favorable results in athletes with early return to activity and rare reports of complications.[104,165,302] Early results with the use of electrical stimulation are also promising; however, prospective studies are needed to better define the role of this modality in managing stress fractures of the proximal fifth metatarsal distal to the tuberosity.[23,123]

7. Sesamoid Bones

Sesamoid bones of the great toe located within the tendon of the flexor hallucis brevis beneath the head of the first metatarsal bone may be sites for stress fractures. Stress fractures are thought to affect the medial sesamoid bone more often. These fractures have been reported in runners, basketball players, gymnasts, and dancers.[127,189,244,288] The main symptom is pain in the region of the metatarsophalangeal joint of the great toe, characteristically accompanying the activity (e.g., running) and disappearing on resting. Physical examination reveals painful tenderness over the plantar side of the first metatarsophalangeal joint, and mere passive dorsiflexion of the great toe provokes pain. Radiographs should include weight-bearing AP and lateral views as well as an axial view centered on the sesamoids. Sesamoid stress fracture is characterized by a specific fissure form, i.e., a transverse fracture line (or possibly two lines) that has jagged margins and sharp corners, but the sesamoid bone can sometimes be splintered into several fragments. When stress fracture of the sesamoid bone is only clinically suspected but not seen on radiographs, a bone scan should be performed to confirm the diagnosis and radiographs should be repeated in 3 weeks. In differential diagnosis of the sesamoid bone stress fracture, the following conditions should be taken into account: congenital variations and anomalies of the sesamoid bones, sesamoiditis, osteochondritis, nonunion of previous fractures, metatarsalgia, podagra (gout), and arthritis of the first metatarsophalangeal joint. Initial treatment of sesamoid bone stress fracture is invariably non-operative. Treatment consists of a short-leg non-weight-bearing cast that extends to the distal tip of the toe to prevent dorsiflexion for 6 weeks. As these fractures show a tendency for delayed union, nonunion, or recurrence, surgery may often be necessary. Partial or complete excision of the sesamoid is recommended, although bone grafting without excision also provides satisfactory results.

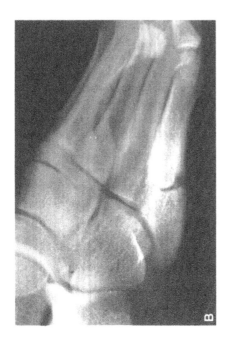

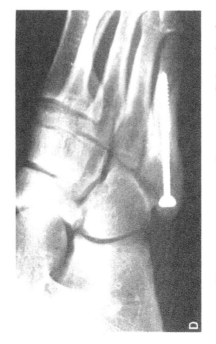

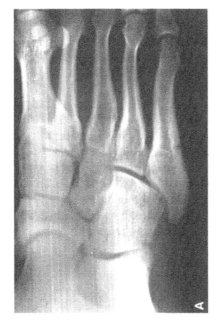

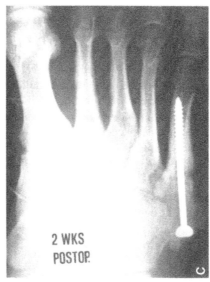

2 WKS
POSTOP.

FIGURE 12.11 Stress fracture of the fifth metatarsal bone (Jones fracture). (A) Initial roentgenogram; (B) roentgenogram preceding surgery; (C) 2 weeks after surgery; (D) 8 weeks after surgery when athlete resumed full sports activities.

REFERENCES

1. **Abbot, A.E. and Hannafin, J.A.** Stress fracture of the clavicle in a female lightweight rower. A case report and a review of the literature. *Am. J. Sports Med.*, 2001; 29: 370–372.
2. **Abel, M.A.** Jogger's fractures and other stress fractures on the lumbar sacral spine. *Skel. Radiol.*, 1985; 13: 221–227.
3. **Adolfsson, L. and Lysholm, J.** Case report: clavicular stress fracture in a javelin thrower. *Clin. Sports Med.*, 1990; 2: 41–45.
4. **Ahluwalia, R., Datz, F.L., Morton, K.A. et al.** Bilateral fatigue fractures of the radial shaft in gymnast. *Clin. Nucl. Med.*, 1994; 19: 665–667.
5. **Alfred, R.H., Belhobek, G, and Bergfeld, J.A.** Stress fractures of the tarsal navicular. A case report. *Am. J. Sports Med.*, 1992; 20: 766–768.
6. **Allen, M.E.** Stress fracture of the humerus. A case study. *Am. J. Sports Med.*, 1984; 12: 244–245.
7. **Ammann, W. and Matheson, G.O.** Radionuclide bone imaging in the detection of stress fractures. *Clin. J. Sport Med.*, 1991; 1: 115–122.
8. **Arendt, E.A.** Stress fractures and the female athlete. *Clin. Orthop.*, 2000; 372: 131–138.
9. **Arendt, E.A. and Griffiths, H.J.** The use of MR imaging in the assessment and clinical management of stress reactions of bone in high-performance athletes. *Clin. Sports Med.*, 1997; 16: 291–306.
10. **Aro, H. and Dahlstrom, S.** Conservative management of distraction-type stress fractures of the femoral neck. *J. Bone Joint Surg.*, 1986; 68B: 65–67.
11. **Atwell, E.A. and Jackson, D.W.** Stress fractures of the sacrum in runners. Two case reports. *Am. J. Sports Med.*, 1991; 19: 531–533.
12. **Barbaix, E.J.** Stress fracture of the sternum in a golf player. *Int. J. Sports Med.*, 1996; 17: 303–304.
13. **Barrett, G.R., Shelton, W.R., and Miles, J.W.** First rib fractures in football players: a case report and literature review. *Am. J. Sports Med.*, 1988; 16: 674–676.
14. **Barrick, E.F. and Jackson, C.B.** Prophylactic intramedullary fixation of the tibia for stress fracture in a professional athlete. *J. Orthop. Trauma*, 1992; 6: 241–244.
15. **Barrow, G.W. and Saha, S.** Menstrual irregularity and stress fractures in collegiate female distance runners. *Am. J. Sports Med.*, 1988; 16: 209–216.
16. **Bartsokas, T.W., Palin, W.D., and Collier, B.D.** An unusual stress fracture site: midhumerus. *Phys. Sportsmed.*, 1992; 20: 119–122.
17. **Batt, M.E., Kemp, S., and Kerslake, R.** Delayed union stress fractures of the anterior tibia: conservative management. *Br. J. Sports Med.*, 2001; 35: 74–77.
18. **Beaman, D.N., Roeser, W.M., Holmes, J.R. et al.** Cuboid stress fractures: a report of two cases. *Foot Ankle*, 1993; 14: 525–528.
19. **Belkin, S.C.** Stress fractures in athletes. *Orthop. Clin. North Am.*, 1980; 11: 735–742.
20. **Bell, R.H. and Hawkins, R.J.** Stress fracture of the distal ulna: a case report. *Clin. Orthop.*, 1986; 209: 169–171.
21. **Bellah, R.D., Summerville, D.A., Treves, S.T. et al.** Low-back pain in adolescent athletes: detection of stress injury to the pars interarticularis with SPECT. *Radiology*, 1991; 180: 509–512.
22. **Benazzo, F., Barnabei, G., Ferrario, A. et al.** Stress fractures in track and field athletes. *J. Sports Trauma. Relat. Res.*, 1992; 14: 51–65.
23. **Benazzo, F., Mosconi, M., Beccarisi, G. et al.** Use of capacitive coupled electric fields in stress fractures in athletes. *Clin. Orthop.*, 1995; 310: 145–149.
24. **Bennell, K.L. and Brukner, P.D.** Epidemiology and site specificity of stress fractures. *Clin. Sports Med.*, 1997; 16: 179–196.
25. **Bennell, K.L., Malcolm, S.A., Thomas, S.A. et al.** Risk factors for stress fractures in female track-and-field athletes. A retrospective analysis. *Clin. J. Sport Med.*, 1995; 5: 229–235.
26. **Bennell, K.L., Malcolm, S.A., Thomas, S.A. et al.** The incidence and distribution of stress fractures in competitive track and field athletes. A twelve-month prospective study. *Am. J. Sports Med.*, 1996; 24: 211–217.
27. **Black, K.P. and Ehlert, K.J.** A stress fracture of the lateral process of the talus in a runner. *J. Bone Joint Surg.*, 1994; 76A: 441–443.
28. **Blank, S.** Transverse tibial stress fractures. A special problem. *Am. J. Sports Med.*, 1987; 15: 597–602.

29. **Blatz, D.J.** Bilateral femoral and tibial shaft stress fractures in a runner. *Am. J. Sports Med.,* 1981; 9: 322–325.

30. **Blickenstaff, L.D. and Morris, J.M.** Fatigue fracture of the femoral neck. *J. Bone Joint Surg.,* 1966; 48A: 1031–1047.

31. **Boden, B.P. and Speer, K.P.** Femoral stress fractures. *Clin. Sports Med.,* 1997; 16: 307–317.

32. **Boden, B.P. and Osbahr, D.C.** High-risk stress fractures: evaluation and treatment. *J. Am. Acad. Orthop. Surg.,* 2000; 8: 344–353.

33. **Boden, B.P., Osbahr, D.C., and Jimenez, C.** Low-risk stress fractures. *Am. J. Sports Med.,* 2001; 29: 100–111.

34. **Bojanić, I. and Pećina, M.M.** Traitement conservateur des fractures de contrainte du scaphoide tarsien chez le sportif. *Rev. Chir. Orthop.,* 1997; 83: 133–138.

35. **Bojanić, I. and Desnica, N.** Stress fracture of the sixth rib in an elite athlete. *Croat. Med. J.,* 1998; 39: 458–460.

36. **Bojanić, I., Pećina, H.I., and Pećina, M.** Prijelomi zamora. *Arh. Hig. Rada Toksikol.,* 2001; 52: 471–482.

37. **Bollen, S.R., Robinson, D.G., Crichton, K.J. et al.** Stress fractures of the ulna in tennis players using a double-handed backhand stroke. *Am. J. Sports Med.,* 1993; 21: 751–752.

38. **Bottomley, M.B.** Sacral stress fracture in a runner. *Br. J. Sports Med.,* 1990; 24: 243–244.

39. **Boyer, B.W., Jr.** Trapshooter's shoulder: stress fracture of the coracoid process. Case report. *J. Bone Joint Surg.,* 1975; 57A: 862.

40. **Bradshaw, C., Khan, K., and Brukner, P.** Stress fracture of the body of the talus in athletes demonstrated with computer tomography. *Clin. J. Sport Med.,* 1996; 6: 48–51.

41. **Brahms, M.A., Fumich, R.M., and Ippolito, V.D.** Atypical stress fracture of the tibia in a professional athlete. *Am. J. Sports Med.,* 1980; 8: 131–132.

42. **Branch, T., Partin, C., Chamberland, P. et al.** Spontaneous fractures of the humerus during pitching. A series of 12 cases. *Am. J. Sports Med.,* 1992; 20: 468–470.

43. **Breithaupt, M.B.** Zur Pathologie des menschlichen Fusses. *Med. Z.,* 1855; 24: 169–177.

44. **Brogle, P.J., Eswar, S., and Denton, J.R.** Propagation of a patellar stress fracture in a basketball player. *Am. J. Orthop.,* 1997; 26: 782–784.

45. **Brooks, A.A.** Stress fractures of the upper extremity. *Clin. Sports Med.,* 2001; 20: 613–620.

46. **Brudvig, T.J.S., Gudger, T.D., and Obermeyer, L.** Stress fractures in 295 trainees. A one-year study of incidence as related to age, sex, and race. *Mil. Med.,* 1983; 148: 666–667.

47. **Brukner, P., Bradshaw, C., Khan, K. et al.** Stress fractures: a review of 180 cases. *Clin. J. Sport Med.,* 1996; 6: 85–89.

48. **Brukner, P. and Bennell, K.** Stress fractures in female athletes. Diagnosis, management and rehabilitation. *Sports Med.,* 1997; 24: 419–429.

49. **Brukner, P.** Stress fractures of the upper limb. *Sports Med.,* 1998; 26: 415–424.

50. **Brukner, P., Bennell, K., and Matheson, G.O.** *Stress Fracture.* Carlton, Victoria: Blackwell Science Asia, 1999.

51. **Brunet, M.E., Cook, S.D., Brinker, M.R. et al.** A survey of running injuries in 1505 competitive and recreational runners. *J. Sports Med. Phys. Fitness,* 1990; 30: 307–315.

52. **Buckwalter, J.A. and Brandser, E.A.** Stress and insufficiency fractures. *Am. Fam. Physician,* 1997; 56: 175–182.

53. **Butler, J.E., Brown, S.L., and McConnell, B.G.** Subtrochanteric stress fractures in runners. *Am. J. Sports Med.,* 1982; 10: 228–232.

54. **Carek, P.J. and Fumich, R.M.** Stress fracture of the distal radius. Not just a risk for elite gymnasts. *Phys. Sportsmed.,* 1992; 20: 115–118.

55. **Carter, S.R. and Aldridge, M.J.** Stress injury of the distal radial growth plate. *J. Bone Joint Surg.,* 1988; 70B: 834–836.

56. **Chang, P.S. and Harris, R.M.** Intramedullary nailing for chronic tibial stress fractures. A review of five cases. *Am. J. Sports Med.,* 1996; 24: 688–692.

57. **Chen, J.B.** Cuboid stress fracture. A case report. *J. Am. Podiatr. Med. Assoc.,* 1993; 83: 153–155.

58. **Chen, W.-C., Hsu, W.-Y., and Wu, J.-J.** Stress fracture of the diaphysis of the ulna. *Int. Orthop.,* 1991; 15: 197–198.

59. **Christiansen, E. and Kanstrup, I.L.** Increased risk of stress fractures of the ribs in elite rowers. *Scand. J. Med. Sci. Sports*, 1997; 7: 49–52.

60. **Christiansen, E.** Rib stress fractures in elite rowers. A case series and proposed mechanism. *Am. J. Sports Med.*, 2000; 28: 435–436.

61. **Ciullo, J.V. and Jackson, D.W.** Pars interarticularis stress reaction, spondylolysis, and spondylolisthesis in gymnasts. *Clin. Sports Med.*, 1985; 4: 95–110.

62. **Clapper, M.F., O'Brien, T.J., and Lyons, P.M.** Fractures of the fifth metatarsal: analysis of a fracture registry. *Clin. Orthop.*, 1995; 315: 239–241.

63. **Clark, R.J., Sizer, P.S., Jr., and Slauterbeck, J.** Stress fracture of the ulna in a male competitive polo player. *Am. J. Sports Med.*, 2002; 30: 130–132.

64. **Clayer, M., Krishnan, J., Lee, W.K. et al.** Longitudinal stress fracture of the tibia: two cases. *Clin. Radiol.*, 1992; 46: 401–404.

65. **Clement, D.B., Taunton, J.E., Smart, G.W. et al.** A survey of overuse running injuries. *Phys. Sportsmed.*, 1981; 9: 47–58.

66. **Clement, D.B., Ammann, W., Taunton, J.E. et al.** Exercise-induced stress injuries to the femur. *Int. J. Sports Med.*, 1993; 14: 347–352.

67. **Coady, C.M. and Micheli, L.J.** Stress fractures in the pediatric athlete. *Clin. Sports Med.*, 1997; 16: 225–238.

68. **Congeni, J., McCulloch, J., and Swanson, K.** Lumbar spondylolysis. A study of natural progression in athletes. *Am. J. Sports Med.*, 1997; 25: 248–253.

69. **Creighton, R., Sonoga, A., and Gordon, G.** Stress fracture of the tarsal middle cuneiform bone: a case report. *J. Am. Podiatr. Med. Assoc.*, 1990; 80: 489–495.

70. **Crockett, H.C., Wright, J.M., Madsen, M.W. et al.** Sacral stress fracture in an elite college basketball player after the use of a jumping machine. *Am. J. Sports Med.*, 1999; 27: 526–528.

71. **DeLee, J.C., Evans, J.P., and Julian, J.** Stress fracture of the fifth metatarsal. *Am. J. Sports Med.*, 1983; 11: 349–353.

72. **Deutsch, A.L., Coel, M.N., and Mink, J.H.** Imaging of stress injuries to bone: radiography, scintigraphy and MR imaging. *Clin. Sports Med.*, 1997; 16: 275–290.

73. **Devas, M.B. and Sweetnam, R.** Stress fractures of the fibula. A review of fifty cases in athletes. *J. Bone Joint Surg.*, 1956; 38B: 818–829.

74. **Devas, M.B.** Stress fractures of the patella. *J. Bone Joint Surg.*, 1960; 42B: 71–74.

75. **Devas, M.B.** Stress fractures in children. *J. Bone Joint Surg.*, 1963; 45B: 528–541.

76. **Devas, M.B.** Stress fractures of the femoral neck. *J. Bone Joint Surg.,* 1965; 47B: 728–738.

77. **Devas, M.B.** Stress fractures in athletes. *Proc. R. Soc. Med.*, 1969; 62: 933–937.

78. **Devas, M.B.** *Stress Fractures.* Edinburgh: Churchill-Livingstone, 1975.

79. **Dickson, T.B. and Kichline, P.D.** Functional management of stress fractures in female athletes using a pneumatic leg brace. *Am. J. Sports Med.*, 1987; 15: 86–89.

80. **Dufek, P., Ostendorf, V., and Thormahlen, F.** Stress fracture of the ulna in a table tennis player. *Sportverletz. Sportschaden*, 1999; 13: 62–64.

81. **Dugowson, C.E., Drinkwater, B.L., and Clark, J.M.** Nontraumatic femur fracture in an oligomenorrheic athlete. *Med. Sci. Sports Exerc.*, 1991; 23: 1323–1325.

82. **Edwards, T.B. and Murphy, C.** Nonunion of a dominant side first rib stress fracture in a baseball pitcher. *Orthopaedics*, 2001; 24: 599–600.

83. **Egol, K.A., Koval, K.J., Kummer, F. et al.** Stress fractures of the femoral neck. *Clin. Orthop.*, 1998; 348: 72–78.

84. **Eller, D.J., Katz, D.S., Bergman, A.G. et al.** Sacral stress fractures in long-distance runners. *Clin. J. Sport Med.*, 1997; 7: 222–225.

85. **Engel, A. and Feldner-Busztin, H.** Bilateral stress fracture of the scaphoid. A case report. *Arch. Orthop. Trauma Surg.*, 1991; 110: 314–315.

86. **Escher, S.A.** Ulnar diaphyseal stress fracture in a bowler. *Am. J. Sports Med.,* 1997; 25: 412–413.

87. **Fallon, K.E. and Fricker, P.A.** Stress fracture of the clavicle in a young female gymnast. *Br. J. Sports Med.*, 2001; 35: 448–449.

88. **Featherstone, T.** Magnetic resonance imaging in the diagnosis of sacral stress fracture. *Br. J. Sports Med.*, 1999; 33: 276–277.

89. **Fehlandt, A.F. and Micheli, L.J.** Lumbar facet stress fracture in a ballet dancer. *Spine*, 1993; 18: 2537–2539.

90. **Fernandez Fairen, M., Guillen, J., Busto, J.M. et al.** Fractures of the fifth metatarsal in basketball players. *Knee Surg. Sports Traumatol. Arthrosc.*, 1999; 7: 373–377.

91. **Fitch, K.D.** Stress fractures of the lower limbs in runners. *Aust. Fam. Physician*, 1984; 13: 511–515.

92. **Fitch, K.D., Blackwell, J.B., and Gilmour, W.N.** Operation for non-union of stress fracture of the tarsal navicular. *J. Bone Joint Surg.*, 1989; 71B: 105–110.

93. **Fragniere, B., Landry, M., and Siegrist, O.** Stress fracture of the ulna in a professional tennis player using a double-handed backhand stroke. *Knee Surg. Sports Traumatol. Arthrosc.*, 2001; 9: 239–241.

94. **Fredericson, M., Bergman, A.G., Hoffman, K.L. et al.** Tibial stress reaction in runners: correlation of clinical symptoms and scintigraphy with a new magnetic resonance imaging grading system. *Am. J. Sports Med.*, 1995; 23: 472–481.

95. **Frey, C.** Footwear and stress fractures. *Clin. Sports Med.*, 1997; 16: 249–257.

96. **Friberg, O.** Leg length asymmetry in stress fractures. *J. Sports Med. Phys. Fitness*, 1982; 22: 485–488.

97. **Fullerton, L.R., Jr. and Snowdy, H.A.** Femoral neck stress fractures. *Am. J. Sports Med.*, 1988; 16: 365–377.

98. **Fullerton, L.R., Jr.** Femoral neck stress fractures. *Sports Med.*, 1990; 9: 192–197.

99. **Gardner, L.I., Jr., Dziados, J.E., Jones, B.H. et al.** Prevention of lower extremity stress fractures: a controlled trial of a shock absorbent insole. *Am. J. Public Health*, 1988; 78: 1563–1567.

100. **Georgen, T.G., Venn-Watson, E.A., Rossman, D.J. et al.** Tarsal navicular stress fractures in runners. *Am. J. Roentgenol.*, 1981; 136: 201–203.

101. **Geyer, M., Sander-Beuermann, A., Wegner, U. et al.** Stressreaktionen und Stressfrakturen beim Leistungssportler. Ursachen, Diagnostik und Therapie. *Unfallchirurg*, 1993; 96: 66–74.

102. **Giladi, M., Milgrom, C., Simkin, A. et al.** Stress fractures and tibial bone width: a risk factor. *J. Bone Joint Surg.*, 1987; 69B: 326–329.

103. **Giladi, M., Milgrom, C., Simkin, A. et al.** Stress fractures. Identifiable risk factors. *Am. J. Sports Med.*, 1991; 19: 647–652.

104. **Glasgow, M.T., Naranja, R.J., Jr., Glasgow, S.G. et al.** Analysis of failed surgical management of fractures of the base of the fifth metatarsal distal to the tuberosity: the Jones fracture. *Foot Ankle*, 1996; 17: 449–457.

105. **Godshall, R.W., Hansen, C.A., and Rising, D.C.** Stress fractures through the distal femoral epiphysis. *Am. J. Sports Med.*, 1981; 9: 114–116.

106. **Goldberg, B. and Pecora, C.** Stress fractures. A risk of increased training in freshmen. *Phys. Sportsmed.*, 1994; 22: 68–78.

107. **Goodman, P.H., Heaslet, M.W., Pagliano, J.W. et al.** Stress fracture diagnosis by computer-assisted thermography. *Phys. Sportsmed.*, 1985; 13: 114–132.

108. **Graff, K.H., Krahl, H., and Kirschberger, R.** Stressfrakturen des Os Naviculare Pedis. *Z. Orthop.*, 1986; 124: 228–237.

109. **Green, N.E., Rogers, R.A., and Lipscomb, A.B.** Nonunions of stress fractures of the tibia. *Am. J. Sports Med.*, 1985; 13: 171–176.

110. **Gregory, P.L., Biswas, A.C., and Batt, M.E.** Musculoskeletal problem of the chest wall in athletes. *Sports Med.*, 2002; 32: 235–250.

111. **Guha, A.R. and Marynissen, H.** Stress fracture of the hook of the hamate. *Br. J. Sports Med.*, 2002; 36: 224–225.

112. **Guille, J.T., Lipton, G.E., Bowen, J.R., and Uthaman, U.** Delayed union following stress fracture of the distal fibula secondary to rotational malunion of lateral malleolar fracture. *Am. J. Orthop.*, 1997; 26: 442–445.

113. **Gurtler, R., Pavlov, H., and Torg, J.S.** Stress fracture of the ipsilateral first rib in a pitcher. *Am. J. Sports Med.*, 1985; 13: 277–279.

114. **Hallel, T., Amit, S., and Segal, D.** Fatigue fractures of tibial and femoral shaft in soldiers. *Clin. Orthop.*, 1976; 118: 35–43.

115. **Hamilton, B.H., Colsen, E., and Brukner, P.** Stress fracture of the ulna in a baseball pitcher. *Clin. J. Sport Med.*, 1999; 9: 231–234.

116. **Hamilton, H.K.** Stress fracture of the diaphysis of the ulna in a body builder. *Am. J. Sports Med.*, 1984; 12: 405–406.

117. **Hanks, G.A., Kalenak, A., Bowman, L.S. et al.** Stress fractures of the carpal scaphoid. A report of four cases. *J. Bone Joint Surg.,* 1989; 71A: 938–941.
118. **Harrington, T., Crichton, K.J., and Anderson, I.F.** Overuse ballet injury of the base of second metatarsal. A diagnostic problem. *Am. J. Sports Med.,* 1993; 21: 591–598.
119. **Hershman, E.B. and Mailly, T.** Stress fractures. *Clin. Sports Med.,* 1990; 9: 183–214.
120. **Hershman, E.B., Lombardo, J., and Bergfeld, J.A.** Femoral shaft stress fractures in athletes. *Clin. Sports Med.,* 1990; 9: 111–119.
121. **Hill, P.F., Chatterji, S., Chambers, D. et al.** Stress fracture of the pubic ramus in female recruits. *J. Bone Joint Surg.,* 1996; 78B: 383–386.
122. **Holden, D.L. and Jackson, D.W.** Stress fracture of the ribs in female rowers. *Am. J. Sports Med.,* 1985; 13: 342–348.
123. **Holmes, G.B., Jr.** Treatment of delayed unions and nonunions of the proximal fifth metatarsal with pulsed electromagnetic fields. *Foot Ankle,* 1994; 15: 552–556.
124. **Horwitz, B.R. and DiStefano, V.** Stress fracture of the humerus in a weight lifter. *Orthopaedics,* 1995; 18: 185–187.
125. **Howard, C.B., Lieberman, N., Mozes, G. et al.** Stress fracture detected sonographically. *Am. J. Roentgenol.,* 1992; 159: 1350–1351.
126. **Hulkko, A., Orava, S., and Nikula, P.** Stress fracture of the fifth metatarsal in athletes. *Ann. Chir. Gynaecol.,* 1985; 74: 233–238.
127. **Hulkko, A., Orava, S., Pellinen, P. et al.** Stress fractures of the sesamoid bones of the first metatarsophalangeal joint in athletes. *Arch. Orthop. Trauma. Surg.,* 1985; 104: 113–117.
128. **Hullko, A., Orava, S., Peltokallio, P. et al.** Stress fracture of the navicular bone. Nine cases in athletes. *Acta Orthop. Scand.,* 1985; 56: 503–505.
129. **Hulkko, A., Orava, S., and Nikula, P.** Stress fractures of the olecranon in javelin throwers. *Int. J. Sports Med.,* 1986; 7: 210–213.
130. **Hulkko, A. and Orava, S.** Stress fractures in athletes. *Int. J. Sports Med.,* 1987; 8: 221–226.
131. **Hunter, L.Y.** Stress fractures of the tarsal navicular. More frequent than we realize? *Am. J. Sports Med.,* 1981; 9: 217–219.
132. **Ilahi, O.A. and Kohl, H.W., III.** Lower extremity morphology and alignment and risk of overuse injuries. *Clin. J. Sport Med.,* 1998; 8: 38–42.
133. **Inagaki, H. and Inoue, G.** Stress fracture of the scaphoid combined with distal radial epiphysiolysis. *Br. J. Sports Med.,* 1997; 31: 256–257.
134. **Ishibashi, Y., Okamura, Y., Otsuka, H. et al.** Comparison of scintigraphy and magnetic resonance imaging for stress injuries of bone. *Clin. J. Sport Med.,* 2002; 12: 79–84.
135. **Israeli, A., Engel, J., and Ganel, A.** Possible fatigue fracture of the pisiform bone in volleyball players. *Int. J. Sports Med.,* 1982; 3: 56–57.
136. **Ivkovic, A., Bojanić, I., and Ivkovic, M.** Trijas sportašica. *Liječ. Vjesn.,* 2001; 123: 200–206.
137. **Iwaya, T. and Takatori, I.** Lateral longitudinal stress fractures of the patella: report of three cases. *J. Pediatr. Orthop.,* 1985; 5: 73–75.
138. **Jackson, D.W., Wiltse, L.L., Dingeman, R.D. et al.** Stress reactions involving the pars interarticularis in young athletes. *Am. J. Sports Med.,* 1981; 9: 304–312.
139. **Jerosch, J.G., Castro, W.H.M., and Jantea, C.** Stress fracture of the patella. *Am. J. Sports Med.,* 1989; 17: 579–580.
140. **Jeske, J.M., Lomasney, L.M., Demos, T.C. et al.** Longitudinal tibial stress fracture. *Orthopaedics,* 1996; 19: 263.
141. **Johanson, A.W., Weiss, C.B., Jr., Stento, K. et al.** Stress fractures of the sacrum. An atypical cause of low back pain in the female athlete. *Am. J. Sports Med.,* 2001; 29: 498–508.
142. **Johansson, C., Ekenman, I., Tornkvist, H. et al.** Stress fractures of the femoral neck in athletes: the consequence of a delay in diagnosis. *Am. J. Sports Med.,* 1990; 18: 524–528.
143. **Johnson, A.W., Weiss, C.B., Jr., and Wheeler, D.L.** Stress fractures of the femoral shaft in athletes — more common than expected. A new clinical test. *Am. J. Sports Med.,* 1994; 22: 248–256.
144. **Jones, B.H., Harris, J.M., Vinh, T. et al.** Exercise-induced stress fractures and stress reactions of bone: epidemiology, etiology, and classification. *Exerc. Sport Sci. Rev.,* 1989; 17: 379–422.
145. **Jones, B.H., Bovee, M.W., Harris, J.M. et al.** Intrinsic risk factors for exercise-related injuries among male and female army trainees. *Am. J. Sports Med.* 1993; 21: 705–710.

146. **Jowett, A. and Brukner, P.** Fifth metacarpal stress fracture in a female softball pitcher. *Clin. J. Sport Med.,* 1997; 7: 220–221.

147. **Kadel, N.J., Teitz, C.C., and Kronmal, R.A.** Stress fractures in ballet dancers. *Am. J. Sports Med.,* 1992; 20: 445–449.

148. **Kanstrup, I.L.** Bone scintigraphy in sports medicine: a review. *Scand. J. Med. Sci. Sports,* 1997; 7: 322–330.

149. **Karlson, K.A.** Rib stress fractures in elite rowers. A case series and proposed mechanism. *Am. J. Sports Med.,* 1998; 26: 516–519.

150. **Kavanaugh, J.H., Browe, T.D., and Mann, R.V.** The Jones' fracture revisited. *J. Bone Joint Surg.,* 1978; 60A: 776–782.

151. **Keating, J.F., Beggs, I., and Thorpe, G.W.** 3 cases of longitudinal stress fracture of the tibia. *Acta Orthop. Scand.,* 1995; 66: 41–42.

152. **Keating, T.M.** Stress fracture of the sternum in a wrestler. *Am. J. Sports Med.,* 1987; 15: 92–93.

153. **Khan, K.M., Fuller, P.J., Brukner, P.D. et al.** Outcome of conservative and surgical management of navicular stress fracture in athletes. Eighty-six cases proven with computerized tomography. *Am. J. Sports Med.,* 1992; 20: 657–666.

154. **Khan, K.M., Brukner, P.D., and Bradshaw, C.** Stress fracture of the medial cuneiform bone in a runner. *Clin. J. Sport Med.,* 1993; 3: 262–264.

155. **Khan, K.M., Brukner, P.D., Kearney, C. et al.** Tarsal navicular stress fracture in athletes. *Sports Med.,* 1994; 17: 65–76.

156. **Kiss, Z.A., Khan, K.M., and Fuller, P.J.** Stress fractures of the tarsal navicular bone. CT findings in 55 cases. *Am. J. Roentgenol.,* 1993; 160: 111–115.

157. **Kiuru, M.J., Pihlajamaki, H.K., Hietanen, H.J. et al.** MR imaging, bone scintigraphy, and radiography in bone stress injuries of the pelvis and the lower extremity. *Acta Radiol.,* 2002; 43: 207–212.

158. **Knapp, T.P. and Garrett, W.E., Jr.** Stress fractures: general concepts. *Clin. Sports Med.,* 1997; 16: 339–356.

159. **Korpelainen, R., Orava, S., Karpakka, J. et al.** Risk factors for recurrent stress fractures in athletes. *Am. J. Sports Med.,* 2001; 29: 304–310.

160. **Koskinen, S.K., Mattila, K.T., Alanen, A.M. et al.** Stress fracture of the ulnar diaphysis in a recreational golfer. *Clin. J. Sport Med.,* 1997; 7: 63–65.

161. **Kottmeier, S.A., Hanks, G.A., and Kalenak, A.** Fibular stress fracture associated with distal tibiofibular synostosis in an athlete. A case report and literature review. *Clin. Orthop.,* 1992; 281: 195–198.

162. **Krivickas, L.S.** Anatomical factors associated with overuse sports injuries. *Sports Med.,* 1997; 24: 132–146.

163. **Lacroix, H. and Keeman, J.N.** An unusual stress fracture of the fibula in a long-distance runner. *Arch. Orthop. Trauma. Surg.,* 1992; 111: 289–290.

164. **Lankenner, P.A.J. and Micheli, L.J.** Stress fracture of the first rib: a case report. *J. Bone Joint Surg.,* 1985; 67A: 159–160.

165. **Larson, C.M., Almekinders, L.C., Taft, T.N. et al.** Intramedullary screw fixation of Jones fractures. Analysis of failure. *Am. J. Sports Med.,* 2002; 30: 55–60.

166. **Lassus, J., Tulikoura, I., Konttinen, Y.T. et al.** Bone stress injuries of the lower extremity: a review. *Acta Orthop. Scand.,* 2002; 73: 359–368.

167. **Lehman, T.P., Belanger, M.J., and Pascale, M.S.** Bilateral proximal third fibular stress fractures in an adolescent female track athlete. *Orthopaedics,* 2002; 25: 329–332.

168. **Leinberry, C.F., McShane, R.B., Stewart, W.G. et al.** A displaced subtrochanteric stress fracture in a young amenorrheic athlete. *Am. J. Sports Med.,* 1992; 20: 485–487.

169. **Letts, M., Smallman, T., Afanasiev, R. et al.** Fracture of the pars interarticularis in adolescent athletes: a clinical-biomechanical analysis. *J. Pediatr. Orthop.,* 1986; 6: 40–46.

170. **Lombardo, S.J. and Benson, D.W.** Stress fractures of the femur in runners. *Am. J. Sports Med.,* 1982; 10: 219–227.

171. **Loosli, A.R. and Leslie, M.** Stress fractures of the distal radius. A case report. *Am. J. Sports Med.,* 1991; 19: 523–524.

172. **Lord, M.J., Ha, K.I., and Song, K.S.** Stress fractures of the ribs in golfers. *Am. J. Sports Med.,* 1996; 24: 118–122.

173. **Mabit, C. and Pecout, C.** Non-union of a midshaft anterior tibial stress fracture: a frequent complication. *Knee Surg. Sports Traumatol. Arthrosc.,* 1994; 2: 60–61.

174. **Macera, C.A., Pate, R.R., Powell, K.E. et al.** Predicting lower-extremity injuries among habitual runners. *Arch. Intern. Med.,* 1989; 149: 2565–2568.

175. **Maffulli, N., Chan, D., and Aldridge, M.J.** Overuse injuries of the olecranon in young gymnasts. *J. Bone Joint Surg.,* 1992; 74B: 305–308.

176. **Maitra, R.S. and Johnson, D.L.** Stress fractures. Clinical history and physical examination. *Clin. Sports Med.,* 1997; 16: 259–274.

177. **Major, N.M. and Helms, C.A.** Sacral stress fractures in long-distance runners. *Am. J. Roentgenol.,* 2000; 174: 727–729.

178. **Markey, K.L.** Stress fractures. *Clin. Sports Med.,* 1987; 6: 405–425.

179. **Martin, A.D. and McCulloch, R.G.** Bone dynamics: stress, strain and fracture. *J. Sports Sci.,* 1987; 5: 155–163.

180. **Marymont, J.H., Mills, G.O., and Merritt, W.D.** Fracture of the lateral cuneiform bone in the absence of severe direct trauma. *Am. J. Sports Med.,* 1980; 8: 135–136.

181. **Mata, S.G., Grande, M.M., and Ovejero, A.H.** Transverse stress fracture of the patella. *Clin. J. Sport Med.,* 1996; 6: 259–261.

182. **Matheson, G.O., Clement, D.B., McKenzie, D.C. et al.** Stress fractures in athletes. A study of 320 cases. *Am. J. Sports Med.,* 1987; 15: 46–58.

183. **Matheson, G.O., Clement, D.B., McKenzie, D.C. et al.** Scintigraphic uptake of 99mTc at non-painful sites in athletes with stress fractures: the concept of bone strain. *Sports Med.,* 1987; 4: 65–75.

184. **Matin, P.** Basic principles of nuclear medicine techniques for detection and evaluation of trauma and sports medicine injuries. *Semin. Nucl. Med.,* 1988; 18: 90–112.

185. **Mazione, M. and Pizzutillo, P.D.** Stress fracture of the scaphoid waist. A case report. *Am. J. Sports Med.,* 1981; 9: 268–269.

186. **McBryde, A.M., Jr. and Bassett, F.H.** Stress fracture of the fibula. *GP,* 1968; 38:120–123.

187. **McBryde, A.M., Jr.** Stress fractures in athletes. *J. Sports Med.,* 1976; 3: 212–217.

188. **McBryde, A.M., Jr.** Stress fractures in runners. *Clin. Sports Med.,* 1985; 4: 737–752.

189. **McBryde, A.M., Jr. and Anderson, R.B.** Sesamoid foot problems in the athlete. *Clin. Sports Med.,* 1988; 7: 51–60.

190. **McFarland, E.G. and Giangarra, C.** Sacral stress fractures in athletes. *Clin. Orthop.,* 1996; 329: 240–243.

191. **McKenzie, D.C.** Stress fracture of the rib in an elite oarsman. *Int. J. Sports Med.,* 1989; 10: 220–222.

192. **Micheli, L.J., Sohn, R.S., and Soloman, R.** Stress fractures of the second metatarsal involving Lisfranc's joint in ballet dancers: a new overuse of the foot. *J. Bone Joint Surg.,* 1985; 67A: 1372–1375.

193. **Mikawa, Y. and Kobori, M.** Stress fracture of the first rib in a weightlifter. *Arch. Orthop. Trauma. Surg.,* 1991; 110: 121–122.

194. **Milgrom, C., Finestone, A., Shlamkovitch, N. et al.** Youth is a risk factor for stress fracture. A study of 783 infantry recruits. *J. Bone Joint Surg.,* 1994; 76B: 20–22.

195. **Mindrebo, N., Shelbourne, K.D., Van Meter, C.D. et al.** Outpatient percutaneous screw fixation of the acute Jones fracture. *Am. J. Sports Med.,* 1993; 21: 720–723.

196. **Mintz, A.C., Albano, A., Reisdorf, E.J. et al.** Stress fracture of the first rib from serratus anterior tension. An unusual mechanism of injury. *Ann. Emerg. Med.,* 1990; 19: 411–414.

197. **Moeller, J.L. and Rifat, S.F.** Spondylolysis in active adolescents. *Phys. Sportsmed.,* 2001; 29: 27–32.

198. **Monteleone, G.P., Jr.** Stress fracture in the athlete. *Orthop. Clin. North Am.,* 1995; 26: 423–432.

199. **Morita, T., Ikata, T., Katoh, S. et al.** Lumbar spondylolysis in children and adolescents. *J. Bone Joint Surg.,* 1995; 77B: 620–625.

200. **Moss, A. and Mowat, A.G.** Ultrasonic assessment of stress fractures. *Br. Med. J.,* 1983; 286: 1479–1480.

201. **Motto, S.G.** Stress fracture of the lateral process of the talus — a case report. *Br. J. Sports Med.,* 1993; 27: 275–276.

202. **Murakami, Y.** Stress fracture of the metacarpal in an adolescent tennis player. *Am. J. Sports Med.,* 1988; 16: 419–420.

203. **Mutoh, Y., Mori, T., Suzuki, Y. et al.** Stress fractures of the ulna in athletes. *Am. J. Sports Med.,* 1982; 10: 365–367.

204. **Nagle, C.E. and Freitas, J.E.** Radionuclide imaging of musculoskeletal injuries in athletes with negative radiographs. *Phys. Sportsmed.*, 1987; 15: 147–155.

205. **Nattiv, A. and Armsey, T.D.** Stress injury to bone in the female athlete. *Clin. Sports Med.*, 1997; 16: 197–224.

206. **Nelson, B.J. and Arciero, R.A.** Stress fractures in female athletes. *Sports Med. Arthrosc. Rev.*, 2002; 10: 83–90.

207. **Noakes, T.D., Smith, J.A., Lindenberg, G. et al.** Pelvic stress fractures in long distance runners. *Am. J. Sports Med.*, 1985; 13: 120–123.

208. **Nordin, M. and Frankel, V.H.** *Basic Biomechanics of the Musculoskeletal System*, 2nd ed. Philadelphia: Lea & Febiger, 1989.

209. **Nuber, G.W. and Diment, M.T.** Olecranon stress fractures in throwers. A report of two cases and a review of the literature. *Clin. Orthop.*, 1992; 278: 58–61.

210. **Nunley, J.A.** Fractures of the base of the fifth metatarsal. The Jones fracture. *Orthop. Clin. North Am.*, 2001; 32: 171–180.

211. **Okada, K., Senma, S., Abe, E. et al.** Stress fractures of the medial malleolus: a case report. *Foot Ankle*, 1995; 16: 49–52.

212. **O'Malley, M.J., Hamilton, W.G., Munyak, J. et al.** Stress fractures at the base of the second metatarsal in ballet dancers. *Foot Ankle*, 1996; 17: 89–94.

213. **Orava, S.** Stress fractures. *Br. J. Sports Med.*, 1980; 14: 40–44.

214. **Orava, S., Jormakka, E., and Hulkko, A.** Stress fractures in young athletes. *Arch. Orthop. Trauma. Surg.*, 1981; 98: 271–274.

215. **Orava, S. and Hulkko, A.** Stress fracture of the mid-tibial shaft. *Acta Orthop. Scand.*, 1984; 55: 35–37.

216. **Orava, S. and Hulkko, A.** Delayed union and nonunions of stress fractures in athletes. *Am. J. Sports Med.*, 1988; 16: 378–382.

217. **Orava, S., Jakkola, L., and Kujala, U.M.** Stress fracture of the seventh rib in a squash player. *Scand. J. Med. Sci. Sports*, 1991; 1: 247–248.

218. **Orava, S., Karpakka, J., Hulkko, A. et al.** Diagnosis and treatment of stress fractures located at the mid-tibial shaft in athletes. *Int. J. Sports Med.*, 1991; 12: 419–422.

219. **Orava, S., Kallinen, M., Aito, H. et al.** Stress fracture of the ribs in golfers: a report of five cases. *Scand. J. Med. Sci. Sports*, 1994; 4: 155–158.

220. **Orava, S., Karpakka, J., Taimela, S. et al.** Stress fracture of the medial malleolus. *J. Bone Joint Surg.*, 1995; 77A: 362–365.

221. **Orava, S., Taimela, S., Kvist, M. et al.** Diagnosis and treatment of stress fracture of the patella in athletes. *Knee Surg. Sports Traumatol. Arthrosc.*, 1996; 4: 206–211.

222. **Orloff, A.S. and Resnick, D.** Fatigue fracture of the distal part of the radius in a pool player. *Br. J. Accident Surg.*, 1986; 17: 418–419.

223. **O'Toole, M.L.** Prevention and treatment of injuries to runners. *Med. Sci. Sports Exerc.*, 1992; 24: S360–S363.

224. **Pavlov, H., Nelson, T.L., Warren, R.F. et al.** Stress fracture of the pubic ramus. A report of twelve cases. *J. Bone Joint Surg.*, 1982; 64A: 1020–1025.

225. **Pećina, M., Bojanić, I., and Ribarić, G.** Stres fraktura baze pete metatarzalne kosti — Jonesov prijelom. *Acta Orthop. Iugosl.*, 1988; 19: 118–123.

226. **Pećina, M., Bojanić, I., and Dubravčić, S.** Stress fractures in figure skaters. *Am. J. Sports Med.*, 1990; 18: 277–279.

227. **Pester, S. and Smith, P.C.** Stress fractures in the lower extremities of soldiers in basic training. *Orthop. Rev.*, 1992; 21: 297–303.

228. **Petsching, R., Wurning, C., Rosen, A. et al.** Stress fracture of the ulna in a female table tennis tournament player. *J. Sports Med. Phys. Fitness*, 1997; 37: 225–227.

229. **Pietu, G. and Hauet, P.** Stress fracture of the patella. A case report. *Acta Orthop. Scand.*, 1995; 66: 481–482.

230. **Plasschaert, V.F., Johnsson, C.G., and Micheli, L.J.** Anterior tibial stress fracture treated with intramedullary nailing: a case report. *Clin. J. Sport Med.*, 1995; 5: 58–61.

231. **Polu, K.R., Schenck, R.C., Jr., Wirth, M.A. et al.** Stress fracture of the humerus in a collegiate baseball pitcher. A case report. *Am. J. Sports Med.*, 1999; 27: 813–816.

232. **Pozderac, R.V.** Longitudinal tibial fatigue fracture: an uncommon stress fracture with characteristic features. *Clin. Nucl. Med.*, 2002; 27: 475–478.

233. **Prather, J.L., Nusynowitz, M.L., Snowdy, H.A. et al.** Scintigraphic findings in stress fractures. *J. Bone Joint Surg.*, 1977; 59A: 869–874.

234. **Quill, G.E., Jr.** Fractures of the proximal fifth metatarsal. *Orthop. Clin. North Am.*, 1995; 26: 353–361.

235. **Rao, P.S., Rao, S.K., and Navadgi, B.C.** Olecranon stress fracture in a weight lifter. A case report. *Br. J. Sports Med.*, 2001; 35: 72–73.

236. **Read, M.T.F.** Stress fracture of the distal radius in adolescent gymnasts. *Br. J. Sports Med.*, 1981; 15: 272–276.

237. **Read, M.T.F.** Case report — stress fracture of the rib in a golfer. *Br. J. Sports Med.*, 1994; 28: 206–207.

238. **Reed, W.J. and Mueller, R.W.** Spiral fracture of the humerus in a ball thrower. *Am. J. Emerg. Med.*, 1998; 16: 306–308.

239. **Reeder, M.T., Dick, B.H., Atkins, J.K. et al.** Stress fractures. current concepts of diagnosis and treatment. *Sports Med.*, 1996; 22: 198–212.

240. **Reider, B., Falconiero, R., and Yurkofsky, J.** Nonunion of a medial malleolus stress fracture. A case report. *Am. J. Sports Med.*, 1993; 21: 478–481.

241. **Rettig, A.C.** Stress fracture of the ulna in an adolescent tournament tennis player. *Am. J. Sports Med.*, 1983; 11: 103–106.

242. **Rettig, A.C. and Beltz, H.F.** Stress fracture in the humerus in an adolescent tennis tournament player. *Am. J. Sports Med.*, 1985; 13: 55–58.

243. **Rettig, A.C., Shelbourne, K.D., McCarroll, J.R. et al.** The natural history and treatment of delayed union stress fractures of the anterior cortex of the tibia. *Am. J. Sports Med.*, 1988; 16: 250–255.

244. **Richardson, E.G.** Hallucal sesamoid pain: causes and surgical treatment. *J. Am. Acad. Orthop. Surg.*, 1999; 7: 270–278.

245. **Riel, K.-A. and Bernett, P.** Ermüdungsbruche im Sport. Eigene Erfahrungen und Literaturüberblick. *Z. Orthop.*, 1991; 129: 471–476.

246. **Robbins, S. and Gouw, G.** Athletic footwear: unsafe due to perceptual illusions. *Med. Sci. Sports Exerc.*, 1991; 23: 217–224.

247. **Robertsen, K., Kristensen, O., and Vejen, L.** Manubrium sterni stress fracture: an unusual complication of non-contact sport. *Br. J. Sports Med.*, 1996; 30: 176–177.

248. **Rolf, C.** Pelvis and groin stress fractures: a cause of groin pain in athletes. *Sports Med. Arthrosc. Rev.*, 1997; 5: 301–304.

249. **Rosenberg, G.A. and Sferra, J.J.** Treatment strategies for acute fractures and nonunions of the proximal fifth metatarsal. *J. Am. Acad. Orthop. Surg.*, 2000; 8: 332–338.

250. **Roset-Llobet, J. and Salo-Orfila, J.M.** Sports-related stress fracture of the clavicle: a case report. *Int. Orthop.*, 1998; 22: 266–268.

251. **Roy, S., Caine, D., and Singer, K.M.** Stress changes of the distal radial epiphysis in young gymnasts. A report of twenty-one cases and a review of the literature. *Am. J. Sports Med.*, 1985; 13: 301–308.

252. **Ruggles, D.L., Peterson, H.A., and Scott, S.G.** Radial growth plate injury in a female gymnast. *Med. Sci. Sports Exerc.*, 1991; 23: 393–396.

253. **Rupani, H.D., Holder, L.E., Espinola, D.A. et al.** Three-phase radionuclide bone imaging in sports medicine. *Radiology*, 1985; 156: 187–196.

254. **Sacchetti, A.D., Beswick, D.R., and Morse, S.D.** Rebound rib. Stress-induced first rib fracture. *Ann. Emerg. Med.*, 1983; 12: 177–179.

255. **Saillant, G., Noat, M., Benazet, J.P. et al.** Les fractures de fatigue du scaphoide tarsien (os naviculaire) A propos de 20 cas. *Rev. Chir. Orthop.*, 1992; 78: 566–573.

256. **Saxena, A., Fullem, B., and Hannaford, D.** Results of treatment of 22 navicular stress fractures and a new proposed radiographic classification system. *J. Foot Ankle Surg.*, 2000; 39: 96–103.

257. **Schils, J. and Hauzeur, J.P.** Stress fracture of the sacrum. *Am. J. Sports Med.*, 1992; 20: 769–770.

258. **Schils, J.P., Freed, H.A., Richmond, B.J. et al.** Stress fracture of the acromion. *Am. J. Radiol.*, 1990; 155: 1140–1141.

259. **Schils, J.P., Andrish, J.T., Piraino, D.W. et al.** Medial malleolar stress fractures in seven patients: review of the clinical and imaging features. *Radiology*, 1992; 185: 219–221.

260. **Scully, T.J. and Besterman, G.** Stress fracture: a preventable training injury. *Mil. Med.*, 1982; 147: 285–287.

261. **Shabat, S., Sampson, K.B., Mann, G. et al.** Stress fractures of the medial malleolus — review of the literature and report of a 15-year-old elite gymnast. *Foot Ankle*, 2002; 23: 647–650.

262. **Shah, M.M. and Stewart, G.W.** Sacral stress fractures: an unusual case of low back pain in an athlete. *Spine*, 2002; 27: E104–108.

263. **Shearman, C.M., Brandser, E.A., Parman, L.M. et al.** Longitudinal tibial stress fractures: a report of eight cases and review of the literature. *J. Comput. Assist. Tomogr.*, 1998; 22: 265–269.

264. **Shelbourne, K.D., Fisher, D.A., Rettig, A.C. et al.** Stress fracture of the medial malleolus. *Am. J. Sports Med.*, 1988; 16: 60–63.

265. **Shin, A.Y. and Gillingham, B.L.** Fatigue fractures of the femoral neck in athletes. *J. Am. Acad. Orthop. Surg.*, 1997; 5: 293–302.

266. **Shin, A.Y., Morin, W.D., Gorman, J.D. et al.** The superiority of magnetic resonance imaging in differentiating the cause of hip pain in endurance athletes. *Am. J. Sports Med.*, 1996; 24: 168–176.

267. **Sinha, A.K., Kaeding, C.C., and Wadley, G.M.** Upper extremity stress fractures in athletes: clinical features of 44 cases. *Clin. J. Sport Med.*, 1999; 9: 199–202.

268. **Spitz, D.J. and Newberg, A.H.** Imaging of stress fractures in the athlete. *Radiol. Clin. North Am.*, 2002; 40: 313–331.

269. **Stanitski, C.L., McMaster, J.H., and Scranton, P.E.** On the nature of stress fractures. *Am. J. Sports Med.*, 1978; 6: 391–396.

270. **Stechow, A.W.** Fussoedem und Roentgenstrahlen. *Dtsch. Mil.-Aerztl. Z.*, 1897; 26: 465–471.

271. **Sterling, J.C., Calvo, R.D., and Holden, S.C.** An unusual stress fracture in a multiple sport athlete. *Med. Sci. Sports Exerc.*, 1991; 23: 298–303.

272. **Sterling, J.C., Edelstein, D.W., Calvo, R.D. et al.** Stress fractures in the athlete. Diagnosis and management. *Sports Med.*, 1992; 14: 336–346.

273. **Strudwick, W. and Goodman, S.B.** Proximal fibular stress fracture in an aerobic dancer. A case report. *Am. J. Sports Med.*, 1992; 20: 481–482.

274. **Sullivan, D., Warren, R.F., Pavlov, H. et al.** Stress fractures in 51 runners. *Clin. Orthop.*, 1984; 187: 188–192.

275. **Suzuki, K., Minami, A., Suenaga, N. et al.** Oblique stress fracture of the olecranon in baseball pitchers. *J. Shoulder Elbow Surg.*, 1997; 6: 491–494.

276. **Swenson, E.J., DeHaven, K.E., Sebastienelli, W.J. et al.** The effect of a pneumatic leg brace on return to play in athletes with tibial stress fractures. *Am. J. Sports Med.*, 1997; 25: 322–328.

277. **Sys, J., Michielsen, J., Bracke, P. et al.** Nonoperative treatment of active spondylolysis in elite athletes with normal x-ray findings: literature review and results of conservative treatment. *Eur. Spine J.*, 2001; 10: 498–504.

278. **Taimela, S., Kujala, U.M., and Orava, S.** Two consecutive rib stress fractures in a female competitive swimmer. *Clin. J. Sport Med.*, 1995; 5: 254–257.

279. **Tanabe, S., Nakahira, J., Bando, E. et al.** Fatigue fracture of the ulna occurring in pitchers of fast-pitch softball. *Am. J. Sports Med.*, 1991; 19: 317–321.

280. **Taunton, J.E., Clement, D.B., and Webber, D.** Lower extremity stress fractures in athletes. *Phys. Sportsmed.*, 1981; 9: 77–86.

281. **Teitz, C.C. and Harrington, R.M.** Patellar stress fracture. *Am. J. Sports Med.*, 1992; 20: 761–765.

282. **Thorne, D.A. and Datz, F.L.** Pelvic stress fracture in female runners. *Clin. Nucl. Med.*, 1986; 11: 828–829.

283. **Ting, A., King, W., Yocum, L. et al.** Stress fractures of tarsal navicular in long distance runners. *Clin. Sports Med.*, 1988; 7: 89–101.

284. **Torg, J.S. and Moyer, R.A.** Non-union of a stress fracture through the olecranon epiphyseal plate observed in an adolescent baseball pitcher. A case report. *J. Bone Joint Surg.*, 1977; 59A: 264–265.

285. **Torg, J.S., Pavlov, H., Cooley, L.H. et al.** Stress fractures of the tarsal navicular. A retrospective review of twenty-one cases. *J. Bone Joint Surg.*, 1982; 64A: 700–712.

286. **Torg, J.S., Balduini, F.C., Zelko, R.R. et al.** Fractures of the base of the fifth metatarsal distal to the tuberosity: classification and guidelines for non-surgical and surgical management. *J. Bone Joint Surg.*, 1984; 66A: 209–214.

287. **Towne, L.C., Blazina, M.E., and Cozen, L.N.** Fatigue fracture of the tarsal navicular. *J. Bone Joint Surg.*, 1970; 52A: 376–378.

288. **Van Hal, M.E., Keene, J.S., Lange, T.A. et al.** Stress fractures of the great toe sesamoids. *Am. J. Sports Med.*, 1982; 10: 122–128.

289. **Veluvolu, P., Kohn, H.S., Guten, G.N. et al.** Unusual stress fracture of the scapula in a jogger. *Clin. Nucl. Med.*, 1988; 13: 531–532.

290. **Verma, R.B. and Sherman, O.** Athletic stress fractures: Part I. History, epidemiology, physiology, risk factors, radiography, diagnosis, and treatment. *Am. J. Orthop.*, 2001; 30: 798–806.

291. **Verma, R.B. and Sherman, O.** Athletic stress fractures: Part II. The lower body. Part III. The upper body — with a section on the female athlete. *Am. J. Orthop.*, 2001; 30: 848–860.

292. **Walter, N.E. and Wolf, M.D.** Stress fractures in young athletes. *Am. J. Sports Med.*, 1977; 5: 165–170.

293. **Walter, S.D., Hart, L.E., McIntosh, J.M. et al.** The Ontario cohort study of running-related injuries. *Arch. Intern. Med.*, 1989; 149: 2561–2564.

294. **Waninger, K.N. and Lombardo, J.A.** Stress fracture of index metacarpal in an adolescent tennis player. *Clin. J. Sport Med.*, 1995; 5: 63–66.

295. **Waninger, K.N.** Stress fracture of the clavicle in a collegiate diver. *Clin. J. Sport Med.*, 1997; 7: 66–68.

296. **Ward, W.G., Bergfeld, J.A., and Carson, W.G., Jr.** Stress fracture of the base of the acromial process. *Am. J. Sports Med.*, 1994; 22: 146–147.

297. **Warden, S.J., Gutschlag, F.R., Wajswelner, H. et al.** Aetiology of rib stress fractures in rowers. *Sports Med.*, 2002; 32: 819–836.

298. **Weinfeld, S.B., Haddad, S.L., and Myerson, M.S.** Metatarsal stress fractures. *Clin. Sports Med.*, 1997; 16: 319–338.

299. **Whitelaw, G.P., Wetzler, M.J., Levy, A.S. et al.** A pneumatic leg brace for the treatment of tibial stress fractures. *Clin. Orthop.*, 1991; 270: 302–305.

300. **Wilkerson, R.D. and Johns, J.C.** Nonunion of an olecranon stress fracture in an adolescent gymnast. A case report. *Am. J. Sports Med.*, 1990; 18: 432–434.

301. **Wiltse, L.L., Widell, E.H., Jr., and Jackson, D.W.** Fatigue fracture: the bone lesion in isthmic spondylolisthesis. *J. Bone Joint Surg.*, 1975; 57A: 17–22.

302. **Wright, R.W., Fischer, D.A., Shively, R.A, et al.** Refracture of proximal fifth metatarsal (Jones) fracture after intramedullary screw fixation in athletes. *Am. J. Sports Med.*, 2000; 28: 732–736.

303. **Wu, C.D. and Chen, Y.C.** Stress fracture of the clavicle in a professional baseball player. *J. Shoulder Elbow Surg.*, 1998; 7: 164–167.

304. **Young, C.C., Raasch, W.G., and Geiser, C.** Ulnar stress fracture of the nondominant arm in a tennis player using a two-handed backhand. *Clin. J. Sport Med.*, 1995; 5: 262–264.

305. **Zeni, A.I., Street, C.C., Dempsey, R.L. et al.** Stress injury to the bone among women athletes. *Phys. Med. Rehabil. Clin. North Am.*, 2000; 11: 929–947.

306. **Zogby, R.G. and Baker, B.E.** A review of non-operative treatment of Jones' fracture. *Am. J. Sports Med.*, 1987; 15: 304–307.

307. **Zwas, S.T., Elkanovitch, R., and Frank, G.** Interpretation and classification of bone scintigraphic findings in stress fractures. *J. Nucl. Med.*, 1987; 28: 452–457.

13 Nerve Entrapment Syndromes

Long-term repetitive microtrauma can lead to nerve entrapment syndromes, which is the reason they are included among overuse injuries. Contemporary medical literature includes numerous reports on various nerve entrapment syndromes. Acute trauma and especially long-term repetitive microtrauma have been indicated as possible instigating agents.[12,14,30,40,71,72,110,134,135,144] Certain sports or physical activities that have been mentioned lead to specific nerve entrapment syndromes, e.g., cyclist's palsy and bowler's thumb. Nerve entrapment syndromes in athletes are not as rare as they were once considered to be. It is also evident that when athletes have pain, the possibility of nerve entrapment syndromes must always be considered. Diagnosis relies on a detailed history and physical examination with modern diagnostic equipment. In most cases, non-operative treatment is sufficient, and surgery is therefore seldom recommended. The purpose of this chapter is to present currently available information about nerve entrapment syndromes in athletes.

I. UPPER LIMB

A. SPINAL ACCESSORY NERVE

The spinal accessory nerve is the cranial nerve most susceptible to injury (Figure 13.1). The clinical picture is primarily characterized by loss of power of trapezius muscle and difficulty in lifting the arm. During sports, the spinal accessory nerve may be injured by blunt stretching trauma.[80] Stretch injuries can also be caused by lifting heavy objects, or by vigorous training programs that include floor pushups.[88] The nerve may be damaged by a direct blow, for example, with a hockey stick or as a result of direct contact between athletes. Another mechanism that has been described is depression of the shoulder with the head forced in the opposite direction.[80] Such an injury occurs most commonly in wrestling, the result of a cross-face maneuver.

B. THORACIC OUTLET SYNDROME

The syndrome of upper limb comprising pain, paresthesias, vascular insufficiency, and motor dysfunction secondary to compression of the brachial plexus, subclavian artery, or subclavian vein before their division and separation bears the name *thoracic outlet syndrome.* Thoracic outlet syndrome has been described in the athletic population, especially with regard to certain sports such as swimming and other activities that require swing motion of the arm (i.e., throwing).[67,68,76,140] Compression in the outlet may occur at any one of three levels: (1) interscalene triangle, (2) costoclavicular space, and (3) pectoralis minor muscle insertion on the coracoid process. Abnormal structural variations (cervical rib, fibrous band, "abnormal" scalene muscle development) may compress or cause friction of the plexus or vessels at the level of the interscalene triangle. Compression of neurovascular structures through the costoclavicular space is usually caused by dynamic changes, especially in shoulder girdle mechanics, i.e., functional anatomy of the shoulder girdle.[116] The coracoid process and pectoralis minor muscle insertion act as a fulcrum over which the neurovascular structures change direction when the arm is elevated. This site has been implicated as a source of neurovascular compression among athletes who repetitively hyperabduct the arm,

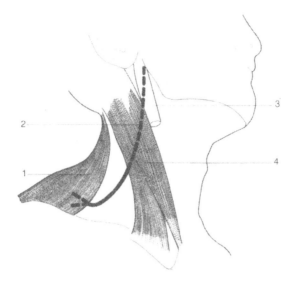

FIGURE 13.1 The spinal accessory nerve may be compressed at multiple sites along its course from the base of the skull along the lateral side of the neck to its endings in the region of the trapezius muscle. (1) trapezius muscle; (2) spinal accessory nerve; (3) internal jugular vein; (4) sternocleidomastoideus muscle.

i.e., swimmers, tennis players, and pitchers. In swimmers, neurovascular compression in this area may develop as a result of the pectoralis minor muscle hypertrophy.[66]

Different patterns of clinical presentations are seen depending on where and which neurovascular structures are compressed. The majority of patients' symptoms are created by neurological compression.[67] Typical symptoms are pain, numbness, or paresthesias. Sensory loss and muscle atrophy are rare but can occur. Vascular symptoms of thoracic outlet syndrome are quite rare. Venous obstruction may cause arm edema, cyanotic discoloration, and venous collateralization across the shoulder and chest wall, whereas arterial obstruction produces symptoms of coolness, numbness, ischemic pain, and external fatigue. A very common symptom pattern in thoracic outlet syndrome is that of "mixed involvement." In the mixed symptom pattern, patients have symptoms of both upper and lower trunk compression, along with variable degrees of vascular insufficiency. Thoracic outlet syndrome remains a clinical diagnosis, based almost entirely on the history and physical examination.[67] Therefore, thoracic outlet syndrome should be a diagnosis of exclusion.

Initial treatment should be non-operative, including rest from athletic activities.[67,76,110] Surgical treatment is indicated in patients with significant neurological or vascular involvement that does not respond to non-operative treatment. [67,76,110]

C. Brachial Plexus

Compression of the brachial plexus may arise from both intrinsic and extrinsic factors. Both of these mechanisms may occur in association with athletic activity. The most common external agent creating compression of the brachial plexus is a knapsack.[53,75,150] In Hirasawa and Sakakida's series,[53] most of the observed brachial plexus lesions were described as *backpack paralysis*. Brachial plexus compression results when large, heavy backpacks are carried for long periods. The axillary straps create a compression force around the plexus with the clavicle as a firm strut against which compression can occur. The shoulder girdle is pulled posteriorly by the heavy pack, adding a component of traction. Treatment of backpack paralysis consists of avoidance of mechanisms thought to have caused it and participation in physical therapy. Physical therapy restores the patient's strength, allowing complete recovery.

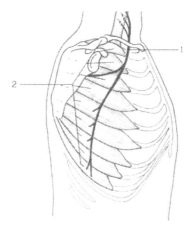

FIGURE 13.2 The long thoracic nerve (1) runs in the lateral and caudal direction along musculus serratus anterior, innervating its indentations (2).

D. Long Thoracic Nerve

Long thoracic nerve entrapment (Figure 13.2) has been described in a wide variety of sports, including tennis, golf, cycling, gymnastics, soccer, bowling, weight lifting, basketball, and football.[49,81,105,133,151] Clinical features may include pain around the shoulder girdle, decreased active shoulder motion, and a winged scapula (Figure 13.3). Electromyography and nerve conduction studies can be used to exclude other causes of scapular winging and confirm the diagnosis. Treatment involves physical therapy and cessation of the instigating activity. Prognosis is quite favorable, but recovery could take as long as 2 years.[49,81,133,151]

E. Axillary Nerve

Entrapment of the axillary nerve in the quadrilateral space is rare in athletes,[5] but has been described in baseball pitchers.[121] Paladini et al.[106] described two cases of isolated neuropathy, not consequent to acute trauma, of the axillary nerve of young volleyball players. The lesion site is thought to be in the quadrilateral space. The quadrilateral space syndrome also has been seen in tennis players.[78]

F. Suprascapular Nerve

Suprascapular nerve entrapment is an infrequently observed disorder and is often misdiagnosed. The manner of presentation of this syndrome depends on the anatomical site of compression. Entrapment usually occurs at the suprascapular notch (Figure 13.4). Patients, mostly throwing athletes, suffer from poorly localized shoulder pain, intact sensation, weakness of external rotation and abduction, and atrophy of the supraspinatus and infraspinatus muscle.[56,64,79,94,115,126,145] Occasionally, entrapment occurs distally, at the spinoglenoid notch. Patients may be asymptomatic or may describe mild pain and weakness of the shoulder because of denervation of the infraspinatus.[13,19,28,39,44,46,98,146] Ferretti et al.[39] found 12 top-level volleyball players with an isolated asymptomatic paralysis of the infraspinatus muscle. Sandow and Ilić[130] describe the suprascapular nerve rotator cuff compression syndrome in volleyball players. Ganzhorn et al.[44] describe the case of a weight lifter who noted wasting in the region of the dorsal scapula while posing in the mirror. Zeiss et al.[156] and Zuckerman et al.[159] also describe suprascapular entrapment neuropathy in weight lifters. We present a weight lifter with suprascapular nerve syndrome, lateral axillary hiatus syndrome and syndrome of the musculocutaneous nerve in the shoulder region in Figure 13.5. When the entrapment is localized at the suprascapular or spinoglenoid notch, restraint from athletic activities,

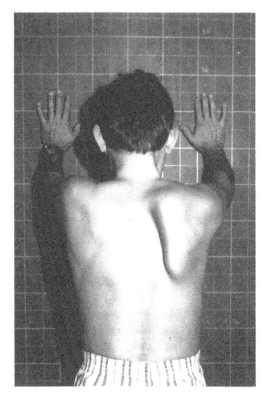

FIGURE 13.3 Scapular winging results from paralysis of the serratus anterior because of long thoracic nerve palsy. Results of the wall test are characteristic clinical signs.

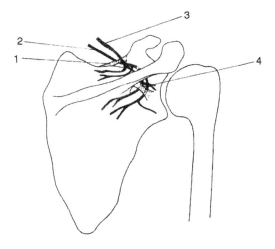

FIGURE 13.4 Suprascapular notch and pertinent anatomical relationship of the scapula and ligament to the neurovascular bundle. (1) Transverse scapular ligament; (2) suprascapular nerve; (3) suprascapular artery; (4) spinoglenoid ligament.

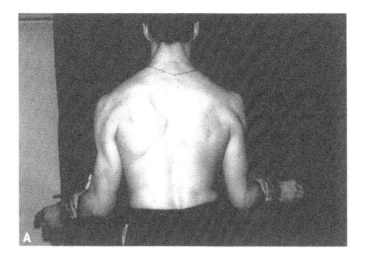

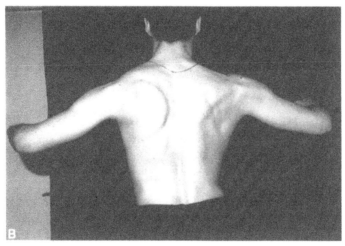

FIGURE 13.5 After intensive weight lifting for a period of several weeks, a 24-year-old athlete noticed a weakness of the right biceps brachii and hypotrophy of the right shoulder muscles. Clinical and electrographic tests proved the presence of suprascapular nerve syndrome, lateral axillary hiatus syndrome, and syndrome of the musculocutaneous nerve in the shoulder region. (A) During external rotation in the shoulder against force, hypotrophy of the supraspinatus, infraspinatus, teres minor, and the posterior part of the deltoideus muscles is visible. (B) Hypotrophy of the supraspinatus and the deltoid muscles during abduction of the upper arm is visible.

nonsteroidal anti-inflammatory medication, and local steroid injections may be useful.[11,94,115] If such non-operative measures are unsuccessful, surgical exploration is indicated.

G. MUSCULOCUTANEOUS NERVE

Musculocutaneous nerve entrapment in the shoulder region does not occur frequently, but several cases have been reported among athletes after heavy physical activity.[15,70,90,112,113] This syndrome was initially described by Braddom and Wolfe[15] in 1978 who based their experience on two weight lifters. Musculocutaneous nerve compression leads to biceps brachii muscle wasting and weakness (Figure 13.6). Sensory complaints are referred to the radial aspect of the forearm. Typically, no pain is associated. Neurological findings include absent biceps reflex, decreased biceps tone, and hypesthesias and paresthesias in the radial aspect of the forearm. This syndrome usually resolves spontaneously with cessation of the strenuous activity.[112] Compression of the musculocutaneous nerve

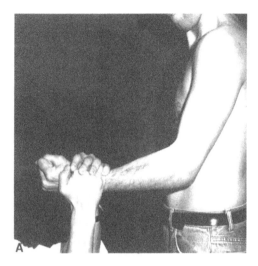

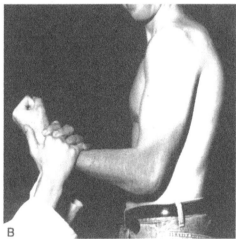

FIGURE 13.6 Musculocutaneous nerve entrapment syndrome. (A) Weakness of the biceps brachii muscle. (B) Return of strength and breadth to the biceps muscle 6 weeks after ceasing strenuous physical work.

at the elbow, i.e., of the lateral antebrachial cutaneous nerve, may occur when the nerve passes below the tendon of the biceps muscle before piercing the brachial fascia. According to Bassett and Numley,[4] the lateral free margin of the biceps aponeurosis compresses the nerve against the brachial fascia with elbow extension, and pronation further increases nerve compression. This entity has been described in racquetball and tennis players, and in a windsurfer.[4,60,81] Symptoms include pain, paresthesias, and numbness over the radial aspect of the forearm. Treatment consists of rest, nonsteroidal anti-inflammatory medication, and a posterior elbow splint that prevent full extension. After 12 weeks of unsuccessful non-operative treatment, surgical decompression is indicated.[4,143]

H. RADIAL NERVE

Entrapment of the radial nerve above the elbow is rare in athletes.[114] Cases have been described after throwing a discus and serving in tennis.[118] The site of compression is in the region of the lateral intermuscular septum, which the radial nerve pierces as it enters the anterior aspect of the arm. It has been reported in weight lifting following strenuous muscular activities.[96,139] Patients develop a complete radial nerve palsy. Treatment is rest and cessation of all strenuous activities.

In most cases, the symptoms will disappear within several weeks. Persistent or progressive symptoms suggest the need for surgical decompression.[82,114]

I. RADIAL TUNNEL SYNDROME

In their study of a group of patients with chronic tennis elbow, Roles and Maudsley[128] recognized the compression of the radial nerve within its tunnel and called it *radial tunnel syndrome*. The syndrome differs from a posterior interosseous nerve syndrome in which the problem is localized to compression of the nerve at one particular site, the arcade of Frohse, and results in only a motor deficit.[93,99,122,148] In radial tunnel syndrome, there may be a spectrum of complaints, including pain, paresthesias, and weakness.[100] A motor deficit is not nearly as common as in a posterior interosseous nerve syndrome. There are five potential sites of compression within the radial tunnel: (1) fibrous bands at its proximal portion, (2) fibrous medial edge along the extensor carpi radialis brevis, (3) "fan" of radial recurrent vessels, (4) arcade of Frohse, and (5) fibrous band at the distal edge of the supinator muscle. The radial tunnel syndrome occurs most commonly in tennis players, but may also be seen in rowers and weight lifters.[114] Non-operative measures should be the first form of treatment. Such measures include rest of the elbow and wrist from repetitive stressful activity and a course of anti-inflammatory medication. Surgical exploration with neurolysis is indicated if non-operative treatment fails.[65,114,127]

J. WARTENBERG'S DISEASE

Athletes involved in sports requiring repetitive pronation supination ulnar flexion activities may acquire Wartenberg's disease — entrapment of the superficial sensory branch of the radial nerve in the forearm.[31,123] The wearing of wristbands, as in racket sports, has also been implicated as a cause of this syndrome; this is also known as *handcuff neuropathy*.[35,89,93] The patient's main complaints are burning pain or numbness and tingling over the dorsoradial aspect of the wrist, thumb, and web space, usually aggravated by wrist movement. If the syndrome occurs from external compression, non-operative therapy can be successful. It may take several months for the symptoms to resolve. Surgical exploration is necessary if non-operative therapy fails.[31,123]

K. DISTAL POSTERIOR INTEROSSEOUS NERVE

The distal posterior interosseous nerve syndrome occurs when the nerve becomes compressed or irritated traveling in the fourth extensor compartment. The repetitive dorsiflexion activities in the wrist can result in irritation or in compression of the nerve. In the statistics of Carr and Davis,[22] ten patients were employed in occupations or engaged in vigorous athletic activities, such as gymnastics, that required repetitive dorsiflexion of the wrist. The patients presented with dull ache, which could be reproduced by dorsiflexion of the wrist and by pressure over the fourth extensor compartment.

L. ULNAR NERVE

Ulnar nerve entrapment at the elbow is most frequently encountered by throwing athletes, such as baseball pitchers, tennis players, and javelin throwers, but is also observed in skiing, weight lifting, and stick-handling sports.[23,32,43,47,124,152,155] Because of its position in the cubital tunnel (Figure 13.7), the ulnar nerve is vulnerable to repetitive "tension" or "traction" stresses in athletes. This may also be compounded by subluxation or instability of the nerve. Childress[24] reported that 16.2% of the population demonstrated recurrent dislocation of the ulnar nerve when the elbow was flexed and extended. Repeated stress and injury may lead to inflammation, adhesions, and progressive compressive neuropathy. The intermittent nature of the athletic endeavors may confuse the presentation of the athlete with entrapment of the ulnar nerve at the elbow. Sometimes, the first symptom will

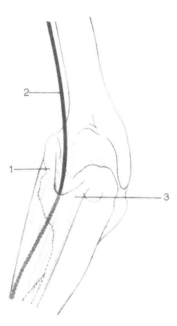

FIGURE 13.7 Compression of the ulnar nerve, distal to the elbow, by the heads of the flexor carpi ulnaris muscle. (1) Humeral head of the flexor carpi ulnaris muscle; (2) ulnar nerve; (3) ulnar head of the flexor carpi ulnaris muscle.

consist of pain along the medial joint line either associated with or exacerbated by overhead activities. As the inflammation of the nerve progresses, pain and paresthesias will be noted down the ulnar aspect of the forearm to the hand. Sensory changes definitely precede motor changes; however, a careful evaluation of the intrinsic musculature of the hand is essential to detect any weakness. Quite often, recalcitrant ulnar nerve entrapment at the elbow requires surgery. However, many transient episodes can be treated non-operatively.[47] Del Pizzo et al.[32] reported 19 baseball players with ulnar nerve entrapment at the elbow who underwent surgery. The surgery consisted of anterior transfer of the nerve deep into the origin of the flexor muscles.

M. Ulnar Tunnel Syndrome

Entrapment of the ulnar nerve in Guyon's canal (ulnar tunnel syndrome) is seen in cyclists and racquetball players as a result of chronic external compression. The first report of ulnar neuropathy as a complication of long-distance cycling was published in 1896.[33] Several reports have since described this complication, called *cyclist's* or *handlebar palsy*.[20,27,38,42,61,87,137,147] Factors reported in the literature as contributing to the development of neuropathies in cyclists include the use of worn-out gloves, unpadded handlebars, prolonged grasping of dropped handlebars, riding an improperly adjusted bicycle, and vibratory trauma from rough roads. Jackson[61] studied 20 cyclists with riding experience of more than 100 miles per week and found that 9 of 20 cyclists complained of either hand or finger numbness during cycling, which disappeared after completion of the ride. They reported that their hand numbness or pain was reduced after adjusting their hand position. Conventional treatment for nerve compression syndrome at the wrist consists of changes in cycling technique, including frequently varying hand position; the use of properly padded gloves and handlebars; and changes in the bicycle to ensure a proper fit.[61,87] These changes frequently will relieve symptoms in most cases without need for surgical decompression of the Guyon's canal.

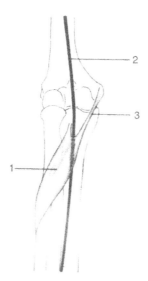

FIGURE 13.8 The median nerve can run through the pronator teres muscle or between its heads during its course into the hand. (1) Pronator teres muscle; (2) median nerve; (3) humeral head of the pronator teres muscle.

N. Hypothenar Hammer Syndrome

Repetitive trauma to the heel of the palm can cause ulnar artery spasm, thromboses, or aneurysms and thus compromise the ulnar nerve function with a more vascular type of presentation. This condition, known as *hypothenar hammer syndrome,* has been described in conjunction with several sports, including karate, judo, tennis, and lacrosse.[26,54,103,123] Nonunion of the hook of the hamate or of the pisiform, which may be fractured during a tennis, baseball, or golf swing, can also cause entrapment within the ulnar tunnel (Guyon's canal).[93] It is also important to keep in mind the possibility of a double crush injury of the ulnar nerve with coexistence of the syndrome of the flexor carpi ulnaris muscle (cubital tunnel syndrome) and ulnar tunnel syndrome.[57,61]

O. Median Nerve

Entrapment of the median nerve at the elbow is termed *pronator teres syndrome* and may result from repetitive exercise and hypertrophy of the flexor-pronator muscle group (Figure 13.8).[25,57,149] This entity has been seen in baseball players and weight lifters.[84] Patients complain of pain and tenderness in the volar aspect of their forearms over the area of compression, which worsens with exertional activities. Sensory complaints are common, consisting of numbness and paresthesias in part or all of the median nerve distribution of the hand. The pronator teres syndrome is often a difficult diagnosis and must be distinguished from carpal tunnel syndrome. Because the majority of cases are intermittent and mild, non-operative treatment should be tried first.[57,61] Persistent or progressive symptoms suggest the need for surgical intervention.[57,149]

P. Anterior Interosseous Nerve

The anterior interosseous nerve syndrome (Kiloh–Nevin syndrome) has been described in association with repetitive activities such as throwing, racket sports, or weight lifting.[104,114] It is characterized by a vague feeling of discomfort in the proximal forearm, which may mimic pronator teres syndrome. However, because the anterior interosseous nerve is a pure motor division of the median nerve, there are no sensory complaints or deficits as in pronator teres syndrome. The classic finding is that the patient loses the ability to pinch between his or her thumb and index finger. However, this symptom is not always present. Initial treatment should be non-operative because in many cases spontaneous improvement will occur. However, if there is no improvement after 8 to 12 weeks, surgical decompression and neurolysis should be performed.[57,110]

Q. CARPAL TUNNEL SYNDROME

The incidence of carpal tunnel syndrome as a sports-related problem is surprisingly low when compared with the incidence in the general population. Carpal tunnel may be seen in sports secondary to gripping, throwing, cycling, repetitive wrist flexion/extension activity, as well as direct trauma.[25,53,57,93,99,110,123,129,147,153] Because carpal tunnel syndrome is so rare in the athlete, unusual causes must be suspected when the diagnosis is entertained.

R. DIGITAL NERVES

In athletes, digital nerve entrapment syndromes are less common than those occurring at the wrist level. Digital nerves may be compressed during their course in the distal palm or at the proximal digit level. *Bowler's thumb* is the most common syndrome, involving the digital nerve in the hand.[25,34,37,58,93,95,99,123,136,147,153] Repetitive compression of the ulnar digital nerve to the thumb secondary to direct pressure on the nerve from the thumb hole of a bowling ball has been implicated as a cause of bowler's thumb. Bowler's thumb has also been reported incidentally in a baseball player.[93] On physical examination, the patients have tenderness over the ulnar volar aspect of the metacarpophalangeal joint of the thumb and a positive Tinel's sign in this area with paresthesias radiating to the ulnar aspect of the tip of the thumb. There is no motor involvement; however, grip strength may be somewhat diminished secondary to pain. Bowler's thumb should be treated non-operatively with rest, cessation of activity, nonsteroidal anti-inflammatory medication, and modification of equipment and technique.[34,123] In advanced cases, a molded plastic thumb guard is recommended to prevent trauma. Surgical treatment is indicated for those with persistent significant symptoms.[34,95,123] Surgical options include resection of the neuroma and primary repair of the nerve, neurolysis, and transfer to a new location.

Compression of digital nerves in tennis players has recently been reported.[102,104] Symptoms include numbness along the volar surface of the index finger of the racket hand and an abnormal sweat pattern, especially in players who have recently started playing or who have recently increased their amount of playing. Physical findings usually include calluses over the second metacarpal head, which implies rubbing of the digital nerve between the fixed bone and the racket handle. Early recognition, improved technique, better equipment, and protective measures are helpful in treating this problem.[102,104] Surgery is very rarely indicated.

II. LOWER LIMB

A. GROIN PAIN

Groin pain in athletes can be a consequence of nerve entrapment syndrome.[1,16,17,85] According to Akita et al.[1] chronic groin pain, especially in athletes, has been diagnosed in various ways. In Europe, recently, the concept of "sports hernia" has been advocated. Entrapment of the ilioinguinal nerve and the genitofemoral nerve may play a very important role in chronic groin pain produced by groin hernia. Bradshaw et al.[16,17] describe a case of obturator nerve entrapment, a previously unreported cause of chronic groin pain in athletes. They report 32 cases of "obturator neuropathy," a fascial entrapment of the obturator nerve where it enters the thigh. There is a characteristic clinical pattern of exercise-induced medial thigh pain commencing in the region of the adductor muscle origin and radiating distally along the medial thigh. Needle electromyography demonstrates denervation of the adductor muscles. Surgical neurolysis treatment provides the definitive cure for this problem, with athletes returning to competition within several weeks of treatment. The surgical

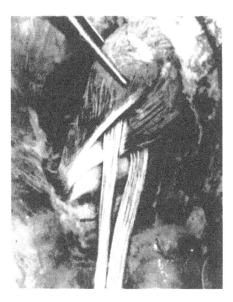

FIGURE 13.9 One of the variations in the form of the sciatic nerve. This specimen shows the common peroneal nerve as it courses between tendinous portions of the piriformis muscle.

findings are entrapment of the obturator nerve by a thick fascia overlying the short adductor muscle. The role of conservative treatment in the management of this condition is unknown at present.[17] Ziprin et al.[157] have described the results of surgical exploration in 25 male athletes presenting with groin pain. According to their findings athletes' groin pain may be due to nerve entrapment in the external oblique aponeurosis. An awareness of this injury may reduce delays in operating, leading to an earlier return to sport. Of 23 evaluated patients, 20 described the operation as good or excellent.[157]

B. PIRIFORMIS MUSCLE SYNDROME

Piriformis muscle syndrome is not discussed with specific reference to athletes although athletic activities may cause changes that significantly contribute to the development of the syndrome. Basic anatomical relationships of the muscle and sciatic nerve, direct and indirect trauma, muscular hypertrophy or anatomical nerve variations, inflammation, and local ischemia probably combine to induce the piriformis muscle syndrome (Figure 13.9 and Figure 13.10).[85,109,110,144] The piriformis

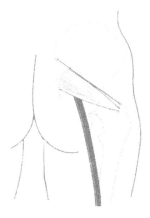

FIGURE 13.10 Projection of the piriformis muscle on the surface anatomy of the gluteal region.

syndrome has many similarities to (and overlaps with symptoms of) low back pain, ischialgias, vascular disease, and lower extremity pathologies.[59,110] Pain in the sacral or gluteal region remains the most constant symptom. The pain increases with sitting, walking, or running and decreases with lying supine. Frequently, diagnosis requires eliminating other causes of sciatic pain. Nonoperative treatment includes physiotherapy, nonsteroidal anti-inflammatory medication, and local steroid injection.[30,110] Surgical treatment consists of sectioning the piriformis muscle at its tendinous origin and external neurolysis of sciatic nerve.[110] Kouvalchouk et al.[73] report four athletic patients (two cyclists, two long-distance runners) who have been treated surgically by section of the piriformis muscle and neurolysis of the sciatic nerve. Pećina treated several athletes (soccer players, track and field athletes, fencers) with piriformis muscle syndrome conservatively and surgically.

C. PUDENDUS NERVE

Pudendus nerve syndrome is caused by compression of the nerve when it passes through the foramen infrapiriforme, foramen ischiadicum minus, and especially in the region of Alcock's canal situated in the lateral wall of the ischiorectal fossa. Compression of the nerve results in sensitive disturbances, often of the neuralgic type, in the innervation field of the nerve. The etiology of pudendus nerve syndrome includes some sports activities, such as bicycling, motor cycling, and horseback riding or all three, causing pressure, blows, or vibration in the pelvic region.[10] Perineal numbness is well known among cyclists and often is attributable to fixing the saddle in a "nose-up" position. This can be alleviated by using a softer saddle and placing it either horizontally or "nose-down."[21] Impotence and nerve entrapment in long-distance amateur cyclists was reported by Andersen and Bovim.[2]

D. MERALGIA PARESTHETICA

Meralgia paresthetica is an entrapment syndrome of the lateral femoral cutaneous nerve as it enters the thigh through or under the superolateral end of the inguinal ligament, causing burning sensations, paresthesias, and dysesthesias of the anterior and lateral thigh. This entrapment could be due to direct or repetitive trauma. Among athletes, it has been found primarily in gymnasts.[86] Meralgia paresthetica usually responds to non-operative treatment, including avoidance of repetitive trauma or pressure sources, nonsteroidal anti-inflammatory medications, and steroid injections.[30,86,144] Resistant cases require surgical intervention, neurolysis, or nerve resection.

E. SAPHENOUS NERVE

In athletes, the saphenous nerve may be compressed within the adductor canal (Hunter's or subsartorial canal) or where it exits the fascia (Figure 13.11) during strong contraction of the surrounding musculature, such as may occur with knee extensions or squats.[30,36,154] Hemler et al.[51] reported saphenous nerve entrapment caused by pes anserine bursitis. Entrapment of the saphenous nerve causes medial knee pain, dysesthesia, and hypesthesia in the distal distribution of the nerve. Relief is usually obtained with non-operative measures, but surgical exploration and neurolysis may be necessary.[30,154]

F. SURAL NERVE

Sural nerve entrapment may occur anywhere along its course. In the athletic population, it is most often described in runners.[30,131,132] Recurrent ankle sprains may lead to fibrosis and subsequent nerve entrapment.[117] Patients complain of shooting pain and paresthesias along the lateral border of the foot, sometimes extending proximally to immediately behind the lateral malleolus and up the posterior lateral aspect of the lower leg. Non-operative treatment usually is successful.[30,131,132] Several cases of sural nerve entrapment have been described in athletes who sustained avulsion

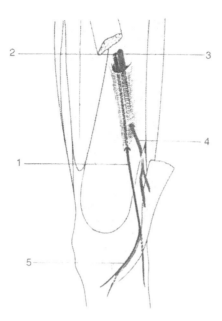

FIGURE 13.11 Compression of the saphenous nerve typically occurs in the region shown. (1) Saphenous nerve; (2) femoral vein; (3) femoral artery; (4) descending genicular artery; (5) infrapatellar branch of the saphenous nerve.

fractures of the base of the fifth metatarsal bone.[48] In these cases, persisting symptoms and nonunion of the fracture made surgical excision of the nonunited fragment and a neurolysis of the sural nerve necessary.

G. COMMON PERONEAL NERVE

There were only a few case reports about common peroneal nerve entrapment in runners.[97,138] Leach et al.[74] reported eight athletes, seven runners, and one soccer player with common peroneal nerve entrapment. In all reported patients, running induced pain and numbness. Examination after running revealed muscle weakness and a positive Tinel's test where the nerve winds around the fibular neck. As a result of the failure of various non-operative treatments, all of the patients were treated surgically by neurolysis of the peroneal nerve as it travels under the sharp fibrous edge of the peroneus longus muscle origin. Leach et al.[74] reported that seven of eight operated athletes returned to their previous level of activity without any further symptoms.

H. SUPERFICIAL PERONEAL NERVE

Superficial peroneal nerve entrapment occurs most commonly in runners, but may also be seen in soccer players, hockey players, tennis players, bodybuilders, and dancers.[69,83,92,141,142] According to clinical and anatomical studies, the point of entrapment of the nerve is at its exit point from the deep fascia — 12 cm above the tip of the lateral malleolus (Figure 13.12). Loss of or disturbances in sensation during exercise over the outer border or distal calf and over the dorsum of the foot, including the second to fourth toes, is a common sign of the entrapment. Occasionally, patients complain of pain only at the junction of the middle and distal third of the leg, with or without the presence of local swelling. The symptoms typically worsen with any physical activity, including walking, jogging, running, or squatting. Relief by conservative measures is uncommon. Decompression by local fasciectomy and fasciotomy of the lateral compartment have been reported to give good results.[141,142] One wrestler was successfully operated on in our department in Zagreb. Daghino et al.[29] describe the fascial entrapment of the superficial peroneal nerve in a 16-year-old

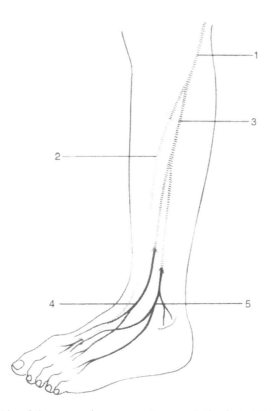

FIGURE 13.12 Relationship of the peroneal nerves as they reach the foot. (1) Common peroneal nerve; (2) deep peroneal nerve; (3) superficial peroneal nerve; (4) medial dorsal cutaneous nerve; (5) intermediate dorsal cutaneous nerve.

female athlete. MR imaging confirmed the diagnosis of this neuropathy. Limited fasciotomy, at the point where the nerve becomes subcutaneous, relieved all symptoms.

I. Deep Peroneal Nerve (Anterior Tarsal Tunnel Syndrome)

Entrapment of the deep peroneal nerve (syndrome of the anterior tarsal tunnel) has been described in runners, soccer players, skiers, and dancers (Figure 13.13).[30,131,132] Patients frequently have a history of recurrent ankle sprains or previous trauma. Tight, high-heeled shoes or ski boots have also been implicated as inciting factors.[45,77] An osteophyte on the dorsum of the talus or of the intermetatarseum at the tarsometatarsal joint can also press on the nerve.[101] Baxter and co-workers[30,101,131,132] described this entrapment in joggers who put keys under the tongue of their running shoes and in athletes who did sit-ups with their feet hooked under a metal bar. The patients complained of dorsal foot pain, numbness, and paresthesias over the first web space. The pain usually occurs during athletic activities. Most patients respond well to non-operative therapy with local steroid injections, alteration of footwear, and orthotic devices.[131,132,158] Occasionally, when these measures fail, a patient may require surgical decompression.

J. Tarsal Tunnel Syndrome

Tarsal tunnel syndrome is an uncommon condition in the athletic population, although it has been described in runners, ballet dancers, and basketball players.[3,62,63,91,119] The most common etiology is alteration of the normal spatial relationships stemming from space-occupying lesions, such as lipomas, ganglion cysts, neurilemomas, neurofibromas, varicose veins, and enlarged venous plexus

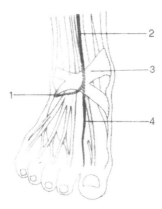

FIGURE 13.13 The deep peroneal nerve may be compressed as it enters the dorsum of the foot under the extensor retinaculum. (1) Lateral branch of the deep peroneal nerve; (2) deep peroneal nerve; (3) inferior extensor retinaculum (cruciform ligament); (4) medial branch of the deep peroneal nerve.

(Figure 13.14). Other causes include severe pronation of the hindfoot, chronic flexor tenosynovitis, post-traumatic scarring, and inflammatory collagen vascular disease. According to the literature, many cases are idiopathic. Athletes usually suffer burning, sharp pain at the medial malleolus radiating into the sole of the foot, the heel, and sometimes the calf. They may also notice numbness and burning paresthesias on the plantar aspect of the foot and in the toes, which also may radiate up the calf. Initially, symptoms may be intermittent but may become more constant over time. The symptoms are accentuated by prolonged standing, walking, and especially prolonged running. Treatment should be directed toward identifying and correcting the etiology of the syndrome. Non-operative treatment of the athlete with tarsal tunnel syndrome includes rest, nonsteroidal anti-inflammatory medication, local steroid injection, flexibility exercises, well-fitting shoes, and

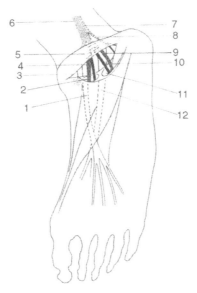

FIGURE 13.14 The complex anatomy of the tarsal tunnel. (1) Flexor digitorum muscle; (2) upper (medial) tarsal tunnel; (3) medial plantar nerve; (4) medial plantar artery; (5) ligamentum lacinatum; (6) posterior tibial artery; (7) tibial nerve; (8) calcaneal branches of the tibial nerve; (9) lateral plantar artery; (10) lateral plantar nerve; (11) lower (lateral) tarsal tunnel; (12) flexor hallucis longus muscle.

custom-made foot orthotics to help control abnormal mechanics.[3,62,63,91,119] Failure of non-operative treatment necessitates surgical exploration and decompression of the nerve.

K. FIRST BRANCH OF THE LATERAL PLANTAR NERVE

One of the most commonly overlooked causes of chronic heel pain in athletes is entrapment of the first branch of the lateral plantar nerve (nerve to the abductor digiti quinti muscle). Although runners and joggers account for the overwhelming majority of cases, this entrapment has been reported in athletes who participate in soccer, dance, tennis, and other track and fields events.[6,8,41,52,132] Entrapment occurs between the heavy deep fascia of the abductor hallucis muscle and the medial caudal margin of the medial head of the quadratus plantae muscle. Athletes complain of chronic heel pain intensified by walking and especially by running. Tenderness over the course of the nerve, maximal in the area of entrapment, is a characteristic and pathognomonic finding. In plantar fasciitis, tenderness is localized at the calcaneal origin of the plantar fascia. Infrequently, the patient may experience paresthesias along the course of the nerve. Park and Del Toro[108] describe a case of an isolated neuropathy of the first branch of the lateral plantar nerve proven with electrodiagnosis. Treatment is similar to that of other forms of heel pain: rest, nonsteroidal anti-inflammatory medication, heel cups, stretching programs, and occasionally local steroid injections.[6,8,52,132] If 6 to 12 months of non-operative therapy fail to relieve the symptoms and other possible causes of heel pain have been ruled out, then surgical intervention is indicated.[7]

L. MEDIAL PLANTAR NERVE (JOGGER'S FOOT)

Medial plantar nerve entrapment, or medial plantar nerve compression syndrome is known as "jogger's foot" and occurs in the region of the master knot of Henry (Figure 13.15).[101,120,132] The patients, usually middle-aged joggers, complain of aching or shooting pain in the medial aspect of their arch during running.[9] Most characteristically, the onset of pain is associated with the use of a new arch support. Physical examination reveals point tenderness of the plantar aspect of the medial arch in the region of the navicular tuberosity. The pain may be reproduced by everting the heel or having the patient stand on the ball of the foot. Park and Del Toro[107] describe a nerve conduction technique for study of the medial plantar nerve. Differentiation from posterior tibial tendinitis should be considered. Non-operative treatment is usually sufficient.[101,120,132] At surgery, the area of maximum tenderness should be addressed by releasing the fascia over the nerve in the affected zone.[132]

M. INTERDIGITAL NEUROMAS (METATARSALGIA)

Interdigital neuromas (metatarsalgia) are not uncommon in athletes, especially in runners and dancers.[30,55,81,101,111,131,132] Patients characteristically complain of plantar or forefoot pain associated with sprints or long-distance running. The pain is described as burning or sharp and frequently radiates to the toes. Patients may also notice numbness or tingling in the affected toes. They often give a history of many shoe changes in an attempt to seek relief. Typically, the pain is relieved by rest, removal of the shoes, and massage of the forefoot. A variety of metatarsal pads and orthotic devices have been suggested, but they are usually uncomfortable and are rejected by athletes. A small percentage of interdigital neuromas respond to local steroid injections. Most of them require surgical excision of the neuroma.[30,81,101,111,131,132]

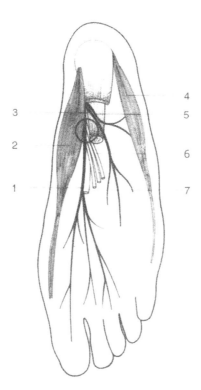

FIGURE 13.15 Medial plantar nerve compression may occur when the nerve passes through an osseo-fibromuscular tunnel between the abductor hallucis muscle and the navicular tarsal bone. (1) Medial plantar nerve; (2) abductor hallucis muscle; (3) lateral plantar nerve; (4) abductor digiti quinti muscle; (5) the first branch of the lateral planar nerve; (6) flexor digitorum longus muscle; (7) flexor hallucis longus muscle.

REFERENCES

1. **Akita, K. et al.** Anatomic basis of chronic groin pain with special reference to sports hernia. *Surg. Radiol. Anat.,* 1999; 21: 1–5.
2. **Andersen, K.V. and Bovim, G.** Impotence and nerve entrapment in long distance amateur cyclists. *Acta Neurol. Scand.,* 1997; 95: 233–240.
3. **Antonini, G., Gragnani, F., and Vichi, R.** Tarsal tunnel syndrome in skiers. Case report. *Ital. J. Neurol. Sci.,* 1993; 14: 391–392.
4. **Bassett, H.F. and Numley, A.J.** Compression of the musculocutaneous nerve at the elbow. *J. Bone Joint Surg.,* 1982; 64A: 1050–1052.
5. **Bateman, J.E.** Nerve injuries about the shoulder in sports. *J. Bone Joint Surg.,* 1967; 49A: 785–792.
6. **Baxter, D.E., Pfeffer, G.B., and Thigpen, M.** Chronic heel pain: treatment rationale. *Orthop. Clin. North Am.,* 1989; 20: 563–269.
7. **Baxter, D.E. and Pfeffer, G.B.** Treatment of chronic heel pain by surgical release of the first branch of the lateral plantar nerve. *Clin. Orthop.,* 1992; 279: 229–236.
8. **Bazzoli, A.S. and Polina, F.S.** Heel pain in recreational runners. *Phys. Sportsmed.,* 1989; 17: 55–61.
9. **Beskin, J.L.** Nerve entrapment syndromes of the foot and ankle. *J. Am. Acad. Orthop. Surg.,* 1997; 5: 261–269.
10. **Bisschop, G.D.E, Bisschop, E., and Commandre, F.** *Les Syndromes Canalaires.* Masson: Paris, 1997.
11. **Biundo, J.J. and Harris, M.A.** Peripheral nerve entrapment, occupation-related syndromes and sports injuries, and bursitis. *Curr. Opin. Rheumatol.,* 1993; 5: 224–229.
12. **Biundo, J.J., Mipro, R.C., and Djurić, V.** Peripheral nerve entrapment, occupation-related syndromes, sports injuries, bursitis, and soft-tissue problems of the shoulder. *Curr. Opin. Rheumatol.,* 1995; 7: 151–155.

13. **Black, K.P. and Lombardo, J.A.** Suprascapular nerve injuries with isolated paralysis of the infraspinatus. *Am. J. Sports Med.,* 1990; 18: 225–228.

14. **Bora, F.W. and Osterman, A.L.** Compression neuropathy. *Clin. Orthop.,* 1982; 163: 20–32.

15. **Braddom, R.L. and Wolfe, C.** Musculocutaneous nerve injury after heavy exercise. *Arch. Phys. Med. Rehabil.,* 1978; 59: 290–293.

16. **Bradshaw, C. and McCrory, P.** Obturator nerve entrapment. *Clin. J. Sports Med.,* 1997; 7: 217–219.

17. **Bradshaw, C. et al.** Obturator nerve entrapment. A case of groin pain in athletes. *Am. J. Sports Med.,* 1997; 25: 402–408.

18. **Braithwaite, I.J.** Bilateral median nerve palsy in a cyclist. *Br. J. Sports Med.,* 1992; 26: 27–28.

19. **Bryan, W.J. and Wild, J.J.** Isolated infraspinatus atrophy: a common cause of posterior shoulder pain and weakness in throwing athletes. *Am. J. Sports Med.,* 1989; 17: 130–131.

20. **Burke, E.R.** Ulnar neuropathy in bicyclists. *Phys. Sportsmed.,* 1981; 9: 53–56.

21. **Campbell, A.** Cycle saddles. *Lancet,* 1994; 344: 695–697.

22. **Carr, D. and Davis, P.** Distal posterior interosseous nerve syndrome. *J. Hand Surg.,* 1985; 10(6): 873–878.

23. **Caldwell, G.L. and Safran, M.R.** Elbow problem in the athlete. *Orthop. Clin. North Am.,* 1995; 26: 465–485.

24. **Childress, H.M.** Recurrent ulnar nerve dislocation at the elbow. *J. Bone Joint Surg.,* 1956; 38A: 978–984.

25. **Collins, K., Storey, M., Peterson, K., and Nuttler, P.** Nerve injuries in athletes. *Phys. Sportsmed.,* 1988; 16: 92–100.

26. **Conn, J., Bergan, J.J., and Bell, J.L.** Hypothenar hammer syndrome. Posttraumatic digital ischemia. *Surgery,* 1970; 68: 1122–1128.

27. **Converse, T.A.** Cyclist palsy (letter). *N. Engl. J. Med.,* 1979; 301: 1397–1398.

28. **Cummins, C.A. et al.** Suprascapular nerve entrapment at the spinoglenoid notch in a professional baseball pitcher. *Am. J. Sports Med.,* 1999; 27: 810–812.

29. **Daghino, W., Pasquali, M., and Falletti, C.** Superficial peroneal nerve entrapment in a young athlete: the diagnostic contribution of magnetic resonance imaging. *J. Foot Ankle Surg.,* 1997; 36: 170–172.

30. **Deese, J.M., Jr. and Baxter, D.E.** Compressive neuropathies of the lower extremity. *J. Musculoskel. Med.,* 1988; 5: 68–91.

31. **Dellon, A.L. and Mackinnon, S.E.** Radial sensory nerve entrapment in the forearm. *J. Hand Surg.,* 1986; 11A: 199–205.

32. **Del Pizzo, W., Jobe, F.W., and Norwood, L.** Ulnar nerve entrapment syndrome in baseball players. *Am. J. Sports Med.,* 1977; 5: 182–185.

33. **Destot, M.** Paralysie cubitale per l'usage de la bicyclette. *Gaz. Hop. Civ. Mil.,* 1896; 69: 1176–1177.

34. **Dobyns, J.H., O'Brien, E.T., and Linscheid, R.L.** Bowler's thumb, diagnosis and treatment: review of 17 cases. *J. Bone Joint Surg.,* 1972; 54A: 751–755.

35. **Dorfman, L.J. and Jayoram, A.R.** Handcuff neuropathy. *J. Am. Med. Assoc.,* 1978; 239: 957.

36. **Dumitru, D. and Windsor, R.E.** Subsartorial entrapment of the saphenous nerve of a competitive female bodybuilder. *Phys. Sportsmed.,* 1989; 17: 116–125.

37. **Dunham, W., Haines, G., and Spring, J.M.** Bowler's thumb. (Ulnovolar neuroma of the thumb). *Clin. Orthop.,* 1972; 83: 99–101.

38. **Eckman, P.B., Perlstein, G., and Altrocchi, P.H.** Ulnar neuropathy in bicycle riders. *Arch. Neurol.,* 1975; 32: 130–131.

39. **Ferretti, A., Cerullo, G., and Russo, G.** Suprascapular neuropathy in volleyball players. *J. Bone Joint Surg.,* 1987; 69A: 260–263.

40. **Fischer, M.A. and Gorelick, P.B.** Entrapment neuropathies: differential diagnosis and management. *Postgrad. Med.,* 1985; 77: 160–174.

41. **Fredericson, M., Standage, S., Chou, L., and Matheson, G.** Lateral plantar nerve entrapment in a competitive gymnast. *Clin. J. Sports Med.,* 2001; 11: 111–114.

42. **Frontera, W.R.** Cyclist palsy: clinical and electrodiagnostic findings. *Br. J. Sports Med.,* 1983; 17: 91–93.

43. **Fulkerson, J.P.** Transient ulnar neuropathy from Nordic skiing. *Clin. Orthop.,* 1980; 153: 230–231.

44. **Ganzhorn, R.W. et al.** Suprascapular nerve entrapment. *J. Bone Joint Surg.,* 1981; 63A: 492–494.

45. **Gessini, L., Jandolo, B., and Pietrangeli, A.** The anterior tarsal syndrome: report of four cases. *J. Bone Joint Surg.,* 1984; 66A: 786–787.
46. **Glennon, T.P.** Isolated injury of the infraspinatus branch of the suprascapular nerve. *Arch. Phys. Med. Rehab.,* 1992; 73: 201–202.
47. **Glousman, R.E.** Ulnar nerve problems in the athlete's elbow. *Clin. Sports Med.,* 1990; 9: 365–377.
48. **Gould, N. and Trevino, S.** Sural nerve entrapment by avulsion fracture of the base of the fifth metatarsal. *Foot Ankle,* 1981; 2: 153–155.
49. **Gregg, J.R., Labosky, D., and Harry, M.** Serratus anterior paralysis in the young athlete. *J. Bone Joint Surg.,* 1979; 61A: 825–832.
50. **Hainline, B.** Nerve injuries. *Med. Clin. North Am.,* 1994; 78: 327–343.
51. **Hemler, D.E., Ward, W.K., Karstetter, K.W., and Bryant, P.M.** Saphenous nerve entrapment caused by pes anserine bursitis mimicking stress fracture of the tibia. *Arch. Phys. Med. Rehabil.,* 1991; 72: 336–337.
52. **Henricson, A.S. and Westlin, N.E.** Chronic calcaneal pain in athletes: entrapment of the calcaneal nerve? *Am. J. Sports Med.,* 1984; 12: 152–154.
53. **Hirasawa, Y. and Sakakida, K.** Sports and peripheral nerve injury. *Am. J. Sports Med.,* 1983; 11: 420–426.
54. **Ho, P.K., Dellon, A.L., and Wilgis, E.F.S.** True aneurysms of the hand resulting from athletic injury. *Am. J. Sports Med.,* 1985; 13: 136–138.
55. **Hockenbury, R.T.** Forefoot problems in athletes. *Med. Sci. Sports Exerc.,* 1999; 31(7 Suppl.): 448.
56. **Holzgraefe, M., Kukowski, B., and Eggert, S.** Prevalence of latent and manifest suprascapular neuropathy in high-performance volleyball players. *Br. J. Sports Med.,* 1994; 28: 177–179.
57. **Howard, F.M.** Controversies in nerve entrapment syndromes in the forearm and wrist. *Orthop. Clin. North Am.,* 1986; 17: 375–381.
58. **Howell, A.E. and Leach, R.E.** Bowler's thumb: perineural fibrosis of the digital nerve. *J. Bone Joint Surg.,* 1970; 52A: 379–381.
59. **Hunter, S.C. and Poole, R.M.** The chronically inflamed tendon. *Clin. Sports Med.,* 1987; 6: 371–388.
60. **Jablecki, C.K.** Lateral antebrachial cutaneous neuropathy in a windsurfer. *Muscle Nerve,* 1999; 22: 944–945.
61. **Jackson, D.L.** Electrodiagnostic studies of median and ulnar nerves in cyclists. *Phys. Sportsmed.,* 1989; 17: 137–148.
62. **Jackson, D.L. and Haglund, B.** Tarsal tunnel syndrome in athletes. Case reports and literature review. *Am. J. Sports Med.,* 1991; 19: 61–65.
63. **Jackson, D.L. and Haglund, B.L.** Tarsal tunnel syndrome in runners. *Sports Med.,* 1992; 13: 146–149.
64. **Jackson, D.L. et al.** Suprascapular neuropathy in athletes: case reports. *Clin. J. Sports Med.,* 1995; 5: 134.
65. **Jalovaara, P. and Lindholm, R.V.** Decompression of the posterior interosseous nerve for tennis elbow. *Arch. Orthop. Trauma Surg.,* 1989; 198: 243.
66. **Johnson, D.C.** The upper extremity in swimming, in *Symposium on Upper Extremity Injuries in Athletes,* Pettrone, F.A., Ed. St. Louis: C.V. Mosby, 1986; 36–46.
67. **Karas, S.E.** Thoracic outlet syndrome. *Clin. Sports Med.,* 1990; 9: 297–310.
68. **Katirji, B. and Hardy, R.W., Jr.** Classic neurogenic thoracic outlet syndrome in a competitive swimmer: a true scalenus anticus syndrome. *Muscle Nerve,* 1995; 18: 229–233.
69. **Kernohan, J., Levack, B., and Wilson, J.N.** Entrapment of the superficial peroneal nerve: three case reports. *J. Bone Joint Surg.,* 1985; 67B: 60–61.
70. **Kim, S.M. and Goodrich, J.A.** Isolated proximal musculocutaneous nerve palsy: case report. *Arch. Phys. Med. Rehabil.,* 1984; 65: 735–736.
71. **Komar, J.** *Alagut — Szindromak.* Budapest: Medicina–Konyvkiado, 1977.
72. **Kopel, H.P. and Thompson, W.A.L.** Peripheral entrapment neuropathies of the lower extremity. *N. Engl. J. Med.,* 1960; 262: 55–60.
73. **Kouvalchouk, J.F., Bonnet, J.M., and deMondenard, J.P.** Le syndrome de du piramidal. *Rev. Chir. Orthop.,* 1996; 82: 647–657.
74. **Leach, R.E., Purnell, M.B., and Saito, A.** Peroneal nerve entrapment in runners. *Am. J. Sports Med.,* 1989; 17: 287–291.
75. **Leffert, R.D.** Brachial plexus injuries. *N. Engl. J. Med.,* 1974; 291: 1059–1066.

76. **Leffert, R.D.** Thoracic outlet syndrome and the shoulder. *Clin. Sports Med.,* 1983; 2: 439–452.
77. **Lindenbaum, B.L.** Ski boot compression syndrome. *Clin. Orthop.,* 1979; 140: 19–23.
78. **Linker, C.S., Helms, C.A., and Fritz, R.C.** Quadrilateral space syndrome: findings at MR imaging. *Radiology,* 1993; 188: 675–676.
79. **Liveson, J.A., Bronson, M.J., and Pollack, M.A.** Suprascapular nerve lesions at the spinoglenoid notch: report of three cases and review of the literature. *J. Neurol. Neurosurg. Psychiatr.,* 1991; 54: 241–243.
80. **Logigian, E.L. et al.** Stretch induced spinal accessory nerve palsy. *Muscle Nerve,* 1988; 11: 146–150.
81. **Lorei, M.P. and Hershman, E.B.** Peripheral nerve injuries in athletes. Treatment and prevention. *Sports Med.,* 1993; 16: 130.
82. **Lotem, M., Fried, A., and Levy, M.** Radial palsy following muscular effort: a nerve compression syndrome possibly related to a fibrous arch of the lateral band of the triceps. *J. Bone Joint Surg.,* 1971; 53B: 500–506.
83. **Lowdon, I.M.R.** Superficial peroneal nerve entrapment: a case report. *J. Bone Joint Surg.,* 1985; 67B: 58–59.
84. **Lubahn, J.D. and Cermak, M.B.** Uncommon nerve compression syndromes of the upper extremity. *J. Am. Acad. Orthop. Surg.,* 1998; 6: 378–386.
85. **McCrory, P. and Bell, S.** Nerve entrapment syndromes as a cause of pain in the hip, groin and buttock. *Sports Med.,* 1999; 27: 261–274.
86. **McGregor, J. and Moncur, J.A.** Meralgia paresthetica — a sports lesion in girl gymnasts. *Br. J. Sport Med.,* 1977; 11: 16–19.
87. **Maimaris, C. and Zadeh, H.G.** Ulnar nerve compression in the cyclist's hand: two case reports and review of the literature. *Br. J. Sport Med.,* 1990; 24: 245–246.
88. **Mariani, P.P., Santorielo, P., and Maresca, G.** Spontaneous accessory nerve palsy. *J. Shoulder Elbow Surg.,* 1998; 7: 545–546.
89. **Massey, E.W. and Pleet, A.B.** Handcuffs and cheiralgia paresthetica. *Neurology,* 1978; 28: 1312–1313.
90. **Mastiglia, F.L.** Musculocutaneous neuropathy after strenuous physical activity. *Med. J. Aust.,* 1986; 145: 153–154.
91. **Mattalino, A.J., Deese, J.M., Jr., and Campbell, E.D., Jr.** Office evaluation and treatment of lower extremity injuries in runners. *Clin. Sports Med.,* 1989; 8: 461–475.
92. **McAuliffe, T.B., Fiddian, N.J., and Browett, J.P.** Entrapment neuropathy of the superficial peroneal nerve: a bilateral case. *J. Bone Joint Surg.,* 1985; 67B: 62–63.
93. **McCue, F.C., III, and Miller, G.A.** Soft-tissue injuries of the hand, in *Symposium on Upper Extremity Injuries in Athletes,* Pettrone, F.A., Ed. St. Louis: C.V. Mosby, 1986; 79–94.
94. **Mendoza, F.X. and Main, K.** Peripheral nerve injuries of the shoulder in the athlete. *Clin. Sports Med.,* 1990; 9: 331–342.
95. **Minkow, F.V. and Basset, F.H., III.** Bowler's thumb. *Clin. Orthop.,* 1972; 83: 115–117.
96. **Mitsunanga, M.M. and Nakano, K.** High radial nerve palsy following strenuous muscular activity. A case report. *Clin. Orthop.,* 1988; 234: 39.
97. **Moller, B.N. and Kadin, S.** Entrapment of the common peroneal nerve. *Am. J. Sports Med.,* 1987; 15: 90–91.
98. **Montagna, P. and Colonna, S.** Suprascapular neuropathy restricted to infraspinatus muscle in volleyball players. *Acta Neurol. Scand.,* 1993; 87: 248–250.
99. **Mosher, J.F.** Peripheral nerve injuries and entrapment of the forearm and wrist, in *Symposium on Upper Extremity Injuries in Athletes,* Pettrone, F.A., Ed. St. Louis: C.V. Mosby, 1986; 174–181.
100. **Moss, S.H. and Switzer, H.E.** Radial tunnel syndrome. A spectrum of clinical presentations. *J. Hand Surg.,* 1983; 8: 414–420.
101. **Murphy, P.C. and Baxter, D.E.** Nerve entrapment of the foot and ankle in runners. *Clin. Sports Med.,* 1985; 4: 753–763.
102. **Naso, S.J.** Compression of the digital nerve: a new entity in tennis players. *Orthop. Rev.,* 1984; 13: 47.
103. **Nuber, G.W., McCarthy, W.J., Yao, J.S.T., Schafer, M.F., and Suker, J.R.** Arterial abnormalities of the hand in athletes. *Am. J. Sports Med.,* 1990; 18: 520–523.
104. **Osterman, L.A., Moskow, L., and Low, D.W.** Soft-tissue injuries of the hand and wrist in racquet sports. *Clin. Sports Med.,* 1988; 7: 329–348.

105. **Packer, G.J., McLatchie, G.R., and Bowden, W.** Scapula winging in a sports injury clinic. *Br. J. Sports Med.,* 1993; 27: 90.
106. **Paladini, D. et al.** Axillary neuropathy in volleyball players: report of two cases and literature review. *J. Neurol. Neurosurg. Psychiatr.,* 1996; 6: 345–347.
107. **Park, T.A. and Del Toro, D.R.** Isolated inferior calcaneal neuropathy. *Muscle Nerve,* 1996; 19: 106–108.
108. **Park, T.A. and Del Toro, D.R.** The medial calcaneal nerve: anatomy and nerve conduction technique. *Muscle Nerve,* 1995; 18: 32–38.
109. **Pećina, M.** Contribution to the etiological explanation of the piriformis syndrome. *Acta Anat.* (Basel), 1979; 105: 181–187.
110. **Pećina, M., Krmpotić-Nemanić, J., and Markiewitz, A.D.** *Tunnel Syndromes. Peripheral Nerve Compression Syndromes,* 3rd ed. Boca Raton, FL: CRC Press, 2001.
111. **Pećina, M., Bojanić, I., and Markiewitz, A.D.** Nerve entrapment syndrome in athletes. *Clin. J. Sport Med.,* 1993; 3: 36–43.
112. **Pećina, M. and Bojanić, I.** Nervus musculocutaneous entrapment syndrome in the shoulder region. *Int. Orthop. (SICOT),* 1993; 17: 232–234.
113. **Pećina, M. and Bojanić, I.** Musculocutaneous nerve entrapment in athlete. *Period. Biol.,* 1994; 96: 63–64.
114. **Posner, M.A.** Compressive neuropathies of the median and radial nerves at the elbow. *Clin. Sports Med.,* 1990; 93: 34–63.
115. **Post, M. and Mayer, J.** Suprascapular nerve entrapment. *Clin. Orthop.,* 1987; 223: 126–136.
116. **Priest, J.D.** A physical phenomenon: shoulder depression in athletes. *Sports Care Fitness,* 1989; 3/4: 20–24.
117. **Pringle, R.M., Protheroe, K., and Mukherjee, S.K.** Entrapment neuropathy of the sural nerve. *J. Bone Joint Surg.,* 1974; 56B: 465–467.
118. **Prochaska, V., Crosby, L.A., Murphy, R.P.** High radial nerve palsy in a tennis player. *Orthop. Rev.,* 1993; 22: 90–92.
119. **Radin, E.L.** Tarsal tunnel syndrome. *Clin. Orthop.,* 1983; 181: 167–170.
120. **Rask, E.L.** Tarsal plantar neuropraxia (jogger's foot): report of three cases. *Clin. Orthop.,* 1978; 134: 193–198.
121. **Redler, M.R., Ruland, L.J., and McCue, F.C., III.** Quadrilateral space syndrome in a throwing athlete. *Am. J. Sports Med.,* 1986; 14: 511–513.
122. **Regan, W.D.** Lateral elbow pain in the athlete: a clinical review. *Clin. J. Sport Med.,* 1991; 1: 53–58.
123. **Rettig, A.C.** Neurovascular injuries in the wrist and hands of athletes. *Clin. Sports Med.,* 1990; 9: 389–417.
124. **Rettig, A.C. and Ebben, J.R.** Anterior subcutaneous transfer of the ulnar nerve in the athlete. *Am. J. Sports Med.,* 1993; 21: 836–849.
125. **Richmond, D.R.** Handlebar problems in bicycling. *Clin. Sports Med.,* 1994; 13: 165.
126. **Ringel, S.P. et al.** Suprascapular neuropathy in pitchers. *Am. J. Sports Med.,* 1990; 18: 80–86.
127. **Ritts, G.D., Wood, M.B., and Linscheid, R.L.** Radial tunnel syndrome: a ten-year surgical experience. *Clin. Orthop.,* 1987; 219: 201–205.
128. **Roles, N.C. and Maudsley, R.H.** Radial tunnel syndrome. Resistant tennis elbow as a nerve entrapment. *J. Bone Joint Surg.,* 1972; 54B: 499–508.
129. **Ruby, L.K.** Common hand injuries in the athlete. *Orthop. Clin. North Am.,* 1980; 11: 819–839.
130. **Sandow, M.J. and Ilić, J.** Suprascapular nerve rotator cuff compression syndrome in volleyball players. *J. Shoulder Elbow Surg.,* 1998; 7: 516–521.
131. **Schon, L.C. and Baxter, D.E.** Neuropathies of the foot and ankle in athletes. *Clin. Sports Med.,* 1990; 9: 489–509.
132. **Schon, L.C.** Nerve entrapment, neuropathy, and nerve dysfunction in athletes. *Orthop. Clin. North Am.,* 1994; 25: 47–59.
133. **Schultz, J.S. and Leonard, J.A., Jr.** Long thoracic neuropathy from athletic activity. *Arch. Phys. Med. Rehabil.,* 1992; 73: 87–90.
134. **Sheon, R.P.** Peripheral nerve entrapment, occupation-related syndromes, and sports injuries. *Curr. Opin. Rheumatol.,* 1992; 4: 219–225.

135. **Sicuranza, M.J. and McCue, F.C., III.** Compressive neuropathies in the upper extremity of athletes. *Hand Clin.,* 1992; 8: 263–273.

136. **Siegel, I.M.** Bowling thumb neuroma (letter). *J. Am. Med. Assoc.,* 1965; 192: 263.

137. **Smail, D.F.** Handelbar palsy (letter). *N. Engl. J. Med.,* 1975; 292: 322.

138. **Stack, R.E., Bianco, A.J., and MacCarty, C.S.** Compression of the common peroneal nerve by ganglion cysts. *J. Bone Joint Surg.,* 1965; 47A: 773–778.

139. **Streib, E.** Upper arm radial nerve palsy after muscular effort. Report of three cases. *Neurology,* 1992; 42: 1632–1634.

140. **Strukel, R.J. and Garick, J.G.** Thoracic outlet compression in athletes. *Am. J. Sports Med.,* 1978; 6: 35–39.

141. **Styf, J.** Entrapment of the superficial peroneal nerve: diagnosis and results of decompression. *J. Bone Joint Surg.,* 1989; 71B: 131–135.

142. **Styf, J.** Chronic exercise-induced pain in the anterior aspect of the lower leg: an overview of diagnosis. *Sports Med.,* 1989; 7: 331–339.

143. **Swain, R.** Musculocutaneous nerve entrapment: a case report. *Clin. J. Sport Med.,* 1995; 5: 196–198.

144. **Tackmann, W., Richter, H.P., and Stohr, M.** *Kompressionssyndrome peripherer Nerven.* Berlin: Springer-Verlag, 1989.

145. **Tardif, G.S.** Nerve injuries. Testing and treatment tactics. *Phys. Sportsmed.,* 1995; 23: 61–65.

146. **Wang, D.H. and Koehler, S.M.** Isolated infraspinatus atrophy in a collegiate volleyball player. *Clin. J. Sports Med.,* 1996; 6: 225–228.

147. **Weinstein, S.M. and Herring, S.** Nerve problems and compartment syndromes in the hand, wrist, and forearm. *Clin. Sports Med.,* 1992; 11: 161–188.

148. **Werner, C.O.** Lateral elbow pain and posterior interosseous nerve entrapment. *Acta Orthop. Scand. (Suppl.),* 1979; 174:1–62.

149. **Wilhelm, A.** Unklare Schmerzzustände an der oberen Extremität. *Orthopadie,* 1987; 16: 458–464.

150. **White, H.H.** Pack palsy: a neurological complication of scouting. *Pediatrics,* 1968; 41: 1001–1003.

151. **White, S.M. and Witten, C.M.** Long thoracic nerve palsy in a professional ballet dancer. *Am. J. Sports Med.,* 1993; 21: 626.

152. **Wojtys, E.M., Smith, P.A., and Hankin, F.M.** A cause of ulnar neuropathy in a baseball pitcher: a case report. *Am. J. Sports Med.,* 1986; 14: 522–524.

153. **Wood, M.B. and Dobyns, J.H.** Sports-related extraarticular wrist syndromes. *Clin. Orthop.,* 1986; 202: 93–102.

154. **Worth, R.M., Kettelkamp, D.B., Defalque, R.J., and Duane, K.V.** Saphenous nerve entrapment. A case of medial knee pain. *Am. J. Sports Med.,* 1984; 12: 80–81.

155. **Yocum, L.A.** The diagnosis and nonoperative treatment of elbow problems in the athlete. *Clin. Sports Med.,* 1989; 8: 39–51.

156. **Zeiss, J. et al.** MRI of suprascapular neuropathy in a weight lifter. *J. Comput. Assist. Tomogr.,* 1993; 17: 303–308.

157. **Ziprin, P., Williams, P., and Foster, M.E.** External oblique aponeurosis nerve entrapment as a cause of groin pain in the athlete. *Br. J. Surg.,* 1999; 86: 566–568.

158. **Zongzhao, L., Jiansheng, Z., and Li, Z.** Anterior tarsal tunnel syndrome. *J. Bone Joint Surg.,* 1991; 73B: 470–473.

159. **Zuckerman, J.D., Polonsky, L., and Edelson, G.** Suprascapular nerve palsy in a young athlete. *Bull. Hosp. Joint Dis.,* 1993; 53: 11–12.

14 Overuse Injuries in Young Athletes*

The past few decades have witnessed a dramatic increase in top-level, world-ranked results achieved by young athletes between the ages of 8 and 16. Although most notable in swimming and gymnastics, the trend of people entering serious training and organized competition at ever-decreasing ages now pervades most athletic activities. High expectations and the imperative of a good result, combined with extremely competitive surroundings, often place very young athletes under enormous physical and psychological pressure, driving them not only toward the fulfillment of their own dreams and ambitions, but often to the point of assuming responsibility for their parents' and coaches' ambitions as well. Consequently, young athletes undertake prolonged and intensive training schedules, often under the supervision of private coaches.

At the same time, their growing musculoskeletal system is particularly susceptible to injuries, with the risk of injury peaking during the adolescent growth spurt. Even though acute injuries such as fractures, sprains, or strains are not uncommon in the general population at this age, heavy athletic training, coupled with ongoing growth, causes an increasing number of specific problems that often result in athletic injuries belonging to the overuse group. Although a child subjected to repetitive training is susceptible to many of the same overuse injuries adults can sustain, there are several overuse injuries unique to the growing child.[4-6,15,17,24-26] This chapter offers an overview of these specific, growth-related overuse injuries in the young athlete.

I. EPIDEMIOLOGY

In the U.S., 50% of males and 25% of females between the ages of 8 and 16 engage in some type of competitive, organized sport activity in the course of the school year. An additional 20% of children in this age range are involved in community sports programs, and 75% of U.S. primary and secondary schools have significant competitive sports programs. However, this increased rate of participation by children and adolescents in organized sports and fitness activities does not come without risk of injury. Available data show that the incidence of sporting injuries accounts for 36 to 53% of all injuries sustained in childhood and adolescence.[51,74,77] Comparison of these data with statistics on the impact of macrotrauma injuries reveals no clear evidence that organized sports are in any way more dangerous, or safer, than free play.

However, overuse injuries, such as osteochondroses, stress fractures, patellofemoral stress syndrome, and bursitis,[40,46,48,50,59,61,64,68,84] are a whole new genre of injuries occurring in children engaged in organized sports, rarely occurring in the context of free play. It is difficult to estimate the true magnitude of this problem, as the existing epidemiological data reported in literature vary significantly in terms of parameters used in analysis (population, methodology, types of injuries, etc.).

Recent data show that 30 to 50% of all childhood and adolescent sports injuries are due to overuse.[3,19,90] The relative incidence of overuse injuries varies by type of sport and athletic activity. Participants in contact sports, such as football, soccer, or wrestling, have a much higher overall probability of sustaining injuries, mostly minor acute trauma. In contrast, young athletes participating in swimming, running, gymnastics, and figure skating have low overall risk of injury, but

---

* Co-authored by Alan Ivković.

most of the injuries they sustain are associated with overuse. These athletes lose 54% more time from training and competition.[3,21,82]

II. SPECIAL CONSIDERATIONS FOR GROWING INDIVIDUALS

The process of growth is the key factor that differentiates children and adolescent athletes from their adult peers. From birth to the end of adolescence, the human body goes through remarkable changes in terms of height, weight, and proportions. Over this period, body weight will increase 25-fold, body height 3.5-fold, and muscle mass 7-fold.[88] Growth is particularly intense during the adolescent growth spurt that occurs during the ages of 10 to 14 in girls, and 13 to 17 in boys.

It is well known that a certain level of physical activity is necessary for the normal growth and development of the musculoskeletal system. However, immature musculoskeletal systems have many unique traits that must be taken into consideration to establish musculoskeletal balance and prevent overuse injuries in young athletes.[37,75] A growing bone is more porous and has lower trauma tolerance than its adult counterpart.[28] Furthermore, an immature bone is characterized by a comparatively high degree of elasticity and plasticity, so that bone deformation without fracture may occur. Luckily, the periosteum of a child's bone is thicker, stronger, and more vascularized than its adult counterpart, which properties give the immature bone remarkable healing and regenerative potential.

The most important difference between immature and mature musculoskeletal systems is the presence of growth cartilage. Growth cartilage presents at three locations (Figure 14.1): the epiphyseal growth plate, the joint surface, and the apophyseal insertion of the musculotendinous unit to the bone. Each of these sites may sustain injury, and is particularly susceptible to repetitive microtraumas. Several reports have shown that growth cartilage is vulnerable to two kinds of stress: acute macrotrauma or repetitive microtrauma.[1,9,16,23] Therefore, it is growth cartilage that is the "weakest link" in an immature musculoskeletal system.

Longitudinal and appositional growth of long bones occurs between epiphyses and metaphyses. Owing to its anatomical and biomechanical features, the epiphyseal growth plate is particularly susceptible to injury during the adolescent growth spurt. However, overuse injuries of the epiphyseal growth plate are not very common, except for two entities called Little League elbow (medial epicondyle) and Little League shoulder (proximal humerus). Overuse injuries to physes were also reported — at the proximal tibia in runners and at the distal radius in gymnasts.[12,14]

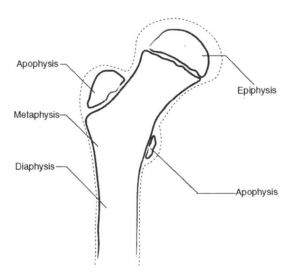

FIGURE 14.1 Growth cartilage in proximal femur (longitudinal, latitudinal, and appositional growth).

A growing individual's articular cartilage contains growth cartilage. Osteochondritis dissecans is the most commonly encountered disorder, with knee, ankle, and elbow the most frequently injured regions. Although the etiology of these disorders remains unclear, a strong relationship between repetitive microtrauma and osteochondral lesions is apparent.

Apophyseal growth plates serve as insertions for muscle–tendon units into the bone. Consequently, they are subjected to strong traction forces. During the adolescent growth spurt, the relative imbalance in flexibility between musculotendinous structures and the adjacent bone can cause repetitive tensile microtraumas to the apophyses. When the reparatory mechanisms of the bone are exhausted, the inflammatory process causes pain, and a clinical picture of traction apophysites develops. The most frequent entities in this group of overuse injuries include Osgood-Schlatter disease (the tibial tubercle), Sever disease (the calcaneus), and Sinding-Larsen-Johansson disease (the lower part of patella).

III. RISK FACTORS

When assessing the occurrence of overuse injuries in a young athlete, it is of utmost importance to be aware of the gamut of factors that may contribute to the probability of injury. Forming an understanding of potential risk factors is also the most effective way to prevent injury. The risk factors have traditionally been divided into two main groups: extrinsic and intrinsic. Intrinsic factors (growth-related, anatomical, physiological, psychological, history-related) may be viewed as inherent to the individual in question, and it can be difficult to influence or change them. Extrinsic factors, on the other hand (schedule and technique, equipment and environment), reflect external influences and can be modified more easily.

A. INTRINSIC FACTORS

1. Growth-Related Factors

As already mentioned, the growth process is a unique characteristic of a young athlete. There are two main aspects of this process that need to be taken into consideration: the presence of growth cartilage and musculoskeletal imbalance.[57] Susceptibility of growth cartilage to injury, the first aspect, has already been discussed above. The second growth-related factor occurs as a result of rapid changes in the relative length of the long bones, and the resulting strain on the adjacent musculotendinous unit. During the adolescent growth spurt, long bones grow faster than muscle–tendon units, resulting in inflexibility and dynamic muscle imbalance. Short tendons and muscles can produce strong traction forces on apophyses (traction apophysites), as well as stress to the articular cartilage (patellofemoral pain syndrome).

2. Anatomic Malalignment

Anatomic malalignment commonly occurs in growing individuals and can play an important role in the development of overuse injuries. Femoral neck anteversion, patella alta, genu valgum or varum, external tibial rotation, and excessive foot pronation are all shown to be predisposing factors for overuse injuries.[32] The mentioned anatomic malalignments relating to lower extremities are strongly associated with the occurrence of patellofemoral pain.[22] Another example are stress fractures of the pars interarticularis in ballet dancers.[31,33,34] To compensate for hip movement reductions due to femoral neck anteversion, young dancers may exaggerate lumbar lordosis.[72,78]

3. Physiological Factors

It is not sufficient to define the maturation process in adolescents only in terms of height, weight, and body proportions, without taking into account the underlying physiological changes unfolding at this time. To develop into a mature individual, a young body goes through a series of significant changes in its endocrinological status.[62] This is particularly true for young girls who are starting to experience menstrual cycles due to stabilizations of the reproductive hormonal axis. Low calorie intake coupled with vigorous training may induce amenorrhea or delay menarche in young athletes.[89] This may lead to hypoestrogenism and a decrease in bone mineral content, predisposing these athletes to stress fractures. This syndrome is known as the female athlete triad and is described in more detail in Chapter 15.

Musculoskeletal maturity is another important factor and should always be assessed in preparticipation physical evaluation of the young athlete.[2,8] Some of the indicators include Tanner staging criteria for genital development, date of menarche, and secondary sexual development.[80,88] This kind of assessment is useful to ensure that the young individual chooses an appropriate sport and sporting environment.

4. Psychological Factors

Participation in competitive sports has a positive influence on personal and social development of children and adolescents. It provides young athletes with an opportunity to develop self-esteem, self-discipline, self-confidence, independence, and interpersonal skills. However, professional sport has come to a point where it is financial interests that dictate the rules of the game. These days, sport is a highly lucrative business, far removed from Pierre de Coubertain's idea of Olympic excellence. Recent studies have shown that that adolescents perceive professional athletes as rich, famous, and glorified, and rank enhancement of status and financial gain as more important factors in a decision to become an athlete than pure desire to play sports.[85] Furthermore, enormous pressure exerted by parents, coaches, managers, media, and even peers can have an impact on the young athlete's psychological development processes. Some young athletes define their value to their parents or coaches only in terms of athletic success, and this may cause severe anxiety and depression. This kind of pressure can induce eating disorders in young female athletes, the first step of the female athlete triad mentioned earlier. For the same reasons, a young athlete may also be reluctant to report pain when it first occurs. This may aggravate an injury that would have otherwise been preventable or treatable. On the other end of the spectrum, demotivated young athletes may feel that reported injury is a justifiable excuse to discontinue athletic activity, which leads to instances of hypochondriac behavior.

5. Inadequate Conditioning and Prior Injury

Poor preparation and inadequate conditioning can substantially increase the incidence of overuse injuries. First-time introduction of a young individual to organized sporting activity should be careful and gradual. Warming and stretching prior to any activity are compulsory and must not be waived under any circumstances. Athletes with a history of prior injury should be checked for established errors in training approach or technique. Repeated injury may also signal that the previous injury had received inadequate treatment or rehabilitation.

B. Extrinsic Factors

1. Training Schedule and Sporting Technique

Improper training is probably the most important risk factor for the occurrence of overuse injuries in young athletes. Fortunately, it is also the one most easily corrected. Intensive, prolonged training schedules designed with adults in mind are not suitable for immature athletes. Training programs should be as individualized as possible, and all the risk factors listed above taken into consideration at the time of design. The usual scenario for the development of overuse injuries is a steep increase in the intensity of training ("too much, too soon"). This usually occurs during summer camps, pre-season training programs, or at the beginning of competition at a higher rank or league. The frequency and duration of the training should be commensurate with the individual's capabilities.

Incorrect technique, especially in contact, racket, and throwing sports, is another important factor contributing to development of overuse injuries. The syndrome known as Little League elbow is an example of overuse injury that can be avoided if proper technique is used. Repetitive valgus stress can injure humeral epiphyses in young baseball or handball players, and much attention should be devoted to ensure that correct pitching or throwing technique is adopted.

2. Sporting Equipment and Environment

Faulty and inappropriately fitted individual equipment is another risk factor. Footwear needs to fit well and have an appropriate sole. Sports shoes should be replaced regularly, as they can lose more than 40% of their shock-absorbing capacity after 250 to 500 miles.[18] The equipment should be of an appropriate size, especially in upper-limb and kicking sports (tennis, baseball, soccer, football). Changes in training surface may also trigger overuse injuries. This is particularly true for those athletes who switch from outdoor surfaces to indoor, artificial facilities.

IV. OVERVIEW OF THE MOST FREQUENT OVERUSE INJURIES IN CHILD AND ADOLESCENT ATHLETES

Overuse injuries occur when tissue is exposed to repetitive submaximal loading. A group of unique overuse injuries characteristic of the adolescent athlete can be identified. As previously described, these unique overuse injuries are associated with the presence of growth cartilage and, additionally, with the growth process itself (Table 14.1).

TABLE 14.1
The Most Common Overuse Injuries in Young Athletes

Site	Overuse Injury	Sport
Shoulder	Little League shoulder Impingement syndromes	Baseball, handball, water polo
Elbow	Little League elbow	Baseball, handball, water polo
Hand	Distal radial growth plate injury	Gymnastics
Spine	Scheuermann disease Spondylolysis	Gymnastics, volleyball, backstroke swimming
Hip and pelvis	Iliac apophysitis Rectus femoris apophysitis Sartorius apophysitis Iliopsoas apophysitis Apophysis of greater trochanter (Mandl)	Soccer, football, weight lifting, skiing, running, rowing, track and field
Knee	Osgood-Schlatter disease Sinding-Larsen-Johansson disease Patellofemoral stress syndrome	Soccer, football, basketball, track and field
Ankle and foot	Sever disease Accessory navicular syndrome Iselin disease Medial malleolus apophysitis Köhler disease Freiberg disease	Football, soccer, tennis, track and field, figure skating, ballet

---

TABLE 14.2
Siffert's Classification of Osteochondroses[81]

I. Articular Osteochondroses
    a. Primary involvement of articular and epiphyseal cartilage and subjacent
       enchondral ossification (e.g., Freiberg disease)
    b. Secondary involvement of articular and epiphyseal cartilage as a consequence of
       avascular necrosis of subjacent bone (osteochondritis dissecans, Köhler disease)
II. Nonarticular Osteochondroses
    a. At tendon attachments (e.g., Osgood-Schlatter disease)
    b. At ligament attachments (Little League elbow)
    c. At impact sites (Sever disease)
III. Physeal Osteochondroses
    a. Long bones (e.g., Blount disease)
    b. Vertebrae (e.g., Scheuermann disease)

A. OSTEOCHONDROSES

Osteochondrosis is a term used to describe a group of disorders characterized by a disturbance of enchondral ossification, including chondrogenesis and osteogenesis, in a previously normal enchondral growth region. This process has been observed in virtually every growth center of the skeleton, and more than 50 locations have been reported in literature. Traditionally, osteochondroses tend to be named after the first individual who described their clinical and radiological characteristics.

The etiology of osteochondroses remains unclear. Many authors believe that repetitive stress is the major, or at least one of the major contributing factors.[19,36] Vigorous physical activity combined with growth-related musculoskeletal imbalance in the adolescent athlete may produce excessive stress at the bone–ligament junctions or articular surfaces. However, hormonal, genetic, and metabolic factors also contribute to the vulnerability of certain areas to mechanical stress.

Siffert[81] proposed the classification of osteochondroses based on anatomical localization of involved growth cartilage into three major groups: nonarticular (apophyses), physeal, and articular osteochondroses (Table 14.2).

1. Apophyseal Injuries (Traction Apophysites)

This group of disorders is characterized by irritation of apophyses due to excessive tensile forces at the point of attachment of a musculotendionous unit to the bone.[36,44,58,71] They occur during the adolescent growth spurt as a consequence of musculoskeletal imbalance. Previously believed to be inflammatory in nature (thus the name apophys*ites*), they are now considered a series of microavulsions at the bone–cartilage junction, whereas inflammation is the body's response to trauma. The process most frequently involves patellar tendon insertion at the tibial tubercle (Osgood-Schlatter disease), Achilles tendon insertion at the calcaneus (Sever disease) and the insertion of the wrist pronators and flexors at the medial epicondyle of the humerus (Little League elbow). Other common localizations include the base of the fifth metatarsal (Iselin disease), pelvis, and olecranon.

Osgood-Schlatter disease (OSD) was first reported in 1903, by Osgood[66] in Boston and Schlatter in Zurich, respectively and independently. OSD is strongly associated with sporting activity in adolescent athletes between the ages of 11 and 15, and is predominant in disciplines that involve jumping, kicking, and running. During the adolescent growth spurt, bones grow much faster than muscles and tendons. The comparatively slower elongation of the musculotendinous extensor apparatus of the knee (m. quadriceps) inflicts very strong tensile forces on the relatively small site of insertion of the patellar tendon to the tibial tubercle. These forces cause microavulsions of the tibial tubercle, and the prominence of the tibial tubercle occurs as a consequence of the process of

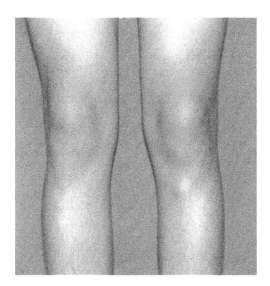

FIGURE 14.2 Prominence of the left tibial tuberosity in a young athlete with Osgood-Schlatter disease.

healing and ossification of these microavulsions. A clinical examination reveals pain, tenderness, and, at times, swelling over the tibial tubercle, prominence of the tubercle, and tightness of the quadriceps muscle (Figure 14.2). Pain is the leading symptom and is typically present several weeks to months before seeking medical care. It is aggravated during running, jumping, and walking up and down the stairs, and is relieved by rest. Typically, fragmented or irregular apophysis is shown on lateral radiographs; however, ossicle separated from the tibial tubercle may also present (Figure 14.3). Treatment should begin with rest, icing, and nonsteroidal anti-inflammatory drugs, and focus on stretching and strengthening exercises not only for the quadriceps and hamstrings but also for all lower extremity muscles. Braces, tape, or a slip-on knee support with an infrapatellar pad or strap may be useful if the athlete proposes to continue with the sporting activity. OSD is self-limited and will generally improve without any serious consequences or impairment of function. Rarely, a small ossicle may remain painful and this requires surgical extirpation.

Sinding-Larsen-Johansson disease (described by Sinding-Larsen and Johansson independently in 1921 and 1922, respectively) resembles OSD, and, at times, these two conditions may coexist.[52] Osteochondrosis of the lower part of the patella develops as a result of persistent traction from a tight patella tendon (Figure 14.4). It usually appears in active boys aged 9 to 12, and girls aged 7 to 10 years, especially in those participating in sports requiring stooping, sitting, or squatting. Pain and tenderness are localized over the lower part of the patella and quadriceps muscle tightness is usually present as well. Treatment is similar to that used for OSD and prognosis is very good.

Sever disease (first described by Sever in 1912) or calcaneal apophysites develops as a result of a repetitive force produced by a tight Achilles tendon and plantar fascia, in 61% of cases with bilateral involvement.[60,63] This disorder is frequent in field sports involving running, hiking, jumping, and kicking, presenting in athletes between the ages of 9 and 12. Clinical examination reveals a point of tenderness at the posterior aspect of the heel, and dorsiflexion of the ankle is limited. Typically, no tenderness over the plantar fascia is elicited. Tightness of the Achilles tendon may be noted. Swelling is not common and may indicate bursitis or stress fracture. The onset of Sever disease is usually associated with the beginning of the season, or with changes in footwear and training surface. Initially, it is present only during the sporting activity and improves with rest, but with continued activity it may persist throughout the day. Plain radiographs show some type of disorderly ossification of the calcaneal apophysis, either as fragmentation, incomplete appearance, or complete formation with increased sclerosis (Figure 14.5). Differential diagnosis includes other possible causes of heel pain such as stress fractures, calcaneal cyst, and posterior ankle

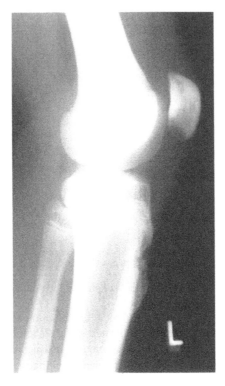

FIGURE 14.3 Lateral radiograph of the knee demonstrates Osgood-Schlatter disease in a 12-year-old soccer player.

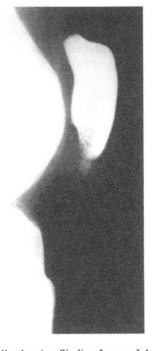

FIGURE 14.4 Lateral radiograph of the patella showing Sinding-Larsen-Johansson disease.

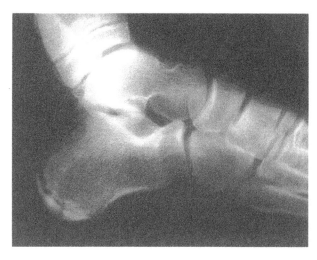

FIGURE 14.5 Lateral radiograph of the foot with typical findings of Sever disease in a 11-year-old soccer player.

impingement. Treatment depends on the severity of the symptoms and should begin with rest and icing, followed by stretching and strengthening exercises of the gastrocnemius-soleus muscle.[79,83] Heel lift (1 to 2 cm) is another important measure to relieve calf muscle tension. The disorder is self-limiting and generally heals in a period of 12 to 18 months, during which exacerbation of the symptoms shows a sinusoidal pattern.

Iselin disease (first described by Iselin in 1912) is the osteochondrosis of the base of the fifth metatarsal. Tightness of the peroneus brevis tendon produces recurrent microtears of the apophyses, and a low-grade inflammatory response occurs.[42] The condition is usually seen in adolescents participating in sports that involve running, jumping, or skating. Inversion stress is a mechanism that produces repetitive microstress to the apophyses. The pain over the base of the fifth metatarsal is the leading symptom, and usually there is no history of trauma. Plain radiographs may show irregular apophyses, slightly larger and minimally separated from the rest of the metatarsal when compared with the contralateral side. Bone scan scintigraphy is usually positive. Treatment includes rest, icing, and physical therapy for stretching and strengthening of the peroneal musculature. Although the prognosis is good and bony union eventually occurs, bony overgrowth can sometimes result in slightly larger base of fifth metatarsal that may be a problem for shoe fitting.

Little League elbow (LLE) is a syndrome resulting from lateral compression and medial tension to the elbow. This group of disorders is frequently seen in athletes participating in throwing sports such as baseball, handball, water polo, and badminton, and develops as a result of repetitive valgus strain on the elbow.[7,11,20,29,38] The term was first used in 1960 by Brogden to describe a case of apophyseal avulsion of the medial epicondyle in a young baseball pitcher. Since then, many other conditions have been included in the general classification of LLE. The most frequently encountered component of the LLE syndrome is *medial epicondylitis* or Adams disease (named after Adams who reported it in 1968 as a part of LLE). Strong, repetitive traction forces produced by wrist pronators and flexors can result in microavulsions and fragmentation of the medial epicondyle apophyses. Symptoms include pain and tenderness over the medial side of the elbow and are usually present weeks before medical care is sought. Hypertrophy of the affected arm, valgus deformity, and flexion contracture are also common findings in LLE. Plain roentgenographs may reveal fragmentation, sclerosis, and widening of the epicondylar apophysis. Treatment consists of the cessation of activity, icing, and stretching and strengthening exercises. Lateral compression injuries of the capitellar ossification center include two entities: *Panner disease* and *osteochondritis dissecans* (Figure 14.6). Panner disease is a disorder of unknown origin that affects children aged

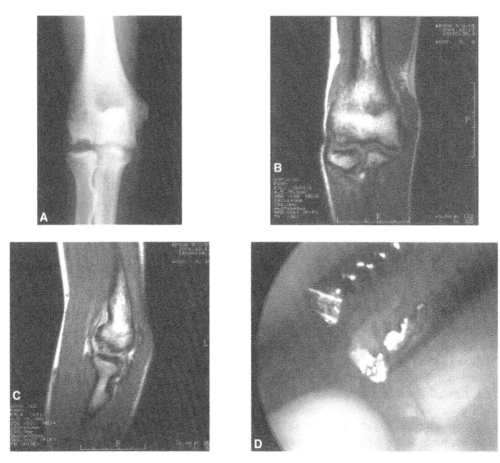

FIGURE 14.6 Osteochondritis dissecans of the elbow in a 15-year-old gymnast. (A) Anteroposterior radiograph; (B) coronal T1-weighted MR image; (C) sagittal T1-weighted MR image; (D) arthroscopic removal of the loose body of the same patient.

7 to 12 years. It affects capitellar ossification centers in terms of degeneration and necrosis followed by regeneration and recalcification. Symptoms include dull pain in the elbow, aggravated by activity, accompanied by swelling and inability to fully extend the elbow. Plain radiography shows fragmentation, subchondral radiolucency, and sometimes loose body formation. Treatment consists of rest and immobilization until symptoms have subsided. Throwing activity should not be reintroduced before radiographic resolution occurs. Osteochondritis dissecans is described further in this chapter.

2. Physeal Injuries

In this group of disorders, repetitive stress causes injuries of the growth cartilage plate or physes. These types of overuse injuries are not very common but two entities should be mentioned: proximal humerus physeal injury in throwers and pitchers (also known as Little League shoulder) and distal radius physeal injury in gymnasts.

Little League shoulder is the condition most frequently seen in young baseball pitchers, badminton players, and athletes participating in throwing sports (water polo, handball).[70,73,91] It occurs between ages 12 and 15 with gradual or sudden onset of pain in the throwing shoulder. Clinical examination reveals no abnormalities except tenderness over the proximal humerus. Diagnosis is based on plain radiography that shows widening of the proximal humeral physis.

The treatment includes rest and icing, followed by strength, endurance, and flexibility conditioning. Sporting activity may be resumed after the resolution of the physeal changes has been radiologically demonstrated.

Distal radial growth plate injuries are common in competitive gymnasts.[92] Repetitive compression forces applied over the distal radial growth plate during training and competition may result in injury.[14,29,41] Clinical examination reveals a point tenderness and pain over the distal radius and a decreased range of motion in the radiocarpal joint. Plain radiographs show widening and failure of the proximal radial physes calcification zone. Treatment consists of rest and, if necessary, short-term cast immobilization for rest compliance. The prognosis is usually very good, although a decrease in the growth of distal radius with continued growth of ulna might result in relative overgrowth of ulna with respect to the radius.[49]

3. Articular Cartilage Injuries

Osteochondritis dissecans (OCD) is a condition where focal avascular necrosis occurs in subchondral bone as the primary pathologic process, with secondary involvement of overlying cartilage. Sometimes the involved osteochondral fragment separates from its bed, forming a loose body. The etiology of this condition is not yet fully understood. Primary vascular insult of the subchondral bone was originally thought to be the most important cause of OCD. However, several researchers recently proposed repetitive microtrauma or acute macrotrauma to be more likely causes.[16] There are three most common localizations where OCD occurs: medial femoral condyle of the knee, posterior medial surface of the talus, and anterolateral portion of the humeral capitellum (Figure 14.7 and Figure 14.8).[43,63,87] Patients typically present with vague, poorly localized symptoms, which include activity-related pain, catching, swelling, and instability. More often than not, no single trauma preceding the onset of symptoms is identifiable. Instead, a recent increase in the intensity of sporting activity is a common anamnestic indicator. Physical examination may reveal signs of internal derangement with effusion and restricted joint motion. Depending on the stage of the injury, plain radiography ranges from well-demarcated hyperlucent areas to irregular areas of ossification representing isolated osteochondral fragments. Bilateral findings occur in 25 to 30% of cases.[51] Computerized tomography (CT) and magnetic resonance (MR) with/without contrast may delineate the extent of the bony and cartilage involvement, but are not routinely used in diagnosis of OCD.[39] Treatment for OCD may be conservative or surgical. Non-operative treatment is recommended for young athletes whose articular surface has remained intact, and treatment should include rest from activity and use of crutches during the acute phase, followed by recreational cycling and swimming once symptoms subside. Stretching and strengthening exercises should be introduced in the final phase, as a part of rehabilitation. Surgical treatment is indicated when conservative treatment fails to show any progression, or when the articular cartilage is damaged. Operative treatment options include arthroscopic internal fixation with metallic or bioresorbable pins or screws, filling the defect with a paste of mortilized autologous cartilage and bone taken from the joint, core autographs harvested with one of the commercially available systems, or autologous cell culture grafting.[10,30,86] The status of the physis is the most important prognostic factor. If the physis is still open, as is the case in children and young adolescents, there is a higher probability of healing without degenerative changes.[43]

Köhler disease is ischemic necrosis of the tarsal navicular. Repetitive microtrauma is thought to be the main etiological factor, and there is a large predominance in active, male children ages 4 to 7. The main symptom is activity-related pain over the medial aspect of the foot. Plain radiography shows collapse and narrowing of the navicular with occasional fragmentation. The condition is self-limiting and does not require surgical treatment.[35] Initial treatment includes decreased activity and use of orthotics to support the medial section of the foot. A leg cast for a period of 3 to 6 weeks may be helpful in promoting relief.

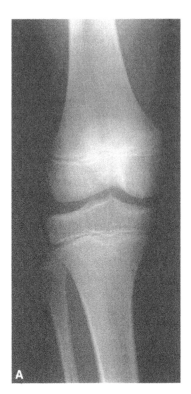

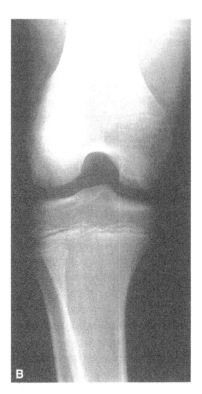

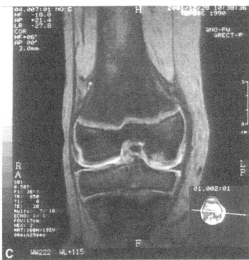

FIGURE 14.7 Osteochondritis dissecans of the knee in a 12-year-old track-and-field athlete. (A) Anteroposterior radiograph; (B) tunnel radiograph; (C) coronal STIR magnetic resonance (MR) image.

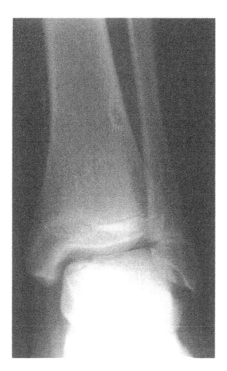

FIGURE 14.8 Anteroposterior radiograph showing osteochondritis dissecans of the posteromedial talar dome in a 15-year-old basketball player.

Frieberg disease is avascular necrosis of the second metatarsal epiphysis. There is female predomination and the average age of presentation is 13.[63] Repetitive stress and a short first metatarsal are thought to be main contributing factors. Clinical examination reveals pain and tenderness over the metatarsophalangeal joint and a decreased range of motion. Plain radiography shows irregularity and collapse, as well as a narrowing of joint space. The treatment is conservative and includes rest, application of orthosis, and occasionally a leg cast for a brief period of time.

B. STRESS FRACTURES

Stress fractures occur when repetitive stress overpowers the bone's ability to repair itself. Repetitive microstrains produce microdamage to the tissue, and the subsequent reparatory processes induce the symptoms. Chapter 12 contains a detailed description of the etiology, epidemiology, diagnostics, treatment, and rehabilitation of stress fractures. The female athlete triad and the strong connection between eating disorders, amenorrhea, and osteoporosis (resulting in stress fractures) are described in Chapter 15. Here, we briefly discuss specific aspects of stress fractures in the adolescent athlete.

Stress fractures are less frequent in children and adults, but the incidence increases throughout late childhood and adolescence. In a series of 368 patients, Orava and Hulkho found an incidence of 10% in children under 15 years and 32% in adolescents between 16 and 19 years of age.[65] Furthermore, increased participation of adolescents in top athletic activities contributes to the rise in the incidence of stress fractures in this population segment. In addition, stress fractures are distributed somewhat differently in adolescent athletes. As is the case with adults, tibia represents approximately half of the pediatric and adolescent stress fractures, followed by fibula (20%). Pars interarticularis of the lumbar vertebrae is the next localization (15%), and this injury is more common in adolescents, particularly among gymnasts and football players.[27] Other localizations that seem to be more common in children and adolescents are distal femur (Figure 14.9) and metatarsal stress fractures (Figure 14.10).[67,69]

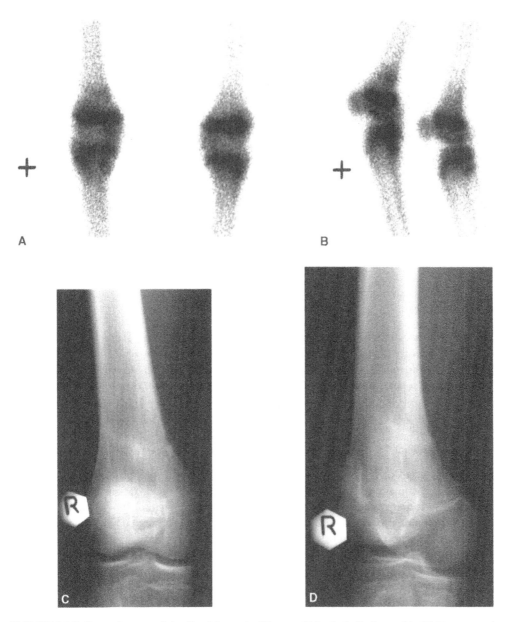

FIGURE 14.9 Stress fracture of the distal femur in 15-year-old basketball player. (A, B) Bone scan demonstrating increased radioisotope uptake; (C, D) AP and LL radiographs taken at presentation; (E, F) AP and LL radiographs after 6 weeks; (G, H) AP and LL radiographs after 12 weeks before resuming sports activities.

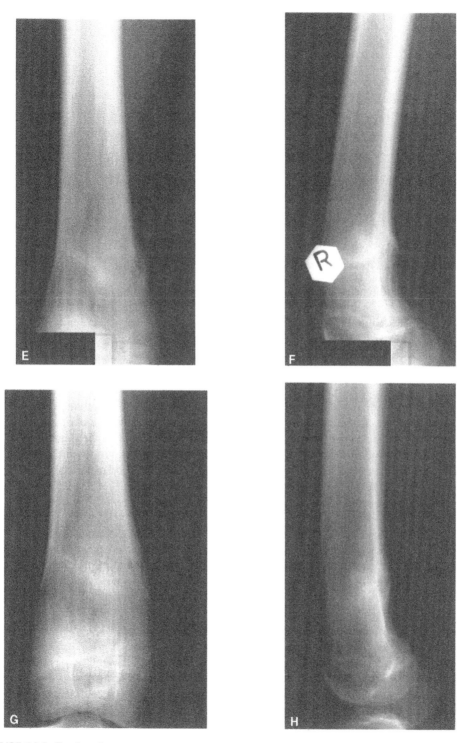

FIGURE 14.9 Continued.

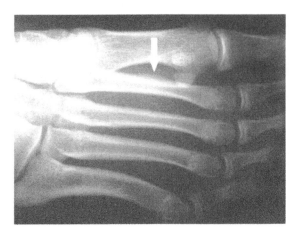

FIGURE 14.10 Lateral radiograph of the foot demonstrating stress fracture of the second metatarsal in a 13-year-old female basketball player.

C. ARTICULAR MALALIGNMENT AND INSTABILITY

This group of overuse injuries is characterized by osseous malalignment or imbalance of muscular and ligamentous soft tissues about the joint. These abnormalities cause biomechanical alterations that result in pain and instability syndromes. Most frequently affected are patellofemoral and glenohumeral joints described in more detail in the relevant chapters of this book.

V. CONCLUSION

With the increasing participation of children and adolescents in organized sporting activity, overuse injuries in this age group are becoming increasingly common. Of all the factors contributing to this situation discussed in this chapter, it is training malpractice — particularly a "too much, too soon" approach — that has the most significant impact.[47] Young athletes must never be treated as undersized adults, and their training schedules must be adjusted to the level of maturity of their musculoskeletal system.[53,76] Prevention is the key word in matters concerning overuse injuries in this age group, and the most important measures include preparticipation in physical evaluation and prehabilitation programs.

Preparticipation physical evaluation (PPE) should be carried out 4 to 6 weeks prior to initiation of athletic activity, and revisited once a year. Its purpose is to determine the young athlete's general health and maturity level, as well as to uncover any disqualifying conditions.[8,45,54,55] The most important part of the PPE is the athlete's history, followed by basic and focused physical examination.

Prehabilitation is a term used to describe the process of pre-season conditioning of young athletes. Its aim is to address and correct potential strength and flexibility shortfalls, as well as to prepare the athlete for more intensive and strenuous activity during the upcoming season. Pre-season conditioning can reduce the injury rate to up to 63%.[13]

In conclusion, a good relationship and understanding among the young athlete, coach, parents, and the treating physician are essential in the prevention of acute and overuse injuries alike. Physical and psychological health benefits — the main objective for childhood and adolescent participation in organized sport — must never be disregarded.

REFERENCES

1. **Aegter, E. and Kirkpatrick, J.A.** *Orthopaedic Diseases*, 4th ed. Philadelphia: W.B. Saunders, 1975.
2. **Bar-Or, O.** The young athlete: some physiological considerations. *J. Sports Sci.*, 1995; 13: S31–33.
3. **Baxter-Jones, A., Maffuli, N., and Helms, P.** Low injury rates in elite athletes. *Arch. Dis. Child*, 1993; 68(1): 130–132.
4. **Benezis, C., Simeray, J., and Simon, L.** *Muscles, Tendon et Sport.* Paris: Masson, 1990; 187–197.
5. **Bernhardt, D.T. and Landry, G.L.** Sports injuries in young athletes. *Adv. Pediatr.*, 1995; 42: 465–500.
6. **Best, T.M.** Muscle-tendon injuries in young athletes. *Clin. Sports Med.*, 1995; 14(3): 669–686.
7. **Blohm, D., Kaalund, S., and Jakobsen, B.W.** "Little League elbow" — acute traction apophysitis in an adolescent badminton player. *Scand. J. Med. Sci. Sports*, 1999; 9: 245–247.
8. **Bratton, R.L.** Preparticipation screening of children for sports. Current recommendations. *Sports Med.*, 1997; 24(5): 300–307.
9. **Bright, R.W., Burstein, A.H., and Elmore, S.M.** Epiphyseal plate cartilage: a biochemical and histological analysis of failure models. *J. Bone Joint Surg.*, 1974; 56A: 688–705.
10. **Brittberg, M., Lindahl, A, Nilsson, A. et al.** Treatment of deep cartilage defects in the knee with autologous chondrocyte transplantation. *N. Engl. J. Med.*, 1994; 331: 889–895.
11. **Bylak, J. and Hutchinson, M.R.** Common sports injuries in young tennis players. *Sports Med.*, 1998; 26(2): 119–132.
12. **Cahill, B.R.** Stress fracture of the proximal tibia epiphysis: a case report. *Am. J. Sports Med.*, 1977; 5(5): 186–187.
13. **Cahill, B.R. and Griffith, E.H.** Effect of preseason conditioning on the incidence and severity of high school football injuries. *Am. J. Sports Med.*, 1978; 6: 180–184.
14. **Cain, D., Roy, S., Singer, K.M. et al.** Stress changes of the distal radial growth plate: a radiographic survey and review of the literature. *Am. J. Sports Med.*, 1992; 20(3): 290–298.
15. **Clain, M.R. and Hershman, E.B.** Overuse injuries in children and adolescents. *Phys. Sportsmed.*, 1989; 17: 111–123.
16. **Clanton, T.O. and Dellee, J.C.** Osteochondritis dissecans: history, pathophysiology and current treatment concepts. *Clin. Orthop.*, 1982; 167: 50–64.
17. **Cohen, A.R. and Metzl, J.D.** Sports-specific concerns in the young athlete: basketball. *Pediatr. Emerg. Care*, 2000; 16(6): 462–468.
18. **Cook, S.D., Brinker, M.R., and Poche, M.** Running shoes: their relationship to running injuries. *Sports Med.*, 1998; 6: 427–466.
19. **Dalton, S.E.** Overuse injuries in adolescent athletes. *Sports Med.*, 1992; 13: 58–70.
20. **DaSilva, M.F., Williams, J.S., Fadale, P.D., Hulstyn, M.J., and Ehrlich, M.G.** Pediatric throwing injuries about the elbow. *Am. J. Orthop.*, 1998; 27(2): 90–96.
21. **Dubravšić-Šimunjak, S., Pećina, M., Kuipers, H., Moran, J., and Hašpl, M.** The incidence of injuries in elite junior figure skaters. *Am. J. Sports Med.*, 2003; 31: in press.
22. **Dugdale, T.W. and Barnett, P.R.** Historical background: patellofemoral pain in young people. *Orthop. Clin. North. Am.*, 1986; 17: 211–219.
23. **Dupuis, J.M.** Croissance et sport. *Actual. Sport Med.*, 1992; 18: 10–16.
24. **Đapić, T., Antićević, D., and Čapin, T.** Overuse injuries in children and adolescents. *Arch. Hyg. Indust. Toxicol.*, 2001; 52: 483–489.
25. **Emery, H.M.** Considerations in child and adolescent athletes. *Rheum. Dis. Clin. North. Am.*, 1996; 22(3): 499–513.
26. **Fricker, P.** The young athlete. *Aust. Fam. Physician.*, 1999; 28(6): 543–547.
27. **Gerbino, P.G., II and Micheli, L.J.** Back injuries in the young athlete. *Clin. Sports Med.*, 1995; 14(3): 571–590.
28. **Gerrard, D.F.** Overuse injury and growing bones: the young athlete at risk. *Br. J. Sports. Med.*, 1993; 27(1): 14–18.
29. **Gill, T.J., IV and Micheli, L.J.** The immature athlete. Common injuries and overuse syndromes of the elbow and wrist. *Clin. Sports Med.*, 1996; 15(2): 401–423.
30. **Hangody, L., Kish, G., Karpati, Z. et al.** MosaicPlasty for the treatment of reticular cartilage defects: application in clinical practice. *Orthopaedics*, 1998; 21: 751–756.

31. **Harvey, J. and Tanner, S.** Low back pain in young athletes. A practical approach. *Sports Med.,* 1991; 12(6): 394–406.

32. **Hawkins, D. and Andersson, H.L.** Overuse injuries in youth sports: biomechanical considerations. *Med. Sci. Sports Exerc.,* 2001; 33: 1701–1707.

33. **d'Hemecourt, P.A., Gerbino, P.G., II, and Micheli, L.J.** Back injuries in the young athlete. *Clin. Sports Med.,* 2000; 19(4): 663–679.

34. **Ikata, T., Morita, T., Katoh, S., Tachibana, K., and Maoka, H.** Lesions of the lumbar posterior end plate in children and adolescents. An MRI study. *J. Bone Joint Surg.,* 1995; 77: 951–955.

35. **Ippolito, E., Ricciari-Pollini, P.T., and Falez, F.** Koehler's disease of tarsal navicular. Long-term follow up of 12 cases. *J. Pediatr. Orthop,* 1984; 4(4): 416–417.

36. **Katz, J.F.** Nonarticular osteochondroses. *Clin. Orthop.,* 1981; 158: 70–76.

37. **Khan, K., McKay, H.A., Haapasalo, H., Bennell, K.L., Forwood, M.R., Kannus, P., and Wark, J.D.** Does childhood and adolescence provide a unique opportunity for exercise to strengthen the skeleton? *J. Sci. Med. Sport,* 2000; 3(2): 150–164.

38. **Kibler, W.B. and Safran, M.R.** Musculoskeletal injuries in the young tennis player. *Clin Sports Med.,* 2000; 19(4): 781–792.

39. **Kramer, J., Stiglbauer, L., Engle, A., Prayer, K., and Imhof, H.** MR contrast artrography (MRA) in osteochondritis dissecans. *J. Comput. Assist. Tomogr.,* 1992; 16: 254–260.

40. **Lai, A.M., Stanish, W.D., and Stanish, H.I.** The young athlete with physical challenges. *Clin. Sports Med.,* 2000; 19(4): 793–819.

41. **Le, T.B. and Hentz, V.R.** Hand and wrist injuries in young athletes. *Hand Clin.,* 2000; 16(4): 597–607.

42. **Lehman, R.C., Gregg, J.R., and Torg, E.** Iselin's disease. *Am. J. Sports Med.,* 1986; 14: 494–496.

43. **Linden, B.** Osteochondritis dissecans of the femoral condyle: a long-term follow-up study. *J. Bone Joint Surg.,* 1977; 59(6): 769–776.

44. **Longis, B., Surzur, P., and Moulies, D.** Apophysites de croissance. *Actual. Sport Med.,* 1992; 19: 9–10.

45. **Lysens, R.J., Ostyn, M.S., Auweele, Y.V., Lefevre, J., Vuylsteke, M. et al.** The accident-prone and overuse-prone profiles of the young athlete. *Am. J. Sports Med.,* 1989; 17: 612–619.

46. **Maffulli, N.** Injuries in young athletes. *Eur. J. Pediatr.,* 2000; 15: 959–963.

47. **Maffulli, N.** Intensive training in young athletes. The orthopaedic surgeon's viewpoint. *Sports Med.,* 1990; 9: 229–243.

48. **Maffulli, N. and Baxter-Jones, A.D.** Common skeletal injuries in young athletes. *Sports Med.,* 1995; 19(2): 137–149.

49. **Mandelbaum, B.R., Bartolozzi, A.R., Davis, C.A. et al.** Wrist pain syndrome in the gymnast. Pathogenic, diagnostic and therapeutic considerations. *Am. J. Sports Med.,* 1989; 17: 305–317.

50. **Marsh, J.S. and Daigneault, J.P.** The young athlete. *Curr. Opin. Pediatr.,* 1999; 11(1): 84–88.

51. **McCoy, R.L., II, Dec, K.L., McKeag, D.B., and Honing, E.W.** Common injuries in the child or adolescent athlete. *Primary Care,* 1995; 22(1): 117–144.

52. **Medlar, R.C., Lyne, E.D., and Sohn, R.S.** Sinding-Larsen-Johansson disease: etiology and natural history. *J. Bone Joint Surg.,* 1978; 60A: 1113–1116.

53. **Metcalf, J.A. and Roberts, S.O.** Strength training and the immature athlete: an overview. *Pediatr. Nurs.,* 1993; 19(4): 325–332.

54. **Metzl, J.D.** Preparticipation examination of the adolescent athlete: part 1. *Pediatr. Rev.,* 2001; 22(6): 199–204.

55. **Metzl, J.D.** Preparticipation examination of the adolescent athlete: part 2. *Pediatr. Rev.,* 2001; 22(7): 227–239.

56. **Metzl, J.D. and Micheli, L.J.** Youth soccer: an epidemiologic perspective. *Clin. Sports Med.,* 1998; 17(4): 663–673.

57. **Micheli, L.J.** Overuse injuries in children's sports: the growth factor. *Orthop. Clin. North Am.,* 1983; 14: 337–359.

58. **Micheli, L.J.** The traction apophysitis. *Clin. Sports Med.,* 1987; 6: 389–404.

59. **Micheli, L.J.** Sports injuries in children and adolescents. Questions and controversies. *Clin. Sports Med.,* 1995; 14: 727–745.

60. **Micheli, L.J. and Ireland, M.L.** Prevention and management of calcaneal apophysitis in children: an overuse syndrome. *J. Pediatr. Orthop.,* 1987; 7: 34–38.

61. **Moreland, M.S.** Special concerns of the paediatric athlete. In *Sports Injuries: Mechanism, Prevention, Treatment*, 2nd ed., Fu, F.H. and Stone, D.A., Eds. Philadelphia: Lippincott/Williams & Wilkins, 2002.

62. **Naughton, G., Farpour-Lambert, N.J., Carlson, J., Bradney, M., and Van Praagh, E.** Physiological issues surrounding the performance of adolescent athletes. *Sports Med.*, 2000; 30(5): 309–325.

63. **Omey, M.L. and Micheli, L.J.** Foot and ankle problems in the young athlete. *Med. Sci. Sports Exerc.*, 1999; 31: 470–486.

64. **O'Neill, D.B. and Micheli, L.J.** Overuse injuries in the young athlete. *Clin. Sports Med.*, 1988; 7: 591–610.

65. **Orava, S. and Hulkko, A.** Stress fractures in young athletes. *Arch. Orthop. Trauma Surg.*, 1981; 98: 271–274.

66. **Osgood, R.B.** Lesion of the tibial tubercle occurring during adolescence. *Boston Med. Surg. J.*, 1903; 148: 114.

67. **Ostlie, D.K. and Simons, S.M.** Tarsal navicular stress fracture in a young athlete: case report with clinical, radiologic, and pathophysiologic correlations. *J. Am. Board Fam. Pract.*, 2001; 14(5): 381–385.

68. **Outerbridge, A.R.** Overuse injuries in the young athlete. *Clin. Sports Med.*, 1995; 14: 503–515.

69. **Paletta, G.A., Jr. and Andrish, J.T.** Injuries about the hip and pelvis in the young athlete. *Clin. Sports Med.*, 1995; 14(3): 591–628.

70. **Paterson, P.D. and Waters, P.M.** Shoulder injuries in the childhood athlete. *Clin. Sports Med.*, 2000; 19(4): 681–692.

71. **Peck, D.M.** Apophyseal injuries in the young athlete. *Am. Fam. Physician.*, 1995; 51(8): 1891–1898.

72. **Pizzutillo, P.D.** Spinal considerations in the young athlete. *Instr. Course. Lect.*, 1993; 42: 463–472.

73. **Podesta, L., Sherman, M.F., and Bonamo, J.R.** Distal humeral epiphyseal separation in a young athlete: a case report. *Arch. Phys. Med. Rehabil.*, 1993; 74(11): 1216–1218.

74. **Proctor, M.R. and Cantu, R.C.** Head and neck injuries in young athletes. *Clin. Sports Med.*, 2000; 19(4): 693–715.

75. **Roemmich, J.N. and Rogol, A.D.** Physiology of growth and development. Its relationship to performance in the young athlete. *Clin. Sports Med.*, 1995; 14(3): 483–502.

76. **Rooks, D.S. and Micheli, L.J.** Musculoskeletal assessment and training: the young athlete. *Clin. Sports Med.*, 1988; 7(3): 641–677.

77. **Saperstein, A.L. and Nicholas, S.J.** Pediatric and adolescent sports medicine. *Pediatr. Clin. North Am.*, 1996; 43(5): 1013–1033.

78. **Sassmannshausen, G. and Smith, B.G.** Back pain in the young athlete. *Clin Sports Med.*, 2002; 21(1): 121–132.

79. **Sever, J.W.** Apophysites of the os calcus. *N.Y. Med.*, 1912; 95: 1025–1029.

80. **Shaffer, T.E.** The uniqueness of the young athlete: introductory remarks. *Am. J. Sports Med.*, 1980; 8(5): 370–371.

81. **Siffert, R.** Classification of osteochondroses. *Clin. Orthop.*, 1981; 158: 10–18.

82. **Smith, A.D.** The young skater. *Clin. Sports Med.*, 2000; 19(4): 741–755.

83. **Stanish, W.D.** Lower leg, foot, and ankle injuries in young athletes. *Clin. Podiatr. Med. Surg.*, 1997; 14(3): 559–578.

84. **Stanitski, C.L.** Management of sports injuries in children and adolescents. *Orthop. Clin. North Am.*, 1988; 19: 689–697.

85. **Stiles, D.A., Gibbons, J.L., Sebben, D.J., and Wiley, D.C.** Why adolescent boys dream of becoming professional athletes. *Psychol. Rep.*, 1999; 84: 1075–1085.

86. **Stone, K. and Walgenback, A.** A surgical technique for articular cartilage transplantation to full thickness cartilage defects in the knee joint — operative techniques. *Orthopaedics*, 1997; 7: 305–310.

87. **Stubbs, M.J., Field, L.D., and Savoie, F.H., III.** Osteochondritis dissecans of the elbow. *Clin. Sports Med.*, 2001; 20(1): 1–9.

88. **Tanner, J.M., Whitehouse, R.H., and Takashi, M.** Standards from birth to maturity for height, weight, height velocity, and weight velocity: British children. *Arch. Dis. Child.*, 1966; 41: 613–635.

89. **Van de Loo, D.A. and Johnson, M.D.** The young female athlete. *Clin. Sports Med.* 1995; 14(3): 687–707.

90. **Watkins, J. and Peabody, P.** Sports injuries in children and adolescents treated at a sports injury clinic. *J. Sports Med. Phys. Fitness*, 1996; 36(1): 43–48.

91. **Yen, K.L and Metzl, J.D.** Sports-specific concerns in the young athlete: baseball. *Pediatr. Emerg. Care,* 2000; 16(3): 215–220.
92. **Zetaruk, M.N.** The young gymnast. *Clin. Sports Med.,* 2000; 19: 757–780.

15 Overuse Injuries in Female Athletes*

In ancient Greek society only men were allowed to participate in the Olympic Games; this held true for the first modern Olympic Games in Athens in 1896, as well. However, some 100 years later in Sydney 2000, 4096 women from all around the world competed in the majority of the 300 official Olympic events. Apart from top-level and professional sport, there has been also a dramatic increase of women's sports participation on the recreational and amateur level. In the U.S., a crucial turning point was the passage of Title IX of the Educational Assistance Act in 1972, which required institutions receiving federal funds to offer women equal opportunities in all areas.[61] Since that time, high school and collegiate female participation has increased by >600% to a total of 1.9 million female athletes.[95]

The tremendous increase in female sport participation during the last two decades has offered scientists and clinicians valuable data concerning the physiologic and pathological issues of the exercising female. This chapter provides basic information on the most frequent overuse injuries and syndromes in female athletes in a context of the anatomic, physiologic, and psychological differences between genders.

I. EPIDEMIOLOGY

In the past, most studies were male oriented, and the majority of epidemiological data concerning female sport participation has been gathered in the last 20 years. Since 1982, *National Collegiate Athletic Association Surveillance System* has been published with detailed injury information in 16 sports, and many other studies have compared male and female incidence of injury in similar sports.[19,76,94] According to the limited available data two main conclusions may be drawn. First, women appear to suffer the same kind of injuries as men, i.e., athletic injuries tend to be sport and not gender related, and second, it appears that overuse injuries occur more often in women than in men.[80]

Some overuse injuries such as patellofemoral pain syndrome, stress fractures, or lateral epicondylitis are especially prevalent in female athletes. For example, it was reported that the incidence of lateral epicondylitis in women between the ages of 42 and 46 is 10%, compared with 1 to 5% in the general population.[1] The incidence of patellofemoral pain syndrome in women is 20%, compared with 7.4% in men, and the incidence of recurrent patellar dislocation is six times higher in women than in men.[19] Several series have reported increased incidence of stress fractures among female military personnel and athletes.[51,59,64,70]

II. SPECIAL CONSIDERATIONS OF THE FEMALE ATHLETE

A. ANATOMIC CONSIDERATIONS

Bones and joints. Women have shorter and smaller limbs relative to body length than men. For example, men have longer lower extremities, comprising 56% of their total height compared to 51.2% in women.[35] Longer bones act as more powerful levers, producing more force when striking

---

* Co-authored by Alan Ivković.

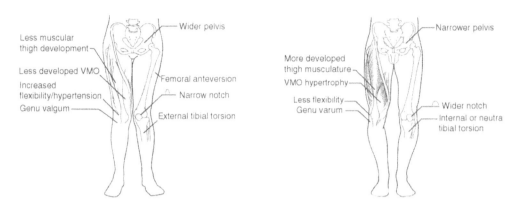

FIGURE 15.1 Figures show lower extremity anatomic differences between genders (female, left; male, right) that may predispose females to certain overuse injuries. Note wider pelvis, femoral anteversion, genu valgum, external tibial torsion, increased Q angle, less developed musculature, and narrow femoral notch.

or kicking.[40] Shorter limbs along with narrower shoulders and elbow valgus can contribute to altered mechanics when throwing or pitching. Because of their shorter stature and wider pelvis, women have a lower center of gravity, which gives them substantial advantage in some athletic disciplines where balance control is essential (e.g., gymnastics).[36] Additionally, a wider pelvis can produce varus of the hips, increased femoral anteversion, and genu valgum, resulting in increased Q angle, which is known to be a predisposing factor for patellofemoral problems. Abnormal values for Q angle are considered to be more than 10° in men and 15° for women (Figure 15.1).[45]

Muscles. Before puberty, muscle mass is pretty much the same in boys and girls, but during puberty, through the influence of the testosterone, boys accumulate greater muscle mass. In adults, total cross-sectional area of muscles in women is 60 to 80% that of men.[18] Further, there are gender differences in the balance between muscle groups. Women have decreased muscle strength ratios between the quadriceps and hamstrings group than men. Also, the quadriceps is the predominant stabilizer of the knee joint in women, whereas the hamstring group is more important in men.[43] However, the importance of this observation is not fully understood and requires additional investigation.

Ligaments. The widely accepted belief that women have increased ligamentous laxity and are, therefore, more prone to injuries is only partially true. It is known that increased levels of relaxin during pregnancy and puerperium increase ligamentous laxity to facilitate changes in sacroiliac joints and the pubic symphysis. This is important for enlargement of the pelvic outlet during childbirth. The role of cyclical estrogen and progesterone production is yet to be determined.

B. PHYSIOLOGIC CONSIDERATIONS

During the prepubertal years boys and girls do not differ much in terms of height, weight, heart size, or aerobic capability. After the onset of puberty, the principal gender differences are due to stabilization of the reproductive hormonal axis. Proper estrogen serum levels are necessary for women to obtain maximum peak bone mass during the second and third decade.

Adult females have 22 to 26% fat per body weight and males have 12 to 16%. Androgens are responsible for greater lean body weight in males, and estrogen contributes to the greater amount of fat weight.[96] Also, women have a higher amount of essential fat (9 to 12%) than men (3%) because of the fat in sex-specific tissues.[60] It was previously thought that there was a critical level of body fat necessary to maintain normal menstrual function. Although this theory is not supported in the literature, it should be kept in mind that possibly there is an individual threshold of body fat necessary for normal menstrual cycle.

For the same body weight, female athletes have smaller heart sizes, lower diastolic and systolic pressures, and smaller lungs, which decreases female athlete effectiveness in both aerobic and anaerobic activities. Maximum oxygen consumption (VO_2 max) reflects the body's ability to extract and utilize oxygen and is used as a measure for aerobic metabolism; women have a lower VO_2 max baseline.[17,34,85]

C. PSYCHOLOGICAL CONSIDERATIONS

In all Western cultures athletic participation was traditionally considered a man's thing. Aggressiveness, achievement, fortitude, and desire to win and conquer were masculine, not feminine qualities. Thus, it is sadly true that "the winning male athlete has just proved his masculinity, whereas the winning female often needs to justify her femininity."[10] This kind of prejudice may lead to depression and anxiety episodes because the female athlete feels she is not meeting the perceived expectations of her sex. In addition, women have been found to be lower in dominance and confidence and higher in impulsiveness, tension, and general anxiety. Outlined characteristics are known to be contributing psychological factors to development of eating disorders as part of the female athlete triad syndrome, which is discussed later in this chapter.

III. THE FEMALE ATHLETE TRIAD

Disordered eating, amenorrhea, and osteoporosis are the main constituents of the syndrome described in 1992 by the American College of Sports Medicine and termed the *female athlete triad*.[100] Although each of the three problems may develop independently, the syndrome is in fact a cascade of interrelated pathophysiological events, resulting in the clinical picture of the female athlete triad. By acting synergistically, strenuous exercise and disordered eating induce menstrual disorders and hypoestrogenism, which is responsible for decreased bone mineral density (BMD) and osteoporosis.[47] The obvious consequence of this vicious circle is greater risk of stress fractures.

A. DISORDERED EATING

This arm of the triad encompasses a wide spectrum of disorders ranging from occasional meal skipping and calorie avoiding to anorexia and bulimia nervosa. The main question is: Why do young female athletes become so obsessed with their physical appearance?

Risk factors for development of disordered eating include *Western sociocultural norms*, which attribute thinness to beauty, power, and control; *psychologic factors* such as poor coping skills, low self-esteem, general anxiety, and depression; and *gender*: 90% of patients suffering from disordered eating are women.[50] Furthermore, it is known that there are certain athletic disciplines, such as ballet, figure skating, gymnastics, distance running, etc., that emphasize low body weight and thinness of the competitors (Table 15.1).[15] For example, both the age and weight of gymnasts and ice skaters competing in the Olympics have been decreasing. In 1976, the mean weight of female gymnasts was 48.1 kg and, in 1992, it was 37.6 kg. The mean height during the same period decreased from 1.61 m to 1.44 m, as did the mean age, which fell from 18 years to 16 years.[79]

TABLE 15.1
Sports That Emphasize Low Body Weight and Body Image of Participants

Sport in which performance is subjectively scored	Dance, figure skating, and gymnastics
Endurance sports favoring participants with low body weight	Distance running, cycling, cross-country skiing
Sports in which body contour-revealing clothing is worn for competition	Volleyball, swimming, diving, running
Sports using weight categories for participation	Horse racing, martial arts, rowing
Sports in which prepubertal body habitus favors success	Figure skating, gymnastics, diving

Engaging in complete fasting, stimulants and laxative abuse, and self-induced vomiting is a consequence of desire to achieve the "degree of thinness" required from judges, coaches, and trainers, or even parents and peers. The incidence of disordered eating among female athletes is between 15 and 62%.[27,28,50,77,92] By contrast, the incidence in the general population is 1%.

Disordered eating may impair athletic performance and increase risk of injury. Decreased strength, endurance, reaction time, and concentration are just some of the negative consequences of decreased caloric and mineral intake and fluid and electrolyte imbalance. Inadequate calcium intake is very common in female athletes and various studies have showed that they consume less than two thirds of recommended daily allowances (RDA).[25,54] Along with strenuous exercise, a low-calorie diet will induce amenorrhea and potentially irreversible loss of bone mass.

B. MENSTRUAL DYSFUNCTION

Normal menstrual function is dependent on intact function of the pituitary gland, hypothalamus, ovaries, and endometrium. The cyclic nature of the process is maintained by precise secretion of both *luteinizing hormone* (LH) and *follicle-stimulating hormone* (FSH) from the anterior pituitary, in response to *gonadotropin releasing hormone* (GnRH) arising in hypothalamus. The normal menstrual cycle lasts 25 to 35 days and occurs 10 to 13 times per year. The average age of menarche is 12.7 years in the U.S. and 13.5 years in some parts of Europe.

Delay of menarche, the time when a female first starts menstruating, is related to athletic activity. Athletes who begin strenuous training before menarche occurs may experience a later menarche and have increased incidence of menstrual dysfunction when compared with athletes who begin their training after menarche.[30,63,91] It seems that each year of intensive training before menarche delays the onset of menarche for 5 months.[20] This is very important because bone mass accumulation is most intensive during puberty and those athletes with delayed menarche will have lower BMD and increased risk of scoliosis and stress fractures in years to follow.

There are three main types of menstrual dysfunction: *oligomenorrhea, amenorrhea,* and *luteal phase deficiency.* Amenorrhea is the most frequent type of dysfunction found in athletes and its prevalence varies from 3.4 to 66%, compared with 2 to 5% in general population.[73] Amenorrhea is the absence of menstrual bleeding and can be classified as either primary or secondary. *Primary amenorrhea* is defined as an absence of menarche by age 16 and *secondary amenorrhea* is defined as no menstrual cycles in a 6-month period in a female who has had at least one episode of menstrual bleeding.

Exercise-associated amenorrhea (EAA) is a subset of hypothalamic amenorrhea and is usually induced by synergism of low caloric intake and intense training.[29,32,69,93] Other factors such as weight, body composition, fat distribution, and mental stress must be considered as well. Suppression and disorganization of pulsatile LH release and complete suppression of leptin diurnal rhythm are thought to be underlying pathophysiologic mechanisms of EEA.[55,62] EEA is a diagnosis of exclusion, and all necessary diagnostic steps must be undertaken before it is made (Table 15.2). Nevertheless, it remains the most frequent cause of amenorrhea in athletes.

TABLE 15.2
Differential Diagnosis of Exercise-Associated Amenorrhea

- Pregnancy
- Hyperprolactinemia
- Primary ovarian failure
- Virilization syndromes including misuse of anabolic steroids
- Thyroid disease
- Genetic disorders
- Anatomical abnormalities

Because of the resulting hypoestrogenic state, amenorrhea may affect many different functions (cardiovascular, reproductive), and the main concern is premature bone loss and increased risk of both acute fractures and stress fractures.[57] Estrogen seems to affect the mechanism controlling the balance between the amount of bone formed by osteoblasts and the amount of bone resorbed by osteoclasts. It is hypothesized that estrogen promotes bone formation by inhibiting the rate of appearance of new resorption sites in the skeleton.[39]

C. Osteoporosis

Osteoporosis, the third part of the triad, is defined as inadequate bone formation and/or premature bone loss, resulting in low bone mass and increased risk of fracture. Most bone mass is acquired during the adolescent years, and by the age of 18 most women have reached 95% of their peak bone mass. After peak mass is achieved, both men and women lose bone at a rate of 0.3 to 0.5% per year. At menopause, women experience rate acceleration to 3% per year.

When amenorrheic, young athletes may fail to lay down sufficient bone mass or may lose already accumulated bone mass.[56] It is known that an amenorrheic athlete may lose 2 to 6% of bone mass per year, and develop the bone structure profile similar to that of a 60-year-old woman. Several studies have shown that, when compared with healthy athletes, amenorrheic athletes have significantly lower BMD at the lumbar spine, femoral neck, greater trochanter, Ward triangle, intertrochanteric region, femoral shaft, and tibia.[23,24,66,74] This kind of weakened bone places the athlete at threefold risk of stress fracture.[101] Although BMD can be partially restored on resumption of menses, studies have shown that it still remains lower than in healthy athletes.[23,24,58] Because of this partial irreversibility, it is crucial to identify all athletes at risk as early as possible.

D. Clinical Evaluation and Treatment of the Female Athlete Triad

Prevention and early detection are crucial in matters concerning the female athlete triad. The ideal time to screen for the triad is during the preparticipation physical evaluation (PPE) prior to sports participation or, in the case of professional athletes, at the beginning of the season.

History. The history should be detailed and focused on menstrual, nutritional, and body weight history, which are the most important aspects. The menstrual history should include age at menarche, frequency and duration of menstrual periods, the date of the last menstrual period, and use of hormonal therapy. The nutritional history should include eating habits such as number of meals per day, 24-hour recall of the food intake, list of any forbidden foods, calorie counting, etc.[71,90] The body weight history should include the highest and the lowest weights since menarche and the athlete's satisfaction with her present weight.

Physical examination. General physical examination including basic anthropometric measures such as weight, height, and subcutaneous fat thickness should be taken. Inspection should be focused on external signs of androgen excess: hirsutism, male pattern alopecia, and acne; thyroid deficiency: dry hair and skin; and stigmata for chromosomal abnormalities, e.g., Turner's syndrome. Fundi, visual fields, thyroid, breasts, and pelvis should be examined, as well.

Laboratory tests. These are discouraged as an integral part of routine examination, but should be performed if there is suspicion of the triad.[81]

Imaging studies. The most precise tool for determination of BMD is dual energy x-ray absorptiometry (DEXA). It should be used for determining the amount of bone loss, as well as for measuring the success of therapy.

Treatment. Treatment should be based on a multidisciplinary team approach and should focus on weight control and menses restoration,[49] which would restore normal serum estrogen concentration and prevent further loss of bone mineral content. The recommended treatment scheme proposed by Benson[8] is as follows: decrease training by 10 to 20%, increase caloric intake, gain 2 to 3% of body weight, add resistance training, supplement calcium (1500 mg/day), and monitor using bone density scans.[84] Estrogen replacement therapy (ERT) in EEA remains a controversial issue. From a theoretical standpoint, administration of estrogen makes sense because in EEA estrogen blood concentrations are lowered, but to date there have been no controlled clinical trials that have examined the efficacy of ERT in treating athletes with EEA.

IV. STRESS FRACTURES IN THE FEMALE ATHLETE

Bone is very dynamic tissue, and it remodels in response to various forms of external stress such as tension, compression, bending, pulling, and torsion.[99] The remodeling process begins with osteoclastic activity and bone resorption, followed by osteoblastic activity and formation of new bone tissue. Stress fractures occur when the equilibrium between bone resorption and formation is temporarily disturbed, i.e., when the load placed on bone overpowers its ability to repair. Stress fractures are considered to be *fatigue fractures* or fractures that occur when abnormal stress is applied to normal bone.[2]

Stress fractures are described in more detail in Chapter 12, and this section briefly outlines specific issues related to stress injuries in female athletes. There are two reasons: first, women in general have a higher incidence of stress fractures and, second, distribution of stress fracture sites seems to differ between genders.[64]

A. EPIDEMIOLOGY

Studies done at West Point in 1976, when women first entered the military academy, showed a higher number of stress fractures in female than in male cadets.[88] Further studies in subsequent years have consistently confirmed that female recruits are at greater risk for stress fractures than are their male counterparts; the relative risk ranges from 1.2 to 10.0.[6,9,37,51–53,65,70,72,75,78,82,86,97] Rates for male recruits are approximately 1 to 3%, and for female recruits are much higher, ranging from 1.1 to 21%. Possible reasons for these observations include lower initial level of physical fitness, endocrine factors, unfavorable biomechanical conditions, lower bone density, and differences in gait.[13]

Although recent literature reports show a higher incidence of stress fractures in the female athletic population, gender differences in stress fracture rates are not as obvious in athletes as in military personnel.[4,12,14,16,22,33,38,41,48] These studies showed no differences between male and female athletes, or a slightly increased risk for women, ranging from 1.5 to 3.5 times that of men. In part, this can be attributed to methodology issues, especially to the difficulty involved in controlling confounding factors such as type, volume, and intensity of training.[13] Bennel et al.[5] suggest that differences in the stress fracture rate between male and female athletes may not be attributable to gender per se, but rather to gender-related causal factors such as diet, menstrual history, and bone density (see above).

B. DISTRIBUTION OF STRESS FRACTURES IN FEMALE ATHLETES

Stress fractures are most common in lower-extremity bones, but they also occur in non-weight-bearing bones such as upper extremities and ribs. The distribution of stress fractures is somewhat different in female than in male athletes. The tibia is the most commonly involved site for both men and women, but fractures of the femoral neck, tarsal navicular, fifth metatarsal (Figure 15.2), and pelvis (Figure 15.3) are seen more commonly in the female athlete.[6,11,42,102] Some of these fractures are particularly troublesome, and may even require operative treatment.

V. PATELLOFEMORAL PAIN SYNDROME

Patellofemoral pain syndrome (PFPS) is the most common complaint among the female athlete population, and the term has been reserved to describe a symptom complex of painful but stable

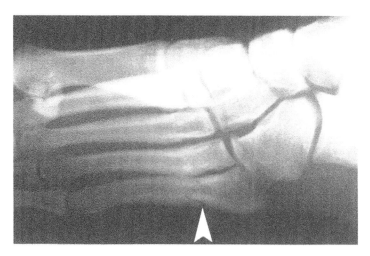

FIGURE 15.2 Jones fracture in an 18-year-old female tennis player.

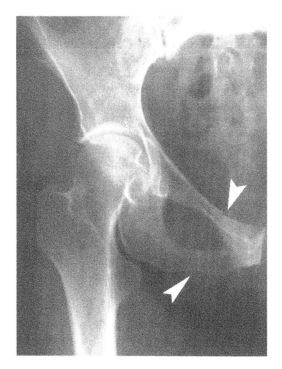

FIGURE 15.3 Stress fracture of the ramus superior and inferior of the pubic bone in a senior female runner (arrowheads).

patella. Other terms used in the literature to describe pain-related problems in the anterior portion of the knee include patellofemoral arthralgia, patellar pain, patellar pain syndrome, and patellofemoral stress syndrome.[89] The diagnosis of PFPS is made by exclusion of intra-articular pathologies, patellar tendinopathy, peripatellar bursitis, the plica syndrome, and Sinding-Larsen-Johansson and Osgood-Schlatter lesions.[31,87]

The increased incidence of PFPS in females compared to males is thought to be related to structural, biomechanical, sociological, and hormonal differences between genders.[3,31,44,46,67] Despite its high incidence, the etiology of PFPS remains unclear. There is no single factor causing PFPS; instead, it is considered a result of numerous different etiologic factors. They are usually classified

---

TABLE 15.3
Risk Factors Contributing to Development of the
Patellofemoral Pain Syndrome

Extrinsic Factors	Intrinsic Factors
Excessive exercise	Lower limb malalignment
Overtraining	Patellofemoral malalignment
Training errors	Muscle imbalance and/or weakness
Poor equipment	Joint laxity
Ignorance of the condition	Leg length discrepancy

---

as extrinsic and intrinsic, and three major factors contributing to development of PFPS are lower extremity and patellofemoral malalignment, quadriceps muscle imbalance and/or weakness, and physical overload of the patellofemoral joint (Table 15.3).[7,21,81,98]

More detailed description of etiology, diagnostics, and treatment of anterior knee pain and PFPS is given in Chapter 8.

VI. OTHER FREQUENTLY ENCOUNTERED CONDITIONS

There are several overuse syndromes that may be seen with greater frequency in female athletes, especially in those unconditioned who are just beginning sporting activities.[26] All these conditions are described in more detail elsewhere in this book; they are just briefly mentioned here.

Lateral epicondylitis. In this condition, commonly called *tennis elbow,* the origin of the extensor carpi radialis brevis is afflicted. It usually manifests between the ages of 30 and 50, and women are more at risk than men. The main symptoms consist of pain and tenderness over the lateral humeral epicondyle. Treatment is usually non-operative and consists of pain relief, inflammation control, and activity monitoring. Operative treatment is required in 5 to 10% of patients (see Chapter 4).

Iliotibial band friction syndrome. This syndrome results from activity comprising many repetitive flexion and extension movements of the knee, during which rubbing of the band against lateral femoral epicondyle occurs. The dominant symptom is pain at the lateral side of the knee. The treatment is usually non-operative and is based on modification of athletic activity, stretching exercises, nonsteroidal anti-inflammatory drugs, and correction of predisposing factors (see Chapter 8).

Tibiotalar impingement syndrome. Repeated maximal dorsal flexion of the foot leads to the development of bony exostoses on the anterior edge of the tibia, the neck of the talus, and occasionally the navicular bone. The syndrome occurs most frequently in soccer players and ballet dancers. Symptoms include pain, swelling, and localized tenderness during palpation of the area between the medial malleolus and the tibialis posterior muscle tendon, and between the lateral malleolus and the extensor digitorum muscle tendon. Conservative treatment consists of avoiding maximal dorsal flexion of the foot, rising the heels of the shoes, physical therapy, and use of anti-inflammatory drugs. Surgical procedures (which can be performed arthroscopically) are aimed at removing the bony exostosis (see Chapter 9).

Spondylolysis. Spondylolysis is a term used to describe a break in bone continuity resulting in a defect in the junction between the superior and inferior processus articularis (the most common localization is the fourth and fifth lumbar vertebra). It is more common in female athletes, especially in gymnasts. It is caused by trauma and may also develop as a consequence of overuse — from stress fractures. The condition is, in most of cases, asymptomatic and is detected by roentgenographic examination. Special slanted oblique projections of the spine are taken, which in positive cases show the figure of a "Scottish terrier" with an abnormally extended neck, indicating a defect in the isthmus of the vertebral arch (Figure 15.4). Treatment is conservative, and surgical fixation and bone transplantation of the vertebral arch are very rarely indicated[68] (see Chapter 6).

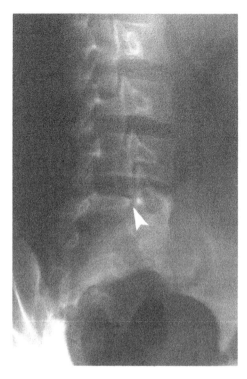

FIGURE 15.4 Roentgenogram of spondylolysis in a top-level rhythmic gymnast. Note the "Scottish terrier" figure (arrowhead).

VII. CONCLUSION

The dramatic increase of female sport participation in the last two decades demonstrates that women can be as competitive and successful as their male peers. Clearly, regular exercise is very important for general health, positive lifestyle behavior, and positive self-image, and sport teaches such skills as teamwork, commitment, and goal setting.

Education remains the most important tool for prevention of overuse injury. Female athletes, both professional and recreational, should be encouraged to learn how their body works and the nature of the possible health risks of sport participation. In addition, preparticipation physical evaluation (PPE) is the ideal time to identify athletes at risk and screen for any problems that may predispose an athlete to injury.

The differences between genders outlined in this chapter represent average values only, and there is significant variability within each sex. Moreover, these differences should not be used as means of discrimination or to catalog the abilities of each sex. Instead, they should be used to design individualized training programs and schedules that will bring health benefits and good athletic results to each sex.

REFERENCES

1. **Allander, E.** Prevalence, incidence and remission rates of some common rheumatic diseases or syndromes. *Scand. J. Rheumatol.,* 1974; 3: 145–153.
2. **Arendt, E.A.** Stress fractures and the female athlete. *Clin. Orthop.,* 2000; 372: 131–138.
3. **Baker, M.M. and Juhn, M.S.** Patellofemoral pain syndrome in the female athlete. *Clin. Sports Med.,* 2000; 19: 315–329.

4. **Bennel, K.L., Malcolm, S.A., Thomas, S.A. et al.** Risk factors for stress fractures in female track-and-field athletes: A twelve month prospective study. *Am. J. Sports. Med.*, 1996; 24: 810–818.
5. **Bennel, K.L., Malcolm, S.A., Thomas, S.A. et al.** The incidence and distribution of stress fractures in competitive track-and-field athletes. *Am. J. Sports Med.*, 1996; 24: 211–217.
6. **Bennel, K.L. and Brukner, P.D.** Epidemiology and site specificity of stress fractures. *Clin. Sports Med.*, 1997; 16(2): 179–196.
7. **Bennet, W. et al.** Insertion and orientation of terminal vastus lateralis obliquus and vastus medialis obliquus muscle fibers in human knees. *Clin. Anat.*, 1993; 6: 129–134.
8. **Benson, J.E.** Nutritional aspects of amenorrhea in the female athlete triad. *Int. J. Sport Nutr.*, 1996; 6: 134–145.
9. **Bijur, P.E., Horodyski, M., Egerton, W. et al.** Comparison of injury during cadet basic training by gender. *Arch. Pediatr. Adolesc. Med.*, 1997; 151: 456–461.
10. **Birell, S.** The psychological dimension of female athletic participation, in *The Sporting Women*, Boutilier, M. and SanGiovanni, L., Eds. Champaign, IL: Human Kinetics, 1984; 49–91.
11. **Bradley, J.N. and Robert, A.A.** Stress fractures in female athlete. *Sports Med. Arthrosc. Rev.*, 2001; 10(1): 83–90.
12. **Brukner, P.D. and Bennell, K.L.** Stress fractures in female athletes: diagnosis, management, and rehabilitation. *Sports Med.*, 1997; 24: 419–429.
13. **Brukner, P., Bennell, K., and Matheson, G.** The epidemiology of stress fractures, in *Stress Fractures*, Doyle, D., Ed. Victoria: Blackwell Science Asia, 1999; chap. 2.
14. **Brunet, M.E., Cook, S.D., Brinker, M.R. et al.** A survey of running injuries in 1505 competitive and recreational runners. *J. Sports Med. Phys. Fitness*, 1990; 30: 307–315.
15. **Byrne, S. and McLean, N.** Elite athletes: effects of the pressure to be thin. *J. Sci. Med. Sport*, 2002; 5(2): 80–94.
16. **Collins, K. et al.** Overuse injuries in triathletes: a study of the 1989 Seafair Triathlon. *Am. J. Sports Med.*, 1989; 17: 675–680.
17. **Corbin, C.B.** Self-confidence of females in sports and physical activity. *Clin. Sports Med.*, 1984; 3: 895–908.
18. **Cureton, K.J. et al.** Muscle hypertrophy in men and women. *Med. Sci. Sports Exerc.*, 1990; 20: 338–344.
19. **DeHaven, K.E. and Lintner, D.M.** Athletic injuries: comparison by age, sport and gender. *Am. J. Sports Med.*, 1986; 14: 218–224.
20. **Deuster, P.A., Kyle, S.B., Moser, P.B. et al.** Nutritional intakes and status of highly trained amenorrheic and eumenorrheic women runners. *Fertil. Steril.*, 1986; 46: 636–643.
21. **Devereaux, M.D. and Lachmann, S.M.** Athletes attending a sports injury clinic: a review. *Br. J. Sports Med.*, 1983; 17:137–142.
22. **Dixon, M. and Fricker, P.** Injuries to elite gymnasts over 10 years. *Med. Sci. Sports Exerc.*, 1993; 25: 1322–1329.
23. **Drinkwater, B.L., Nilson, K., Ott, S. et al.** Bone mineral content of amenorrheic and eumenorrheic athletes. *N. Engl. J. Med.*, 1984; 311: 277–281.
24. **Drinkwater, B.L., Breummer, B., and Chesnut, C.H., III.** Menstrual history as a determinant of a current bone density in young athletes. *J. Am. Med. Assoc.*, 1990; 263: 545–548.
25. **Druss, R.G.** Body image and perfection of ballerinas: comparison and contrast with anorexia nervosa. *Gen. Hosp. Psychiatr.*, 1979; 2: 115–121.
26. **Dubravčić, S., Pećina, M., Bojanić, I. et al.** Common orthopaedic problems in female athletes. *Croat. Sports Med. J.*, 1991; 6: 38–46.
27. **Dummer, G.M., Rosen, L.W., Heusner, W.W. et al.** Pathogenic weight-control behaviours of young competitive swimmers. *Phys. Sports. Med.*, 1987; 15: 75–84.
28. **Dummer, G.M., Rosen, L.W., and Heusner, W.W.** Pathogenic weight control behaviours of female college gymnasts. *Phys. Sports. Med.*, 1987; 15: 85–86.
29. **Dućek, T.** Influence of high intensity training on menstrual cycle disorders in athletes. *Croat. Med. J.*, 2001; 42: 79–92.
30. **Frisch, R.E., Gotz-Welbergen, A.V., McArthur, J.W. et al.** Delayed menarche and amenorrhoea of college athletes in relation to age and onset of training. *J. Am. Med. Assoc.*, 1981; 246: 1559–1563.
31. **Fulkerson, J.P. and Arendt, E.A.** Anterior knee pain in females. *Clin. Orthop.*, 2000; 372: 69–73.

32. **Gidwani, G.P.** Amenorrhoea in the athlete. *Adolesc. Med.*, 1999; 10(2): 275–290.
33. **Goldberg, B. and Pecora, C.** Stress fractures: a risk of increased training in freshmen. *Physician Sports Med.*, 1994; 22: 68–78.
34. **Griffin, L.Y.** The female athlete, in *Orthopedic Sports Medicine*, DeLee, J.C. and Drez, D., Eds. Philadelphia: W.B. Saunders, 1994; 356–373.
35. **Hale, R.W.** Factors important to women engaged in vigorous physical activity, in *Sports Medicine*, Strauss, R., Ed. Philadelphia: W.B. Saunders, 1984; 250–269.
36. **Hale, R.W.** Differences and similarities between the sexes, in *Caring for Exercising Women*, Hale, R.W., Ed. New York: Elsevier Science 1991; 31–37.
37. **Heir, T. and Glosmaker, P.** Epidemiology of musculoskeletal injuries among Norwegian conscripts undergoing basic military training. *Scand. J. Med. Sci. Sports*, 1996; 6: 186–191.
38. **Hickey, G.J., Fricker, P.A., and McDonald, W.A.** Injuries to elite rowers over a 10-year period. *Med. Sci. Sports Exerc.*, 1997; 29: 1567–1572.
39. **Highet, R.** Athletic amenorrhoea. An update on aetiology, complications and management. *Sports Med.*, 1989; 7: 82–108.
40. **Hoffman, T., Stauffer, R., and Jackson, A.** Sex differences in strength. *Am. J. Sports Med.*, 1979; 7(4): 265–267.
41. **Holden, D.L. and Jackson, D.W.** Stress fractures of the ribs in female rowers. *Am. J. Sports Med.*, 1985; 13(5): 342–348.
42. **Hulkko, A. and Orava, S.** Stress fractures in athletes. *Int. J. Sports Med.*, 1987; 8: 221–226.
43. **Huston, L.J. and Wojtys, E.M.** Neuromuscular performance characteristics in elite female athletes. *Am. J. Sports Med.*, 1996; 24(4): 427–436.
44. **Hutchinson, M.R. and Irelan, M.L.** Knee injuries in female athletes. *Sports Med.*, 1995; 19(4): 288–302.
45. **Hvid, I., Anderson, L.B., and Shmidt, H.** Chondromalacia patellae: the relation to abnormal joint mechanics. *Acta Orthop. Scand.*, 1981; 52: 661–666.
46. **Ireland, M.L. and Wall, C.** Epidemiology and comparison of knee injuries in elite male and female United States basketball athletes. *Med. Sci. Sports Exerc.*, 1990; 22(2): 582.
47. **Ivković, A., Bojanić, I., and Ivković, M.** Trijas sportaćica. *Lijeć. Vjes.*, 2001; 123: 200–206.
48. **Johnson, A.W., Weiss, C.B., and Wheeler, D.L.** Stress fractures of the femoral shaft in athletes — more common than expected: a new clinical test. *Am. J. Sports Med.*, 1994; 22: 248–256.
49. **Johnson, M.D.** Tailoring the participation exam to female athletes. *Phys. Sportsmed.*, 1992; 20: 61–72.
50. **Johnson, M.D.** Disordered eating in active and athletic women. *Clin. Sports Med.*, 1994; 13: 355–369.
51. **Jones, B.H., Bovee, M.W., Harris, J.M. et al.** Intrinsic risk factors for exercise-related injuries among male and female army trainees. *Am. J. Sports Med.*, 1993; 21: 705–710.
52. **Jones, B.H. et al.** Epidemiology of injuries associated with physical training among young men in the army. *Med. Sci. Sports. Exerc.*, 1993; 25: 197–203.
53. **Jordaan, G. and Schwellnus, M.P.** The incidence of overuse injuries in military recruits during basic military training. *Mil. Med.*, 1994; 159: 421–426.
54. **Kasenbaum, S. et al.** Nutrition, physiology and menstrual status of female distance runners. *Med. Sci. Sports Exerc.*, 1989; 21: 2–7.
55. **Laughlin, G.A. and Yenn, S.S.** Hypoleptinemia in women athletes: absence of a diurnal rhythm with amenorrhea. *J. Clin. Endocrinol. Metabol.*, 1997; 82: 318–321.
56. **Lebrun, C.M.** The female athlete triad: disordered eating, amenorrhea and osteoporosis. *Orthop. In. Ed.*, 1994; 2: 519–526.
57. **Lebrun, C.M.** Female athlete triad, in *Sports Medicine for Specific Ages and Abilities*, Maffuli, N. et al., Eds. London: Churchill Livingstone, 2001; 177–185.
58. **Lindberg, J.S., Powel, M.R., Hunt, M.M. et al.** Increased vertebral bone mineral density in response to reduced exercise in amenorrheic women. *West. J. Med.*, 1987; 146: 39–42.
59. **Lloyd, T.** Diet and menstrual status as determinants of injuries in the athletic female, in *The Athletic Female*, Pearl, A.J., Ed. Champaign, IL: Human Kinetics, 1993; 61–80.
60. **Lohman, T.G. et al.** Methodological factors and the prediction of body fat in female athletes. *Med. Sci. Sports Exerc.*, 1984; 16: 92–96.
61. **Lopiano, D.A.** Modern history of women in sports: twenty-five years of Title IX. *Clin. Sports Med.*, 2000; 19: 167–173.

62. **Loucks, A.B. et al.** Alternations in the hypothalamic-pituitary-ovarian and hypothalamic-pituitary-adrenal axes in athletic women. *J. Clin. Endocrinol. Metab.*, 1989; 68: 402–411.

63. **Malina, R.M.** Menarche in athletes: a synthesis and hypothesis. *Ann. Hum. Biol.*, 1983; 246: 1559–1563.

64. **Matheson, G.O., Clement, D.B., McKenzie, D.C. et al.** Stress fractures in athletes: a study of 320 cases. *Am. J. Sports Med.*, 1987; 15(1): 34–58.

65. **Milgrom, C., Finestone, A., Shlamkowitch, B. et al.** Youth is a risk factor for stress fracture: a study of 783 infantry recruits. *J. Bone Joint Surg.*, 1994; 76B: 20–22.

66. **Myburg, K., Bachrach, L.K., Lewis, B. et al.** Low bone mineral density at axial and appendicular sites in amenorrheic athletes. *Med. Sci. Sport. Exerc.*, 1993; 25: 1197–1202.

67. **Neely, F.G.** Intrinsic risk factors for exercise-related lower limb injuries. *Sports Med.*, 1998; 26(4): 253–263.

68. **Omey, M.L., Micheli, L.J., and Gerbino, P.G., II.** Idiopathic scoliosis and spondylolisis in the female athlete. Tips for treatment. *Clin. Orthop.*, 2000; 372: 74–84.

69. **Otis, C.L.** Exercise-associated amenorrhea. *Clin. Sports Med.*, 1992; 23: 351–356.

70. **Pester, S. and Smith, P.C.** Stress fractures in the lower extremities of soldiers in basic training. *Orthop. Rev.*, 1992; 21: 297–303.

71. **Powers, P.S.** Eating disorders: initial assessment and early treatment options for anorexia nervosa and bulimia nervosa. *Psychiatr. Clin. North Am.*, 1996; 19: 639–655.

72. **Protzman, R.R. and Griffis, C.** Stress fractures in men and women undergoing military training. *J. Bone Joint Surg.*, 1977; 59A: 825–830.

73. **Putukian, M.D.** The female athlete triad. *Clin. Sports Med.*, 1998; 17: 675–696.

74. **Rencken, M.L., Chesnut, C.H., III, and Drinkwater, B.L.** Bone density at multiple skeletal sites in amenorrheic athletes. *J. Am. Med. Assoc.*, 1996; 276: 238–240.

75. **Renker, K.A. and Ozbourne, S.** A comparison of male and female orthopaedic pathology in basic training. *Mil. Med.*, 1979; 144: 532–536.

76. **Ritter, M.A., Goie, T.J., and Albohn, M.** Sport-related injuries. *Wom. Col. Health.*, 1980; 28: 267–268.

77. **Rosen, L.W. and Hough, D.O.** Pathogenic weight-control in behaviours of female college athletes. *Phys. Sports Med.*, 1988; 16: 141–144.

78. **Rudzki, S.J.** Injuries in Australian army recruits. Part II: Location and cause of injuries seen in recruits. *Mil. Med.*, 1997; 162: 477–480.

79. **Sabatini, S.** The female athlete triad. *Am. J. Med. Sci.*, 2001; 322(4): 193–195.

80. **Sallis, R.E, Jones, K., Sunshine, S. et al.** Comparing sports injuries in men and women. *Int. J. Sports Med.*, 2001; 22: 420–423.

81. **Sanborn, C. et al.** Disordered eating and the female athlete triad. *Clin. Sports Med.*, 2000; 19: 199–213.

82. **Sanchis-Alfonso, V., Rosello-Sastre, E., and Martinez-Sanjaun, V.** Pathogenesis of anterior knee pain and functional patellofemoral instability in the active young. *Am. J. Knee Surg.*, 1999; 12(1): 29–40.

83. **Shwayhat, A.F., Linenger, J.M., Hofherr, L.K. et al.** Profile of exercise history and overuse injuries among United States Navy Sea, Air, and Land (SEAL) recruits. *Am. J. Sports. Med.*, 1994; 22: 835–840.

84. **Snow-Harter, C.M.** Bone health and prevention of osteoporosis in active and athletic women. *Clin. Sports Med.*, 1994; 13: 389–404.

85. **Stark, J.A. and Toulouse, A.** The young female athlete: psychologic consideration. *Clin. Sports Med.*, 1984; 3: 909–921.

86. **Taimela, S. et al.** Risk factors for stress fractures during physical training programs. *Clin. J. Sports Med.*, 1992; 2: 105–108.

87. **Thomee, R., Augustsson, J., and Karlsson, J.** Patellofemoral pain syndrome: a review of current issues. *Sports Med.*, 1999; 28: 245–262.

88. **Tomasi, L.F. et al.** Women's response to army training. *Phys. Sports Med.*, 1977; 5(2): 32–35.

89. **Tumia, N. and Maffuli, N.** Patellofemoral pain in female athletes. *Sports Med. Arthrosc. Rev.*, 2002; 10(1): 69–75.

90. **Van de Loo, D.A. and Johnson, M.D.** The young female athlete. *Clin. Sports Med.*, 1995; 14: 687–707.

91. **Warren, M.P.** The effects of exercise on pubertal progression and reproductive function in girls. *J. Clin. Endocrinol. Metab.*, 1980; 51: 1150–1157.

92. **Warren, B.J., Stanton, A.L., and Blessing, D.L.** Disordered eating in competitive female athletes. *Int. J. Eat. Disord.*, 1990; 9: 565–569.

93. **Weimann, E.** Gender-related differences in elite gymnasts: the female athlete triad. *J. Appl. Physiol.*, 2002; 92(5): 2146–2152.

94. **Whiteside, P.A.** Men's and women's injuries in comparable sports. *Phys. Sportsmed.,* 1980; 8: 130–136.

95. **Wiggins, D.L. and Wiggins, M.E.** The female athlete. *Clin. Sports Med.,* 1997; 17: 593–603.

96. **Wilmore, J.H.** The application of science to sport: physiological profiles of male and female athlete. *Can. J. Appl. Sport Sci.,* 1979; 4(2): 103–115.

97. **Winfield, A.C., Bracker, M., Moore, J. et al.** Risk factors associated with stress reactions in female marines. *Mil. Med.,* 1997; 162: 698–702.

98. **Witrouw, E. et al.** Intrinsic risk factors for the development of anterior knee pain in an athletic population. *Am. J. Sports Med.,* 2000; 28: 480–488.

99. **Wolf, J.** *Das Gesetz der Transformation der Knochen.* Berlin: Verlag August Hirschwald, 1892.

100. **Yager, K.K.** American College of Sports Medicine ad Hoc Task Force on Women's Issues in Sports Medicine, June, 1992.

101. **Yurth, E.** Epitome, female athlete triad. *West. J. Med.,* 1995; 162: 149–150.

102. **Zeni, A.I. et al.** Stress injury to the bone among women athletes. *Phys. Med. Rehabil. Clin. North Am.,* 2000; 3: 929–947.

Index

C

Printed and bound by CPI Group (UK) Ltd, Croydon, CR0 4YY

23/10/2024

01778246-0016